SURGERY
FOR NURSES

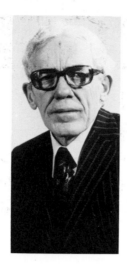

James Moroney
24TH JULY 1916–29TH JULY 1981

The Publishers are sad to have
to report the sudden death of
James Moroney. At the time of
his death he had already
completed the work for this
fifteenth edition of *Surgery for
Nurses*, which now becomes a
fitting memorial to him.

SURGERY FOR NURSES

THE LATE

James Moroney MBChB FRCS(Eng) LRCP(Lond)

Honorary Consultant Surgeon, Liverpool Area Health
Authority (Teaching).
Formerly Consultant Surgeon, Broadgreen Hospital, Liverpool
and Clatterbridge Hospital, Wirral, Merseyside. Clinical
Lecturer in Surgery, Clinical Sub Dean and Chairman, Board
of the Faculty of Medicine, University of Liverpool. Examiner
in Surgery, General Nursing Council for England and Wales.
Hunterian Professor, Royal College of Surgeons of England.

FIFTEENTH EDITION

CHURCHILL LIVINGSTONE
EDINBURGH LONDON MELBOURNE AND NEW YORK 1982

CHURCHILL LIVINGSTONE
Medical Division of Longman Group Limited

Distributed in the United States of America by Churchill
Livingstone Inc., 19 West 44th Street, New York, N.Y. 10036,
and by associated companies, branches and representatives
throughout the world.

First Edition 1950   Eleventh Edition 1967
Second Edition 1952   Twelth Edition 1971
Third Edition 1955   ELBS Edition first published 1971
Fourth Edition 1956   Thirteenth Edition 1975
Fifth Edition 1958   ELBS Edition of Thirteenth Edition 1975
Sixth Edition 1959   Fourteenth Edition 1978
Seventh Edition 1961   Hindi translation 1979
Eighth Edition 1962   Fifteenth Edition 1982
Ninth Edition 1964   ELBS Edition of Fifteenth Edition 1982
Tenth Edition 1966

ISBN 0 443 02241 0

British Library Cataloguing in Publication Data
Moroney, James
   Surgery for nurses. — 15th ed.
   1. Surgery
   I. Title
   617'.0024613   RT65

Library of Congress Catalog Card Number 81–67469

Printed in Great Britain by
William Clowes (Beccles) Limited, Beccles and London

Preface to the Fifteenth Edition

This book has been almost rewritten. The space devoted to nursing care has been increased and new chapters or sections include those on stoma care, the pathophysiology of the gastrointestinal tract, surgical nutrition and incontinence. All the chapters on the surgical specialties have been rewritten and those on more basic subjects such as infection, inflammation, haemorrhage and microbiology have required much revision to reflect contemporary surgical practice.

Elsewhere I express my gratitude to all who have been so generous with their help. Mr Ken Biggs, who undertook the onerous task of reillustrating the book with such artistic skill and clarity and Mrs Joan Bowstead, who not only typed the manuscript but correlated the efforts of my colleagues, deserve my special thanks.

The publishers have responded magnificently to the challenge which so extensive a revision presented by designing what is virtually a new book with a format, page layout and a type all of which are new. In addition it is a pleasure to thank them for their constant help and advice.

The aim of the book to provide a simple, well-illustrated, up-to-date text for the student nurse remains unchanged.

1981   J.M.

Extract from
the Preface to
the First Edition

In writing this book for nurses I have had constantly in mind the difficulties and anxieties which confront the student nurse preparing for the Final State Examination and at the same time undertaking an increasing amount of responsible work in the wards.

The subject matter is based on the syllabus of the General Nursing Council, and in each section I have endeavoured to include an account of the nursing care which is so inseparable a part of the treatment of every surgical condition.

Without unduly sacrificing the space devoted to general surgery, sections on the more specialised branches of surgery have been included.

While it is written primarily for the student I hope that the trained nurse may find it a useful book of reference.

1949   J.M.

Contributors

The author gratefully acknowledges his indebtedness to all who have helped in the preparation of all editions of this book. In many cases it is impossible to identify their contribution by chapter reference since it has always been the aim of this work to coordinate the nursing care with the surgical condition.

Nursing advisors and contributors

Miss E.E. Fenn SRN, SCM, RFN, RNT
Formerly Principal Tutor, Broadgreen Hospital, Liverpool

Mrs M.E. Jackson SRN, SCM, RNT
Senior Tutor, Broadgreen Hospital, Liverpool

N.J. Lawrence BA, SRN, BTA, RNT
Principle Tutor, Noble's Isle of Man Hospital, Isle of Man

Miss E.M. Oliver SRN, SCM
Ward Sister, Broadgreen Hospital, Liverpool

H.H. Rose SRN, RFN, RNT, MITO
Assistant Director of Nurse Education, Liverpool Area Health Authority (Teaching) School of Nursing

Mrs J. Twentyman SRN, SCM, JBCNS
Stoma Care Nurse, Broadgreen Hospital, Liverpool

Miss E. Wilkinson SRN
Nursing Officer, Operating Theatres, Broadgreen Hospital, Liverpool

Medical contributors

H.M. Alty BDS, MB, ChB, FDSRCS
Consultant Faciomaxillary Surgeon, Broadgreen Hospital, Liverpool
Clinical Lecturer in Dental Surgery, University of Liverpool

T.R. Beatson MB, BS, FRCS
Consultant Orthopaedic Surgeon, Noble's Isle of Man Hospital, Isle of Man

D.M.J. Burns MA, MB, BChir, FRCS
Consultant Surgeon, St. Paul's Eye Hospital, Liverpool
Clinical Lecturer in Ophthalmology, University of Liverpool

John A. Campbell BA, MB, BCh, BAO, DCP, FRCPath
Consultant Haematologist, Broadgreen Hospital, Liverpool
Clinical Lecturer in Pathology, University of Liverpool

M.R. Colmer MA, MB, MChir, FRCS, JP
Consultant Surgeon, Whiston Hospital, Merseyside

J.M. Dhorajiwala MB, FRCS
Senior Surgical Registrar, Broadgreen Hospital, Liverpool

R.J. Donnelly MB, FRCSEd
Consultant Cardiothoracic Surgeon, Regional Cardiothoracic Unit, Liverpool
Clinical Lecturer in Cardiothoracic Surgery, University of Liverpool

R.A. Gregory CBE, FRCP, FRS
Holt Professor of Physiology, University of Liverpool

W. Lloyd-Jones ChM, FRCS
Consultant Surgeon, Broadgreen Hospital, Liverpool
Clinical Lecturer in Surgery, University of Liverpool

J.B. Meade MCh, BAO, FRCSI
Consultant Cardiac Surgeon, Regional Cardiothoracic Unit, Liverpool
Director of Cardiothoracic Studies, University of Liverpool

J.C. Richardson MB, ChB, DA, FFARCS
Consultant Anaesthetist, Broadgreen Hospital, Liverpool
Lecturer in Anaesthesia, University of Liverpool

J.B. Rogers MA, BM, BCh, FRCS, DLO
Consultant Ear, Nose and Throat Surgeon, Liverpool Area Health Authority (Teaching)
Clinical Lecturer in Otorhinolaryngology, University of Liverpool

A.B. Semple CBE, MD
Emeritus Professor of Community Medicine, University of Liverpool

G.P. Walker MB, ChB, FRCOG
Consultant Gynaecologist and Obstetrician, Mill Road Maternity Hospital
and Royal Liverpool Hospital
Clinical Lecturer in Gynaecology, University of Liverpool

Charles West MA, MB, BChir, FRCS
Consultant Neurosurgeon, Salford Area Health Authority (Teaching)

Illustrations
Ken Biggs BA

Overall editing and collation
Mrs Joan Bowstead, Mark Moroney

Clinical photographs
Dr Trevor Bayley
Dr J.C. Davis
Dr Michael Garret
Dr Julian Verbov

Contents

1
Surgery, the nurse and the patient

Surgery is one of the most ancient arts in the world. Its oldest branch, obstetric surgery, is almost as old as the world itself. The daring and manual dexterity of the barber-surgeon were surpassed only by the courage and forbearance of his conscious patient. Survival of such an ordeal was followed by many months in bed, during which time 'laudable' pus drained from the wound. A century ago the surgeon of that day operated without even washing his hands, and was clad in a top hat and a frock coat well stained with blood and pus. For convenience, he carried his ligature and suture materials in the buttonhole of his lapel!

The discovery of anaesthetics and the appreciation of the importance of eliminating infection in the patient's wound have transformed the surgical art. Each year adds much to the vast store of knowledge, even to the knowledge of such fundamentals as the sciences of anaesthetics and asepsis. The comparatively recent advances of blood transfusion and chemotherapy are examples of some of the outstanding achievements of contemporary scientists.

A century ago there were few skilled nurses as we know them today. The nurse's predecessor was often an illiterate, rough, dirty handywoman, and in many institutions a patient was in great measure dependent on what help he could secure from the patient in the adjoining bed.

Surgery, surgeons, and nurses have changed considerably in a century, but the plea for relief from suffering has remained essentially the same.

Every patient is a man, woman, or child living and working in different surroundings and in different spheres of activity. They are all different — different in outlook, different in character, different in their reaction to the same disease. Appreciation of the importance of this individual variation is a fundamental principle of good nursing.

Surgical treatment is usually undertaken away from the patient's own home. The advantages are overwhelming, but there is one serious disadvantage, however, in that hospital staffs have few opportunities of visiting ill patients in their own homes. It is surprising at times to see what 'home' means, and the advice given to a patient on leaving hospital must be considered against this background. The current trend of nursing education aims at a 'wider basic training' with secondment of the student to the community nurse.

The patient's mental outlook, his fears, his hopes, and his will, may play a part equal in importance to the purely physical treatment of his disease. To ignore, to be unaware of, or to neglect these factors may make a patient prefer death to a struggle, and then no amount of effort may be able to regain the valuable ground which has been lost or opportunities which have been cast away.

As medicine, of which surgery is a branch, becomes more specialised and complex, certain procedures are undertaken in specially equipped centres. Some of these may be comparatively large, such as those for cardiothoracic or neurosurgery, while others may be very small. Where patients suffering from identical or similar diseases meet in the ward or at repeated attendances at a clinic, their conversation inevitably turns to an evaluation of their progress and treatment. Not surprisingly most patients at an artificial limb centre have a very poor opinion of the results of arterial surgery! Nor can one expect a patient who has undergone surgery and perhaps radiotherapy to be enthusiastic about repeated courses of cytotoxic therapy for malignancy.

In other circumstances, a patient of suitable disposition may be most helpful to another sufferer who has, or is about to, undergo a procedure like a colostomy or ileostomy. The nurse has to exercise considerable judgement in all these situations — aware at one moment of the conflicts and despair in the patient's mind, at another of the opportunity where one patient can help another.

THE PATIENT'S CONCEPTION OF DISEASE

The term disease has a wider connotation to the nurse and the doctor than it has to the public, many of whom conceive the term as restricted to an infection or, even more narrowly, as an infectious disease. Most patients have little appreciation of the nature of their illness and still less of what measures its cure or control may entail.

As far as possible, making due allowance for intelligence and language difficulties, the patient is encouraged to interest himself in everything that is happening to him so that the reason for every procedure is understood and that it is not transformed into a ritual. In some units there is a check list to ensure that this has been carried out by the nurses and medical staff.

The reason for an investigation, a preoperative procedure like shaving the skin, preoperative medication and its effects or intravenous infusion and the nature of the fluid infused are given. It makes them all the more acceptable and encourages the patient to ask questions and perhaps reveal his anxieties. The nature of the operation and its effects are explained by the surgeon, but a nurse who knows the patient's response to procedures already undertaken by her, can brief the surgeon more fully before he explains the operation he advises.

The nurse can do much to allay and alleviate the inevitable anxieties of the surgical patient, on arrival, and throughout his stay in the ward. Success, or failure, will be determined by:

The application of professional knowledge

There can be no substitute for knowledge gained by study and experience. Since its projection is ultimately on human beings, its first impact is on the patient's mind.

It is obvious that the patient's confidence will be gained and maintained only by a combination of knowledge and understanding.

Appreciation of the aims of modern surgical treatment

Without a high order of technical competence and anatomical knowledge, in surgeon and nurse alike, no operation could be a success. The operation, however, is only a part, albeit an important part, of treatment. To the patient it is dominant and likely to be most feared. While a scar may be the only visible anatomical distortion, physiological and psychological changes may be profound and with the passage of time may cause increasing disability. To diminish or alleviate these disabilities requires the exercise of sympathy and judgment at least equal to the operative skill.

An operation is not an inevitable sequel of admission to a surgical ward, because many conditions subside without operative treatment. An operation may be:

1. An emergency. This is performed only when there is an immediate threat to life from haemorrhage, respiratory or intestinal obstruction, or a spreading infection not likely to be controlled by conservative measures alone.

2. Planned (elective). Strategically this is the most desirable, because it can be undertaken when the patient's general and local conditions are controlled to the maximal degree.

3. Multistaged. This may be necessary because:

(a) The patient's condition is not good enough to do all that is necessary at once, or

(b) The first operation may be designed to rest or drain an organ or cavity, so that subsequent curative measures can be safely undertaken.

(c) There is a need for reoperation due to a complication. This is particularly distressing to the patient and disappointing to the surgeon and nurse.

The aim of surgery is to assist and not to usurp the place of natural healing. For this reason timing may be as important as the nature and extent of the operation.

Human sympathy and understanding

It is a fair presumption that one becomes a nurse because one is activated by a desire to help others in distress. In addition, one must have an imaginative mind and considerable tact and patience. Good powers of observation and an ability to listen are essential. Only by imagining oneself in the patient's position can it be realised how he is feeling and how one can help. The background of professional knowledge and detailed care is discussed in Chapter 4. The following aspects of some of these subjects are discussed from the point of view of the nurse—patient relationship.

Reception

The relationship must be established at once—it is that of the good hostess and the welcome guest—natural, kind, and cheerful. Questions should be answered simply and there is no place for dramatisation. Many questions can be answered only by the sister of the ward who will refer all questions on diagnosis and prognosis to the medical staff. Arrangements should be made for the patient to see his relatives, the medical social worker, and a minister of religion if he so desires—all of whom have a part to play in assisting him to settle down peacefully and quietly.

Preparation of the patient

The patient may be admitted for an emergency operation, or for one where time is a less urgent factor. Where there are several days in hand, the nurse can get to know the patient as an individual and consider how he will react to the various preparations, and how they are best undertaken. It is now customary to admit a patient the evening before or even on the day of operation. Many preliminary preparations are undertaken as an outpatient.

1. *Consent form.* This has to be signed by the patient before any operative procedure can be undertaken. It is a medical responsibility to see that this is done.

2. *Collection of specimens.* Blood may have to be taken by the doctor or by the phlebotomist for examination or for cross-matching. This is the first experience of a hospital procedure.

The reason given for the procedure, and how it is performed, may well determine the patient's future attitude. An efficient vein tourniquet and really sharp needles, with an adequate choice to ensure that the smallest possible needle is used, are important in fulfilling the promise that it is really 'only a little prick'. Urine is tested without the patient's knowledge, but it is usually better that he should be told about it.

3. *Dental hygiene* may have been poor and require correction. When referring the patient for dental advice the doctor and nurse should remember that they are not qualified to express an opinion, and a remark to the patient that he should have his teeth extracted may be as erroneous as it is unprofessional.

4. *Physiotherapy* may be necessary to improve pulmonary function.

5. *Skin preparation.* This is discussed fully in Chapter 4. Plenty of soap and hot water are used and good foam raised if the skin is to be shaved. Disposable razors are cheap and hygienic. A quiet unhurried preparation with the patient engaged in conversation may well increase his confidence.

6. *Bowel.* In the few cases where an enema or washout is necessary the patient will require reassurance, and a simple explanation makes the nurse's task easier.

Special points to bear in mind in the postoperative period

The nurse must always look beyond the operation to the postoperative period and anticipate how her own difficulties may be diminished by a judicious word beforehand. The patient is made to feel that everything will be done to minimise the discomfort.

Pain and sleep. The patient quite rightly desires reassurance that he will not be kept awake by pain.

Diet. While everyone may appear very satisfied with the patient, he may be wondering how he will recover on a diet of fluids alone. A simple reassurance of the importance of a fluid diet at this stage can often allay these fears.

Blood transfusion. If a postoperative blood transfusion is likely to be running, it is as well to say beforehand that this is usual. The patient will feel that he is being well cared for and not that some unexpected complication has arisen.

Oxygen therapy may be particularly alarming, as many patients consider it to be a last desperate measure. If it is to be used postoperatively he should be accustomed to it before operation.

Breathing exercises are important but may be painful, and special care must be taken if the best result is to be achieved. Arrangements may be made for him to see the physiotherapist preoperatively.

Fear of bursting a wound. This is a point on which all patients desire reassurance, because this is exactly the sensation that arises from distension of viscera beneath an abdominal wound. The patient should be shown how to support his wound while coughing.

Drainage tubes. Their removal causes some discomfort, and an analgesic one or two hours beforehand may be given but is not usually necessary.

Care of wound. A clean wound is usually kept covered, and no special treatment is necessary unless there is reason to suspect that it has become infected. Drainage tubes are usually sited away from the main wound. Daily dressing of the drainage tube site and cleansing should be performed. Not unnaturally, the patient, who is encouraged to move his legs and his chest, may think that his wound has been forgotten and a word of explanation is necessary to ease what may be a suppressed anxiety on this account.

Removal of stitches. Anticipation always worries the patient. It can be quietly explained that it is only the stitch that is cut.

Early mobilisation avoids pressure sores and as muscular strength is not lost, weary legs and painful feet are avoided. The risk of venous thrombosis is diminished, chest movement is improved and bowel action facilitated. The slight change of scene and wider contact, even in the ward, provides relief from the monotony of the patient's bed and improves sleep.

Any other postoperative procedure which may worry the patient should be anticipated in advance, for example, the cuff of the sphygmomanometer can be put on the patient's arm preoperatively if frequent postoperative blood-pressure estimations are required. In special circumstances these readings may be monitored.

The patient in whom a gross mutilation has to be undertaken requires more than ordinary care, as well as special sympathy, and the nurse cannot know too much about the various devices and treatment to help these patients. The patient, when he leaves hospital, should feel that, in his misfortune, be it minor or serious, everything possible was done to rehabilitate him. At least he should have no reason to feel that they — 'they' in this case being the hospital staff — never realised what they had done to him.

Relationship of disease to emotion and of emotion to disease

With experience, these relationships become well known to the nurse, but there is always the proviso that if they are taken too much for granted as a routine the patient's complaint may be neglected.

Certain lesions, such as thyrotoxicosis, peptic ulcer, and ulcerative colitis, are conditions where stress seems to play a part in their aetiology or their aggravation. All patients suffering from these conditions are anxious but, of course, there are other causes of anxiety.

The overanxious patient is liable to a higher incidence of complications which a more phlegmatic character may avoid. They include:

1. *Retention of urine.* In many cases, where there is no mechanical obstruction, retention may be purely nervous in origin, particularly following operations on the perineum and anus or on any occasion when the recumbent position has to be assumed postoperatively.

2. *Air swallowing.* Air swallowing (aerophagy) sometimes results in dilatation of the stomach and again is a nervous reaction.

3. *Deep venous thrombosis.* This is more liable to occur in the patient who lies stiff and immobile in bed and movement must be encouraged.

4. *Tachycardia.* Many patients develop postoperative tachycardia in the absence of haemorrhage or toxaemia, and it can in itself be very wearisome. Sedation is usually indicated.

5. *General exhaustion* from:
   (a) Lack of rest and inadequate sleep;
   (b) Failure to take adequate nourishment because of nervous upset of digestion;
   (c) Persistent hiccough which is particularly difficult to control.

The mind and body are an integrated whole, and any attempt to manage them in isolation from one another is doomed to failure. The patient may be shy, reserved, taciturn and resent loss of dignity — he may be worried about his job or his family.

In addition to some of the detailed points which have been discussed above, the following are of considerable importance to the patients:

The pattern of his day. The more normal this can be the more normally we can expect the patient to react. Most patients are not accustomed to being awakened in the early hours of the morning, and if this can be avoided it is a great advantage.

The elimination of noise. It is unfortunately true that the hospital environment is often noisy and disturbed rather than quiet and peaceful.

Explanation. A simple explanation of what is happening is too often avoided.

THE ECONOMICS OF MEDICAL CARE

The demand for health care is far in excess of the resources from which it can be provided. The cost may be defrayed by:

1. The patient. The majority of the world's population is extremely poor and even in the more prosperous countries the number who can bear the full cost of treatment, directly or indirectly, through insurance provision is negligible.

2. The state, which has no money except what can be raised by taxation and borrowing. In spending this money health services are in competition with facilities for education, housing and the many complex services which a modern state has to try to provide.

3. Voluntary contributions and voluntary service is the oldest, and for so long in the United Kingdom, the only provision for the sick, and in many parts of the world is still the only source. Even where the state bears almost all the cost, there will always be ample scope for voluntary effort. The donation of sophisticated equipment from the efforts of charitably disposed contributors may be welcome, but the cost of operating it with the constant attendance of skilled nurses or technicians may be prohibitive.

The task of all engaged in health care is to stretch the available resources to get the maximal value by the elimination of waste and good management. The patient under treatment must not suffer but waste prevents or delays other patients being treated. While the cost of drugs and dressings requires no stressing other sources of misuse are easily overlooked. Excessive investigation, the necessity to repeat investigations because of inadequate preparation or failure to plan investigations in good time are all a cause of waste. Equipment, whether simple or sophisticated, demands instruction in its use. At all stages in caring for a patient the cost of energy is in itself a constricting factor on a hospital's expenditure. Conservation on this as on so many other items used in patient care enables more patients to be treated from a limited budget.

BIBLIOGRAPHY

Campbell E J, Scadding J G, Roberts R S 1979 British Medical Journal 2: 757
Scadding J G 1967 Lancet 2: 877

2

Surgical diagnosis and the nurse

Accurate diagnosis is the corner-stone of treatment. It is the doctor who makes the diagnosis after he has elucidated all the facts. The nurse's observation may be most important, particularly over a period when the patient's condition is changing.

HISTORY

A careful history is the most important single part of diagnosis. What the patient has observed is nearly always significant. He should have the opportunity of giving his account unhurriedly and without interruption in a room or examination bay. His family history, previous medical history, occupation, and the like are sometimes valuable. For example, a fistula-in-ano may be the first sign of pulmonary tuberculosis, and further inquiry may reveal that someone in the patient's home is a known sufferer from tuberculosis. Another example of the importance of the history is the tendency for some diseases to have a hereditary incidence—carcinoma of the colon is a very striking instance in families suffering from familial polyposis, and haemophilia in males is a well-known example. It is not the nurse's duty to obtain a detailed history as a routine, but patients will often mention to a nurse some fact of great importance which they thought was too trivial to mention to the surgeon. When the nurse is attending to the patient, however, she should always obtain a clear history if the patient complains of a new symptom; the exact complaint, if it is pain, its nature, site, radiation, aggravating and relieving factors, should be obtained at once. Sometimes before the doctor arrives the patient's condition may become such that he is unable to give as clear an account, and in rare cases he may be unconscious. The patient's complaints are known as symptoms, for example pain—what is elicited on examination, such as tenderness or a swelling, is known as a sign.

CLINICAL EXAMINATION

Facts discovered by examination are known as 'signs', and for their orderly elucidation the following plan is advisable.

Inspection reveals what can be observed by looking. It is surprising how much can be missed by impatience or too cursory a glance. For example, in a patient's face may be seen:

Anxiety or distress	Jaundice
Fright	Oedema
Depression	Partial paralysis
Indifference	A swelling
Stupor	A rash
A flush	Exophthalmos
Pallor	Sweat
Cyanosis	

Any of these observations may be informative. The pallor and sweat may be the result of haemorrhage, and cyanosis may signify increasing respiratory obstruction. Jaundice may be due to obstruction of the bile duct or haemolysis from a recent blood transfusion. Facial paralysis may be caused by a draught from lack of care in the ward, an extending intracranial condition, or the spread of middle-ear disease to the brain or mastoid antrum.

Elsewhere similar observations should be made, and in all sites previous scars, dilated veins, or the presence of a swelling are important. Anything abnormal should be reported by the nurse, however trivial it may appear.

Palpation or examination by feeling with the hands is next performed. To be of value the palpation must always be gentle and the hands must be warm. Tenderness, guarding (stiffness or spasm of the underlying muscles), or a swelling may be discovered. It is well to remember that patients who are in hospital for some other condition are not immune to acute abdominal conditions. Hernias still strangulate and peptic ulcers may still perforate. It has been said with no little truth that the most dangerous place for a patient suffering from a peptic ulcer to perforate is in a hospital!

Percussion consists of setting up artificial vibrations in the tissues by means of a sharp tap, usually with the fingers. Considerable experience is required in its interpretation. It is a sign by which a distended bladder gives rise to a dull note on percussion, thus differentiating it from a distended intestine which on percussion is described as being tympanitic (resonant).

Auscultation is particularly valuable to the nurse in the diagnosis and control of atrial fibrillation. It is impossible to control digitalis therapy unless the heart apex rate as well as the pulse rate are counted and charted separately.

The presence of the increased peristaltic sounds of intestinal obstruction may be heard with the stethoscope, but of greater interest is the reappearance of normal peristaltic sounds which signifies that oral feeding can usually be recommenced.

SPECIAL INVESTIGATIONS

Special tests may be necessary to confirm or aid diagnosis, and in carrying out investigations it is important that the regime of preparation is carefully followed.

Radiological diagnosis is based on contrast of shadows, and radio-opacity is proportional to atomic weight. The bones of the skeleton are readily visualised by 'straight' X-rays, and X-ray diagnosis can be almost completely accurate. Soft tissues may be examined by a modification of the type of ray: soft X-rays are used extensively in the diagnosis of chest disease. In general, however, the soft tissues are examined by outlining their cavities by filling them with opaque media. The barium meal, the barium enema, the bronchogram, and the retrograde injection of radio-opaque media into the kidneys are all examples of direct outlining of the interior of organs or tracts. Oral cholecystography for gall-bladder disease and the intravenous pyelogram are indirect methods of outlining organs, and also of testing their function. The examination of the blood vessels and the areas they supply or drain necessitate direct injection of a contrast medium into the vessel. Cine radiography will record the progress of opaque media and allow study at leisure — an image intensifier gives a television account of the conditions in the part X-rayed.

All these examinations depend on the careful co-operation of the nurse. For example, a patient should not take food or drink six hours before a barium meal examination. If a patient vomits the medium taken for a cholecystogram, or diarrhoea follows its ingestion, the radiologist should be informed. Contrast media contain iodide materials to which the patient may be sensitive, so antihistamines, adrenaline and hydro-cortisone, diuretics as well as intravenous equipment should be readily available in case the patient collapses.

Good organisation should reduce to a minimum the necessity to repeat radiological examinations. Diagnostic radiology adds to the hazards from radiation to the individual and the community at large. Amongst the most notable are the genetic effects and the possibility of development of leukaemia.

Radiological examination of women of reproductive age. It has become vitally necessary, in the light of present knowledge, to reduce the possibility of performing a radiological examination on any female patient between the ages of 15 and 50 who might be pregnant. It is, therefore, necessary to restrict certain X-rays in these patients to a time when it should not be possible for them to be pregnant, i.e. in that period of the menstrual cycle prior to ovulation. Therefore it is necessary to enter the date of the last menstrual period on all X-ray request forms in patients of this age or even younger in some communities and it may also be necessary to indicate, for the benefit of a clerk, that the examination should be carried out only between certain dates. These would normally be the ten days commencing with the first day of the period or the first day of the next expected period.

The examinations in question are:
Straight abdomen
Intravenous and retrograde pyelogram, and cystogram
Cholecystogram
Barium meal and enema
Lumbar spine, sacroiliac joints, sacrum and pelvis
Hips

Myelogram

Hysterosalpingogram

Lymphangiogram

It may be justifiable to ignore the above rule (known as the 'ten-day rule'). The grounds for ignoring it are: (1) medical urgency; (2) the patient is taking effective contraceptive precautions and the possibility of pregnancy can be reasonably ignored. If either is applicable it should be indicated on the X-ray request form.

Only by fulfilling the above recommendations can the Code of Practice for those exposed to ionising radiations be observed.

Radioactive isotopes are used to determine the function or the absence of function in many glands and organs. Deep-seated areas of the body may be outlined by such techniques and direct recording by a Geiger counter on a machine produces what is known as a Scintiscan. Radioactive isotopes are discussed in some detail in Chapters 22 and 28. The non-invasive techniques of EMI scanning may well revolutionise the delineation of pathology.

Many laboratory findings are invalidated because the specimens collected are not accurately labelled by the nurse or there has been undue delay in sending them to the laboratory.

Ultrasonic devices, by recording sound waves, give valuable clinical information. The presence of a thrombus in a vein as well as early pregnancy, may be detected by this means. It can also be used to monitor the sounds of the foetal heart.

Visual inspection of the interior of many organs is possible either directly or by indirect means, and these procedures are known as endoscopic inspections. They include cystoscopy, laryngoscopy, bronchoscopy, oesophagoscopy, sigmoidoscopy, gastroscopy, and peritoneoscopy. With all these procedures a biopsy may be taken.

THE NURSE'S SPECIAL CONTRIBUTION TO DIAGNOSIS

Careful observation, accurately recorded, is of great value. The patient in hospital, particularly in a surgical ward, is in highly artificial surroundings. This is greatly exaggerated as treatment progresses, whether by the administration of drugs, artificial feeding, or operation. The patient's physical condition, too, is often quite unstable during the 21 days following an uneventful operation, even though he may have resumed work, and he is more liable to sudden complications — for example, pulmonary embolism. The following examples serve as general illustrations of the care which is necessary:

1. Haemorrhage. An increasing pulse rate, a falling blood pressure and a subnormal temperature together with cold and clammy peripheries are characteristic of haemorrhage. For this reason alone it is important to chart a slight fall of temperature below the normal. Increasing pallor is characteristic, but in jaundiced patients it is unobservable, so particular attention to the pulse is essential.

After many operations — for example, mastectomy or cholecystectomy — a drainage tube is inserted. There is always some bloodstained discharge, which should be measured.

Following prostatectomy, if the drainage is light pink in colour haemorrhage is not excessive.

2. Abnormal discharges. The presence of bile from a gall-bladder wound when the common bile duct has not been opened, or of a faecal discharge from an abdominal wound, should be reported at once.

3. Continuous suction and irrigation apparatus can be very treacherous. The danger is that the cavity is thought to be dry while in fact fluid is welling up and may be causing damage. For this reason intermittent suction of the stomach is usually preferable.

Continuous irrigation is sometimes used after bladder operations and a complete suppression of urine may pass unobserved for days unless a strict check of the volume of fluid run in and the volume recovered has been kept.

4. Analgesics and other measures of symptomatic relief. The patient in severe pain cries out for relief but analgesics should be given only in a dosage to control the pain but of an insufficient dosage to produce narcosis. Following the temporary relief of overwhelming pain, the patient is enabled to co-operate by giving a coherent history and being responsive on clinical examination so that a diagnosis can be made.

5. Patients admitted in coma. These patients present special difficulties because a clear history is not always available, but in all cases the nurse should be alert to the possibility of the presence of associated injuries. Fractures without deformity can easily pass unnoticed in the comatose patient and delayed signs of internal injuries may appear some hours or days after admission. The level of consciousness is noted and assessed regularly.

The size of the pupils, whether they are equal or not, whether they are contracted or dilated, and their reaction to light, are essential observations, and any changes which occur should be written down.

The onset of a fit, its type, spread, duration and other features are frequently seen only by the nurse, and her report of the fit may be decisive in some cases. The appearance of slight weakness (paresis) in any muscles, as well as complete paralysis, is important. If this is done by means of a simple diagram, the right and left side should be clearly labelled.

6. Enemas. Enemas may be prescribed for diagnostic purposes, and the deciding factor as to whether an intestinal obstruction is complete and requires operation, or is incomplete, may be the report of the nurse that no flatus has been passed after an enema.

The passage of flatus by a rectal tube when the patient is suffering from peritonitis or paralytic ileus is a sign that the condition is responding to treatment.

7. General observation when the patient is washed may be very important. A swelling, an ulcer, a rash, oedema, or distension may be noticed when a patient is being washed, and such an observation may be the final clue to the solution of the pathology in an otherwise obscure case.

8. Changes in personality and behaviour should be watched very carefully. The effect of the mind on a patient's bodily ills can be profound, and in a surgical ward it is no less disastrous than elsewhere. Patients with a poor psychological background may break down completely before or, what is worse, after an operation. Chronic alcoholics are bad operative subjects and require special care. Not all mental manifestations have their origin in diseases of the mind and the following are examples of gross organic disease which may be present or appearing:

(a) *Slight confusion* is common preceding cerebral thrombosis.

(b) *Confusion, drowsiness and incoherent speech* may indicate the presence of a cerebral tumour which may be primary or secondary. A considerable amount of major surgery is 'cancer' surgery, and secondary deposits are characteristic of a cancer. The brain is one of the sites where a secondary deposit may lodge, and early recognition is important so that the attempt to remove the primary growth is abandoned, as it would now prove fruitless.

(c) *Polydipsia.* Excessive thirst and polyuria (excessive urinary output) are characteristic of diabetes insipidus. This condition is due to disease or injury of the pituitary body situated in the sella turcica in the middle fossa of the skull. Occasionally the condition is caused by a fracture in this area, with consequent damage to the pituitary gland.

9. Deep venous thrombosis complicated by pulmonary embolism is a condition of which every nurse in every surgical ward in every hospital must be aware. It is the one condition which will kill a fit patient with dramatic suddenness.

THE NURSE AND THE RECOGNITION OF DISEASE

There are times when the gravity of a situation is not recognised. The apparent well-being of the patient may be deceptive and yet it is in such situations that it is vital to act almost reflexly correctly. They may arise from the following:

1. Organisational failure. The failure to communicate the results of routine laboratory tests to monitor the dosage of certain drugs in out-patients constitutes a problem. The failure to act correctly is responsible for a number of deaths each year. The two main categories are:

(a) *The anticoagulant drugs* which are extremely dangerous unless controlled by laboratory tests. Any change in dosage should be communicated quickly to the patient and his doctor.

The patient is given a card and the dosage indicated immediately after the test — both in amount and the colour of the tablet.

(b) *Cytotoxic drugs* require monitoring of the white cell count in the blood. Severe white cell depletion necessitates admission to hospital isolation and the administration of penicillin without delay — both difficult steps to take if the patient has been allowed to leave hospital before the results are to hand! With no resistance to infection a journey home in a public service conveyance exposes him to the very hazards he has no resistance to combat.

2. Adverse drug reactions. An adverse drug reaction has been defined by the WHO as 'one which is noxious, unintended and occurs at doses used in man for prophylaxis, diagnosis or therapy' (WHO 1969). New drugs are released for general use only after clinical trials and after ward controlled trials have been undertaken. Nonetheless, spontaneous reporting by individual clinics of any adverse reaction has been a great help in the central registry issuing an early warning. When a new drug is used, a nurse should be specially observant to note any sign and to listen to and report any unusual symptoms of which the patient may complain.

3. Quiet onset. The failure to pass urine is almost always due to urinary retention, usually a painful condition. Anuria (the failure of the kidneys to secrete urine) is usually painless and the patient may initially look and feel very well. The result is that recognition is delayed 24 hours or longer. Only lynx-eyed observation by a nurse will diagnose the condition earlier, and once suspected all treatment should be stopped until a regime which takes account of the new situation has been designed. Drugs which are excreted in the urine can no longer be eliminated from the body and dangerous concentration may occur in the blood. The whole pattern of drug therapy has to be represcribed. Similarly all fluids are stopped and again the whole situation of fluid balance reconsidered (Ch. 42).

4. Omissions. A notable example of this is a full stomach before the induction of anaesthesia. Of course no one would give an anaesthetic to a patient with a full stomach. There is, however, one situation in which this is liable to occur and every year fatalities are recorded. The fit multiparous woman who has had a good meal may go into labour which may be very short indeed and in the rush to deal with her pressing obstetric problem she is given an anaesthetic in a hurry in unfavourable conditions and no one has remembered to pass a nasogastric tube. It is in just such a situation that a thoughtful nurse has so much to contribute.

Careful observation will always be necessary. The evaluation of findings and history is already in a small way being computerised. In the future the use of computers will be an added aid in the management of a patient.

3
Identification of the patient

The complexity of modern medical practice arises partly from the rapid increase in scientific knowledge and partly from the fact that the application of this knowledge for the patient's benefit demands that a greater and greater number of people are directly or indirectly concerned in his treatment. The amount of scientific equipment and the range of chemical reagents used in the treatment of a single patient can hardly be realised. Well-equipped operating theatres, laboratories and other departments of investigation and treatment are expensive to build and to staff. For this reason alone, the type of work which the acute general hospital undertakes becomes even more complex.

The result is that the treatment of a particular patient has become and will become more specific. That is to say that the treatment will be so well designed for him and his condition that the first essential is that he must be identifiable with certainty. There is greater liability to mistake or to human error today than ever before, and the consequences are liable to be more crippling and more lethal because many drugs and fluids have narrower margins of safety and are more potent in their effects than similar drugs in the past.

For this reason, the nurse must always ask herself two questions:

1. Is this patient William Smith (or whatever his name may be) who was born on 7.10.27?
2. Is this the correct injection, tablet or blood for William Smith?

She must also be able to ask herself these questions in reverse, namely:

1. Is the next patient for the removal of his appendix William Smith?
2. Is this William Smith now being lifted on to the trolley whom I am taking to the theatre for the removal of his appendix?

Certain well-known facts emerge about patients' behaviour in the stress and strain of going to the operating theatre, receiving injections or even in going from the waiting room to the consulting room of a clinic. For example, a patient sometimes thinks that he has been called when in fact another patient's name has been called. Some patients, hard of hearing, do not like to admit it and even though addressed by another patient's name, keep on saying 'yes' to everything!

This is now the paradoxical situation, that as care and treatment become

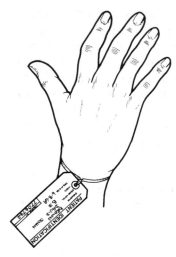

Fig. 3.1 Label attached to patient's wrist for identification.

more specific, more effective and more carefully planned (more personal, in fact), the risk that the plan may misfire through misidentification is greater and more serious.

Many patients have similar names and their place in the ward may be changed, so that identification such as 'third bed from the end on the left' is quite unreliable. A bed card on the wall or locker is certainly useful, but the patient may be moved in the ward and his bed card left, so that this method is not entirely foolproof. The patient's case sheet and records are not suitably kept at the end of the bed so they are not a method of identification. The only safe method is to have a separate identification marked on the bed; either on the bed or on a piece of strapping attached to the crossbar. Addressing machines have been used which produce a sheet of labels stating the patient's name, address, date of birth, sex, ward and unit number. Seriously ill patients and all patients going to the theatre should have their name on their wrist (Fig. 3.1). Ident-A-Band, which is a plastic bracelet, can be used and cannot be removed by the patient. The importance of identification of the patient is even greater when he is unconscious and may require an injection such as insulin, or a transfusion of blood.

IDENTIFICATION OF THE PATIENT'S SPECIMENS

Every specimen for examination taken from a patient either in the ward or operating theatre should be carefully labelled. In the ward there are certain cardinal points to avoid mishap:

1. Everything necessary to collect the specimen should be taken to the bedside.
2. The label should be written out and attached by the person taking the specimen in the presence of the patient and at the bedside.
3. Specimens should never be collected from two patients and then two labels written out together.

Blood specimens from patients suspected of suffering from serum viral hepatitis should carry a warning label.

In the theatre, specimens removed at operations are labelled and sealed after each operation.

THERAPEUTIC FLUIDS, TABLETS, AND OTHER AGENTS

Of all the therapeutic fluids, the one most liable to cause sudden and irreparable damage is incompatible blood. This will be stressed again in the chapter on blood transfusion. The following elementary precautions are essential:

1. The patient must be identified with certainty.
2. The label indicating the cross-match against the patient's blood must be checked against the patient and the bag of blood and also the blood group.

The maze inside a blood refrigerator illustrates how easy it is to pick up the wrong bag.

Other substances particularly liable to cause harm are the anticoagulants, insulin, radium and sedatives. The tragedy of a mistake in the identification of a patient requires no emphasis and in the rush of a busy day it is more likely to occur. Even the coincidence of an identical name, occupation, and disease may play a part, so that the sole identifiable mark may be the patient's home address and his date of birth. If a nurse is in doubt she should never hesitate to share her doubt at once with a more senior member of the staff. No drug or therapeutic substance should be given orally or otherwise without using the correct checking procedure — two persons must always be involved.

The nurse should be able to identify the contents of a medical gas cylinder by its colour. Gas cylinders are now pin indexed — that is, the attachment is so contrived that coupling can be effected only to the correct point on a machine for that particular gas.

4

Perioperative care

The preoperative preparation and the after-care of the patient is a subject to which an increasing amount of attention has been devoted in recent years. Complications once believed to be unavoidable have been reduced to very small proportions, and the convalescence of a larger number of patients has been more comfortable. The final result of an operation is much more likely to be entirely satisfactory in the absence of complications.

The great variation which appears to exist among the methods favoured by different surgeons is undoubtedly a cause of considerable bewilderment and confusion to the junior nurse. However, it must be realised that the differences are not differences of principle but of method.

The principles of preoperative and postoperative care can be readily understood by a moment's reflection on what an operation really means to a patient. In his mind arise thoughts of a wound, loss of blood, an anaesthetic, a period of incapacity in bed, weakness when he gets up, pain and fear of the end result—perhaps of death, perhaps of some incapacity which may prevent him from carrying on his normal life.

Before all operations, but particularly in an emergency, a nurse must inquire if the patient is taking any drugs. (The term drugs covers all medicines including those which are self-prescribed.) Many of these influence the preoperative preparation. Obvious examples are the steroids, the dose of which must always be increased; insulin or other antidiabetic drugs, and anticoagulants. Oestrogens (which are contained in some contraceptive pills) increase the risk of thrombosis. Cytotoxic drugs, or any drug liable to damage the white blood cells, delay healing. Diuretics may lower the blood potassium and prolong the action of muscle relaxants after anaesthesia. Antihypertensive drugs may cause an undesirable fall in blood pressure. Monoamine oxidase inhibitors such as phenelzine (Nardil) react with anaesthetic agents. A note should also be made of any known allergies.

All drug therapy, quite apart from those listed above, should be considered with special reference to its effect on anaesthesia, haemorrhage and all the factors possibly arising in the patient's convalescence.

The principles of treatment, therefore, are:

1. To render safe the administration of an anaesthetic and to ensure that the patient recovers consciousness without mishap.
2. To prevent or treat shock.
3. To achieve healing of the wound as rapidly as possible.
4. To prevent or treat complications which may arise as a result of recumbency in bed.
5. To restore rapidly the function in all the organs of the body as well as in the mind.

The operation should be undertaken when the patient is in the best possible condition and for this reason the planned operation, where the patient can be assessed several days before admission, is preferable to the emergency operation. The chest is X-rayed, the blood haemoglobin level is determined and the blood grouped and crossmatched if necessary. An estimation of the blood urea and electrolytes is undertaken if there is reason to suspect they may be altered. If necessary, pulmonary function tests are performed. A patient of negroid race should be screened for sickle cell disease as those with this disease have unstable red blood cells. This causes aggregation of the haemoglobin inside the cells under conditions of hypoxia.

An electrocardiogram is advisable in patients over 60 years of age.

It is necessary to have the signed permission of the patient before performing an operation, or, if the patient is under 16 years of age, in Great Britain, that of his parent or guardian. Before taking the patient to the theatre the nurse should check that she has the correct patient, his notes and X-ray films. Rings, earrings and hearing aids should be removed or covered with Sellotape so that there can be no contact between metal on the patient's body and diathermy current. The stomach should always be empty before the patient is anaesthetised. Usually this means prohibiting food for six hours previously and fluid for about three/four hours. If a fit patient must have an anaesthetic immediately, such as a sudden labour in a multiparous woman, a stomach tube must be passed without delay. The stomach of patients suffering from intestinal obstruction must be emptied by aspiration — not only must a tube be passed but it must be aspirated continuously until anaesthesia has been induced and the cuff of the endotracheal tube has been inflated. The reason for this is that stomach contents may be aspirated into the bronchial tubes.

The operation bed

The bed is made with clean linen, usually while the patient is having a bath. While the patient is in theatre, the bed is remade. The top bed clothes are double-rolled and then made into a pack. According to the patient's needs, other articles are prepared, e.g.

Post-anaesthetic tray

Oxygen

Charts

Because the preparation for operation, the care of the patient in the theatre and the immediate postoperative treatment are continuous in time they are considered together in this chapter.

THE CARE OF THE PATIENT UNDER ANAESTHESIA

Before the administration of an anaesthetic the patient's heart and lungs are examined and a specimen of urine is tested for the presence of sugar and albumin. The finding of an abnormal constituent in the urine is reported at once. Further preparation of the patient may be necessary and the choice of anaesthetic may be influenced.

Freedom from colds and respiratory infections is desirable, and if the patient suffers from chronic bronchitis the operation should be deferred, if possible, until the warm summer months. He should be persuaded to stop smoking. If a cough is present a corset dressing on the abdominal wound may prevent postoperative complications. Preoperative breathing exercises may also be prescibed with advantage. He must be warmly clad and covered in transit to and from the theatre.

Premedication

This formerly took the form of morphia (10 to 15 mg), pethidine (50 to 100 mg) or omnopon (20 mg) provided that the patient was not taking monoamine oxidase inhibitor drugs. Modern practice tends towards the administration of pure anxietolytic drugs such as Librium 10 mg, Droperidol 10 mg or Valium 10 mg. This helps to avoid the vomiting and nausea which must be attributed to the use of morphia. If a general anaesthetic is to be administered, atropine (0·6 mg) may be prescribed to prevent excessive secretion of mucus in the respiratory tract. With the increasing use of non-irritant anaesthetic techniques it has become quite common to omit the routine administration of atropine before operation. Instead, the drug may be given by the anaesthetist at the same time as anaesthesia is induced. This avoids the unpleasant dry mouth, tachycardia, and blurred vision caused by atropine. It may also avoid rises in temperature, particularly in children, due to the inhibition of sweating.

Anaesthesia

This is a condition in which the patient loses consciousness and is insensible to the proceedings. It can be produced by various routes:

1. Inhalation. Known agents for this purpose are ether, trichlorethlene, (trilene), nitrous oxide, halothane (Fluothane), cyclopropane, methoxyfluorane and enflurane (ethrane). Inhalation may be from:

    (a) An open mask, for example, dripping ether on to a gauze pad.

    (b) A semiclosed circuit—a large flow of gas from an anaesthetic machine is delivered to the patient's airway. With expiration the gases, including CO_2 from the lungs, escape from the apparatus by a one-way valve.

    (c) A closed circuit. A small flow of gas is used. The expired gases are passed through soda lime to absorb CO_2 and the gas is then recirculated.

2. Intravenously. Thiopentone (Pentothal), methohexitone (Brietal) and althesin are well-known examples.

Analgesia

Analgesia is the loss of sensation to pain with or without loss of consciousness. It can be:

1. General. Examples are nitrous oxide, methoxyflurane halothane or trichlorethylene in small dosage. This method is used extensively in dental and obstetric practice. Mixtures of nitrous oxide and oxygen known as Entonox are available in cylinders for use with a demand type machine for self-administered analgesia.

2. Local may be—
   (a) *Regional*, produced by blocking the nerves at a site proximal to the proposed region of operation.
   (b) *Infiltration*, produced by blocking the nerve at the actual site of the operation.
   (c) *Topical*, produced by blocking the nerve endings by the application of an analgesic agent to the surface.

3. Epidural analgesia. Epidural analgesia is induced by the introduction of local anaesthetic into the epidural space.

Muscle relaxants

Muscle relaxation is necessary for many operations, especially upper abdominal procedures, and this can be produced by injecting intravenously certain agents such as d-tubocurarine chloride, Allcuronium, Pavulon (pancuronium bromide), Scoline or succinylcholine, which paralyse the voluntary muscles, including the diaphragm and intercostal muscles. If these drugs are used a perfect airway has to be maintained and the lungs must be artificially ventilated. At the end of the operation the effect of the muscle-relaxant drug has not completely worn off, and the anaesthetist gives the patient a counteracting drug (neostigmine). This is accompanied by an injection of atropine which prevents the undersirable effects of neostigmine, particularly on the heart. Even so a certain amount of weakness may remain in the vital respiratory muscles, so great vigilance is required. There is no antidote to Scoline, but the period of efficacy is short (minutes).

Hypothermia. Hypothermia is now only used in cardiac and neurosurgery. Profound hypothermia to the point of circulatory arrest is used for the correction of congenital heart defects during the first year of life.

Anaesthesia is induced in the usual way. Various drugs are given to diminish metabolism and lower the temperature, and in addition all warm bedclothing is removed and ice-bags placed all over the patient. When a satisfactory fall in temperature to about 32·2°C (90°F) is obtained the operation is performed. The patient's temperature is brought up very slowly postoperatively. For cardiac procedures cooling is induced by cardiopulmonary by pass.

The induction of anaesthesia

General anaesthesia is usually induced by the intravenous injection of one of the barbiturate drugs such as Pentothal (thiopentone).

A peaceful atmosphere in the anaesthetic room comforts the patient and makes the induction of the anaesthetic easier.

If a local or epidural analgesic is used, ear plugs render the patient's ordeal in the theatre less distressing. The patient's eyes should be covered to prevent him from following the course of events by watching the reflection in the lamp. His attention should also be diverted from time to time by engaging him in conversation while the operation is proceeding.

Maintenance of a free airway

The maintenance of a free airway is essential. The clothing should not include any constricting bands around the waist or neck, and if the patient wears dentures they should be removed in the ward and kept in a place of safety.

After operations on the mouth the following complications are particularly liable to occur:
1. Asphyxia due to:
    (a) Blood and mucus running down the trachea.
    (b) Haemorrhage blocking the naso- and oropharynx.
    (c) The tongue falling back.
2. Inhalation pneumonia from the aspiration of pus or other material.

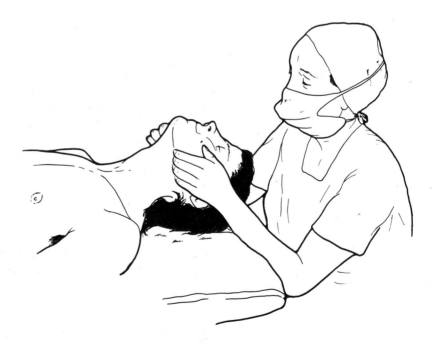

Fig. 4.1 The jaw of the unconscious patient is held forward to prevent his tongue falling back.

After induction of anaesthesia a cuffed endotracheal tube is passed. The patient's throat is packed with a continuing length of gauze. Afterwards he is nursed on his side. The pack must be removed and the nurse must note in writing that this has been done. All swabs and packs used by the anaesthetist are coloured so that they cannot be confused with those used by the surgeon. Exudates of mucus and blood are aspirated and an airway is usually inserted before the patient leaves the theatre.

The jaw of an unconscious patient should always be held well forward; if this is done the tongue cannot slip back (Fig. 4.1). An artificial pharyngeal airway must also be kept on the theatre trolley, and if this instrument is introduced it should not be removed by a nurse until the patient resents its presence.

No patient should be taken from the theatre back to the ward until the anaesthetist has given permission to move him.

The patient is returned to bed accompanied by a nurse who carries a tray containing an airway and gauze swabs. She should note his colour, pulse, breathing, the presence of cyanosis, dyspnoea and coughing.

Anaesthetic deaths occur from:

1. Failure to maintain the airway
2. Failure to maintain ventilation
3. Hypotension — hence the importance of monitoring the blood pressure, the pulse and the heart action by an E.C.G.

Instruction on the timing and amount of postoperative analgesics prescribed should be in writing.

Care of the limbs

While unconscious the patient's legs and arms should be kept in the correct position, and at all times special care should be taken to avoid pressure on the nerves, otherwise paralysis is liable to occur. There is particular danger of radial paralysis if the patient's arm is allowed to hang over the edge of the table. Arms should not be extended over boards whilst the patient is in the head-down position with shoulder supports because of the risk of damage to the brachial plexus. Elastic stockings on the legs reduce the risk of venous thrombosis.

Care of the bladder

For almost all operations the bladder should be empty. The important exceptions are cystoscopic examinations and operations on the bladder.

On return to bed

During transit from the theatre the patient must be warmly clad and, if bald, the head should be covered with a shawl or small blanket. On return to the ward the patient is laid on his side and propped over on his shoulder. Turning the head to one side is not advised as this makes it almost impossible for the patient to vomit (if necessary) and breathing with the twisted neck is very difficult. He should not be left unattended before he is able to speak. When consciousness has returned, the position varies considerably with the nature of the operation which has been performed, but in most cases it is a good rule to allow the patient to assume the position he finds most comfortable. The area of the wound is inspected for bleeding.

It may be noticed that on return to the ward, although the airway is clear, his respiration is unsatisfactory and he is becoming cyanosed. This is particularly liable to occur after the use of the relaxant drugs, where full respiratory function has not been recovered. Oxygen should be given and the anaesthetist summoned at once — further assisted respiration with the anaesthetic machine may be advised. If the pulse is good, the patient sweating and of good colour, respiration may still be unsatisfactory. This failure is due to excessive retention of carbon dioxide in the blood and it is necessary to remove the excess by a carbon-dioxide absorber, using assisted respiration. It is essential to differentiate between respiratory obstruction in which the patient is struggling to breathe and respiratory depression which is caused by relaxant drugs or shock.

However, the anaesthetist will give precise instructions on the management of the patient before the patient leaves the theatre.

Cyanosis in a jaundiced patient as in a member of the coloured races will be detected only if the colour of the lips is noted.

Visiting in open wards on operation days is undesirable and patients recovering from anaesthesia behind screens are in a position of great peril. A better alternative if visiting is allowed, is a recovery area in the ward where constant observation is possible.

Postoperative pain

The reliable relief of postoperative pain remains an unsolved problem. Numerous patients testify to our shortcomings and their friends warn them to expect it. It is impossible to measure pain and two patients who have undergone identical operations, performed by the same surgeon and anaesthetist on the same day, from the same ward, experience quite different degrees of pain. Most patients, because they do not want to appear cowardly, do not complain until their pain is severe. Yet it has been shown that a small dose of an analgesic drug given in good time and repeated frequently is most effective.

In practice, the relief of postoperative pain is largely unsupervised by doctors — the surgeon and the anaesthetist are already immersed in the next operation and the prescription of a specified analgesic after 'an interval' or 'as required' is not the easiest task for the nurse to fulfil. The nurse has a special responsibility as well as an opportunity to acquire special skill in the relief of postoperative pain. She has to make her own assessment of its severity from her own observation and her knowledge of the patient acquired before the operation.

She must, of course, administer the analgesic prescribed. Morphia and pethidine are still the most commonly used. Despite the multiplicity of drugs available, none seems to combine the analgesic qualities of morphia with a comparable degree of mental sedation and a sense of well-being. Its safety has been enhanced by the introduction of naloxine which effectively reverses its depressant effect on the respiratory centre. (It reverses its analgesic effects as well). All analgesic agents have limitations or side effects when given in sufficient dosage to relieve severe pain and the nurse should be familiar with the disadvantages of any drug prescribed on her unit.

The aspiration of gastric contents

Patients who vomit during anaesthesia are liable to inhale gastric contents which are highly acidic.

If this occurs the patient may develop serious pulmonary complications. Such patients are treated by bronchial toilet and the administration of large doses of corticosteroids and antibiotics.

Postoperative vomiting. Postoperative vomiting, if excessive, leads to rapid salt and water depletion. In most cases the vomiting ceases very quickly; if it does not, Maxolon 10 mg or chlorpromazine (Largactil) 25 mg is usually effective. If the vomiting persists, however, the stomach is aspirated with a nasogastric tube. The patient is given only fluid at first until the bowel sounds have returned, after which a normal diet is resumed. If vomiting persists or commences 24 hours postoperatively, the possibilities of intestinal obstruction have to be considered.

Persistent hiccough is sometimes a very distressing complication of an operation. The treatment is to administer CO_2 (carbon dioxide) 5 per cent; if there is no response, 10 per cent CO_2 may be given. Largactil 25 mg is sometimes of value. In intractable cases the administration of hyoscine (0·4 mg) or 'blocking' of the left phrenic nerve in the neck with local anaesthesia may be advisable.

The care of the mouth

After gastric operations fluids by mouth are usually forbidden for 24 hours, and after that the quantity is restricted for a further 24 hours. If a patient who is confined to bed can clean his own teeth, he is given a beaker of water or mouth wash, and a bowl into which to spit.

When a patient is unable to use his hands but is otherwise well, the nurse can clean his teeth for him, using the patient's own toothbrush, and toothpaste, and allow him to rinse his own mouth, spitting into a bowl held by the nurse.

When the patient cannot co-operate in caring for his mouth, a special technique is required along the following lines.

The nurse washes and dries her hands. If possible an explanation is given to the patient. Privacy is ensured. A hand towel is placed over the patient's chest for protection. Using the fingers, a cotton wool swab or a lint square is firmly fixed into the teeth of a pair of forceps which clip, e.g. artery forceps. The swab is dipped into a solution of sodium bicarbonate in water, strength of 1 in 160.

The mouth is opened and is cleaned in a systematic order, e.g. lips, cheeks, gums, teeth, palate, tongue. If necessary the tongue can be depressed using a tongue depressor. Each swab is used only once. It is removed from the forceps using a pair of dissecting forceps, and is discarded into the soiled dressing bag.

After the mouth has been cleaned it can be refreshed using a gauze swab wrapped around a gloved finger dipped into glycothymiline. The lips can be kept moist by a thin film of petroleum jelly of glycerine and borax.

The face is dried, the towel removed and the patient made comfortable. The equipment is removed and discarded.

The nurse washes and dries her hands.

Any unusual condition of the mouth is reported to the Sister or Charge Nurse, who will order any special treatment.

Care of dentures

When a patient can clean his own dentures, he is given a bowl of cold water in which to do so, and also a beaker of water or mouthwash with which to rinse his mouth.

When it is necessary for a nurse to clean the patient's dentures, they are removed and placed into a denture container. Taking the dentures and the patient's toothbrush to the bathroom, she cleans the dentures over a sink using *cold* running water. It is most important for modern dentures that the water used should be cold. They are returned to the patient, who is allowed to rinse his mouth before replacing them.

When a patient does not wish to retain his dentures, or in the case of a very weak or unconscious patient, the dentures are first cleaned and then placed in a denture container labelled with the patient's name, and stored in his locker. Before replacing the dentures which have been stored, they should be rinsed in cold water.

Maintenance of nutrition

If the operation is a short one, such as uncomplicated appendicectomy, no special difficulty arises in feeding. The patient takes fluids shortly after recovering consciousness and soon resumes a normal diet. Following a long period of anaesthesia, the maintenance of nutrition is essential, and of all the constituents of diet, fluid is the most important. Until the patient is able to drink, the fluid balance is maintained by the administration of fluid by other routes.

In severely ill patients or following extensive resections of the intestinal tract where it is clear that there is no likelihood of maintaining nutrition by eating within a couple of days, nitrogen imbalance (Ch. 15) has to be restored. An elemental diet may be given through a nasogastric tube or if this is not possible, feeding by the intravenous route is established. (Ch. 15).

Deep-breathing exercises

Deep-breathing exercises, particularly in the 48 hours following the operation, do much to eliminate pulmonary complications. These should be taught by the physiotherapist in the preoperative waiting period if possible.

THE WOUND

The diminution or elimination of infection at the site of the disease

A wound will heal rapidly only if it is non-infected. The wound includes not only the incision in the skin, fascia and muscles, but in all the deeper organs which have been opened. If infection is present in the organ to be operated on it should, if possible, be controlled before the operation takes place. Not only is the operation easier and safer, but the patient's convalescence is smoother.

In some cases several weeks' preparation may be necessary before the operation is undertaken. To illustrate this principle, operations at the following sites may be taken as examples:

1. The lungs. In Chapter 30 this problem is considered in detail. In the condition known as bronchiectasis, for which a lobe of the lung is removed, every effort is made to empty the cavities of pus and render their walls as clean as possible. Expectorant mixtures, antibiotics, postural drainage, breathing exercises, and physiotherapy are all prescribed for this purpose.

2. The stomach and duodenum. Operation is commonly undertaken for chronic gastric and duodenal ulceration which has failed to respond to medical treatment, or because the ulcer has produced an obstruction to the outlet of the stomach (pyloric stenosis). If the emptying of the stomach is defective, gross infection results in the stagnant food. The stomach must be washed out repeatedly.

3. The intestine. It is impossible to sterilise the intestinal contents, but the degree of infectivity can be reduced considerably. The incision and suture of a septic swollen intestine are fraught with considerable danger. The stitches may cut out, resulting in leakage of the intestinal contents. Before an operation on the intestine, the diet should consist of food which leaves no residue, so that faecal accumulation is diminished. Antibacterial drugs are administered systematically in the anaesthetic room. Attempts to sterilise the bowel by oral administration have been less effective.

4. The urinary tract. A wound communicating with the urinary tract will be very slow to heal in the presence of grossly infected urine. The consumption of about 3000 ml of fluid daily is adequate to ensure elimination of waste products and not too excessive to dilute the concentration of antibacterial drugs in the kidneys.

The same principle applies to all sites where an operation may be performed, whether it be the mouth, the eye, the ear, or the joints. The methods of controlling infection will be discussed in detail (p. 56). Some surgeons like to operate under an 'antibiotic umbrella' if there is a risk of infection, but experience has shown that this is not as effective as one may think.

The preparation of the skin

The preparation of the skin is a procedure common to almost all operations. The skin should be shaved, and if the patient is fit a bath or better a shower is given to remove loose hairs. The skin is then washed with soap and water and dried on a clean towel. After this preparation the patient is put into a theatre gown and goes to bed in freshly laundered sheets. No antiseptic, towelling or dressings are applied in the ward.

The skin of the thighs of a patient who is incontinent of faeces requires special preparation if anaerobic infections are to be avoided after operations such as amputation or nailing operations for fracture of the femoral neck.

The importance of adequate vitamin C in the body

If vitamin C is deficient the healing of the wound may be delayed or fail to occur, but in the United Kingdom vitamin C deficiency is now uncommon except in the elderly who live alone.

The care of the wound

This is considered in Chapter 11.

Prevention and treatment of shock

This subject is considered in detail in Chapter 14.

Usually until 4 hours before the operation the patient may drink freely. If drinking is difficult or the patient is vomiting, fluids must be administered by the intravenous route. In pyloric stenosis, or intestinal obstruction, as fluid cannot leave the stomach, fluid by mouth is prohibited for hours or even days preoperatively. A patient depleted of salt and water becomes collapsed very rapidly. Severe purgation, once thought to be a good preoperative measure, is now known to be harmful since it produces severe dehydration and loss of electrolytes. In most cases a reduction of diet is all that is necessary.

An anaemic patient collapses very easily, and slight haemorrhage increases this tendency. A preliminary blood transfusion is given and may be continued during the operation. Fear predisposes to shock and sedatives and hypnotics may be useful. The relief of pain and the promotion of sleep are important. Analgesic and hypnotic drugs are administered, but an uncomfortable bandage or an awkward position in bed should be corrected. The patient must be returned to a warm bed, but excessive warming only increases the degree of shock.

After operation the nurse should note carefully the patient's colour and the state of his skin, any increase in the rate of the pulse, its quality, and any irregularity, and a strict check on the blood pressure is also indicated. In more serious cases a half-hourly check is recorded or the heart rate is monitored. Basically the treatment is relief of pain, elevation of the foot of the bed, and blood transfusion.

The prevention and treatment of complications which arise as a result of recumbency in bed

With very few exceptions no patient should be confined to bed before operation. The principal exception is a patient suffering from thyrotoxicosis and even in this condition confinement to bed to secure complete rest to the heart is now rarely necessary as modern antithyroid drugs control the toxicity so effectively.

The complications which may arise are:

1. Difficulty with micturition. Many patients find it difficult to pass urine while lying flat in bed and the difficulty is increased if there is an abdominal wound. The patient may sit or stand up or use a commode. Relaxation is necessary and the relief of pain essential. The treatment of this condition is discussed in Chapter 43. Catheterisation is not resorted to until all other measures have failed. A patient suffering from a minor degree of prostatic obstruction should have a catheter passed in the theatre after any operation which may precipitate retention. It can be removed in a day or two when he is up and about and pain has diminished.

2. Difficulty with defaecation. Difficulty in defaecation arises from conditions similar to those which interfere with micturition. The main factor in this condition, however, is intestinal distension with gas causing pain, and in all cases it should be relieved at regular intervals by the passage of a flatus tube — otherwise the heart and lungs may be embarrassed and the onset of the condition known as paralytic ileus may be encouraged.

Distension may be induced by an unsuitable diet during the two days before operation. Foods likely to cause residue and flatulence, such as vegetables, pastries, and large quantities of milk, should be avoided. The immediate preoperative care of the bowel has been discussed, but if the bowel is the site of the operation, as in removal of a portion of the colon, extra precautions are necessary (Ch. 39).

3. Respiratory complications. Respiratory complications are very common. Many anaesthetic mixtures are irritant and produce excessive secretion. This may result in bronchitis, retained secretions or massive lobar collapse of the lungs. Pneumonia is an occasional complication. Many patients are afraid to take deep breaths because of fear of damage to their wounds. Lack of movement and shallow breathing increase the liability to pulmonary complications. They need help and supervision. The patient is encouraged to use his hands to support the abdominal wound.

Inhalations, of which steam is the most important, are sometimes of value. Alternatively an ultrasonic nebuliser producing 'cold steam' or an electric nebuliser may be used. Nebulisers may be fitted to the oxygen supply. The moisture produced by either method reaches the smaller bronchioles and liquefies the mucus.

Pulmonary complications following operation are much commoner after interference in the upper abdomen and in all operations are more closely related to pre-existing bronchitis rather than the type of anaesthetic. Preoperative assessment and treatment with antibiotics, bronchial dilators, breathing exercises and, if necessary, steroids, diminish the risk. In addition

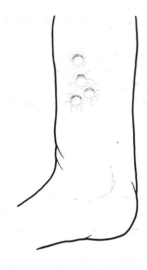

Fig. 4.2 Pitting oedema and swelling of the leg due to thrombosis.

of course the patient should stop smoking. Good postoperative physiotherapy is essential.

4. Thrombosis. Inactivity from rest in bed and an increase in the number of platelets in the blood as the result of a wound are conditions which favour the occurrence of a blood clot (or thrombus) in the veins of the legs (Fig. 4.2). Movement of the clot into the general circulation (embolism) may give rise to sudden death. Measures to diminish thromboembolism are discussed in Chapter 13. Preoperative oestrogens have already been mentioned as likely to increase thrombosis. Operating on the patient, with the heels slightly elevated off the table and continued slight bed elevation post-operatively, diminish the risk of thrombosis by taking pressure off the calves. In high-risk patients prophylactic heparin therapy may be prescribed (Ch. 13).

5. Pressure. Great care should be taken to prevent pressure sores after operations and in any severe illness. Their treatment is described in Chapter 21.

6. Muscular disuse and deformity. Muscular disuse and deformity have to be carefully guarded against, especially in orthopaedic conditions where they are most likely to occur, but they are none the less important in all conditions where the patient has been confined to bed for a considerable period.

7. Mental inactivity. Many patients tend to deteriorate mentally during a long stay in bed, and occupational therapy has a useful part to play.

Postoperative mania may occur in unstable subjects after operation. Old people are liable to develop mental changes. This is also liable to occur in toxic conditions. Paraldehyde (7 to 10 ml) is usually prescribed if the patient is otherwise uncontrollable.

Delirium tremens may occur in chronic alcoholics.

8. Diminution in circulating blood volume. This occurs with bed rest and increases the risk of circulatory collapse (shock) during operation. It may be further aggravated by the vasodilatation produced by many anaesthetic agents in current use.

9. Postoperative pyrexia. Following operation many patients develop a rise in temperature which usually subsides after 24 hours. If it persists the following steps are advisable:

(a) The wound should be inspected for swelling or tenderness, which may be due to haematoma formation or infection.

(b) The urine is examined for pus and organisms.

(c) The legs are inspected for signs of thrombosis (Ch. 13).

(d) The chest is examined and a radiograph may show a segment of collapse.

(e) After an abdominal operation a residual abscess in the pelvis (detectable by rectal examination) or a subphrenic abscess should be suspected (Ch. 34).

(f) A white blood count for leucocytosis.

Restoration of function

The restoration of function in the organs of the body by rehabilitation, re-education, exercises, and an adequate convalescence are most important.

The advice given to a patient on leaving hospital on such special points as diet, care of his wound, fitness for work, and other activities will do much to ensure a good result. Such advice must however be given against the knowledge of the patient's social background, his psychological attitude, education and personal character.

DAY SURGERY

The patient's general practitioner, together with the community nurse, will be able to continue treatment at home. In some cases where equipment or home help facilities are necessary the social services of the district authority may be used.

Day surgery requires the cooperation of the general practitioner, the community nurse and the hospital. It increases the work of the hospital and good organisation is essential to its smooth running. There is a danger that as the patient has such a short time in contact with the staff he may feel that he has received treatment which was technically competent but that there was no personal concern. A word to show that the nurse who receives and sees him on discharge fully realises this possibility is most welcome. Another difficulty nurses experience in day wards is finding medical staff to come to discharge the patient.

Preoperatively the suitability of the patient's home is assessed, a note is sent to the hospital of any drugs which the patient may be taking, X-rays, blood and urine examination are undertaken before the day of admission but urine must always be examined again on the day of operation. Before the patient is discharged following day surgery he should be—

   (i) seen by the doctor at the hospital and kept in if there is any doubt about his fitness;

  (ii) given analgesics or a note of what treatment is necessary;

 (iii) warned about bleeding;

 (iv) told to report back to the hospital if necessary.

5
Pain

Pain is one of the commonest presenting and continuing symptoms of organic and psychiatric disease. The mechanism of its production and perception are ill understood. It is rarely felt as an isolated sensation — a pin-prick is a mixture of touch and pain. The simple conception of pain receptors conveying impulses along a sensory nerve to a tract in the spinal cord and then to the cerebral cortex which localises the site of the pain is not confirmed by modern physiological research.

Pain arising in the skin can be localised accurately but pain of visceral origin is usually felt in the skin or muscular wall far distant from the organ involved. Conversely, it has been shown that vascular changes and alterations in the tone of a viscus can be produced by stimulating a localised area of skin. Such changes may provide a rational explanation for the use of counter-irritant measures and for acupuncture.

GATE CONTROL THEORY OF PAIN

Melzack and Wall in 1965 postulated the theory of a gate control mechanism. The large 'A' fibres tend to close this gate and the small 'C' fibres tend to open it. If the large 'A' fibres are destroyed, as in herpes zoster, the smaller 'C' fibres have free play and the gate is opened giving rise to pain. Electrical stimulation of the larger nerve fibres in the posterior columns of the spinal cord is effective in the control of some types of pain. Work is at present proceeding to make this a practical possibility.

Pain is protective. It is subjective and cannot be measured or monitored like the temperature or the pulse rate. A nurse will confirm from her own experience on the wards the apparently enormous variation in the degree of pain felt by two different patients from what appears to be an identical clinical lesion. In making this assessment the family doctor with intimate knowledge of a patient and his background has a great advantage over hospital staff. Anxiety and depression are important factors in the causation and escalation of pain. All pain is genuine and real to the patient and it may well be that pain of psychological origin is even more severe. To doubt this is to place oneself at a great disadvantage in the management of the patient. The only pain which is not genuine is one 'produced' for malingering or fraudulent purposes. Pain may be caused by tissue destruction with the release of chemical substances locally as well as by anoxia. The products of the inflammatory reaction are well-recognised sources of the origin of pain although the exact nature of the substances and the mode of action are open to more doubt. That cancer produces so little pain in the earlier stages is an important cause of delay in diagnosis. Lack of oxygen is a well-recognised cause of myocardial pain as it is of intermittent claudication in peripheral arterial disease. Pressure on nerve roots is believed to be a cause of pain and in prolapsed intervertebral disc this is undoubtedly true because removal of the disc cures the pain. It is also believed that collapse of a vertebral body from secondary carcinoma causes pain by compressing the nerve root below, but the fact that removal of even one adrenal gland in a responsive case of breast cancer will relieve the pain immediately provides a nice enigma which baffles explanation on present knowledge. A single dose of oestrogens for a similar pain arising from cancer of the prostate may have the same dramatic effect.

The administration of steroids is effective in relieving susceptible pain but there is a danger that they may mask, exacerbate or reactivate a lesion which in their absence the body would overcome uneventfully. A healed peptic ulcer or a healed focus of pulmonary tuberculosis may become very active.

The endogenous opiates are substances of different structure to the opiates but with apparently similar function. They latch on to the same receptors as morphine and their effects like morphine are reversed by the narcotic antagonist drug Naxolone. There are two groups, the encephalins and the beta-endorphins. Electrode percutaneous stimulation or acupuncture techniques take about twenty minutes before the patient feels any effects, presumably because it requires this time for sufficient quantities of the substances to be released. Beta-endorphin is a neurohormone secreted into the pituitary and Bowsher suggests that its release at the same time as ACTH in stress may explain why soldiers on the battlefield or sportsmen may feel no pain and be unaware at the time that they have been injured.

The prostaglandin PGE$_2$ secreted locally in inflammatory conditions dilates the blood vessels and increases capillary permeability. It is believed that this mechanism is blocked by cortisone or aspirin, with the result that the symptoms may be relieved but not necessarily effecting cure of the disease and in the examples quoted above explains the possibility of reactivation.

CLINICAL MANAGEMENT

The significance of pain as a symptom of disease has to be evaluated by a full examination of the patient so that a diagnosis can be made. Analgesics are restricted in patients suffering from acute abdominal pain until a diagnosis is made. Even in these conditions a sensible explanation will do much to relieve pain by allaying anxiety. In some acute situations an analgesic may have to be administered before transport of the patient to hospital, but the amount should be kept to the minimum and a note made of what has been administered. The dosage and the time of administration should accompany the patient. Obviously the sooner the diagnosis is established and a plan of treatment instituted the better.

The converse situation also holds great danger for the patient. The diagnosis has been clearly established — the patient either complains of repeated pain or the pain suddenly becomes more severe. The alert nurse should ask herself two questions before repeating analgesics — 'Is this the same situation?' or 'Has a complication arisen?' Two examples are:

1. The patient under medical treatment for a peptic ulcer may have repeated pain — one danger is perforation, and it is a regrettable truth that the mortality is higher if the patient in hospital perforates than at home or even on the street! Only awareness of the hazard and re-examination of the patient complaining of repeated or severe pain will enable the diagnosis of perforation to be made when it occurs and prolonged delay by giving analgesics is avoided.

2. Most patients with gall stone colic are treated conservatively. Occasionally a gall stone will obstruct the small intestine — a condition which requires an urgent operation for its relief.

The ultimate relief of pain in acute organic disease is cure of the disease. As this will usually be of short duration the problem of the relief of pain is not a difficult one. Appropriate analgesics are prescribed and the danger of addiction is negligible. None the less, the drugs are chosen after assessment of the pain arising from the local condition, the degree of anxiety or fear and the stability or otherwise of the psychological background. Above all else it must never be suggested to a patient that he or she is too intolerant of pain — pain is never to be equated with an endurance test. In practice the total amount of analgesics can be considerably reduced if they are given in small frequent doses before the pain recurs rather than after the patient has been in pain for some time.

DRUGS

There is an endless variety and combination of drugs but in practice an individual unit will usually use a small number which have been found to be adequate. Rapid and effective absorption is essential for their action. If the patient is unable to eat or drink a parenteral route is essential. The only parenteral route which is effective in the shocked patient is the intravenous one. Subcutaneous or intramuscular injections are not absorbed when the patient is shocked and an undesirable cumulative dosage may arise as recovery occurs.

Analgesic drugs may cause respiratory depression, nausea, constipation or hypotension.

Narcotic analgesics

Patients can tolerate pain better in the morning than in the afternoon and this should be taken into account when prescribing analgesics. The evening doses should be higher than those taken in the morning.

Pethidine (50–100 mg) is an effective analgesic but is less powerful than morphine. It is less likely to cause respiratory depression but lowers blood pressure.

Morphine (10–15 mg) is an excellent analgesic but decreases respiration and is therefore dangerous in bronchitic or asthmatic patients. Many patients complain of nausea and it tends to cause constipation. The action of morphine can be reversed by the administration of naxolone.

Diamorphine (heroin) is the most powerful analgesic agent.

Pentazocine (Fortral) (30–60 mg) is an intermediate between morphine and codeine. It has a low risk of addiction but can cause hallucination.

Dihydrocodeine (DF118) (30–60 mg) is suitable for moderate pain.´

Non-narcotic analgesics

Aspirin is the most widely used analgesic. There is a risk of gastric haemorrhage and it may interfere with blood coagulation by increasing the prothrombin time.

Distalgesic tablets are a mixture of dextropropoxyphene hydrochloride (32·5 mg) and paracetamol (32·5 mg) and are used for mild pain. Paracetamol (500 mg) or Paracodal are also used.

CHRONIC PERSISTENT OR RECURRENT PAIN

Acute pain is fairly easily relieved by analgesics while measures are taken to cure its cause. The pain is protective. In many cases of persistent or recurrent pain the pain is in itself the dominant feature. Such patients may be divided into two categories:

1. Those in whom the expectation of life is short, usually a patient with advanced malignant disease.
2. Sufferers who have a normal life expectancy but persistent pain which is overwhelming. These include arthritics, post-herpetic neuralgia and many other conditions.

The patient with malignant disease can be treated with analgesics and anxiolytic drugs and in severe pain there is a variety of methods listed below which may be effective in a particular case. The patients in the second group present a much more difficult problem. In all it is essential to be certain that pain is the symptom complained of and not just itching or numbness. A careful clinical examination and investigation is indicated to exclude any obvious remedial cause. For intractable pain there are special pain clinics but treatment is always difficult and uncertain.

Methods of treatment

1. Analgesics similar to those administered for acute pain are used — the danger of addiction in non-malignant patients is an overriding consideration and should intensify the efforts to use other methods of control.

2. Anxiolytic drug therapy. Diazepam (Valium) (5–30 mg daily) or chlorpromazine (Largactil) (75–800 mg daily) are widely used for mild anxiety or agitation in combination with analgesics.

3. Local injection of nerves or nerve plexus. Long-acting local anaesthetics are injected.

4. Destruction of nerve routes or tracts by:
  (a) Phenol or alcohol.
  (b) Surgical section.
  (c) Electric coagulation.

Despite such radical measures in time the pain recurs in many patients. Trigeminal neuralgia (Ch. 45) which does not respond to carbamazepine (Tegretol) is treated by injection of the ganglion or nerve section.

5. Radiotherapy is often effective for the relief of secondary malignant deposits in the spine.

6. Hormonal methods including oophorectomy, adrenalectomy or hypophysectomy (Ch. 28).

7. Sympathecomy is indicated for true causalgia — a burning pain which occurs after injury to a peripheral nerve.

8. Posterior-column stimulation. A special electrode is attached to the dura mater and connected by a subcutaneous lead to a button implanted under the skin. The patient controls the button which is attached to a small transmitter on the skin. The patient can press on the button to stimulate the posterior columns.

The control of intractable pain is far from easy and with further understanding of its physiology better methods of control will be discovered.

BIBLIOGRAPHY

Bowsher D 1978 Pain topics. In: Academy News Bulletins Inc, p 3
Melzack R, Walls P D 1965 Science 150: 971
Scottish Health Service Library Bibliography No 14

6

Microbiology

All infections are caused by micro-organisms. These are divided into bacteria, viruses, fungi and protozoa. Bacteria can be seen with the aid of a microscope but viruses are very much smaller and can only be seen with the aid of an electron microscope.

Organisms which cause disease are known as pathogens; those incapable of causing disease non-pathogens.

BACTERIA

Morphology (shape)

Micro-organisms which include bacteria and fungi are described according to their shape, as seen under the microscope:

Bacilli are rod-shaped.
Cocci are rounded.
Spirochaetes are corkscrew-shaped in appearance.
Fungi are much larger in size and branched.
Because organisms are colourless, staining is necessary to make them visible under the microscope.

Physiology

Effect of atmosphere. (1) Aerobic bacteria are organisms which cannot survive without oxygen. (2) Anaerobic organisms can survive only when free oxygen is absent. In the body anaerobic conditions are in practice only created when the blood supply has been cut off so that no oxygen reaches the part, for example, in dead muscle.

Artificial growth of organisms. This is known as culturing. Various substances known as media are used to grow organisms artificially; that most commonly used is agar. Pus containing organisms, swabbed on to an agar plate and kept at body temperature (37°C) overnight, will produce a growth varying in appearance with the strain of the organism. Viewed with the naked eye the effect appears rather like sugar icing on a cake or discrete colonies of the organism may be visible.

Effect of temperature. Conditions favourable to a growth of micro-organisms are warmth, moisture and an adequate supply of nutrients. Cold inhibits the growth of bacteria. It interferes with their ability to divide and multiply, but it never kills them. Some organisms provide for their survival by the formation of spores. A spore is the bacterium in a modified form, modified to protect itself in unfavourable surroundings. A soon as the conditions are most favourable it develops into a normal organism. While moist heat at 100°C (212°F) kills all organisms, spores require a temperature of 116°C (240°F) to 127°C (260°F) for their destruction.

Reaction to Gram's stain. All organisms are divided into those which are Gram-positive or Gram-negative. Organisms which stain and hold the stain are known as Gram-positive. Those in which it disappears after washing with alcohol are known as Gram-negative and require to be counterstained to be visible under the microscope. Since the introduction of the antibiotics this has extended its significance beyond laboratory identification. For example, most Gram-positive cocci are sensitive to penicillin and most Gram-negative bacilli are sensitive to streptomycin.

As bacteria have acquired resistance to antibiotics, this pattern is tending to change, and laboratory sensitivity tests are performed on the infective organisms prior to treatment. Where the patient's condition is such that there is no time for delay, substances such as gentamicin may be prescribed until the results of the sensitivity tests are available.

Sensitivity to organisms. This is determined by adding a particular antibiotic to the culture media and if growth is prevented the organism is described as sensitive.

Enzyme activity. Bacteria produce enzymes one of which, coagulase, spreads a protective fibrin film around the organism. Another is penicillinase which destroys penicillin and is responsible for the development of resistant strains.

Phage typing. Viruses may invade a bacterium like other living cells and susceptible bacteria are classified accordingly. This is known as phage typing.

COMMON PYOGENIC ORGANISMS

The common pyogenic or pus-producing organisms include *staphylococci*, small rounded bacteria which, under the microscope, appear in clusters like bunches of grapes (Fig. 6.1).

The commonest group is the *Staphylococcus pyogenes*. Boils, carbuncles, and many abscesses in the skin and subcutaneous tissues are due to staphylococci. They are the most common cause of bone infection. Less frequently they cause infection elsewhere, for example, a perinephric abscess. Their tendency to acquire antibiotic resistance constitutes a major surgical problem. Sometimes they cause a fulminating enterocolitis which is a major threat to the patient's life.

Streptococci, viewed microscopically, appear in chains (Fig. 6.1). Some strains haemolyse blood on a blood agar plate, and are then known as the haemolytic variety; the remainder as non-haemolytic. The haemolytic

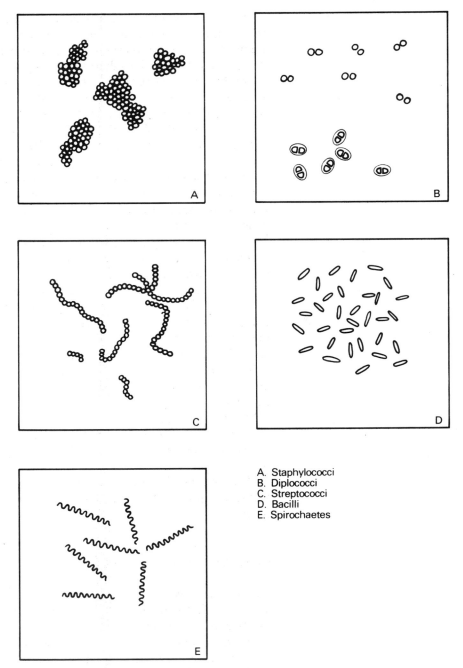

A. Staphylococci
B. Diplococci
C. Streptococci
D. Bacilli
E. Spirochaetes

Fig. 6.1 Microscopic appearance of some micro-organisms.

streptococci, which are much more virulent, are the causal organisms of diseases such as septicaemia, bronchopneumonia, and empyema. A further danger is that they may be harboured in the throat of a healthy individual, causing no harm to the host, who spreads disease to others unknowingly. Such a person is known as a 'carrier'. Haemolytic streptococci are still usually sensitive to penicillin.

Pneumococci are always in pairs (diplococci) (Fig. 6.1). They are the usual cause of lobar pneumonia and occasionally are responsible for arthritis, empyema and meningitis. Pneumococci are usually sensitive to penicillin and the sulphonamides.

Gonococci are also diplococci and are the causal organisms of gonorrhoea.

Escherichia coli (Fig. 6.1) is a rod-shaped organism whose natural habitat is the intestine, where it is non-pathogenic. Like most Gramnegative organisms it produces a powerful endotoxin and may be a cause of septicaemic shock. Perforation of the intestine enables the bacillus to gain access to the peritoneal cavity, where it is pathogenic (disease-causing). Hence it is found in peritonitis secondary to appendicitis and diverticulitis but is greatly outnumbered by organisms of the bacteroides group. Urinary infections such as cystitis and pyelonephritis are frequently due to the *E. coli*. It is penicillin-resistant, but is usually sensitive to the sulphonamide group of drugs, to gentamicin, the cephalosporins or the broad spectrum penicillin deritatives.

Culture: *E. coli*	Penicillin	Gentamicin
	—	+
	Ampicillin	Tetracycline
	—	—
	Kanamycin	
	+	

Fig. 6.2 Laboratory report stating the organism and the antibiotics to which it is sensitive and to which it is resistant.

The *Proteus group* of organisms of which the most common are *Proteus vulgaris* and *Proteus mirabilis* are well-recognised urinary tract pathogens where they cause pyelonephritis as well as infection of the lower urinary tract. They can also contaminate and infect wounds and burns.

Pseudomonas aeruginosa is a pathogenic organism which appears in wounds treated with antibiotics — it may cause persistent urinary infections as well as infection in machines used for assisted respiration. It is noted for the curious bluish-green colour of the pus. The most useful antibiotic is azocillin. It should be used not for the mere presence of the organism but when there is real danger from it. More recently the sulphamino penicillins and gentamicin have been used. The great danger of *Pseudomonas* is that it develops in wounds when the competition from more sensitive bacteria has been removed. The young, the old, the burnt and patients receiving wide spectrum antibiotics or on steroid treatment are liable to develop this infection.

The *bacteroides* are another promiment group of nonspore bearing anaerobes which commonly cause infection and peritonitis. They are the predominant organisms in the large intestine where they outnumber *E. coli*. The bacteroides dominate the bacterial picture in peritonitis caused by perforation of the intestinal tract and in abdominal wound infection.

Anaerobic infections in man are most commonly caused by the nonclostridial anaerobes (Willis). They are part of the normal bacterial flora of the alimentary canal and the lower female genital tract. From their normal habitat they invade tissues debilitated by diabetes, trauma or other pathological conditions. Willis suggests that the use of neomycin (or other aminoglycosides) for preoperative preparation of the large bowel may also be a predisposing factor in colonic surgery since anaerobes are resistant to this group of drugs. The pus produced is foul smelling and copious in contrast to pus produced by *E. coli* which is odourless. While surgical drainage is of the first importance metronidazole is highly effective in treatment.

ORGANISMS WHICH CAUSE SPECIFIC INFECTIONS

Clostridium tetani is an anaerobic spore bearing organism which is very resistant to ordinary methods of sterilisation. As it is a normal inhabitant of the large intestine of several animals, including the sheep, catgut (made from sheep's intestine) is a potential source.

It elaborates a powerful toxin which poisons the motor nerve cells with the result that spasm occurs in the muscles supplied by the corresponding nerves. The disease is known as tetanus.

Clostridium perfringens (*Cl. welchii*) and its associated organisms is also an anaerobic inhabitant of the intestine and proliferates in damaged muscle producing gas and toxins causing gas gangrene. It is a complication of wounding. Contaminated clothing embedded at the time of the accident is commoner than soil as the source of the organism. It is penicillin sensitive but surgical measures are also essential (Ch. 9).

The *Mycobacterium tuberculosis* is an aerobic rod-shaped organism, which causes tuberculosis and, because of certain staining peculiarities, is described by bacteriologists as acid-fast.

Treponema pallidum is a spirochaete (Fig. 6.1) and is the cause of syphilis. It is penicillin sensitive.

VIRUSES

While immunisation for the prevention of viral disease is highly effective, chemotherapy for established infection is almost nonexistent. In addition to causing infection, there is a suspicion that viruses may be the cause of some forms of malignant disease.

Many infectious diseases such as measles, smallpox, mumps, influenza and the common cold are due to a virus. Of special interest to the surgical nurse are:

1. Poliomyelitis (infantile paralysis)
2. Viral hepatitis (Ch. 36) from blood products
3. Rubella (German measles) in the pregnant woman on account of the risk of congenital deformities to the foetus.

Before a virus can cause disease it has to enter and multiply inside the body of a living cell. The cell is stimulated to produce interferon, an antiviral inflammatory substance. Interferon is at present under trial as an anti-cancer agent.

FUNGI

Fungi are large branched organisms. Three groups are of surgical interest.

1. *Tinea pedis* (athlete's foot) causes infection in the web of the toes and *Tinea cruris* infects folds of skin in the thighs and the groin. These lesions are a source of sepsis and when discovered by the nurse should be reported.

2. *Candida albicans* (causing Moniliasis) is a fungus which is normally suppressed by harmless bacteria but may cause a virulent infection following the administration of broad range antibiotics. It is a common cause of infection in the mouth (thrush) or in the vagina.

3. *Actinomycosis* is an infection arising in the floor of the mouth and neck, the lungs, or the ileo-caecal region of the intestine. The organism *Actinomyces israelii* is too large to invade the lymphatic system, but causes destruction of tissue producing typical 'sulphur granules' pus. Small quantities of the pus should be sent in a sterile test tube rather than the usual swab for bacteriological examination if the condition is suspected.

THE PROTOZOA

The protozoa are the cause of a wide spectrum of diseases in the world. The surgical complications of amoebiasis and hydatid disease are the only ones the nurse is likely to encounter in the British Isles and then only very occasionally.

Entamoeba histolytica is the parasite responsible for amoebiasis. While dysentry is the commonest manifestation, surgical complications such as perforation of the intestine, abscess and stricture formation may occur. A liver abscess is a well recognised complication. Metronidazole (Flaygl) is the most effective drug.

Echinococcus granulosa causes hydatid disease which may affect many parts of the body but 80 per cent of lesions occur in the liver as a hydatid cyst. Only surgical treatment is effective. The drug Mebendazole is at present under trial for the treatment of hydatid disease but there are doubts that in the dosage required it is toxic.

ANTIBACTERIAL THERAPY

The antibiotics and chemotherapeutic agents are powerful antibacterial substances which have made surgical procedures safer and increased the scope of surgery. They have not however diminished the need for supportive measures such as good hygiene in the wards or the need for an incision to evacuate pus. Antibiotics are produced by moulds or by bacteria from which they are extracted, while chemotherapeutic agents are produced synthetically from chemical compounds. Some are bactericidal — that is they destroy the organism — penicillin and the aminoglycoside group like streptomycin and neomycin are examples. Others such as tetracycline and chloramphenicol which prevent propagation are known as bacteriostatic.

Before discussing the more important agents briefly, some general principles should be considered:

Choice of agent

Modern chemotherapy has taught us to think not so much in terms of disease but in terms of sensitive organisms. If the organism is known and is sensitive to an antibiotic, cure is certain. This presupposes that the facilities for identification and tests for sensitivity are universally available. It also assumes that the organism can be readily isolated from the patient. Isolation, culture, assessment of sensitivity by the bacteriologist and the administration of the appropriate antibiotic is ideal. Unfortunately this is only possible in certain types of infection and in many cases it has to be assumed that the organism is the one commonly responsible for the condition and the antibiotic to which it is usually sensitive is chosen. The patient's response is used as an indication to sensitivity. If, after 72 hours, there is no response the antibiotic is changed or if, before this period has elapsed, the organism can be isolated and sensitivity tests show that a different antibiotic is indicated, therapy is changed.

When an antibiotic is prescribed it should be:
1. Administered by the *correct route* which may be orally, intramuscularly, intravenously, intrathecally or by local instillation.
2. Given at the stated intervals in the dose prescribed, so that its concentration in the bloodstream is maintained.
3. Continued over a sufficient period of days to cure the infection.

A sufficient quantity of fluid has to be taken so that the antibiotic can be excreted by the kidney if this is its route of elimination, and if used for treatment of urinary infection the fluid intake should not be so great that the concentration of the antibiotic in the urine is so low as to be ineffective. An intake of 3 litres per day is probably the optimum.

It is inadvisable to prescribe antibacterial therapy for mild self-limiting infections. These substances are expensive, not without complications and may produce resistant organisms. It used to be thought that antibiotics given prophylactically would prevent postoperative infection, but experience has shown that this is not so and careful aseptic technique is the best safeguard. There are, however, three conditions where they should be used before operation:
(a) Amputation for gangrene (p. 216).
(b) Operations on patients with congenital or rheumatic heart disease.
(c) Urethral dilatation.

A patient with a resistant organism sensitive to only one antibiotic should be nursed in isolation so that it is not propagated in the ward and may emerge resistant to every known antibiotic. Antibiotic therapy should cease when the period for which it has been prescribed has elapsed.

Complications of antibiotic therapy

1. Resistant organisms. New antibiotics are being developed almost continuously. Penicillin and, in a lesser degree, gentamicin have a margin of safety not possessed by any other antibiotic. The need to use other antibiotics arises only when the organism is insensitive or resistant. One of the problems in hospital is the presence of resistant staphylococci. These arise in the following ways:

(a) Inadequate or too short a dosage of penicillin.
(b) The difficulty of sterilising woollen blankets, which has been overcome by substituting cotton blankets.
(c) Theatres attached to ward blocks are more liable to be infected with these resistant organisms than separate isolated theatre blocks. It is important to be certain that there are no defects in the air-conditioning plant. It is not unknown for defects to result in these organisms being sucked into the theatre from nearby wards and corridors. Even on the foggiest days in winter the atmosphere of an industrial town is sterile. The same cannot be said of the average hospital ward.
(d) Where patients admitted for elective surgery are not admitted to clean units.

The emergence of gram negative organisms resistant to many antibiotics and the increase in this type of infection in hospital is probably due to the widespread use of broad-spectrum antibiotics as well as the increased use of catheters and tubes in the

(i) urinary bladder for drainage
(ii) veins for infusions
(iii) respiratory tract ⎫
(iv) stomach ⎬ for suction

2. *Sensitisation* of the patient or staff may occur with any antibiotic. For this reason antibiotics are not prescribed for trivial infections. Sensitivity reactions take the form of a skin rash or even, in some cases, severe anaphylactic shock may result.

The following precautions are of value in protecting the nurse from sensitivity:

(a) The same needle can be put into the bottle of solution and also used for injection into the patient.
(b) Air in the syringe should be expelled with the needle in the bottle. Spraying it into the atmosphere causes skin reaction on the face and arms.
(c) The overall precaution, of course, is for the nurse to wear gloves.
(d) Hermetically sealed or orally administered capsules of antibiotics prevent skin contact with the antibiotic. Disposable syringes and hand washing to remove any particles after handling antibiotics are probably as important in preventing reactions in the nurse.

Toxic reactions

Toxic reactions are almost unknown with penicillin, but damage to the 8th nerve may occur with the aminoglycoside antibiotics. Streptomycin and gentamicin affect particularly the vestibular branch while neomycin and kanamycin affect the auditory branch and both are more likely to occur in the presence of poor renal function. With local or topical use, neomycin, in addition to damage to the auditory division of the 8th nerve, is dangerous in the presence of hepatic failure as well as when renal function is impaired. It is recommended that inhalation of an aerosol of neomycin in bronchiectasis should be limited to 1 g daily. Similarly topical application to pressure sores should not exceed 1 g daily.

Another well-known toxic reaction is the danger of aplastic anaemia from chloramphenicol. Many antibiotics are so toxic to the kidneys that they are unsuitable for use.

Super infection

Suppression of the normal flora by antibiotics may unleash the activities of organisms which are normally held in check. Examples are monilial infection and staphylococcal enterocolitis.

ANTIBACTERIAL AGENTS

Penicillin

Penicillin was the first and is still the safest of the antibiotics. The original form sodium benzyl penicillin, known as crystalline penicillin, is effective against a large group of organisms of which the more important are:

Streptococcus
Gonococcus
Pneumococcus
Meningococcus
The gas gangrene bacillus, *Clostridium perfrigens* (*welchii*).
Spirochaete of syphilis
Cl. tetani
Bacillus anthracis
B. diphtheria
Some staphylococci

It has no antibacterial action on:

Escherichia coli
Salmonella typhosus
Mycobacterium tuberculosis
Pseudomonas aeruginosa

Administration and dosage

Penicillin may be administered:

1. Systemically. Intramuscular injection is the usual method of systemic administration, but with the present purified penicillin preparations the objection to the subcutaneous route because of painful reactions no longer holds, and this route may have some slight advantage in being followed by slower absorption. Penicillin dissolved in sterile distilled water or saline when injected is excreted by the kidneys in a few hours so that the concentration in the blood falls rapidly. This necessitates repeated injection every three hours. The dosage varies with the severity of the infection; 500 000 to 1 mega units six-hourly or twice daily is usually prescribed, and is continued for four to five days or longer. The dose is readily soluble in 1 ml of sterile water.

The absorption of penicillin may be delayed by dissolving the drug in procaine. The dose is 400 000 units once or twice daily. This preparation, while effective in most cases, is inadequate to maintain a high blood level of penicillin, and in severe infections or persistent infections due to a relatively resistant organism, sodium penicillin in water should be given.

Intramuscular injection. Requirements:

    Receiver
    2 or 5 ml syringe
    Needle—size 23G 1¼ (12) or 21G 1½ (1)
    Needle—19G 2—for drawing up if required
    2 Mediswabs
    Prescription and recording sheet

Disposable gloves should be worn when potentially sensitising drugs are to be injected.

The injection is prepared in the treatment room. Using the aseptic technique the guarded needle and syringe are assembled and placed in the receiver. The drug is checked by two nurses (one of whom is qualified), the ampoule opened, or the cap of a multidose bottle wiped with a mediswab. The needle guard is removed. The drug is drawn up into the syringe, the amount being regulated according to the prescription. The drug is again double checked with the prescription sheet. Air bubbles are expelled, the needle guard is secured, and the syringe and needle are replaced in the receiver together with a mediswab.

The patient is advised of what is to happen. Privacy is ensured and the patient placed in a suitable position. The clothing is arranged so as to expose the site. The site chosen is the lateral aspect of the thigh (Fig. 6.3). If this cannot be used, the ward sister or the unit officer is informed and they may give it into the buttock (Fig. 6.4). The nurse and witness check with the prescription sheet. The nurse cleans the skin with the mediswab.

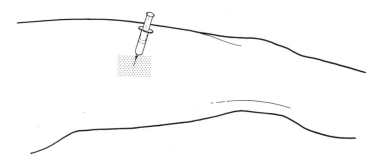

Fig. 6.3. The safest site for intramuscular injection.

The needle is inserted at an angle of 90°, care being taken to avoid touching the bone. The plunger is withdrawn slightly to ensure a blood vessel has not been punctured. If blood is seen entering the syringe, the needle is withdrawn, and firm pressure applied to the puncture site for 10 seconds. An adjacent site is then chosen for the injection. If no blood is

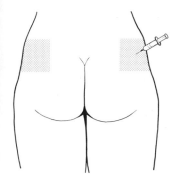

Fig. 6.4 If the buttock is used the upper and outer quadrant is the only safe area.

seen, the fluid is instilled gently. The mediswab is placed over the needle track and the needle withdrawn smoothly. The underlying tissues are massaged, and/or the patient is instructed to carry out 'quadriceps' exercises to aid absorption of the drug and to reduce discomfort. The patient is made comfortable and the recording sheet initialled by the nurse giving the injection. Used equipment is discarded, and the nurse washes and dries her hands.

Subcutaneous or hypodermic injections. Although not used for antibiotics they are necessary for the administration of many drugs. Requirements are:

Receiver
2 ml syringe
Needle — size 25G 1 (17)
Needle — 21G 1½ (1) — for drawing up if required
2 Mediswabs
Prescription and recording sheet

The needle is inserted at an angle of 45°, care being taken not to insert it right up to the hub. The plunger is withdrawn slightly to ensure a vein has not been punctured, depressed gently and the fluid instilled. The mediswab is placed over the needle track and the needle withdrawn smoothly. The skin is massaged gently to aid dispersion of the fluid.

The patient is made comfortable, and the recording sheet initialled by the nurse giving the injection. In the case of a controlled drug, the nurse and the witness sign the register. Used equipment is discarded, and the nurse washes and dries her hands.

2. Locally. Penicillin may be applied locally without the slightest harm to the tissues while killing or preventing the growth of susceptible organisms. It may be injected into the theca, joints, empyema or abscess cavities. However, local penicillin applications should be discouraged as sensitivity often develops.

Apart from a mild skin rash no toxic reactions from systemic penicillin have been reported, but as with any drug an acute sensitivity reaction may accrue. A few reports of fatal collapse following intrathecal penicillin have been reported. It is advisable to enquire if the patient is known to be sensitive to penicillin.

The later penicillins

The basic nucleus of penicillin (6-amino-penicillanic acid) has been isolated, and from this any number of new penicillins can be made. This advance promises penicillins of wider antibacterial activity causing no reactions, together with a fresh approach to the problem of resistant organisms.

1. Phenoxyethyl penicillin (Broxil) has the advantage that it can be given by mouth.
2. Dimethoxyphenyl penicillin (Celbenin). This is invaluable in the treatment of penicillin resistant organisms, but it must be given by injection since, like penicillin, it is destroyed by the gastric acid.

3. Aminophenyl penicillin (Ampicillin, Penbritin) has a broader spectrum than any of the penicillins in use at present and is active against Gram-negative bacilli. It has the advantage that it may be taken by mouth.
4. Cloxacillin (Orbenin) can be given by mouth in the treatment of resistant staphylococcal infection.

Streptomycin

Streptomycin was the first product of intensive research following the demonstration of the powerful antibacterial properties of penicillin. By mouth its action is localised to the intestinal tract, from which it is not absorbed, so for systemic effect it has to be given by intramuscular injection. Its main disadvantages are the risk of damage to the eighth cranial nerve causing vertigo and deafness from prolonged administration, and the extraordinary rapidity with which resistance of bacteria to the drug can develop. For this reason it must be given in adequate doses at once if its use is advisable. It was the antibiotic of most value against the tubercle bacillus but because it requires intramuscular injection, oral antimicrobial drugs which are more acceptable and as effective are now used (Ch. 9).

Dosage. The usual dose is 1 g daily intramuscularly, but always combined with PAS or INAH by mouth in cases of tuberculosis. To diminish bacteria in the colon the usual dose is 1 g three times daily by mouth. It is excreted more slowly than penicillin by the kidneys and reaches a high concentration in the urine, where it is effective in destroying sensitive organisms. The urine must be alkaline for streptomycin to be effective in these infections. Streptomycin given systemically does not reach the cerebrospinal fluid and therefore must be injected intrathecally for meningeal infections.

Gentamicin

This has largely replaced streptomycin as the first choice of powerful broad spectrum antibiotic. It is given in a dosage of 80–120 mg 8 hourly.

The blood level should be monitored to ensure adequate dosage and minimise complications

Chloramphenicol (chloromycetin)

Chloramphenicol which was the first antibiotic to be synthesised, is effective against a wider range of organisms than penicillin and streptomycin together. It is curative in typhoid fever, bacillary dysentery and acute brucellosis. It is effective against some virus diseases. It is administered by mouth or intravenously. The dosage is 250 to 500 mg 6 hourly. Vitamin B complex should be given as well. Nausea, vomiting and diarrhoea as well as agranulocytosis or aplastic anaemia may develop as toxic reactions so its administration should be limited to conditions where other antibiotics are inappropriate.

The tetracyclines

The tetracyclines include chlortetracycline (aureomycin), oxytetracycline (terramycin), tetracycline (achromycin), and dimethylchlortetracycline (ledermycin). They are all antibiotics of wide antibacterial activity and have the advantage that they are effective when taken by mouth but may also be administered intramuscularly or intravenously. Their great value is in conditions in which other antibiotics have failed to effect cure or resistance has developed.

Dosage. Average dosage is 250 mg 6 hourly.

They may produce mild gastrointestinal disturbances, a raw tongue, soreness of the buttocks and anus. Vitamin B complex is administered if treatment is prolonged. Tetracyclines given during pregnancy or in the first year of life cause permanent discoloration of developing teeth. If the prescribing of tretracyclines increases the future population will probably have teeth several shades deeper on average than hitherto. Oxytetracycline causes less discoloration.

Erythromycin

Erythromycin has a similar range of activity to penicillin but its main disadvantage is that bacteria rapidly develop resistance. The dose is 250 to 500 mg 6 hourly.

Fucidin

Fucidin is an antistaphylococcal antibiotic of the 'narrow spectrum' type. It is administered orally only in a dosage of 250 to 500 mg 6 hourly.

Lincomycin (Lincocin)

Lincomycin has recently been introduced as another antibiotic effective against staphylococcus as well as other organisms.

Cephaloridine (Ceporin)

Cephaloridine is an antibiotic effective against many other resistant Gram-negative organisms. It may be given in a dosage of 250 mg 6 hourly intramuscularly. It may also be given by mouth.

Other antibiotics

Other antibiotics include bacitracin, polymyxin, and tobramycin. All are of value in appropriate cases. The main use of these antibiotics is when the organisms are resistant to penicillin or streptomycin.

Metronidazole

Metronidazole which may be given orallly, as a suppository or intravenously, is an old agent long used in the treatment of monilial infection. It is now finding an important place in the treatment of anaerobic organisms in faecal peritonitis, in pelvic sepsis and as a prophylactic agent in colorectal surgery. It is often used in combination with gentamicin. It is also effective in amoebiasis. Some of its metabolites darken the urine and the patient should be warned. Neutropenia and peripheral sensory neuropathy have been reported following prolonged use but are reversible on cessation.

Trimethoprim

Trimethoprim is an antibacterial substance similar in range to the sulphonamides. When combined with a sulphonamide, usually sulphamethoxazole, it has a greatly potentiated and very effective range of activity. Commercially it is supplied as Septrin or Bactrim.

Other antibiotics which are used occasionally are kanamycin, and colomycin.

Bacitracin, polymyxin and neomycin are in the main used as local applications and are combined in a 'polybactrin spray'. Nystatin is effective against monilial infections, for example, *Candida albicans*.

The sulphonamide group of drugs

The sulphonamide group of drugs are, in general, effective against the same organisms as penicillin, with the important exception that *E. coli*, which is insensitive to penicillin, responds to the sulphonamides.

There are several separate sulphonamides which are divisible into two groups:

1. Those absorbable from the intestinal tract. This group includes:

Sulphathiazole and sulphadiazine

Sulphadimidine, sulphamerazine and sulphafurazole (Gantrisin).

They are normally given by mouth. As they pass into the cerebrospinal fluid they are useful for prophylaxis following fractures of the skull. They are also very useful in the treatment of infections of the kidney. The usual dosage is 2 g initially, followed by 1 g 4 hourly for 4 to 5 days or longer. A tablet containing a mixture of three sulphonamides — sulphatriad — was said to be less likely to cause toxic reactions, but investigation has shown that this is not true.

These preparations are insufficiently soluble for parenteral administration and must be given as their sodium salt in 1 ml of normal saline by the intravenous route.

A useful addition to the sulphonamide group of drugs is a long-acting sulphonamide which maintains a therapeutic blood level for at least 24 hours and a single daily dose of 0·5 g is sufficient The untoward effects are, of course, also prolonged. There are three separate long-acting sulphonamides:

Sulphamethoxypyridazine (marketed as Midicel and Lederkyn).

Sulphaphenazole

Sulphadimethozene (Madribon.)

Toxic reactions apart from a skin rash are few. Prolonged dosage with an inadequate fluid intake (3 litres is desirable) can cause crystallisation of the drug in the kidney and lead to anuria (Ch. 42).

Local use of the absorbable sulphonamides. As a powder or cream, sulphathiazole and sulphanilamide are used extensively to combat infection. Sulphacetamide is widely used as eye drops.

2. Those non-absorbable from the intestinal tract. These preparations pass through the gastrointestinal tract almost unchanged, and are used in the treatment of infections such as dysentery. They are of value in surgical practice in diminishing the infectivity of the bowel before and after operations, such as colectomy. Succinyl-sulphathiazole (sulfasuxidine) is the preparation in common use. Its administration, etc. is discussed under Diseases of the Colon (Ch. 39).

Sulphasalazine (Salazopyrin) is taken up selectively by the connective tissue of the intestine; 1 g four or more times daily is the usual dosage. It is strictly speaking an absorbable sulphonamide but is later excreted into the intestinal tract.

OTHER ANTIBACTERIAL AGENTS

Nitrofurantoin is administered orally for urinary infections. Furamide is used in bacillary dysentery, bacillary food-poisoning, and non-specific diarrhoea.

Nalidixic acid (Negram) is an antibacterial agent particularly active against Gram-negative organisms. A side-effect is photo-sensitivity of the skin producing a severe sunburn-like reaction on exposure to sunlight.

Noxythiolin (Noxyflex) is used in local treatment of wounds (aerosol spray) or in the bladder as an instillation.

Griseofulvin is an antifungal agent which is administered orally for tinea and fungal infections of the nail bed.

BIBLIOGRAPHY

Bint A J, Reeves D S 1978 British Journal of Hospital Medicine 19: 335
Willis A T 1977 Anaerobic bacteriology. In: Clinical and laboratory practice, 3rd edn. Butterworths, London
Willis A T 1978 British Journal of Hospital Medicine 20: 579

7

Infection

Infection is the successful invasion and growth of micro-organisms in a body tissue. The severity or mildness of the resulting disease depends upon:

The dosage and virulence of the organisms.

The resistance of the patient.

THE DOSAGE AND VIRULENCE OF ORGANISMS

By dosage we mean number of organisms. Obviously a more severe infection is produced by 10 000 000 organisms than by 1 000 000 of the same strain.

Different strains of the same organism vary in their inherent power to attack the body, and this property is known as virulence; organisms of the same strain vary in virulence under different conditions. The virulence is sometimes a property of the body of the organism when the toxin is known as an endotoxin; and sometimes it is due to a toxin or poison which it produces called an exotoxin. In clinical practice the sensitivity or response to antibacterial drugs may well be decisive in assessing the virulence of the clinical infection.

THE RESISTANCE OF THE PATIENT TO INFECTION

The skin and mucuous membranes, by providing a protective cover, deny organisms access and are the first line of defence. Immune bodies if present in the blood stream and the tissue fluids will prevent the disease developing. The third and final defence is the development of inflammation.

The skin and mucous membranes

Of all the protective coverings, the skin is structurally the best equipped because it has a thick layer of squamous epithelium and organisms on its

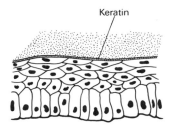

Stratified squamous
epithelial membrane
with keratin

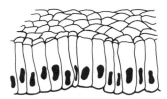

Simple columnar
epithelial membrane

Fig. 7.1 The skin with its many
layers of cells (*top*) is more
resistant to infection and injury
than the more delicate single layer
of cells (*bottom*) lining most
glands and viscera.

surface known as *contaminants* are denied access to the body. In most
surgical procedures the skin is incised, the underlying tissues are exposed
to the air and the skin adjoining the wound, so that the risk of bacterial
invasion is immediate. Single layered mucous membranes are easily damaged and have less strength in combating assault from bacteria (Fig. 7.1).

Types of immune response

Immunity to a particular disease is due to the presence of specific antibodies. Antibodies arise in the body either as a response to the presence of
an antigen or are inherited.

Immunity is a response to previous infection or is created artificially by
the administration of dead or weakened organisms to which there is a
response (active immunisation) or by the administration of gammaglobulin
(passive immunity).

The antibodies are produced by certain lymphocytes in response to an
antigen and form the group of substances known as the immunoglobulins.
The rise in the plasma proteins is due to an increase in gamma globulin
which occurs about 10 days from the onset of infection. A secondary effect
is a rise in the erythrocyte sedimentation rate (ESR) and blood viscosity
which in an obscure case may be used to determine non-specifically the
presence of infection. In established disease like the collagenoses it may be
valuable in monitoring progress. When stimulated to produce antibodies
the lymphocytes change in appearance and are known as plasma cells.

There are also cellular immune reactions in which lymphocytes
embryologically distinct from those which produce antibodies become
sensitised to the patient's own tissue or to implanted tissue. This forms the
basis of a marked inflammatory reaction such as occurs in autoimmune
disease and in the rejection of transplanted organs. It may be rapid, when it
is known as anaphylaxis; or slower, when it is known as rejection.

The degree of immunity

This varies from patient to patient and with different types of organisms.

The following factors may alter, usually unfavourably, the degree of
immunity:

1. Age. In infancy antibody production has not developed because the
infant has not been exposed to latent infection. In extreme old age it may
be depressed like all the other vital functions.

2. Race. The introduction of a new infection to a native race is usually
catastrophic. The inhabitants have no natural immunity to a new disease.
For instance, tuberculosis has almost wiped out the Red Indians in North
America.

3. The following conditions diminish resistance to infection with a resultant lowering of the degree of immunity:

(a) Metabolic diseases, e.g. diabetes mellitus.
(b) Severe anaemias, hypoproteinaemia and blood diseases.
(c) Uraemia.
(d) Cold, exposure, starvation, haemorrhage, and metallic poisoning.

(e) Radioactivity.

(f) A poor blood supply or a wound filled with serum or a haematoma.

Susceptibility to surgical infection

The susceptibility of a patient to infection depends upon the freedom of access of organisms to his body and the degree of immunity which he possesses to the particular organism once it is implanted on his tissues.

Access of organisms. An intact healthy skin or mucosa is the greatest barrier against infection. Organisms may gain access from a wound, or may be inhaled or swallowed.

Great stress has rightly been laid on protecting the patient from infection arising from outside sources (exogenous infection) but insufficient attention has been paid to infection arising from the patient himself (endogenous infection). The importance of eliminating endogenous sources efficiently, particularly in intestinal surgery, is now more widely recognised (Ch. 39).

The whole complex organisation of surgical technique is designed with the sole object of preventing the access of organisms to wounds. This is known as asepsis — literally, no infection.

CLINICAL APPLICATION OF IMMUNITY

Diagnostic

The estimation of the presence of immune bodies in the blood may be of value in diagnosis. The test is usually performed on the blood serum. The specimen of blood should be collected with no anticoagulant in the specimen tube, so that the serum can separate from the clot. The Widal test for the diagnosis of typhoid fever and the Wassermann reaction for the diagnosis of syphilis are examples of its use.

Prophylactic and therapeutic

Tetanus toxoid is administered if the patient has been recently exposed to tetanus. Human antitetanus immunoglobulin is used in treatment of the disease.

Active immunisation is effected to prevent several diseases, for example, tetanus, smallpox, diphtheria, poliomyelitis and tuberculosis.

Active immunisation is undertaken for tetanus, and anyone liable to be at risk, such as agricultural workers, children, and members of the services, are included. The following schedule of active immunisation is advised in children: At twelve weeks the first injection of diphtheria, pertussis and triple antigen is given (0.5 ml) and then the second and third injections are given at 5 months and 11 months respectively. Poliomyelitis vaccine (Sabin type) is given orally at 5 months. After the first year the child is inoculated against measles. A booster dose of diphtheria and tetanus antigen is given when the child starts school and again at the age of 10 years.

B.C.G. (Bacille Calmette-Guerin) immunisation is undertaken when the child is 2 weeks old but only where he is at risk from active tuberculosis in a member of his family. Otherwise B.C.G. is offered to school children found to be Mantoux negative at the age of 13 years. Smallpox vaccination is not recommended in infancy owing to the success of the World Health Organisation smallpox eradication campaign which has practically eliminated smallpox as an infectious disease risk.

Immunisation in older children or adults can, of course, be given by an injection of tetanus toxoid on its own. This is usually given as two injections at four-weekly intervals. For complete protection booster doses should be given each year. There is a tendency to forget or neglect the necessity for immunisation when the disease is rarely seen.

Rubella vaccine is now offered to school girls between 11 and 14 years of age for protection against the risk of congenital foetal malformations in pregnancy. The vaccine can also be given to older women who have been tested and found to have rubella antibodies absent from their blood. The patient of child bearing age should ensure she does not become pregnant for 2 months after rubella vaccination because the vaccine is a living virus.

Serum reactions

Serum reactions may be of three types:

1. Anaphylaxis. This is a state of sensitisation. It does not occur when an injection of serum (the antigen) is given for the first time, but it is liable to occur from the second injection if given after 10 days from the first. For this reason careful inquiry should always be made to elicit whether the patient has had a previous injection of serum or is allergic to foreign protein. If there is any doubt, small doses should be given (desensitisation); that is, an intradermal injection of 0·2 ml and wait for 15 minutes. If there is no reaction the same dose is repeated. Then if, after a further 15 minutes, there is no reaction the remainder of the dose ordered is administered. If there is a reaction doses of 0·5 ml are given at 15-minute intervals until the total amount prescribed has been administered. Anaphylaxis is a frightening condition — the most severe cases collapse and die almost at once in a state of shock and respiratory embarrassment. For this reason an ampoule of adrenalin (1 : 1000 1 ml) and an additional syringe should always be available when serum is to be administered intramuscularly or subcutaneously. Hydrocortisone, 100 mg, by intravenous injection may be given to supplement the action of adrenalin.

2. Serum sickness. An injection of a single dose of antitoxic serum given for the first time may occasionally produce a reaction from foreign protein which comes on seven to 10 days afterwards and is characterised by an urticarial rash, albuminuria, headache, nausea, vomiting, joint pains, and loss of appetite. Antihistamine drugs such as Piriton 4 mg are useful in treatment, and for the skin irritation calamine lotion is applied.

3. Accelerated reaction. This is really serum sickness in a severe form and after a much shorter interval, a few hours after the injection up to 2 or 3 days. It usually, but not invariably, occurs in patients who have had a previous serum injection. The patient is acutely ill with fever, bronchospasm, headache, joint pains, and a rash. He should be admitted for treatment which may include the administration of adrenalin, the antihistamines and, possibly, corticosteroids.

THE PREVENTION AND CONTROL OF INFECTION

Infection is always inimical to the interest of the surgical patient. It adds to his suffering, delays his recovery, and may cause such destruction to his tissues that his last state is worse than his first. If it is severe enough it may cause death.

Many surgical conditions are primarily infective and the prevention of the spread of infecting organisms to other patients is a cause of constant anxiety. In subsequent chapters considerable attention is paid to the practical details of this problem, but certain general principles are worthy of special notice.

1. General measures of hygiene are of the first importance for the patient and the nurse. Cleanliness of the ward, the handling of food, crockery, and personal cleanliness are of the greatest importance. An individual thermometer for each patient commonly stored dry after wiping with a mediswab is an example of the type of measure which it is necessary to take.

2. Control of special local conditions in a surgical wound. Injury or bruising of a wound increases the risk of infection. The patient is instructed not to touch dressings or his skin which may have been contaminated by pus. Hand washing should be frequent and Chlorhexidine soap is used. Masks should not be touched with the fingers, changed frequently and as soon as a dressing has been finished the mask is discarded so that the nurse is able to breathe freely and diminish the risk of infection into her own nose. Naseptin, a mixture of neomycin and hibitane cream, may be used in the nose and is particularly valuable in nasal carriers.

3. Special methods of protection such as immunisation and prophylaxis.

The more specific the action of the organism the more highly developed are the measures to counteract its activity. In hospital it is the common pyogenic organisms which are particularly troublesome, and notable amongst these is the antibiotic-resistant staphylococcus and increasingly gram negative organisms.

4. Recognition. Because some degree of infection is inevitable, it is easy to fail to recognise the outbreak until it has reached serious proportions. Routine recordings of the temperature and pulse rate are invaluable and inspection of the wounds is undertaken. A separate register of any infection which arises in a wound may be kept in each ward; or better, a control of infection sister is appointed to the hospital.

5. Prevention. The following measures are important:

(a) *Bed spacing* should be as generous as possible. A minimum of 2·4 metres is essential.

(b) *Staff* with minor septic lesions should not be on duty in a surgical ward.

(c) *Contaminated dressings and instruments* are treated as appropriate by disinfection or incineration.

(d) *Sterilisation* must be effective and recontamination prevented (Chapter 10).

(e) *Blankets* are a special source of danger, and woollen blankets should be substituted by those made of cotton material or cellulose laundered when each patient is discharged. Gentleness in handling bedclothes reduces the risk of dissemination of infection.

(*f*) *Flies* should be denied access and destroyed without delay if they do break bounds.

(*g*) *Flower vases* are a further source of contamination and require disinfection.

(*h*) *Antibiotics* should be used with care and not indiscriminately (Ch. 6).

(*i*) *The dressing of surgical wounds* requires special care (Ch. 11). The patient should be instructed not to interfere with the dressing and to report if he requires attention for oozing of serum, pus or blood (Ch. 12).

(*j*) *Nothing that is to be put into the bed should be placed on the floor* — back rests, bed cradles and bedpans.

(*k*) *Screen covers and curtains* around the bed require regular laundering.

(*l*) *Isolation*. Where facilities are available, patients with infections due to organisms known to give rise to epidemics, e.g. certain staphylococcal infections, are barrier nursed in an isolation ward.

(*m*) *Indwelling tubes and catheters* are a constant hazard. It has been suggested that 1 in 10 000 patients admitted to hospital dies of septicaemia due to catheterisation of the urinary tract. That would account for 500 deaths in Great Britain yearly (Strong 1980).

6. Control. Patients with an infected wound should, if possible, be isolated. If this is impossible barrier nursing has to be instituted at once. Infection spreads on the hands of the staff, fomites or clothes and through the air or by droplets. Hands should be washed inside the cubicle and *dried outside* to obviate contamination from paper cloths or paper towels stored in the cubicle. Unless gowns are used intelligently they are better not used at all. A surgeon dons a sterile gown before beginning an operation and discards it at the end. Only the same practice must be adopted in barrier nursing — such a practice need not add unduly to the laundry problem since the used gown usually need be only autoclaved and not laundered.

It may be desirable to close the ward to further admissions if the sepsis rate is rising or to empty the ward for cleaning and disinfection if there is a severe outbreak of infection.

Investigations should include bacteriological examination of:
   (a) the wound.
   (b) the mouth, hands, throat and skin of the staff and careful clinical examination to discover any infective lesions in other patients.

BIBLIOGRAPHY

Strong J 1980 Surgical News 9

8

Inflammation

Inflammation is the response of the body to an irritant. The irritant may be a burn, a chemical, a wound, or a micro-organism. It is usually painful; pain warns the patient that the enemy has arrived and is an indication that his body has risen to the attack.

It is only the body tissues which can overcome the irritant. By treatment we can, at best, only aid this struggle. If necessary, the body will sacrifice much of tissue to survive, and when its superiority has been established it will cleanse and repair its wound. The modern conception of inflammation recognises four stages as illustrated in wound healing. Wound healing always follows a regular pattern:

Stage 1. Traumatic inflammation. During this phase the edges of the wound become oedematous and matted together with fibrin. Within a few hours of injury the capillaries dilate and fluid leaks through the damaged endothelium and accumulates in the interstitial space. The body temperature may rise to 37·2 to 37·5°C (99 to 99·5°F) as in acute inflammation elsewhere. Lymphangitis and lymphadenitis occur at this stage.

Stage 2. Destruction, in which necrotic material is removed. It is characterised by the migration of leucocytes and macrophages into the wound. These cells engulf and destroy dead or dying tissue. It is terminated by the formation of pus. If the destructive stage is very severe the process goes on to necrosis, which is death of a small area of tissue as opposed to gangrene, which may also occur and means gross death.

Stage 3. Proliferation. When epithelium and connective tissue develop, new capillaries sprout off the sides of existing wounds. Fibroblasts appear alongside the capillaries. These two together constitute granulation tissue. Fine fibrils soon form in the ground substance and then gradually aggregate into typical collagen fibres. The stage of proliferation starts from the 4th to 14th day. During this phase all the cells forming the surface epithelium undergo rapid division and migrate as a thin film covering the wound. They also grow down as several sprouts into the depth of the wound. It is thought by some pathologists that these tiny growths of epithelial cells stimulate the formation of granulation tissue.

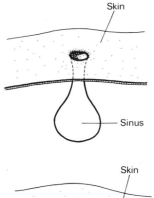

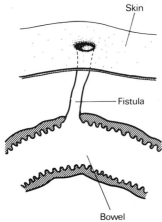

Fig. 8.1 A sinus ends blindly — a fistula connects two epithelial surfaces — in this case the skin and the intestine.

Stage 4. Maturation. During this phase the blood vessels gradually disappear and the number of fibroblasts in relation to fibres diminish. The red elevated recent scar is gradually changed into a thin white line.

Healing by first intention (primary healing) and *healing by second intention* (healing by granulation) were in the past considered to be distinct processes. Healing by granulation is essentially the same as primary healing, the only difference being that usually, as a result of infection, the stage of destruction is greatly prolonged and results in a deep cavity which is filled gradually from the bottom by granulation tissue.

Tissue repair

Repair is the process by which tissue is replaced — the simpler the tissue the more effective repair can be. As tissue, i.e. cells, become highly specialised repair becomes more difficult. Epithelial surfaces and fibrous tissue will regenerate without too much difficulty, but most other cells, and in particular nerve cells and structures like the glomerulus in the kidney, are not replaced but the space they occupy is filled with fibrous tissue. Some apparently highly specialised epithelial tissue is capable of regeneration and this is seen particularly where liver cells may be destroyed by disease.

If granulation tissue is excessive it is raised above the level of the approaching epithelium and forms an insurmountable barrier to the spread of epithelium. This is corrected by cauterising the granulation tissue to the level of the epithelium with silver nitrate (Fig. 11.5).

A blind track which may persist is known as a sinus and is due to the presence of a foreign body such as a knot of unabsorbed catgut or deficient drainage. If the track to the skin surface communicates with another epithelial surface through the granulation tissue the condition is known as a fistula (Fig. 8.1).

THE SPREAD OF INFECTION IN THE TISSUES

According to the form of spread which occurs, special terms are used to describe the process.

1. Cellulitis. It is the direct spread of infection in the tissues, or more strictly in the extracellular spaces. The term cellulitis is really a misnomer, and resolution may occur spontaneously, or pus may form.

2. Lymphangitis. (Fig. 8.2) The lymphatic vessels between the site of infection and the regional lymphatic glands are usually inflamed. Classically they are best seen as red lines on the arm of a patient suffering from a septic finger.

3. Lymphadenitis. The lymphatic glands (syn. nodes) are invaded by organisms carried by the lymph stream in the lymphatic vessels. (Fig. 8.2). The lymphatic glands, which become swollen and tender, are structurally well equipped to deal with infection by their complex network, which filters the organisms.

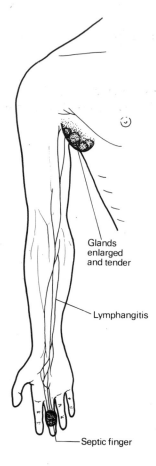

Glands
enlarged
and tender

Lymphangitis

Septic finger

Fig. 8.2 Spread of infection in the lymphatic system.

The common sites for lymphadenitis and the areas from which they are infected are:

Glands	Area of infection
(a) The neck	Face, mouth, tongue and scalp
(b) The axilla	Breast and upper limb
(c) The groin	Lower limb, groin and perineum

4. Bacteraemia. Bacteraemia is the spread of organisms into the blood stream where they are usually destroyed.

5. Septicaemia. Septicaemia is the invasion and multiplication of bacteria in the blood stream, and the onset is usually heralded by a single rigor followed by persistent pyrexia.

6. Pyaemia. Pyaemia is the spread of organisms in the blood stream, with the formation of abscesses at many sites in the body. Although the tissues have failed to contain the process locally, they are still endeavouring to localise it at more distant sites. The great danger is that the abscesses are usually multiple, and are often at sites not only remote from one another but relatively inaccessible to surgical drainage, such as the liver and the brain.

7. Other forms of spread. In the body cavities and the lumen of tubed viscera, infection can spread very rapidly.

Two other terms must be mentioned: *toxaemia*, which is the spread of the toxic products of inflammation from the site of infection into the blood stream; and *suppuration*, which is the process of pus formation (an abscess see Fig. 8.3).

FAILURE OF THE INFLAMMATORY REACTION

In severe infection the inflammatory reaction may fail to develop and the patient succumbs rapidly. More commonly the failure is partial and it is important to recognise at once the factors which may be preventing its full development. They are:

1. Poor arterial blood supply

(a) Age—arteriosclerosis.
(b) Site—the lower third of the leg—gross scarring.
(c) Tight dressings. Tourniquets.
(d) Arterial thrombosis or embolism.
(e) Shock—a poor blood supply diminishes the supply of leucocytes and allows bacteria to multiply.
(f) Gas pressure—gas gangrene.

2. Deficient venous drainage

(a) Venous thrombosis.
(b) Varicose veins.

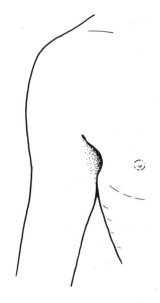

Fig. 8.3   An acute abscess of the arm.

3. Depression or deficiency of the quality of the blood

(a) Anaemia — nutritional.
        haemorrhage.
(b) Leucopenia. Steroids suppress the action of the leucocytes.
(c) Hypoproteinaemia. Plasma protein levels below 5 g per 100 ml are insufficient for a skin graft to take.

4. Malnutrition and dehydration

General.
Vitamin deficiency.
Zinc deficiency.

5. Excess of fluid in the tissues

Oedema

cardiac.
· nephritic.
lymphatic obstruction.
venous obstruction.

6. Metabolic

Diabetes.
Nephritis.
Uraemia.
Portal cirrhosis.
Jaundice.

7. Drugs

ACTH.
Corticosteroids.
Metallic poison.
Cytotoxic drugs.

PATHOPHYSIOLIGAL CHANGES

The blood

The normal count of white blood cells (leucocytes) ranges between 4000 to 10 000/mm³ in the adult and 10 000 to 25 000/mm³ in the infant and consists of:

Granulocytes (polymorphonuclear leucocytes) 40–75 per cent.

Eosinophils	1–6 per cent
Basophils	1 per cent

Lymphocytes 20 to 50 per cent.

Monocytes 1 to 6 per cent

The granulocytes increase in the blood in acute infection, the lymphocytes in viral infections and the monocytes in certain conditions like glandular fever.

The increase in the number of granulocytes in acute infections is rapid and they may account for 95 per cent of the total white cell count. If for any reason this increase fails to occur, the disease takes a more severe course than would otherwise have been expected. Excessive irradiation and the excessive dosage of certain drugs, such as the sulphonamide drugs, some antithyroid drugs, chloramphenicol, and cytotoxic drugs (used in treating malignant disease), depress the production of leucocytes. If the production of granulocytes is markedly depressed the patient is unable to combat even the mildest infection and death results. This condition is known as agranulocytosis (no polymorphonuclear leucocytes), but is more usually a granulocytopenia (diminished number of white cells). Clinically the most obvious feature of agranulocytosis is a destructive condition in the tissues of the mouth and throat because the patient has no resistance to the vast number of organisms he normally inhales and ingests without ill effect each day. The most valuable drugs for this condition are the antibiotics which help to combat infection. ACTH (adrenocorticotrophic hormone), 100 units daily, increases the production of granulocytes and is said to be of value in this condition.

Almost all acute infections result in an increase in the white cells, but there are important exceptions. For example, in typhoid fever, the white cell count is below normal, of the order of 2000 to 3000 mm^3. The term 'leucopenia' is applied to those states in which the *white cells* are fewer than normal.

GENERAL BODILY CHANGES IN INFLAMMATION

Pyrexia. Pyrogens act by the release of a prostaglandin in the temperature regulating centre in the brain. The antipyretic effect of aspirin is due to blocking of the formation of the prostaglandin.

If the infection is mild, the rise in temperature is slight. However, in severe infection and as a result of infection in organs like the kidney or liver where the vascular mass is considerably higher than most, a persistent high temperature may cause dehydration and electrolyte imbalance.

Sometimes the temperature may be the presenting sign and in the absence of an obvious focus a stage one diagnosis of 'pyrexia of unknown origin' is made. Painstaking investigation and observation will be required to reveal the cause. Occasionally a pelvic infection may present with pyrexia without any local symptoms and of course deep seated infection elsewhere in the body may be very difficult to locate.

The rise in temperature increases metabolism and increases the demand for oxygen. A notable exception to a rise in temperature from infection is where the body is flooded rapidly with endotoxins. The temperature is subnormal and the patient in a condition of shock (endotoxic shock).

Metabolism is increased and in prolonged suppuration protein loss is considerable.

Oliguria. The amount of urine secreted is diminished to preserve fluid in the body and is highly concentrated.

Investigations

In the vast majority of infections no investigation is necessary because if the infection is mild, the inflammatory response can be seen or detected on clinical examination. The nature of the infection can be determined and the site localised.

In more severe infections or in conditions where the nature of the disease is obscure investigation will be necessary and include.

1. *White blood cell count* which in acute infection will reveal a leucocytosis.

2. *Bacteriological examination* of material recovered from the site of infection — for example the throat, the urine or a wound as appropriate. The nature and antibiotic sensitivity of organisms discovered is determined. If septicaemia is suspected blood is taken for blood culture. The culture medium should be at hand so that blood is withdrawn when the patient's temperature, if swinging, is at its height or, if rigors are a feature, as soon as the next rigor occurs.

3. *Serum tests for the presence of antibodies* may be valuable in the diagnosis or exclusion of certain infections like syphilis or typhoid fever.

4. *The urine tests* for sugar to exclude diabetes are repeated and albuminuria in prolonged suppuration may herald the onset of amyloid disease.

The signs and symptoms of inflammation

The constitutional symptoms include malaise, loss of appetite, fatigue and sleeplessness. The temperature is elevated and the pulse rate is increased. The urinary output is scanty and the bowel is constipated. All these symptoms are due to the toxins which are liberated by the invading organism into the blood stream. In overwhelming infection the patient may be in septicaemic shock.

Local signs and symptoms

1. Redness is caused by dilatation of capillaries in the inflamed area.

2. Heat is due to the increased blood flow.

3. Swelling occurs because plasma is poured into the surrounding tissues. The degree of swelling is dependent to some extent on the natural laxity or otherwise of the tissues, for example, inflammation below the eyes causes an extreme degree of swelling at a very early stage.

4. Pain is due to the accumulation of toxins which irritate the nerve endings and hormones released locally from stretching of the tiny nerve twigs caused by the excess of fluid in the tissues, which increases as tension becomes greater.

5. Loss of function occurs as a result of pain, swelling and the toxic effect on the tissue itself. The patient's natural desire is to rest and to avoid using any painful part.

The termination of inflammation may be:
  (a) Resolution
  (b) Suppuration
  (c) Ulceration
  (d) Gangrene
  (e) Fibrosis

MANAGEMENT AND NURSING CARE

General Management

Most infections are mild and the patient's resistance is high so that resolution is rapid and only the simplest measures are required. These include rest, a liberal fluid intake, and the avoidance of cold, physical exertion or mental anxiety all of which depress resistance. Antibiotics which are expensive and not without risk are unnecessary in most cases.

The necessary measures and the vigour with which they are pursued depends on the severity, course and site of the disease. They include:

1. Assessment of the patient's resistance. All the factors which may cause the inflammatory reaction to be limited (p. 60) are assessed and as far as possible appropriate action taken. This will include bringing a diabetic condition under control, increasing the dosage of steroids if the patient is on steroid therapy, remedial vitamin therapy if necessary and reviewing the administration of cytotoxic drugs which the patient may be receiving. The presenting picture in leukaemia may be an infection and in a known leukaemic patient infection is a constant hazard.

2. Rest is a fundamental principle.

General rest to the body increases resistance, diminishes strain on the heart which may be poisoned by circulating toxins, and ensures conditions in which sleep can be promoted.

Local rest in addition to diminishing pain relieves the part or organ from the stress and strain of its normal function. It has to be interpreted in relation to the part affected. It consists of a darkened room for an inflamed eye, a bland diet for a gastrointestinal infection or a sling to rest an infected arm.

3. Relief of pain by analgesics enables the patient to sleep.

4. Diet. If the condition is severe or prolonged there is loss of fluid from sweating resulting in dehydration and electrolyte imbalance. A fluid balance chart and electrolyte estimations are necessary so that corrective measures can be taken. The increased metabolism from pyrexia and the breakdown of body protein requires a high protein and high calorie diet. In addition, vitamin supplements are necessary. Vitamin A is antinfective, vitamin B is necessary when administering many antibiotics and vitamin C is required for healing.

5. Antitoxins and antibacterial substances are prescribed as appropriate and have revolutionised the management of infective disease.

6. Pyrexia. Rigors are particularly unpleasant and the patient has to be kept warm with extra blankets if necessary. A temperature of 39·5°C or over is in itself dangerous and described as hyperpyrexia so that every effort is made to prevent it rising further. Frequent tepid sponges, and in severe cases even ice packs, may be advisable.

7. Prevention of further contamination. The nurse should explain to the patient that the skin around a suppurating wound is highly infected and warn him that he can, with his fingers, spread the infection to his eye or ear. The surgical conversion of an open wound into a closed wound, or the deviation of normally infected bowel contents by a colostomy in acute diverticular disease of the colon, are examples of the same principle.

Local Measures

1. Rest has already been mentioned and is the most effective non-operative measure.

2. Increasing the blood supply should help but in practice fomentation and poulticing so long practised are of no value. A cooling lotion applied to the overlying skin is more likely to be soothing. The only measure to increase the blood supply which may be undertaken occasionally for a chronic ulcer of the leg is sympathectomy, and in such patients the arterial supply of blood to the limb is already deficient.

Surgical Measures

Excision of an infected focus is an ideal method of treatment but it is rarely possible — a notable and very effective example being appendicectomy for an acute appendicitis.

Incision and drainage is necessary once an abscess has formed. The incision has to be sufficiently large to allow free drainage. A tube stitched to the skin is usually inserted and the surgeon will give instructions when it has to be shortened or removed. Its removal should be recorded in the patient's notes. If pressure has to be applied to the sides of a wound to express pus, drainage is inadequate and further incision is necessary. The skin surrounding the draining wound is cleansed with an antiseptic when the wound is dressed. A sinus or fistula which persists has to be laid open and dressed as an open wound — a corner of a gauze pack is tucked very lightly into the wound to keep the skin edges apart while healing proceeds from the depths. Tight plugging with gauze is not only painful but also prevents free drainage by acting as a plug.

Failure to heal may be due to the presence of a foreign body including a lost drainage tube. Other causes include all the conditions mentioned on page 60 outlining a failure of the inflammatory reaction. The patient's condition is reviewed with all these in mind and corrective measures undertaken. Prolonged suppuration resulting in hypoproteinaemia may cause a dangerous degenerative condition of the connective tissues in many important organs and is known as amyloid disease. The liver, the kidney and the spleen are particularly liable to be affected. It's appearance may be suggested by the presence of proteinuria and polyuria and further investigation including biopsy of the rectal mucosa may be necessary to confirm it's presence.

A sinus from a wound can discharge for year or a chronic skin ulcer may eventually undergo malignant change.

A persistent sinus or fistula has to be laid open and the management of this is discussed in the section on diseases of the anus, a site in which they are particularly liable to occur.

RESTORATION OF FUNCTION

From the beginning the restoration of full function should be the aim of the nurse and the surgeon and if this is unlikely to be achieved as much function as possible must be preserved. The cooperation of the patient in movement of joints in an affected limb or exercise of muscles liable to waste can be encouraged with sympathy and firmness. A skin graft may be necessary to accelerate healing and diminish scarring and the objective is explained to the patient. The physiotherapist has often an important role. The Social Worker, the patient's family and in some cases the Psychiatrist may have parts to play in the restoration of full function and health.

9

The specific surgical infections

A specific surgical infection is a disease which can be caused only by a particular strain of organism.

TETANUS (LOCK-JAW)

Tetanus is commonly known as lock-jaw, because the muscular spasms which characterise it frequently attack the muscles of the jaw. The discovery of an antitoxin and methods of active immunisation as well as control of the preparation of catgut have made tetanus a rare disease in the West. In the developing countries it is responsible for 500 000 deaths each year.

The organism, the *Clostridium tetani* (Ch. 6), usually gains access through a deep punctured wound but all contaminated wounds are dangerous. In the operating theatre a wound may be contaminated from catgut, improperly sterilised dressings and powders, or from outdoor shoes.

The organism elaborates a powerful toxin which poisons the motor nerve cells, with the result that spasm occurs in the muscles supplied by the corresponding nerves.

Symptoms and signs

The first symptom is slight stiffness of the muscles, particularly those of the jaw. The patient is anxious, but mentally clear. As the disease progresses the classical picture of tetanus appears.

The back is arched and the head may be thrown back (opisthotonos). The facial muscles are in spasm, and the mouth can be opened only with difficulty (trismus). Drawing up of the angle of the mouth gives rise to the characteristic smile (risus sardonicus).

Spasms may affect every muscle in the body, and in severe cases the muscles rupture. Spasm of the sphincter muscles of the body render swallowing, defaecation, and micturition very difficult. Spasm of the respiratory muscles causes long periods of anoxia until death ensues. The temperature is elevated and the pulse rate is increased.

Prognosis. The longer the incubation period the more hopeful is the outlook.

Treatment and nursing care

Prophylactic. Careful surgical toilet and a prophylactic dose of penicillin is the best prevention. If the patient has not been immunised human anti-tetanus immunoglobulin is the ideal.

If an old accidental wound has to be reopened (perhaps years later) tetanus spores may be lying dormant in its substance. Their reactivation may give rise to tetanus. This danger is described as latent tetanus. The best prophylatic treatment is active immunisation against tetanus.

If one can be certain of the patient's immunity status, a patient who has been actively immunised should be given a booster dose of tetanus toxoid, but within three years of immunisation it can be omitted.

Therapeutic — specific treatment. Penicillin is bactericidal and is administered in all cases of tetanus. It is also protective if there is an accompanying pneumonia. Human antiserum is given.

The wound must be excised and irrigated with hydrogen peroxide, because the tetanus bacillus will not grow in the presence of oxygen. The wound is not sutured.

General treatment. Absolute rest and isolation are important, since the slightest noise or flicker increases the spasms. The patient is nursed in a quiet dark room which must be draught-free. The door should be fitted with suitable closing springs to prevent slamming. The nurse should warm her hands before touching the patient to avoid stimulating further spasms.

Most deaths are due to lack of oxygen and pulmonary infection. The toxin infects the bulbar nuclei so that the muscles of the pharynx and larynx are affected; the larynx is no longer the watch-dog for the lungs. Coughing is ineffective and anything that the patient swallows or regurgitates from the stomach is liable to infect the lungs. The important points in treatment are:

1. A nasogastric tube is passed in all but the mildest cases and the stomach is aspirated before each feed if nasogastric feeding is permitted.
2. A tracheostomy is performed and suction applied at regular intervals. Controlled respiration using a mechanical respirator should be used as soon as possible. Regular suction produces sympathetic overactivity with a resultant fall in blood pressure and tachycardia. The pulse should therefore be checked and any alteration reported.
3. Muscle relaxants relieve most of the symptoms. The eyes are protected if curare is used, otherwise conjunctivitis develops.
4. The maintenance of fluid balance by intravenous fluids. The relaxant is injected into the infusion by the anaesthetist.
5. Sedatives are used very sparingly and are almost unnecessary if relaxants are used correctly.

GAS GANGRENE

Wounds which contain lacerated or crushed tissue are those most likely to develop gas gangrene. The organism may be present in a wound but the anaerobic conditions in which a tissue has lost all or most of its blood supply are essential for its proliferation. The organism is *Clostridium perfringens* (*Cl. welchii*) See Chapter 6.

Sources in hospital

The organism is most commonly found in patients incontinent of faeces and infection arises from the patient's own intestinal flora. It is particularly important that, if gas gangrene is to be avoided following amputations or operations on the hip in these patients, the skin should be treated with extra care and care should be taken to exclude faecal matter from the wound. Additionally, penicillin is administered intramuscularly at the beginning of the operation.

Symptoms and signs

Pain in the wound is extremely severe. It is important to remember that the disease may develop in a wound under plaster. Never neglect the pain of a patient in a plaster — it may only indicate a pressure sore but it may also be a symptom of gas gangrene.

The wound, which may be green or black, has a strong 'mouselike' odour. Small bubbles of gas may be seen escaping and the surrounding tissues are swollen and crackle when touched (crepitus). Untreated, deterioration is rapid.

In early cases, radiographic examination may reveal the presence of gas in the tissues.

Treatment

The patient is resuscitated with blood, and penicillin is administered. Anti-gasgangrene serum may be prescribed.

Wide excision of all infected tissue must be performed and the wound left open. The wound is irrigated with hydrogen peroxide and eusol, and the danger has passed only when granulations appear. Complete isolation is essential to prevent infection spreading into the wounds of other patients.

Hyperbaric (i.e. at a pressure greater than the atmosphere) oxygen therapy may save the limb but is of no value until after wound excision has been performed.

SURGICAL TUBERCULOSIS

Tuberculosis is still a prevalent infectious disease in many countries and amongst immigrants from Asia and Africa in the United Kingdom. In one

London Borough 250 out of 290 notifications were immigrants and many lesions were extrapulmonary.

Not common enough to be a major health concern yet not rare enough to be ignored, tuberculosis is still a fatal disease if not diagnosed and managed effectively (Grange, 1979).

The organism may be ingested, inhaled or inoculated through the skin. The pathological reaction of tissues to the bacillus is known as a tubercle which consists of a central necrotic mass of caseous or cheese-like material containing giant cells surrounded by a layer of lymphocytes. It may liquefy to form what is known as a cold or tuberculous abscess which may point on the surface and become infected with organisms on the skin. The result is that chronic infection with pyogenic organisms results in a persistent discharge and this may cause amyloid disease (p. 65). At any stage of the disease healing may occur by fibrosis of the tubercle, and this is sometimes consolidated further by calcification of its substance.

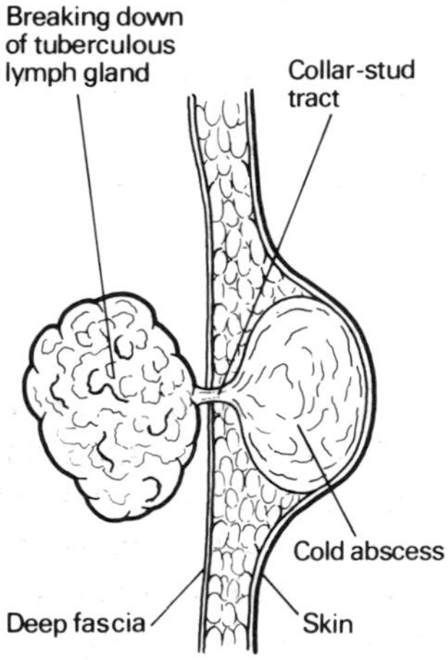

Cold abscess (Fig. 9.1). The tuberculous abscess is described as cold because the skin temperature is not raised. Erythema of the skin and pointing of the abscess develop slowly. Frequently these changes never appear, because resolution occurs and the pus is absorbed.

If pointing is threatened, aspiration is performed through an area of relatively healthy skin. The greatest care is taken to prevent secondary infection. Very rarely are tuberculous abscesses incised, and then only if it is possible to eradicate the underlying focus.

Fig. 9.1 Cold abscess (collar stud type) in the neck.

Treatment

1. Specific treatment. The oral administration of Rifampicin and Isoniaziad for 9 months with the addition of Ethambutol for the first two months is recommended by the British Thoracic and Tuberculous Association. This regime is more acceptable than streptomycin which has to be injected and combined with PAS (para-aminosalicylic acid) which causes nausea.

In almost all cases the patient is cured.

2. Surgical treatment. The scope of surgical treatment has greatly diminished since the advent of chemotherapy, but it still has a place in the excision or partial excision of an organ infected with tuberculosis, and the management of a cold abscess is still an important surgical condition.

THE VENEREAL DISEASES

There are a number of venereal and allied diseases but only two, syphilis and gonorrhoea, are commonly seen in the British Isles. A third disease, chancroid or soft sore, is seen from time to time in the seaports. It is a disease of the tropics caused by Ducrey's bacillus.

Syphilis and gonorrhoea both produce local lesions at the site of infection, usually on the sex organs. The local lesions of gonorrhoea are painful and alarming, and the patient usually seeks advice, while those of syphilis are surprisingly trivial and sometimes so slight that even the patient is unaware of their presence. Both diseases may produce widespread lesions in later years, but the ravages and destruction caused by syphilis in almost every organ of the body culminate in a large variety of lesions which simulate almost every disease. It was for this reason that Osler called it the 'Great Imitator'.

SYPHILIS

Congenital syphilis

The mother may infect her unborn child in utero, and, clinically, this may have the following results:
1. Abortion — usually after the fifth month.
2. The child is rarely born with signs of active disease but may develop them in the first two weeks of life.
3. The child appears to be normal at birth and the signs of congenital syphilis appear in later years.

If treatment is given up to the 28th week of pregnancy the child can be born free from syphilis.

Symptoms and signs

The signs of congenital syphilis are essentially those of acquired syphilis, commencing at the secondary stage. The most characteristic sign is the typical secondary rash, which usually develops in the course of the first fortnight of life. It is a widespread copper-coloured rash affecting almost the whole of the body. Scars may appear around the mouth, known as rhagades, and infection of the nose causes a thick purulent discharge, the typical snuffles of congenital syphilis.

Other signs are:

1. Flattening of the nose from destruction of the nasal septum.
2. Interstitial keratitis and iritis. The cornea is dull and opaque, due to syphilitic thickening, and if the infection is untreated blindness may result.
3. The permanent upper incisor teeth may have concave lower borders (Hutchinson's teeth, Moon's 'turreted' molars are sometimes seen), and are pathognomonic of congenital syphilis.

Other symptoms, such as painless effusion into the knee joints (Clutton's joints), infantile tabes, congenital deafness, and cerebral deterioration, may all appear at a later stage. The bones may be affected by inflammation of the periosteum, which is so painful that the child is unable to move his limbs, and the condition is described as syphilitic pseudoparalysis.

Acquired syphilis

The primary lesion of syphilis is the chancre, or septic sore at the site of infection — in men usually on the penis and in women either on the vulva or the cervix of the uterus. Occasionally chancres are found elsewhere, for example, on the lips, or on the nurse's finger from contact with a syphilitic lesion while in attendance on the patient. The primary lesion has an incubation period of 1 to 3 weeks and is painless; it is highly infectious, and must never be touched with the naked finger. Untreated, it rapidly heals and gives rise later to almost any symptoms in any part of the body. After its disappearance the patient may have no further clinical evidence of syphilis until he develops lesions many years later, or he may pass into the secondary stage 2 to 6 months later.

Secondary syphilis. An extensive rash is the characteristic symptom. It is usually a dull copper-coloured eruption, particularly on the back and face.

A similar lesion occurs in the throat, and the moisture of that area produces what is known as a snail-track ulcer. The presence of secondary syphilitic lesions in the anal region produces large soggy thicknesses known as condylomata.

All the lymphatic glands are very much enlarged. They are rubbery to the touch and are not tender.

Tertiary stage. This may occur years after the primary or secondary lesion. The characteristic lesion is known as a gumma, and may occur in any organ of the body. The tibia and skin overlying it, as well as the palate, are favourite sites. It takes the form of a hard mass which gradually breaks down to form an ulcer, which has a typical punched-out appearance.

Parasyphilitic lesions. These are the most dreaded of all manifestations of syphilis, and include tabes dorsalis, general paralysis of the insane, and lesions of the heart and circulatory system, such as aortic regurgitation and aneurysm of the thoracic aorta.

The diagnosis of syphilis

The finding of the *Treponema pallidum* in the primary lesion is the most certain method of diagnosis. A specimen is taken by the doctor by means of a capillary tube and then examined unstained immediately under a microscope by darkground illumination.

The Kahn or Wassermann reaction is positive on examination of the blood 2 to 3 weeks after the appearance of the primary lesion. The blood collected for this test should not be oxalated, as the test is performed on the serum content. Five millilitres of blood are withdrawn from a vein in the arm.

Treatment

Penicillin is now the drug of choice but penicillin sensitive patients must be treated with tetracycline or erythromycin. In the later stages of the disease potassium iodide is still of value, often in combination with penicillin. Few complications are likely to occur, but some patients are allergic to certain forms of penicillin and care is necessary in such cases.

GONORRHOEA

Gonorrhoea is due to a diplococcus known as the *Gonococcus*. It is an aerobic organism and extremely delicate. The acute symptoms appear after about 3 days from the time of infection. They consist of irritation of the urethra in the male, followed by a copious, yellow, purulent discharge. The patient is toxic, complains of malaise, and has a high temperature. There is frequency of micturition and the patient finds walking uncomfortable. In the female, Bartholin's glands may be swollen and a local abscess or cyst may form.

In pregnant women there is sometimes surprisingly little evidence of infection.

Gonorrhoea may spread through the whole of the genital tract. In the female, infection of the cervix uteri and of the Fallopian tubes (salpingitis) is not uncommon. In the male, the Cowper's glands, the prostate, and sometimes the epididymis may be affected.

Chronic lesions of gonorrhoea

Any of the acute lesions in the urinary tract may become chronic, but, in addition, infection may spread to other regions of the body. Arthritis, particularly of the ankles, is not uncommon. In babies, conjunctivitis and keratitis may be acquired during birth. The treatment of ophthalmia neonatorum is described in Chapter 49. Occasionally gonorrhoea is responsible for infective endocarditis.

The outstanding chronic surgical lesion resulting from gonococcal infection is stricture of the male urethra.

Treatment

The most useful drugs in the treatment of gonorrhoea are penicillin, streptomycin, and the sulphonamides such as sulphathiazole or sulphatriad, either alone or in combination, depending on the stage of the disease when first seen. If resistant strains have developed, spectinomycin or cotrimoxazole may be prescribed.

Repeated examinations by direct smears and cultures are essential before declaring the patient cured.

It is not very uncommon for a patient to be suffering from both gonorrhoea and syphilis. It is important that this should be discovered by the appropriate serological tests as short term penicillin therapy will cure gonorrhoea but only mask syphilis.

NON-SPECIFIC URETHRITIS

This troublesome condition, almost exclusively confined to the male, is becoming increasingly prevalent and it is now commoner than gonorrhoea in the male. It consists of a urethral discharge containing no recognisable organisms and tends, quite often, to run a chronic course. The cause is at present unknown but a virus is suspected in many cases.

It is often associated with various forms of arthritis which may respond to the administration of ACTH or cortisone.

Treatment consists of sulphonamides, the various antibiotics particularly tetracycline, and irrigation of the urethra with a 1 : 8000 oxycyanide of mercury solution.

SOCIAL ASPECTS OF VENEROLOGY

Follow-up contact tracing and publicity campaigns are important in limiting the spread and prevention of disease. The patient is more likely to continue treatment until a cure is effected and to cooperate in tracing contacts if the doctors and nurses treat him with human understanding, tact and compassion.

BIBLIOGRAPHY

British Thoracic and Tuberculous Association 1976 Lancet ii: 1102
Grange J M 1979 British Journal of Hospital Medicine 22: 540

10

The operating theatre

The operating theatre should provide a place in which surgical procedures can be undertaken with maximal safety to the patient. It is a complex of engineering to provide power for lighting, ventilation and the working of machines as well as to meet many demands which are essential for the care of the patient. The prevention of infection which is the most demanding of his requirements is the most difficult to satisfy.

Infection prolongs convalescence, increases morbidity and, if sufficiently severe, will start a chain of events which ultimately may result in death of the patient. Sterilisation and the use of disinfectants will destroy micro-organisms but unfortunately many objects which come in contact with the patient cannot be sterilised. The only course available is to deny the micro-organisms access — a technique called asepsis of which sterilisation is a component. This forms the basis of all theatre procedures and has discipline all of its own and demands constant vigilance.

STERILISATION

Sterilisation is the destruction of all micro-organisms and spores. Most equipment including linen and instruments are supplied already sterilised either from a central sterile supply department or from commercial sources. This saves the nurses time and permits the use of the most efficient methods of sterilisation. The nurses task is to select the correct pack, open it without contamination and dispose of the contents after use so that there is no spread of infection or wastage of recoverable objects. If the container is made of glass or plastic it is examined for cracks or damage and if these are discovered the pack is discarded. Similarly, packages of dressings, operating gowns or instruments wrapped in paper are rejected if tears or dampness are discovered. The high pressure autoclave tape is inspected and any discrepancy in the black lines on the tape indicates that the pack is unsafe to use.

A few objects such as endoscopic instruments may be sterilised in a chemical solution chosen by the theatre team of the nurses own hospital. The instrument should be fully immersed in the solution for the correct time and rinsed before use with sterile water to remove all trace of chemicals which may be irritant to the body tissues. Sterile water is produced by some form of steam distillation, bottled and sterilised in the autoclave (steam under pressure).

Sterilisation undertaken commercially is effected by the use of irradiation, ethylene oxide and ultra violet light while central sterile supply departments use an autoclave.

The provision of materials, already sterile, in a smooth continuous flow is ideal. However, as in all commercial operations, the supply may suddenly cease from a shortage of materials, lack of fuel, transport or industrial disruption and a hospital will then have to rely on its own limited resources and expertise. The least fortunate hospital will be the one where modernisation has removed not only all the water sterilisers but also the autoclave outside its curtilage to a central sterile supply department which may have ceased to function.

Boiling and chemical methods of sterilisation fall short because they do not destroy spores or viruses, but the risk of such infection is smaller than doing nothing for a patient suffering from general peritonitis or from an accidental wound.

The discussion which follows is a bare outline of those methods. Before sterilisation is undertaken by nursing staff whose normal duties do not encompass the mechanisms of sterilisation procedures, they should consult the excellent publications listed at the end of this chapter for detailed information. If an autoclave is available some instruction from an expert will be essential.

Chemical sterilisation

Chemical sterilisation and the methods which are used commercially have been mentioned above. The possible methods likely to be available in hospital all utilise heat.

Dry heat

Dry heat is one of the most efficient methods of sterilisation. The object to be sterilised is sealed in a container and placed in a hot air oven at a temperature of 160°C and this is maintained for 1 hour. The destruction of spores is complete. It is suitable only for glassware, all glass syringes, metal instruments and ointments and powders. In order to prevent reinfection the materials must be sealed in a container.

Moist heat

Moist heat is one of the most important and most universally applicable methods of sterilisation. Autoclaving uses steam under pressure.

Steam-pressure autoclaves

Sterilising times and temperature of steam-pressure autoclaves are always appropriate to the following:

Size of autoclave

Amount of load

Type of material for sterilisation.

The type of autoclave is based on the method of removing air from the autoclave.

Downward displacement autoclave

The DDA can be controlled manually or automatically with a timed cycle. It is run on gas, electricity or from a mains supply. It may be used with or without a drying process, depending on requirements. The downward displacement autoclave destroys bacteria and spores by coagulation. The modern high-vacuum high-pressure steriliser will, after 3 minutes at 143°C, 10 minutes at 126°C and 15 minutes at 121°C and a pressure of 2 kg per cm², sterilise its contents. Less modern autoclaves require a longer period.

The following points, are important:

The containers must be such that adequate penetration of the steam is possible. Suitable material must:

1. Allow steam to penetrate it to sterilise its contents.
2. Afford adequate protection against bacterial contamination and infestation.
3. Be light to transport.
4. Be inexpensive.
5. Have a long shelf life.

Paper, metal, balloon cloth, linen and calico are all used. Packs must be stored on slotted shelves, kept free from dust and dated.

Moist textiles. If dressings or gowns are damp then they should be regarded as unsuitable for use. Gloves should be sterilised at the same pressure, temperature, and time as dressings and textiles. It has been shown that it is quite unsafe to accept a lower standard. In modern rapid autoclaving at high temperature the gloves are not damaged. Most disposable gloves are now sterilised by gamma radiation.

Objects may be unsterile because of:

(a) Incorrect packing.

(b) Incorrect loading of the autoclave.

(c) Mechanical defects such as a blocked air ejector.

Daily testing of the autoclave should eliminate objects being unsterile. The thermocouple is an indicator proving that the correct temperature has been reached and held for the correct time. The thermocouple is inserted into the centre of a load for sterilisation and viewed at the completion of the process.

Autoclaving recording chart. This is a permanent reference of the temperature reached and time held during the cycle of sterilisation.

Sterilisation checks

1. The Bowie-Dick test is a method for testing complete penetration of heat to whole areas of a load and is designed for use in high vacuum high pressure autoclaves. The principle is that high pressure autoclave tape is placed in the centre of a pile of 30 towels. The pile is placed in the centre of the autoclave for the first process of the day. On completion of the cycle the autoclave tape is inspected. Any discrepancy in the black lines on the autoclave tape indicate a faulty cycle.

2. Bacteriological. Spore bearing organisms are put in the centre of a pack of dressings and the bacteriologist determines if the destruction has been complete.

Boiling

Boiling used to be the method in common use but should only be used for surgical procedures when no other means are available. This method destroys bacteria only and not spores. However, it may be the only method available. It is important to ensure:

1. That all instruments are opened before immersing them completely;
2. That the time taken for boiling should commence after the cold instruments have been immersed and the water has started to boil again, the time being 5 minutes or over at a temperature of 100°C.

ASEPSIS AND THEATRE TECHNIQUE

Asepsis is the underlying principle of surgery by which organisms are denied access to the patient. Asepsis has a discipline all its own. From the commencement of her career the nurse must train herself to recognise at once conditions which are at variance with an aseptic technique.

Micro-organisms are to be found everywhere. Objects which can be sterilised and wrapped in sterile containers present the least difficulty provided sterilisation has been adequate, but many objects which come into contact with the patient are either impossible to sterilise or are easily recontaminated.

1. There are particles in the air, i.e. dust and droplets, which are the ideal vehicle for the dissemination of airborne organisms. To lower the bacterial count of the air the following precautions are essential:

(a) Ventilation Ideally air shoud be filtered, moistened, and warmed or cooled to the regular temperature. An air-conditioning plant should be capable of changing the air in the theatre suite 15 or 20 times in each hour. When a wound is exposed movement is kept at a minimum. Doors and windows kept closed. (If the room is air conditioned windows will always be kept closed.)

(b) Speech should be limited to the minimum and masks worn for the elimination of droplets.

(c) Bodily movement should be gentle and unhurried because in so doing the dust particles are kept to the minimum.

(d) Movement of the patient within the theatre suite should be kept to the minimum.

(e) Cleaning procedures should be completed 1 or 2 hours previously with a recommended disinfectant.

(f) The patient is transferred from the trolley to the table in the anaesthetic room or at interchange areas and vice versa at the end of the operation. Patient trolleys and ward blankets should not enter the theatre.

2. Many objects cannot be sterilised
    (a) The patient's skin.
    (b) The hands of the surgeon or nurse. It has been shown, however, that routine baths before operation tend to increase and not diminish infectivity.
    (c) The throat, nose and mouth of the staff.

3. The operating table and floor are easily contaminated from infected material during the operation.

4. Blood stains and pus are excellent media for the propagation of organisms, especially as the temperature is usually fairly high and the atmosphere is kept humid. Cross-infection can occur from anaesthetic apparatus, which should be pasteurised. Theatre staff, as all nursing staff, should be very careful in handling blood and its products since pricking of the skin or abrasions of the finger may be an entry for viruses which are sometimes present not only in stored blood but also in patient's blood.

5. Recontamination of sterile objects may occur because of:
    (a) Inefficient sterilisers or condensation of steam.
    (b) Inefficient air conditioning.
    (c) Poor technique in the handling of sterilised instruments and materials may infect a patient.

6. Faulty packaging of disposable articles and faulty storage may result in infection.

7. Theatre clothing should be laundered daily and footwear cleaned daily.

8. Rings and jewellery should not be worn.

9. Blankets are a source of infection and should be changed after each patient.

Because of the importance of maintaining asepsis, operating theatres should be designed so that they have:
    (a) Air-conditioned ventilation.
    (b) Easily cleanable fabric.
    (c) A one-way traffic circulation from 'clean' area to 'dirty' area.
    (d) Adequate shower facilities for medical and nursing personnel after they have finished a day's operating.

THEATRE TECHNIQUE

The theatre nurse is a member of a team, and unless she and all the theatre staff carefully observe all the principles and technique of asepsis, infection in the patient's wound is an inevitable result of the operation.

Theatre dress

The nurse should be clean in her person, her hands kept free from cracks

and abrasions, and the fingernails kept short, rounded and unvarnished. In
the theatre she should wear the special uniform provided, which usually
consists of an overall-type dress with short sleeves or trousers and top. The
material has a smooth surface and is boilable, so that all germs are destroyed in the laundering process. Mitchell et al have shown that when all
theatre staff, scrubbed as well as unscrubbed, wear suits or dresses made of
a non-woven fabric, air bacterial counts during an operating session are
reduced by 50 per cent. All hair should be concealed under a special cap.
Footwear with antistatic and impervious soles should be kept in the theatre
cloakroom and never worn outside the theatre. It is possible to carry micro-
organisms into the theatre from outside. The nose and mouth are covered
with a mask whilst the operation is in progress and whilst the theatre is
being prepared. Nurses from the ward must change into theatre clothing
like the theatre staff, if they enter the operating theatre.

CONSENT BY PATIENT

I, ...

of ....

hereby consent to undergo the operation of ....

....

the nature and effect of which have been explained to me by
Dr./Mr. ....

I also consent to such further or alternative operative measures as may be
found to be necessary during the course of the operation and to the
administration of a general, local or other anaesthetic for any of these purposes.

No assurance has been given to me that the operation will be performed
by any particular surgeon.

Date .... (Signed) ....
                                                                (Patient)

I confirm that I have explained to the patient the nature and effect of this
operation.

Date .... (Signed) ....
                                                        (Physician/Surgeon)

CONSENT BY RELATIVES

I, ...

of ....

the *husband/wife/parent of the above-named ....

hereby consent to my *wife/husband/child undergoing the operation indicated above.

*delete as necessary.

(Signed) ....

Fig. 10.1 Consent form for operation.

Blankets or blanket substitutes from the ward are not taken into the theatre because they are a source of infection. The patients blanket should be removed on entering the theatre and the patient covered with a clean cotton blanket. Ideally the patient should be visited the night before surgery by the theatre nurse and she should explain what he is to expect when entering the theatre suite.

The ward nurse and the theatre

The ward nurse accompanying the patient to the theatre entrance, must comfort and inspire confidence.

At the theatre entrance the patient is received by the theatre nurse, who accepts the patient from the ward nurse, ensuring that she has the right patient and all documentation is complete, together with any relevant information, e.g. if the patient is deaf, the patient has a stiff hip, etc. The consent form (Fig. 10.1) is checked by the theatre nurse. If it is not signed then the operation must not commence. The theatre nurse accompanies the patient into the anaesthetic room and stays with the patient during induction of anaesthesia. It is most important never to leave the patient prior to induction. The patient may be confused due to drugs and very apprehensive. Each patient should have a label attached to his wrist which is checked by the theatre nurse, the anaesthetist and the surgeon. The final check form (Fig. 10.2) is signed by the anaesthetist.

Patient's
Surname ....

Forenames ....   D.O.B. ....

Ward ....)

Operation ....)   *To be completed by*

Date ....)   *Theatre Sister*

                                                                Tick   *Tick*

Premedication given ....

Dentures removed ....

Urine tested and recorded ....

Signed Consent Form enclosed ....

Signature of   *Signature of*
Ward Sister or   *Anaesthetist*
Staff Nurse

....

Fig. 10.2   Final check form before anaesthesia.

The patient is positioned on the theatre table with the aid of the operating department assistant, and the theatre nurse. The position for an abdominal operation is shown in Figure 10.3 and for other regions in the relevant chapters in this book.

After the operation the patient remains in the theatre suite or recovery area until conscious and fit to return to the ward.

The ward nurse returns to the theatre to collect her patient, ensuring that she is aware of the nature of the anaesthetic, the diagnosis at the operation, and the nature of the operation which has been performed, the number of tubes and drains inserted and any special instructions from the surgeon or anaesthetist about postoperative care.

The ward nurse is entirely responsible for the patient during transit from the theatre to the ward. She must above all keep the airway clear and have with her a receiver with an airway, tongue depressor and gauze swabs. Care must be taken with the intravenous line, and the patient should be kept warm during transit.

The duties of the theatre nurse

It is the scrub nurse who is responsible for the instruments, and she wears a theatre cap which conceals her hair and a mask. The hands and arms are soaped and the nails are scrubbed for 5 minutes with an antiseptic soap. There are many antibacterial agents on the market which may be used for hand washing. The hands and arms are then dried with a sterile towel. The hands are inserted through the armhole of the sterile gown. It is pulled on by the circulating nurse and the back tapes tied. A back wrap gown (Fig. 10.4) has two tapes on the front one of which is handed to another scrubbed nurse or the surgeon who encircles the gown and hands it to the wearer to tie in front. The outside of the gloves and gown must not be touched by the ungloved hand. The hands are powdered and the first glove put on, touching the inside of the cuff only with the bare hand. The second glove is put on, touching the outside of the glove only with the other gloved hand. (Fig. 10.5).

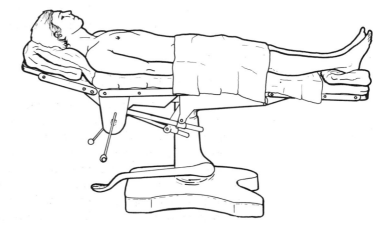

Fig. 10.3 Usual position for abdominal operation. Note elevation of the calves by pads under the heels.

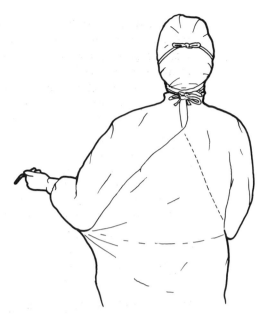

Fig. 10.4 The tapes of a backwrap gown are held by 'scrubbed' member of the staff and one tape is passed to the sister's left hand so that she can tie it in front.

When both gloves are on, the cuffs are pulled over the gown at the wrist. Back wraps on the gown are then tied by another gowned and gloved member of the theatre team. Once scrubbed, hands should be held in front and above waist level. The nurse who has scrubbed up now handles only sterilised materials. Should she inadvertently touch something which is non-sterile she must change her gloves, and gown. She supervises the instruments, threads needles, prepares ligatures, and keeps the surgeon supplied with swabs (which are wrapped in bundles of five), tubes, or anything else which is needed during the operation. She must be quick to respond to the whispered word or gesture, for unnecessary speech is out of place in the theatre.

The instrument nurse takes the soiled swabs from the surgeon and disposes of them into a bucket or container for the circulating nurse to hang on the swab rack (Fig. 10.6).

Duties of the circulating nurse

The circulating nurse is responsible for supplying all additional equipment for the surgical team and for assisting in swab check procedures. She retrieves all the used swabs from the bucket and hangs them in fives on the swab racks to be checked by the scrub nurse. All swabs contain a radio-opaque thread for ease of identification (Figs. 10.7 and 10.8). All materials used in the operation are counted and checked by the two nurses and the Record Book completed and signed by the scrub nurse.

Specimens in a swab tube or test tube for bacteriological examination or in a specimen pot are sealed and labelled so that the patient's identity is unmistakable. The container is then placed in a paper bag for transport to

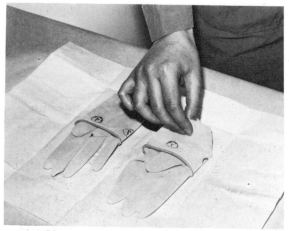

FIG 10.5A

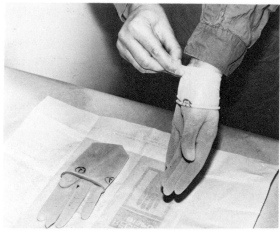

FIG. 10.5B

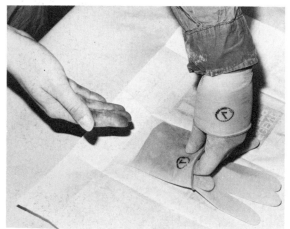

FIG. 10.5C

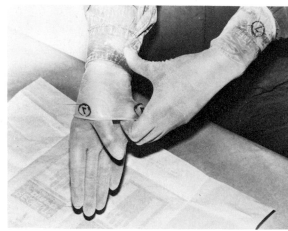

FIG. 10.5D

Fig. 10.5 Correct method of putting on gloves. A. Picking up the first glove. B. Putting on the first glove. C. Picking up the second glove. D. Both gloves drawn over the cuffs. The *outside* surface of the glove is never touched by the skin of the hand.

the laboratory after the surgeon has completed the request form indicating the examination he requires.

Other duties may include checking on pharmacy supplies and the ordering of packs and trays. Each theatre nurse must be aware of the importance of working as a team. She must always maintain a high standard, behave quietly and decorously and never discuss anything which she may see or hear during her theatre duties.

Prevention of infection

Because skin cannot be sterilised this remains one of the most important sources of infection in the theatre. The skin is isolated as soon as the wound has been made. There is considerable difference of opinion as to the best method of covering the skin adjoining the wound. The choice would seem to be:

1. Muslin towelling.
2. Semitransparent sheeting.
3. Adhesive surgical film.
4. Ventile water-repellent material.

An additional precaution is to use a separate sterile needle for every skin stitch.

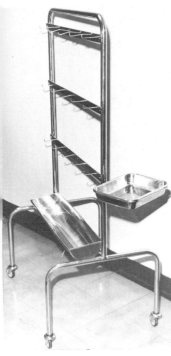

Fig. 10.6 Swab rack on which *all* swabs should be hung and counted.

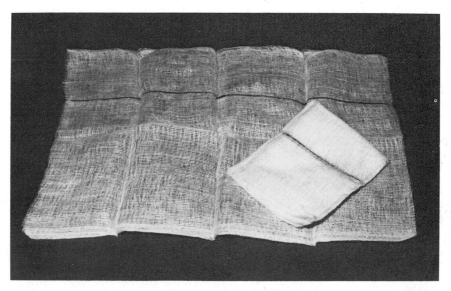

Fig. 10.7 Swabs contain a radio-opaque thread.

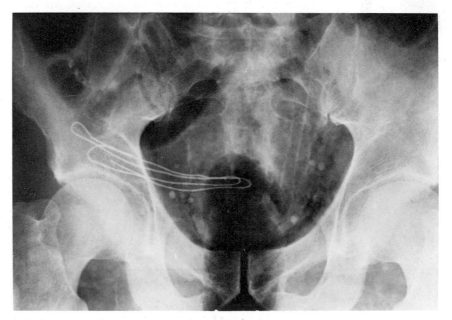

Fig. 10.8 Radiograph of a swab in the abdomen which cannot be closed until it is recovered.

Septic case — clearance of the theatre

The main aim is to confine the infected materials to the one operating room by restricting movement of contaminated staff. All equipment and materials used should be kept to the minimum. Precautions should be taken from the start of the operation contaminated with pathogenic bacteria. Any staff entering the contaminated theatre should be warned of infection, taking the necessary precautions.

1. A towel soaked in a suitable disinfectant is placed on the floor of the theatre entrance as a mat.
2. Any equipment that will not be in use during the operation is removed.
3. Swabs and towels should not be dropped on the floor but put in a plastic bag.
4. The circulating nurse should wear rubber gloves for picking up swabs.
5. At the end of the operation the linen is placed in a plastic bag and sent to the laundry immediately, the laundry having been informed that the linen is infected.
6. Instruments should be returned to the Tray Service Supply Unit immediately, the Tray Service Supply Unit having also been informed that they are infected. If there is no Tray Service Supply Unit, instruments should be left to soak in a bowl filled with strong disinfectant for at least 2 hours. Any adhesive strapping that has come in close proximity with the patient should be discarded. Swabs should be placed in a plastic bag and burnt in the incinerator immediately. Theatre staff then discard their theatre clothing and gloves, and the theatre is thoroughly cleaned with a disinfectant before further use. All staff should change into clean theatre clothing afterwards. Shoes should be disinfected for the recommended period.

Prevention of burns and explosion in the operating theatre

In the operating theatre the patient is vulnerable to burns and explosions which can be avoided by remembering the following:

Anaesthetic explosions. When inflammable agents are used for anaesthetising a patient the presence of a naked flame or sparks from faulty switches can induce violent explosions, extensive burns and death to the patient and theatre staff.

Static electricity. Theatre staff should be aware of static electricity and its dangers. Static electricity is generated when two materials are separated. It may not cause friction. The surface of one material or object becomes positively charged and the other negatively charged, and when these two are separated the static electricity disperses and may produce a spark. Wool and nylon together will build up static electricity.

The following precautions are important:

1. All metal apparatus should be fitted with antistatic rubber wheels.
2. Good earthing of all apparatus.
3. Theatre shoes should be made of a conductive rubber.

4. Theatre staff should wear cotton clothes.
5. Mattresses should be of sorbo and covered with antistatic rubber.
6. All rubber parts of the anaesthetic apparatus should be antistatic type.
7. Floors throughout the suite should have metal strips let in at regular intervals to earth any static electricity.
8. Cotton or flannel sheets should be used on the patients' trolleys.
9. The humidity of the theatre should be checked regularly. The higher the humidity in the theatre the less likely is static electricity to build up. Safe humidity should be 60 per cent.

Surgical diathermy. Surgical diathermy is a very high frequency electric current produced by a diathermy machine. The machine consists of a mains switch, foot pedal, active electrode, indifferent electrode, coagulating and cutting dials.

The active electrode is used by the surgeon, the indifferent electrode is a disposable metal plate which is fixed onto the patient's thigh and bandaged (Fig. 10.9).

The active electrode can coagulate bleeding points or cut through tissue.

To make a complete electrical circuit through the patient the surgeon uses the active electrode and the current passes to the tissues, where heat is generated and the tissues are coagulated.

If the patient is lying on the operating table touching metal, the patient will be burnt at the point of contact if he is not earthed.

Diathermy disposable plates (Fig. 10.9) should be only used once and care should be taken that the whole of the plate is touching skin.

Electrical equipment. All electrical equipment used in the operating theatre should be checked regularly for faults and repaired by a qualified engineer or electrician. Any equipment that is not in good working order should immediately be removed from the theatre and checked.

All theatre staff must make themselves conversant with an electrical failure in the theatre suite as the patient's life will be at risk.

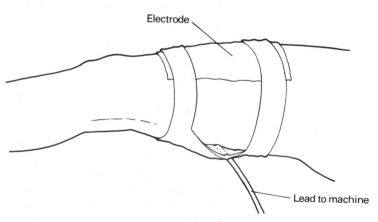

Fig. 10.9 Passive diathermy electrode on the thigh.

ELECTRICITY FAILURE IN HOSPITAL

Sudden failure of electric power becomes increasingly significant as the patient's needs become more dependent on its use. Most people think at once of the theatre lighting and the danger which may ensue for a patient undergoing an operation. In practice, this is usually very well taken care of by the theatre emergency lighting, provided from a 12-volt wet battery. The danger to the patient arises from:

1. Mechanical ventilators (artificial respirators)

This transcends in importance everything in the hospital. The patient whose life is dependent on an artificial mechanical respirator which is powered by electricity is saved by the fact that all machines can be operated manually, and the nurse needs to know how to use those in her own hospital.

2. Blood transfusion

The blood in the refrigerator will usually be safe for some hours but the advice of the blood transfusion officer must be sought. The nurse should consult the medical officer about securing further blood for patients undergoing transfusion or already suffering from haemorrhage.

3. Suction apparatus

For operations such as tonsillectomy, alternative suction should be available in every theatre. This can be provided very simply by syphonage from a water tap or by a foot pump.

Other effects on the hospital are:
- (a) Theatre—sterilisation, diathermy cautery, endoscopic lights, pump for open heart surgery, heating, and even the water supply may be threatened.
- (b) In the laboratory there are no lights, the incubator may be out of action, and microscope lights may be ineffective.
- (c) In the maternity department incubators for premature babies are affected.
- (d) General—X-ray department, kitchen, dispensary, general heating, lighting, laundry, and physiotherapy departments are all affected.

Modern units tend to have a self-starting Diesel alternator as an alternative in case of power failure.

BIBLIOGRAPHY

Brigden R J 1974 Operating theatre technique, 3rd edn. Churchill Livingston, Edinburgh
Cranfield A B 1972 Theatre nurses handbook. Butterworth, London
Dixon E P 1976 An Introduction to the operating theatre. Churchill Livingston, Edinburgh
Mitchell N J, Evans D S, Kerr A 1978 British Medical Journal 1: 696

11

Surgical ward dressings

The provision of a bacteriologically clean atmosphere is one of the greatest of surgical problems. In operating theatres this is attempted at great expense. In the hospital of the future a similar but smaller scale provision will be built on every ward. This would consist of a dressing room which is air conditioned and a 'clean' and 'dirty' room on either side of it. All dressings would be performed in the dressing room, the only exception being infected cases which would be nursed and dressed in their own isolation ward. In the meantime, however, the vast majority of patients will be nursed in large wards and the problems which arise will have to be dealt with as they occur.

It is inevitable that the more patients there are in a ward the greater is the risk of infection, whilst an ideal number of patients from this point of view is one that is economically impossible. However, the situation can be controlled by the separation of clean from infected cases in the ward. A small isolation ward attached to the main ward is a great advantage and glass partitions in the ward diminish cross-infection.

Patients particularly liable to infection are diabetics, amputees and patients on steroid or immunosuppressive drugs.

Where wounds become infected this is most likely to have occurred in the theatre. Other sources of wound infection are:

Dust in the air of the ward

Poor hygiene in nurses or patient

Lack of cleanliness of the ward environment

Infected droplets from mouths and noses

The hands of the dresser or contamination of instruments during procedure

Cross-infection from other infected wounds.

Dressings should ideally be carried out in a room or cubicle specially designed for the purpose. Where this is not practicable the following points should be observed.

1. The air in the ward. The bacterial content of the air in the ward rises to a maximum in the early morning owing, among other factors, to the domestic activities in the ward, including the cleaning of floors, dusting, bed-making, etc. Bacteria are less likely to be scattered if the precautions mentioned on page 56 are observed with the following additional measures:

(a) When making beds the clothes are handled slowly and gently.
(b) Bed-making, floor-cleaning and dusting cease at least 1 hour before the first dressing is uncovered.

When dressings begin the ward is closed to all visitors and all unnecessary personnel. Windows and doors are shut.

2. Droplet infection. To prevent the spread of infection, surgeons, nurses, students, orderlies and domestic workers with respiratory infections or septic lesions should not be on duty in a surgical ward.

3. Hands. Hands cannot be properly sterilised, though thorough washing can remove recent contamination. It is essential, therefore, that during a dressing the hands should not come in contact either with the wound itself or with any material in the vicinity of the wound. The hands should be thoroughly washed, using plenty of soap and water, paying particular attention to the nails, which should be cut short and free of varnish. A Towelmaster or disposable paper towels are used to dry them and the dressing is performed, using sterile forceps.

4. Masks should always be worn during dressings, and efficient masks made of paper are now in use. They should be changed hourly, since after that period they only present a further source of infection, and should not be touched with the fingers during use. As soon as the need has passed, the mask should be removed. To go around all day with a mask covering the nose is to increase the chance of infection because of lack of proper ventilation to the nose.

Nonetheless there are some who advise that masks are unnecessary.

Changing a simple dressing — one nurse

A basic trolley is prepared. The nurse washes and dries her hands, and puts on a mask.

Using Jontex cloth the whole trolley is washed with soap and water and dried. It is then swabbed with a disposable swab soaked in 70 per cent spirit — in some hospitals a similar antiseptic is sprayed over the trolley and allowed to dry.

A basic dressing pack (containing woollen balls, gauze swabs), adhesive tape, recommended antiseptic and any other necessary eqiupment are placed on the bottom shelf. A 'used instrument bag' is attached to one end of the trolley with a strip of Sellotape. Two strips of Sellotape are attached to the rail at the other end for the soiled dressing bag.

The procedure is explained to the patient. Privacy is ensured and nearby windows are closed as necessary. The trolley is then taken to the bedside.

Using her scissors the nurse cuts the sealed end of the pack and tips the inner pack on to the top of the trolley. She attaches the outer pack to the other end of the trolley, for receiving soiled dressings. The patient is placed into an appropriate position and made comfortable. The bedclothes and personal clothing are adjusted as necessary. The nurse loosens the bandage or adhesive holding the dressing. She then thoroughly washes and dries her hands. The inner wrapping is then opened and partially spread by pulling on the first three corners. The fourth corner is lifted carefully with one hand and the nurse picks up the first pair of forceps with the other and continues to spread the final corner. Using the pair of forceps she arranges the sterile field and tray, placing the instruments on the side of the tray. The forceps are then placed at the side of the trolley with the points only on the sterile field. She opens any supplementary packs. She pours out the antiseptic. Using the first pair of forceps she removes the soiled dressing, discarding it into the appropriate bag. The soiled forceps are placed into the used instrument bag. She picks up two pairs of forceps. If towels are necessary, they are arranged around the wound.

With the forceps in her left hand she picks up a swab, dips it into the antiseptic and transfers it to the forceps in her right hand. The wound is cleaned and the swab discarded. As many swabs as necessary are used, each swab being used once only. She discards the forceps in her right hand, and transfers those in her left hand to the right hand. In her left hand she picks up the remaining forceps. Using the two forceps the dressing is applied. Both forceps are discarded. The dressing is secured, using adhesive or bandage as indicated. The patient is made comfortable.

Any unused wool or gauze is saved for suitable unsterile procedures. The tray is then placed into the used instrument bag which is disconnected from the side of the trolley. The sterile field, used towels, and the nurse's mask are placed in the soiled bag, which is also disconnected from the side of the trolley and closed tightly by squeezing the top. The bag containing used instruments is taken to the sluice (or dirty room) and thence to the CSSD. The soiled dressings are also taken in the sealed bag to the sluice and sent for incineration. The trolley is removed and cleaned. The nurse washes and dries her hands. She reports to Sister or Charge Nurse as necessary.

Protective dressings of the wound

Dressings consist of gauze, lint, cotton-wool, and bandage, Airstrip or Dermicel adhesive dressings, Elastoplast, Tubegauz or Netelast, Sellotape and microporous tape.

The advantages of protective dressings for wounds are many, but one disadvantage is that evaporation from the skin surface is hindered. This may be overcome by:

1. No dressings: A little gauze is strapped on the wound for 6 hours until the edges have become sealed off with exudate. After this all dressings are abandoned.

2. A plastic skin dressing. Nobecutane is an acrylic resin dissolved in a mixture of acetic esters. When applied to the skin the solvent evaporates, leaving a transparent, adherent, and elastic film. This film is impervious to bacteria but pervious to evaporation from the skin surface. It must not be used unless haemostasis is perfect. It may be sprayed or spread with a glass rod. A thick layer may be peeled off; a thin layer may be dissolved with ether or acetone.

The advantages are:

(a) The wound is sealed and cannot be infected; this is particularly important if a colostomy or ileostomy is functioning near a fresh wound.

(b) The progress of the wound can be seen without disturbing the dressing.

(c) The patient can take a bath as the dressing is impervious to water.

Clean wounds which have been closed without drainage need not be uncovered until it is time to remove the stitches. Pain in the wound or a rise of temperature may necessitate inspection to see if the wound has become infected. Septic wounds require careful dressing.

Infected discharging wounds require regular dressing, often several times daily. Wound swabs are taken to isolate the causative organism and to enable antibiotic treatment to be instituted.

The stitches

The skin stitches, mersilene, or nylon, are removed when the wound has healed, usually on the 8th to 10th day. It is advisable to remove alternate stitches on one day and the remainder next day, if the wound is sound. In the neck, to avoid stitch marks, they are removed on the fourth or fifth day. Deep sutures (if inserted) which take up the tension of coughing in the case of an abdominal wound are removed on the 12th to 14th day. When removing skin stitches the cut stitch must be extracted from the skin towards the wound — pulling it away from the wound disrupts its edges. Some types of skin sutures are illustrated in Figure 11.1.

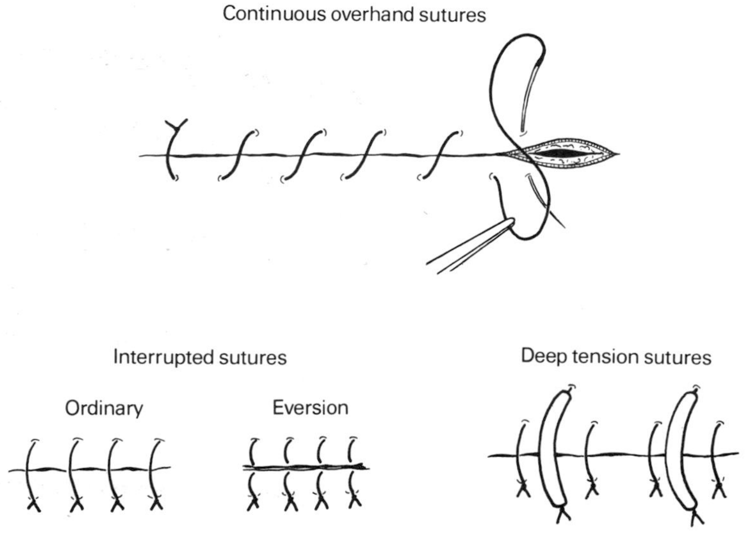

Fig. 11.1 Types of skin sutures.

Michel's clips, Kefa clips or butterfly plasters to hold the skin edges together or Steristrip tape may be used instead of stitches.

A stitch which is cutting through the skin may give rise to considerable pain, and the surgeon's attention should be drawn to this to see if it can be removed earlier than usual.

A stitch abscess is liable to develop if there is slight infection, and to diminish the risk most surgeons paint the skin with antispetic lotion as they are closing the wound before inserting the stitches. If the patient is running a temperature the wound should be examined for a stitch abscess and the stitch removed to provide drainage.

Drains

Drains are used
1. to drain fluid which has collected or is expected to collect, e.g. blood, serum, pus and bile;
2. as a safety valve to an anastomosis or suture line, e.g. the duodenal stump after gastrectomy or the ureter after removal of a stone.

Wherever a drain is inserted it should be covered with an antiseptic dressing. Shortening and rotation of the open tube type of drain are undertaken — shortening so that the cavity can heal from the bottom, and rotation so that the tube does not become adherent to the tissues. A tube should never be removed until clear written instructions have been obtained from the surgeon.

When the original stitch securing the tube has been severed the tube should be fixed with a large safety-pin to a piece of Gamgee so that the tube is not lost in the wound.

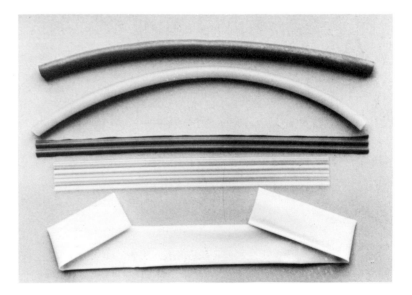

Fig. 11.2 Some types of drains — rubber and plastic tubes and corrugated form — Penrose drain.

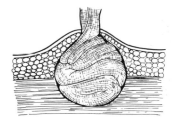

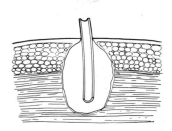

Fig. 11.3 *Above*: Wrong. Gauze plugs the wound, obstructs drainage and is painful.
            Below: Correct. Tube allows free drainage.

The following complications may arise if a tube is left in situ for too long a period:

Infection
Intestinal obstruction
Erosion of a blood vessel causing a secondary haemorrhage
Perforation of an organ causing a fistula
Adhesions
Incisional hernia.

Types of drains

1. Rubber tubing split or fenestrated.
2. Corrugated rubber sheeting.
3. Firm rubber sheeting.
4. Penrose tubing
5. Shaped drains such as catheters or T-tubes for the common bile duct.

Some varieties of drains are illustrated in Figure 11.2.
Gauze is not a drain and, as Figure 11.3 shows, its misuse prevents drainage.

Drainage

Drainage may be:

1. *Open*:
   (a) On to dressings.
   (b) Suction.
2. *Closed*:
   (a) Catheter into a sealed sterile disposable bag.
   (b) Chest under fluid seal (p. 284).
   (c) Vacuum — such as Redivac.

A Redivac drain (Fig. 11.4) is a small bottle in which a vacuum has been created by a high capacity pump attached to the manometric stopper tube. The antennae on the stopper are 100° apart when the vacuum reaches 600 mmHg. When the antennae are in the vertical position the vacuum is only 40–50 mmHg. At this point another prepared bottle has to be used. The catheter is clamped off at the rubber coupling, the exhausted vacuum bottle is removed, and the clamp is released only when a new bottle has been recoupled.

In closed drainage organisms from the air are excluded, the discharge can be measured and it has the further advantage that the main wound can be kept dry.

Open wounds

Sometimes a wound is left open, dressed with petroleum jelly gauze, or insufflated with an antibiotic powder such as Polybactrin.

The edges of a wound must not be allowed to overlap. Unless raw edge is approximated to raw edge, healing is impossible. Similarly, if the edges

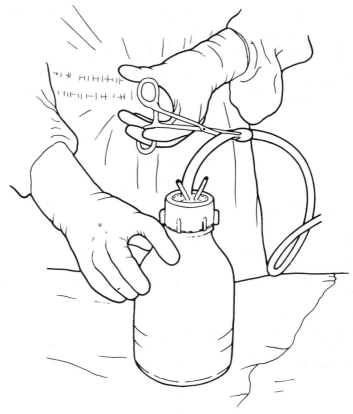

Fig. 11.4   Redivac drain.

of a wound are indrawn or sucked under due to loss of the tissue beneath, delay in healing will result.

   Complications which can occur in a wound are:
Infection
Sloughing
Secondary haemorrhage (p. 100)
Severe pain, which is usually due to infection
A sinus or a fistula
The wound may gape, e.g. 'burst abdomen'
Haematoma (p. 114)
Sinking in of the edges.

Immobilisation of wounds

All wounds heal best when they are immobilised and covered. Daily dressings are not performed. However, the nurse must know when to suspect complications which necessitate inspection of the wound. The following are a guide that all may not be well:

   1. The continued presence of pain.
   2. Persistent rise of temperature and/or an increasing pulse rate.

3. Presence of toxaemia, indicated by the onset of vomiting, diarrhoea, loss of appetite and increasing pallor.
4. Discharge from the wound.
5. Any symptom suggestive of tetanus.
6. Any symptom suggestive of too tight a plaster or dressing, e.g. pain, tingling, or cyanosis of the tips of the fingers or toes.

The healing of wounds

Healing by first intention is the aim in all wounds. The sutures are removed when the wound has healed, usually 8 to 10 days later. When the sutures are about to be removed it may be noticed that there is some tension or swelling of the wound, due to a haematoma. If this is the case, the edges should be separated gently with sinus forceps and a small strip of rubber or plastic drain inserted for 48 hours.

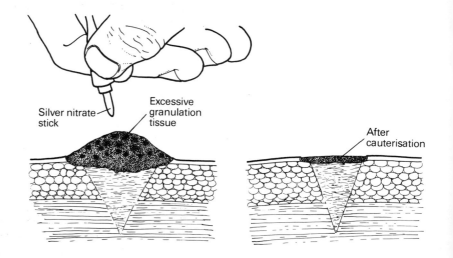

Silver nitrate stick
Excessive granulation tissue
After cauterisation

Fig. 11.5 Cauterisation of excessive granulation tissue.

Gauze packing of the wound for haematoma or a subcutaneous collection of pus delays healing and blocks drainage. It should never be used. If the granulation tissue is excessive (proud flesh) and grows above the level of the skin, the exuberant patches should be burnt down by the careful application of a silver nitrate stick (Fig. 11.5). The nurse must take care not to damage any portion of the patient's skin or her own hands. A wound which is large and septic may require irrigation with antiseptic lotions, such as eusol, Savlon (0·5 per cent) or hydrogen peroxide. The Entonox gas and oxygen machine may be used for producing analgesia when dressing a large infected wound. More usually omnopon 10 mg or pethidine 50 mg is given intramuscularly half an hour previously. When an infected wound has become clean secondary suture of the skin may be performed or a skin graft may be possible.

Chemotherapy

Antibacterial drugs have revolutionised the healing of wounds and are used in almost all traumatic wounds. They may be prescribed locally or systemically.

Prolonged discharge from wounds and consequent loss of protein is liable to give rise to hypoproteinaemia and patients with wounds should have a diet rich in protein and vitamin C, which is an important constituent of the diet in effecting healing.

Complications of wounds. *Prevention of contracture* following a wound is a matter which requires constant attention. It is aided by proper splinting in the early stages and later by active movement. The prevention of oedema and swelling is also aided by movement once sepsis has been controlled. The rehabilitation of a patient who has been wounded is of considerable importance in helping him to overcome any disability, and often dispels any doubts he may have about his capacity to work. The nurse must supervise the movements. They are particularly important following wounds in the hands.

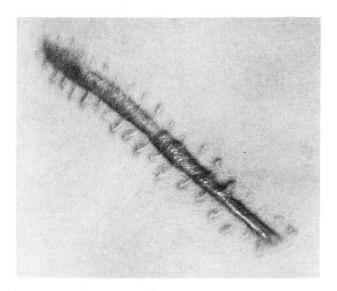

Fig. 11.6 Keloid in abdominal scar.

Keloids. A keloid (Fig. 11.6) is a condition of excessive thickening of a scar. It is particularly liable to develop after operations on tuberculous foci and following wounds in members of the coloured races.

Treatment. Excision is of no value. The use of 'Covermark', a tinted, opaque, non-irritant cream which is water and shower proof, may be advised. Cryotherapy or the local application of steroids may also be used to reduce these blemishes.

12
Haemorrhage

Haemorrhage is the loss of blood from a blood vessel. The blood lost is described as extravasated (outside the vessels) and may lie on the surface of the body, on the patient's clothing or on the floor. Blood which is extravasated into the tissues, a body cavity or the lumen of a hollow organ may in itself be very significant quite apart from any effect which may ensue from loss to the circulation, and the problem is considered at the end of this chapter.

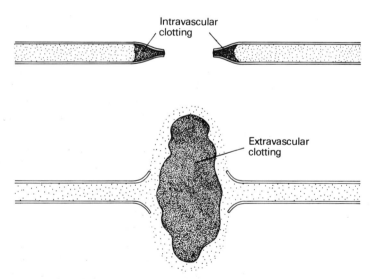

Fig. 12.1 Haemorrhage is arrested by clotting *inside* the vessel but aggravated by clots outside which prevent the severed ends from retracting.

Clotting is the circulatory system's defence mechanism to leakage. Clot formation may be deficient from disease, the absence of essential clotting factors or the use of anticoagulant drugs. To be effective in sealing the leakage the clot has to be inside the lumen of the vessel (intravascular) — clot formation inside a viscus but outside the blood vessels increases the bleeding for reasons given in Figure 12.1. When bleeding occurs and blood is spilt into a receiver or shed on to the floor it is always worth noting whether clots are forming since in conditions of defective clotting or active fibrinolysis the patient bleeds but clots either do not form or are quickly lysed. Replacement of the missing clotting factors, e.g. by fresh frozen plasma, is necessary when there is defective clotting. In conditions of fibrinolysis it may be necessary to give an antifibrinolytic agent such as tranexamic acid, with or without replacement of any clotting factors which may have been depleted by the lysis.

Blood may be lost from all three types of vessel, the arteries, the veins, or the capillaries, and the type of haemorrhage is named accordingly. Bleeding which occurs as soon as the vessel is divided is known as primary haemorrhage. If the patient is collapsed the vessel may not bleed immediately, but as recovery takes place the blood pressure rises and bleeding occurs — this is known as reactionary haemorrhage. If infection is present, the walls of the blood vessels may be eroded and may burst, causing what is known as secondary haemorrhage.

Types:

1. Arterial.
2. Capillary.
3. Venous.

Time:

1. Primary
2. Reactionary or intermediate.
3. Secondary.

Arterial haemorrhage. The blood is bright red and spurts with the heart beat. The escape is from both ends of the vessel and not only from that nearer to the heart. Blood loss is more rapid than from a vein of corresponding size.

Capillary haemorrhage. The blood oozes over the surface and is darkish red in colour. Oozing over several hours can result in considerable blood loss.

Venous haemorrhage. The blood is dark in colour, there is no pulsation, and the rate of loss is much less severe than arterial haemorrhage. Since the large veins are big cave-like structures, injury to them is a serious matter. A further danger is that air may be sucked into the veins, giving rise to fatal air embolism in which the blood and air may form 'foam'.

Increased intravenous pressure with even greater blood loss occurs in rupture of a varicose vein, in portal hypertension and in asphyxia. Blood loss from the pulmonary artery is dark unoxygenated blood while that from the pulmonary vein is fully saturated with oxygen and is, therefore, bright red.

Primary haemorrhage is immediate — a cut finger or an operative incision.

Reactionary haemorrhage occurs in the first 24 hours after operation. The more severe the operation the more likely it is to occur, especially after the patient has recovered from circulatory collapse. Operations on the kidney, the thyroid and the breast as well as total hysterectomy are particularly liable to be followed by reactionary haemorrhage.

Coughing and vomiting by increasing the pressure in the veins are a contributing factor.

Secondary haemorrhage is due to sloughing of the wall of a blood vessel. The commonest cause is bacterial infection, but in the absence of infection it may be caused by the action of an enzyme, for example acid pepsin on a peptic ulcer. The pressure of a drainage tube, a bone fragment and the presence of carcinoma may also be factors. The vessels are eroded. The thinnest walled vessels, the capillaries, burst first and a few specks of blood are found on the dressing, and should be immediately reported. It is a warning that the larger vessels are also being eroded, and in another few days, commonly the 10th after operation, a main artery may burst, giving rise to a torrential, fatal haemorrhage.

Most symptoms of blood loss complained of by patients at diagnostic clinics are in fact small secondary haemorrhages.

The severity of haemorrhage in the body of a healthy individual

There are approximately 5·8 l of blood with a haemoglobin concentration of 14·6 g per dl. If 1·8 l of blood are lost very rapidly — for example in half an hour — death usually results. However should loss occur at the rate of 1 litre over the whole day for several days there would still be very little less than 5·8 l of fluid in the circulation: the haemoglobin concentration, however might be only 2·9 g per dl. The fluid lost from the circulation is replaced by fluid from the tissues, so that the volume of blood is restored, but since vast numbers of red blood cells have been shed, the oxygen carrying power is depleted.

It is always a matter of great surprise to junior nurses to learn that the blood volume of a new born baby is about 350 ml i.e. less than one pint, and consequently a loss of 100 ml is a very serious haemorrhage.

An estimation of the extent of the blood loss is made by clinical observation of the patient (p. 104), records of the pulse, temperature and blood pressure (Figs. 12.2 & 12.3) and the central venous pressure. Blood haemoglobin and packed cell volume (PCV) estimations are essential. In the theatre the weighing of swabs is undertaken and the volume of blood in any suction apparatus is measured. In the ward the quantity of blood vomited or aspirated from the stomach or lost in a bed pan is also measured.

The natural arrest of haemorrhage (Fig. 12.4)

Adequate amounts of calcium and all the clotting factors are essential. The blood in circulation is kept fluid by a fine balance between clotting and fibrinolysis. As a result of a complex series of reactions starting when tissue is damaged, prothrombin is converted to its active form thrombin in the presence of calcium. Fibrinogen is then transformed by thrombin to fibrin, which forms a mesh in which platelets and other blood cells become entangled to form a clot. Alterations of these factors by drugs form the basis of anticoagulant and fibrinolytic therapy.

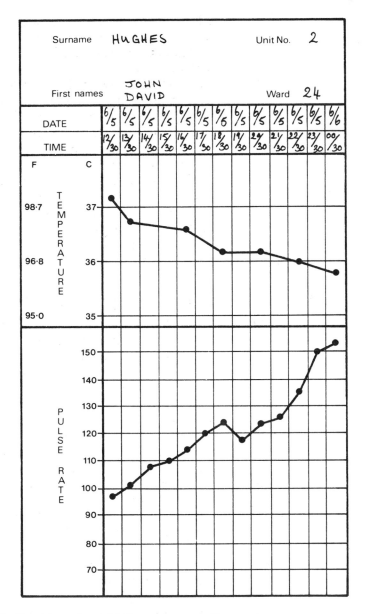

Fig. 12.2 The rising pulse and falling temperature of haemorrhage.

1. Calcium may be displaced from blood by:
(a) A 3·8 per cent solution of sodium citrate.
(b) Acid citrate dextrose solution.
(c) Citrate phosphate dextrose solution.
(d) Oxalate.
(e) Sequestrene (ethylenediamine tetra-acetic acid, or EDTA).

Clinically sodium citrate prevents the formation of clots in the bladder; acid citrate dextrose and acid citrate phosphate solutions are solutions used to prevent clotting in stored blood. Because stored blood has had its

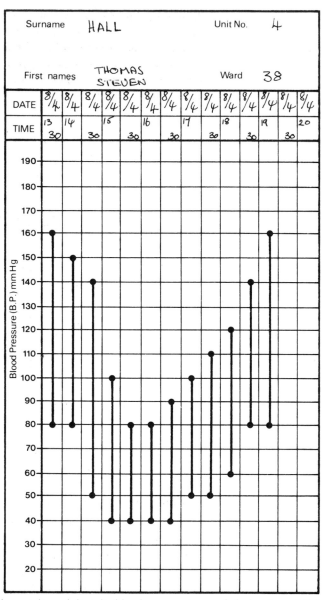

Fig. 12.3 The systolic and diastolic blood pressure is recorded, showing a fall due to haemorrhage.

calcium displaced, a patient receiving blood requires 10 ml of a 10 per cent solution of calcium chloride with every fourth unit of blood.

Oxalate or sequestrene is used in pathological specimen tubes when it is desired to prevent the clotting of blood.

2. Prothrombin is formed from vitamin K, a fat-soluble vitamin absorbed from the small intestine. A patient suffering from obstructive jaundice will not absorb vitamin K and therefore is liable to bleed if operated upon. For this reason vitamin K is given by injection until the prothrombin level of the blood has been restored. Oral anticoagulants like warfarin act by preventing the liver utilising vitamin K and so reducing the formation of prothrombin. The dosage is controlled by the prothrombin time. If it is necessary to reverse the process, vitamin K is given, but it may be too slow to act and a tranfusion of fresh blood may be necessary.

A more immediately acting anticoagulant is heparin given intravenously four- to six-hourly, and its action can be rapidly reversed with protamine sulphate.

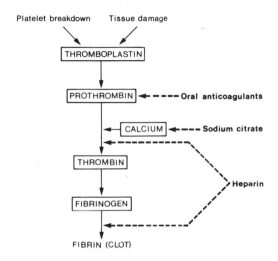

Fig. 12.4 Mechanism of clot formation and the site of action of anticoagulants.

3. Fibrinogen is the precursor of fibrin. In the absence of fibrinogen severe bleeding may occur. Fibrinolysins are substances which dissolve fibrin and the phenomenon is known as fibrinolysis. The fibrinolytic activity of the blood may be increased:

(a) In complicated obstetric cases associated with haemorrhage.
(b) After severe exercise.
(c) In the presence of some malignant new growths.
(d) Occasionally after operations such as prostatectomy, the fibrinolysin being known as urokinase.
(e) In certain streptococcal infections—streptokinase releases an endogenous activator.

Patients suffering from fibrinolysis will show no evidence of clotting and are treated by neutralisation of the fibrinolysins by the administration of tranexamic acid or the administration of fibrinogen. Fibrinolysins such as streptokinase are used in the dissolution of thrombi in cases of deep venous thrombosis and pulmonary embolism.

Fibrinogen is also consumed in the condition known as disseminated intravascular coagulation (D.I.C.). In this condition very small clots are formed inside the blood vessels leading to the development of a haemostatic defect caused by utilization of clotting factors and platelets in the clotting process. There may be secondary activation of the fibrinolytic system in an attempt to keep the vessels patent. Disseminated intravascular coagulation is more common than primary fibrinolysis and may complicate the following conditions:

(a) Obstetric accidents
(b) Surgery, especially that involving the heart and lung.
(c) Gram negative and meningococcal septicaemia.
(d) Haemolytic transfusion reactions.
(e) Widespread carcinoma.
(f) Acute leukaemia.

Patients with D.I.C. must never be given tranexamic acid or the protective fibrinolysis may be inhibited, giving rise to widespread and possibly fatal thrombosis.

The signs and symptoms of haemorrhage

Clinically, haemorrhage may be of two types:
  1. Revealed or external, i.e. the bleeding can be seen.
  2. Concealed or internal. The bleeding occurs in one of the body cavities, such as the abdomen. Since it is less obvious it must be diagnosed on the presence of signs and symptoms alone and these do not develop until a moderate sized bleed has occurred.
  The signs and symptoms are those of a progressive anaemia as well as water and salt depletion when the loss is slow or of acute circulatory collapse when rapid haemorrhage occurs.

Early signs and symptoms

  1. *Restlessness and anxiety*. The patient is conscious that all is not well and feels faint.
  2. *Coldness*. The temperature is slightly subnormal, 36·9°C (98°F).
  3. The *pulse rate* is slightly increased.
  4. The *blood pressure* is lowered.
  5. *Pallor* increases.
  6. The patient is *thirsty*.

Signs and symptoms after severe haemorrhage

  1. *Extreme pallor*. The face may be ashen white, and clammy with cold sweat. The colour as well as the temperature (as palpated with the hand) of the nose and digits are very significant.
  2. *Coldness* is profound and the temperature is of the order of 36°C (97°F) or lower (Fig. 12.2).
  3. *Air hunger*. The patient literally gasps for breath. The respirations are rapid and sighing.
  4. *The pulse* is very rapid in rate, thready in volume and frequently is irregular in rhythm.
  5. *The blood pressure* is extremely low (Fig. 12.3).
  6. *Thirst* is extreme.

7. Blindness, tinnitus (buzzing in the ears) and coma occur in this order prior to death.

8. The volume of urine secreted is diminished — acute renal failure may occur.

9. The central venous pressure is low and often negative (Fig. 14.2).

Diminution of the volume of blood in the circulation with depletion of the supply of oxygen to the tissues is the first and most important result of haemorrhage.

The treatment of haemorrhage

The problems arising from blood loss may be summarised as those of:
1. Its control.
2. Restoration of the blood volume.
3. The fate of the extravasated blood.

THE ARREST OF THE HAEMORRHAGE

EXTERNAL HAEMORRHAGE

Pressure will control all forms of external haemorrhage. According to its severity there is a choice of methods.

1. Pad and bandage. This simple method is applicable to the vast majority of cases. It is effective and causes no damage.

2. Digital Pressure, applied over the pressure point of the artery, will control haemorrhage temporarily. It is particularly valuable in the neck, where other methods are inapplicable.

3. Elevation of the limb will control venous haemorrhage. This is the classical method of dealing with a sudden haemorrhage from a ruptured varicose vein of the leg.

4. Application of a tourniquet. This is rarely required except for the control of a torrential haemorrhage from a limb. *It is not without danger*. A temporary tourniquet may have to be devised in a sudden emergency. A pad, e.g. a handkerchief, is placed over the line of the vessel and a tourniquet — which may be a scarf, a tie, or whatever is available — is bound around the limb and tightened if necessary with a small piece of wood. More usually in hospital three types of tourniquet are used:

The Samway anchor tourniquet

Esmarch's elastic bandage

Inflatable cuff tourniquet.

The great danger of a tourniquet, if left on for more than 30 minutes, is that gangrene of the limb may occur. Damage to the nerves is not infrequent, especially if the skin has not been protected before its application. It is essential, therefore, to slacken the tourniquet and tighten it again if bleeding persists.

The time of application and removal of a tourniquet should be recorded on the theatre blackboard. Some theatres have a stop clock with an alarm which can be set. The limb on which a tourniquet has been used should be kept elevated afterwards to control oedema which may result from venous congestion.

5. Surgical ligation is necessary if the bleeding is persistent.

6. Coagulation of the bleeding point with electrocautery or diathermy may be required.

7. Therapeutic embolisation means the deliberate occulsion of blood vessels by means of emboli introduced through an angiographic catheter in a clinical situation where it is necessary to obliterate local blood flow. The material used ranges from Sterispon (Gelfoam) to lyophilised human dura mater (Lyodura). Haemorrhage from oesophageal varices and gastric ulcers has been controlled by this method (Allison, 1978).

8. A pack will temporarily control very severe haemorrhage. This method is used in the theatre to control temporarily a sudden haemorrhage, and the theatre nurse should always have a pack readily available for this emergency.

9. Styptics, such as snake venom or adrenaline (1 : 1000), may be used locally in certain cases. Thrombin and Gelfoam have their uses in appropriate cases such as low pressure bleeding from venules and capillaries.

INTERNAL OR CONCEALED HAEMORRHAGE

Pressure cannot be employed internally except by surgical ligature or packing. Many internal haemorrhages are secondary in nature, and will cease if the infection can be controlled and the vessels encouraged to contract. The following methods are involved in its control:

1. The organ is emptied of blood clot if possible. In a case of severe bleeding from the bladder a catheter is passed and the bladder emptied. The blood vessels in a dilated paralysed organ are unable to contract.

2. The vessels are encouraged to contract. A lotion of saline or sodium bicarbonate, to which a few drops of adrenaline solution (1 : 1000) have been added, is of great value in washing out the organ. This can be repeated every two hours. The use of ergometrine after the birth of the placenta is an example of stimulating the vessels to contract.

Pitressin intravenously may be effective in the control of bleeding from oesophageal varices (p. 376).

3. The coagulability of the blood is increased. This is not very valuable unless the mechanism of clotting is deficient, due to the absence of an essential constituent of the blood. The parenteral administration of vitamin K is important to a jaundiced patient who is bleeding, because its absorption from the intestine is deficient. In haemophilia, the administration of factor VIII or fresh frozen plasma is indicated and increases coagulability.

4. Packing with gauze soaked in adrenaline is effective at certain sites, and Oxycel, which is absorbable gauze impregnated with fibrin, is used extensively.

5. Surgical ligature e.g. in the case of a ruptured spleen.

6. Antibiotics. A secondary haemorrhage, whether internal or external because it is infective in origin, requires the systemic administration of antibiotics in addition to measures to control the bleeding and restore the blood volume.

7. Internal pressure. May be applied by the balloon of a triluminal tube in bleeding oesophageal varices or by the balloon of a Foley catheter in a prostatectomy cavity.

8. Antifibrinolytic therapy such as tranexamic acid (p. 120).

BLOOD TRANSFUSION

Indications

1. Blood transfusion is undertaken to counteract the effects of severe haemorrhage and replace the blood loss.

2. To prevent shock in operations where blood loss is considerable, such as rectal resection, hysterectomy and arterial surgery.

3. In severe burns to make up for blood lost by burning but only after plasma and electrolytes have been replaced.

4. For severe anaemia from cancer, marrow aplasia and similar conditions.

5. To provide clotting factors normally present in blood which may be absent as a result of disease.

The blood volume can be fairly accurately estimated by a machine using a radio-iodine technique to determine plasma volume and microhaematocrit to estimate red cell volume.

TECHNIQUE OF BLOOD TRANSFUSION

Blood is collected from healthy donors, 420 ml being collected on each occasion. Blood which is administered in the same form as it is collected, apart from the addition of an anticoagulant, is described as whole blood. In some cases 'packed red cells' are given. This consists of the cellular elements left after siphoning off the supernatant plasma. It is used in cases of chronic anaemia where the volume of blood is not substantially diminished and a large volume may induce cardiac failure.

Selection of donors

They should be in good general health. The blood tests for syphilis must be negative, and they must not have had infective hepatitis or malaria.

Blood grouping

All human beings fall into one of four main groups—A, B, AB or O—according to the nature of the blood group antigen which is carried on the red cells. Thus group A persons have A antigen on their red cells, group B, B antigens, group AB both A and B antigens and group O neither A nor B.

A and B antigens have natural antibodies carried in the plasma known as anti-A and anti-B. Anti-A antibody will clump A red cells (and AB) causing a transfusion reaction. Similarly anti-B will clump B cells (and AB). Thus the main groups are made up as follows:

Group	Red cells (antigen)	Plasma (antibodies)
A	A	Anti-B
B	B	Anti-A
AB	A + B	Anti-A and anti-B
O	O	O (none)

In an emergency, where there is doubt as to a patient's blood group, it is safer to cross match a bottle of group O Rh-negative blood than to use another group.

The Rh system

There are six antigens involved in the rhesus blood group. The antigen most frequently involved in incompatibility and haemolysis is D, which is present in 85 per cent of the population. These people are known as rhesus-positive. The 15 per cent of people whose blood does not contain D antigen are known as rhesus-negative. The main problem is the Rh-negative person who if given Rh-positive blood will come to no harm on the first occasion but will produce antibodies against antigen D, and further transfusion with Rh-positive blood will cause haemolysis.

Clarke and others have shown that the production of Rh antibodies in Rh-negative mothers by Rh-positive babies may be prevented by the injection, after the baby is born of 5 ml of gammaglobulin containing high titres of antibodies active against the Rh-positive antigen of the foetus.

In addition to the main groups there are many rare sub-groups which because of their rarity may present great difficulties when blood has to be obtained.

The percentage of the population in the various blood groups is:

| Group AB | 3·0 per cent | Group A | 42·0 per cent |
| Group B | 8·5 per cent | Group O | 46·5 per cent |

Cross matching

The serum of the recipient is matched in tubes against the red cells of the donor and the presence or absence of agglutination is noted to determine compatability. To achieve the high degree of safety necessary in cross matching blood this test is checked under the microscope after 2 hours incubation in tubes.

Collection of blood

Blood is collected into a plastic bag containing either 75 ml acid citrate dextrose (A.C.D.) solution or 63 ml citrate phosphate dextrose (C.P.D.) solution. A needle is inserted into a vein at the elbow after the application of a sphygmomanometer cuff to the arm and 420 ml blood are withdrawn to make a total unit of 495 ml or 483 ml if C.P.D. solution has been used. If the blood is not required for immediate use it is stored in a refrigerator at a temperature from 4° to 6°C.

On the bag containing the blood is marked the group and the latest date for use. It is important that the blood should not be 'outdated' or haemolysed when given. Another important point is that the blood should not be taken out of the refrigerator more than half an hour before use and not over-heated.

Large transfusions of blood may cause citrate intoxication and after every 4 units (2 l) 10 ml 10% calcium chloride should be injected intravenously. The excess of K^+ in banked blood may raise the serum K^+ to dangerous levels, especially with old blood and, to overcome this, an infusion of dextrose and insulin is given as soon as possible.

Transfusion into the patient

Closed infusion

Closed infusion is the usual method of transfusion (Figs. 12.5 and 12.6). The blood is given into the vein of the arm or, very rarely, into a vein of the leg. The arm is the more usual site because in most cases a cannula can be inserted.

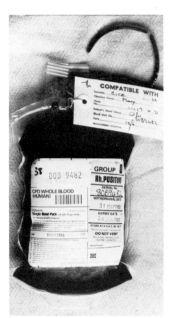

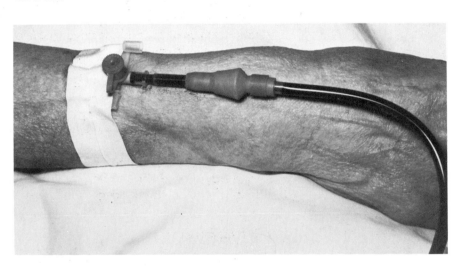

Fig. 12.5 Blood transfusion using the standard gravity drip-giving set.

Fig. 12.6 Teflon cannula in the vein.

Scalp vein drips in infants. An area of the scalp selected by the medical officer is shaved and a special fine scalp vein needle with attached polythene tube is held in position with plaster of Paris.

In young children and babies a special drip set with a graduated burette is used to facilitate the accurate administration of small volumes of blood or other fluids.

The most important precautions to take in preparation for blood transfusion is to check that each bag of blood to be given to the patient is: (a) of the correct group for that patient; (b) that the cross-matching label on each bag bears the full name, date of birth and ward of the patient to whom it is to be given as well as his unit number; (c) that the expiry date on the bag has not been reached; (d) and that the cross-matching label attached to the bag matches the label on the bag. These checks should be done by two persons, one being a qualified nurse or a doctor.

Blood, like plasma, is not normally heated before use but when rapid transfusions are undertaken it is necessary to take measures to warm the blood. This is done by using some form of heating coil which is connected somewhere between the drip set and the patient. Suitable drip heaters set at body temperature are available for this purpose.

The rate of blood flow is carefully regulated on the doctor's instructions by the clip on the delivering tube. The limb is lightly splinted. If the cannula slips out of the vein, blood escapes into the tissues and the patient complains of pain. The tube should be clipped off and the doctor summoned.

In blood transfusion, as in all intravenous injections, the tubing and other portions of the delivery apparatus must be free of air. Air embolism is the danger.

The drip may fail to run because:
(a) The vein is obstructed by too tight a bandage.
(b) The outlet of the cannula is against the wall of the vein. This is corrected by adhesive skin strapping.
(c) The head of pressure is too low (corrected by elevating the container).
(d) The delivery tube is blocked. This can be tested by disconnecting the tube from the shaft of the cannula.
(e) Venospasm. This may be lessened by:
  (i) the injection by the doctor of 2 per cent procaine around the vein.
  (ii) keeping the patient's arm warm. Warmth dilates the vein and is permissible in this strictly localised area.

Other difficulties which may arise are:
1. An airlock which can be cleared by disconnecting the delivery tube from the cannula and running the blood through.
2. The drip-chamber becoming too full. This difficulty can be overcome by turning off the drip and holding the bag upright, i.e. with the neck upwards. Gentle pressure on the drip chamber will cause air to re-enter this chamber.

The drip that is running satisfactorily *may stop* because:
(a) The cannula has come out of the vein.
(b) The bag of blood was allowed to empty before it was changed.
(c) Blood has clotted in the cannula.
The blood running into the patient will not clot because it contains an anticoagulant. The clotting occurs because the patient's blood has been allowed to be siphoned back into the cannula. This can be avoided when changing the bag by:
(a) Clamping off the delivery tube as gently as possible.
(b) Turning off the drip set when changing units of blood.

Fine screen filters. It is now well established that microaggregates in stored blood contribute significantly to many cases of pulmonary insufficiency. These aggregates are not removed by the 170 micron filter supplied with standard blood administration sets. A fine screen filter will remove the aggregates and should be used in the following situations:-

Patients who are likely to require a transfusion of three or more units of blood.

Major trauma, including chest trauma and multiple fractures.

Major obstetric bleeding and surgery.

Gastro-intestinal bleeding.

Vascular surgery.

Previous pulmonary disease.

Patients who have had a febrile reaction during a previous blood transfusion.

Pressure administration pump

This should be used only by medical staff. The Baxter transfusion set (Fig. 12.7) permits either a gravity or pressure pump administration.

The inbuilt blood pump permits the rapid administration of blood. It is always there and obviates the necessity to set up ancillary pumping equipment in an emergency. It eliminates the hazards of positive air pressure systems. It cannot pump air.

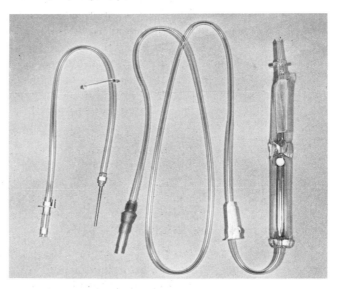

Fig. 12.7 Baxter pressure transfusion set. Note self-sealing rubber (third left) to enable intravenous drugs to be given rapidly into the set.

Pump instructions. When pressure transfusion is required, close the regulating clamp and squeeze the (lower) pump chamber to fill completely, so that the float occludes the inlet. Open the regulating clamp and alternately squeeze and release the pump chamber allowing it to fill completely between each action. Pumping action should be discontinued as soon as the container is empty. To return to gravity tranfusion remove the bag from the stand to the upright position and, by squeezing the pump chamber with tubing clamped off, discharge excess fluid back into the container. Resuspend the bag and tap the set briskly to disperse any froth.

A second type of pressure pump, the Martin's pump, is in use in many hospitals and is of value when rapid transfusion is required. The pump is clamped to the drip-stand and the drip tubing is inserted into a grooved channel. Manual turning of the handle rollers against the tubing produces pressure to force blood into the vein.

Precautions during transfusion

Patients and transfusion apparatus must be kept under constant supervision during the entire period of the transfusion.

The medical officer must inform the nurse of the rate at which the transfusion is to be maintained. Forty drops per minute is the usual rate of transfusion, which means that a bag is transfused in four hours. Patients suffering from haemorrhage may need to be given transfusion at a much greater rate.

Sufferers from cardiac or pulmonary disease, and severely anaemic patients, must be transfused at a slow rate, sometimes as slow as 12 drops per minute or packed cells used.

When a transfusion is in progress half-hourly pulse and hourly temperature records are kept. If the transfusion is for shock the blood pressure and the pulse are recorded after each unit of blood.

Because stored blood contains large amounts of particulate debris, which if infused may cause pulmonary complications by collecting in the lungs, it is wise to insert a special filter into the transfusion system if large quantities of blood are likely to be used.

Patients receiving transfusions should be kept rather warmer than is comfortable, as this reduces the tendency to febrile reactions and circulatory overloading. All patients should be watched for the symptoms of transfusion reactions after the first few ml of blood from each unit of blood. Immediate treatment should be given and the medical officer informed without delay. Measurement of the central venous pressure may be of assistance in assessing the amount of blood required.

Procedure after transfusion

The details of the transfusion, with serial numbers of bags given and the time taken for the transfusion, must be entered in the case records. A note should be made of any untoward reactions.

The used blood bags, containing their residues of blood, should be kept in the ward (preferably in a refrigerator) for 24 hours. The small amount of blood remaining in each bag may be required in the investigation of transfusion reactions.

When 24 hours have elapsed after transfusion, the used bags should be disposed of by incineration. Any unused or partly used bags of blood which have been left at room temperature for one hour or more should be labelled 'dangerous for patients' and returned to the laboratory.

COMPLICATIONS OF BLOOD TRANSFUSION

1. Allergic reactions may occur in patients with a previous history of allergic reactions to transfusion or who have a history of asthma or similar allergic conditions. The reaction tends to occur after about 300 ml of blood have been given. There is no need to stop the transfusion. It is characterised by itching and urticaria. Intravenous antihistamine preparations will usually control it.

2. Pyrexia from pyrogens in the anticoagulant fluid may occur. It is usually due to dirty apparatus and is much rarer since fresh disposable apparatus has been used. Infected blood is another cause of pyrexia.

3. *Haemolysis* gives rise to rigors at an early stage. The transfusion should be stopped and Mannitol infused.

4. Citrate intoxication may manifest itself by an irregular slow pulse. After every fourth unit of blood 10 ml of 10 per cent calcium chloride is injected intravenously.

5. *Overloading* gives rise to signs of right heart failure. It is very rare if the transfusion is controlled by measurement of the central venous pressure.

6. Transmission of infection of which the most important is hepatitis.

7. Air embolism is avoided by keeping air away from the lower portion of the drip chamber and beyond.

8. Thrombophlebitis is an occasional complication.

9. Renal failure is usually caused by mismatched blood.

10. Pulmonary complications may arise (particularly after large amounts of unfiltered blood).

After blood transfusion it is advisable to check the haemoglobin to ensure that the patient has received some benefit. Normally a unit of blood should raise the haemoglobin 1 g per dl. In some cases blood is rapidly destroyed and the patient receives little or no benefit from the transfusion.

Special problems of massive transfusions

The administration of large quantities of blood in a short period gives rise to two special types of problems: haemorrhagic manifestations and metabolic effects.

1. Haemorrhage. Bank blood stored for more than 24 hours contains no functioning platelets and almost no factor VIII (antihaemophilic) factor. A transfusion equal to the blood volume of the patient dilutes the number of circulating platelets and the amount of clotting factor. These are corrected by infusion of concentrated platelets and fresh frozen plasma.

2. Transfusion haemosiderosis. Patients receiving regular blood transfusions for chronic anaemia become iron-overloaded. A litre of blood contains 500 mgs of iron while the normal excretion of iron is only 1 mg. Weatherall et al (1977) have shown that the amount of iron excreted can be increased to 70 to 120 mgs by continuous infusion of desferrioxamine using a small portable pump over 12 hourly periods each week.

CLINICAL USE OF BLOOD AND BLOOD PRODUCTS

Whole blood or some specially prepared constituent of blood may be used in clinical practice.

1. Whole blood is used for replacement in haemorrhage. The usual anticoagulant is citrate phosphate dextrose.

2. Concentrated red cells (packed cells) replace haemoglobin in anaemia without greatly increasing the circulatory volume.

3. Platelets prepared by concentrating the plasma after removal of the red cells may be used in thrombocytopenia.

4. Plasma replaces protein lost in burns and large wounds. Dried pooled plasma has been replaced by plasma protein fraction (PPF) which is supplied as a solution. Whereas dried plasma may transmit the virus of serum hepatitis, plasma protein fraction is heated to inactivate the virus.

5. Fresh frozen plasma (FFP) contains all the clotting factors and is invaluable in bleeding states with loss of coagulation factors.

6. Cryoprecipitate contains a high concentration of factor VIII. It is used for treating patients with haemophilia. Freeze-dried factor VIII is given as soon as possible after bleeding. It arrests haemorrhage and relieves pain. If the patient is unable to give it intravenously himself a competent relation may be taught to administer it.

7. Fibrinogen is used in conditions of hypofibrinogenaemia such as occur in the defibrination syndrome.

8. Gammaglobulin is used for immunisation against such conditions as hepatitis.

Fate of the blood lost in haemorrhage

At the beginning of this chapter it was noted that all the patient's problems may not be resolved when the bleeding ceases or the blood volume has been restored. In some haemorrhages the amount of blood loss is insignificant, but the actual blood lost is highly destructive in specialised tissues such as those of the eye or small but important areas of the brain or spinal cord. In body cavities such as the skull, the brain may be compressed by extravasated blood lying between the bone and the meninges or between the meninges and the brain. In the chest a large effusion of blood and blood clot may interfere with the action of the heart or lungs. In the pharynx, larynx or trachea, blood may seriously obstruct respiration and give rise to a lung infection including an abscess. In more disastrous circumstances the patient may die from flooding of the whole pulmonary field with inhaled blood.

Terms to describe extravasated collections of blood are:

1. *Petechiae* are tiny pinpoint haemorrhages from capillary damage.
2. *An ecchymosis* is a small area of skin bruising.
3. *Haematoma* is a sealed collection of blood and clot. It may be sealed beneath:
   (a) a wound;
   (b) a tissue such as the periosteum (subperiosteal) or beneath the capsule of an organ (subcapsular).
   (c) A tear of a soft organ such as the spleen or liver.

Complications

1. Infection. 'Stale blood' is an ideal medium for the growth of organisms.

2. Rupture. In large haematomas profuse internal 'delayed' haemorrhage may result.

Haemorrhage from special sites

The occurrence of haemorrhage from special sites is designated by special terms.

Epistaxis – bleeding from the nose.

Haemoptysis — the expectoration of blood from the lungs.

Haematemesis — vomiting of blood.

Melaena — the passage of dark blood per rectum from a site high in the intestinal tract.

Haematuria — blood in the urine.

Haemothorax — bleeding into the chest.

Haemoperitoneum — bleeding into the peritoneum.

Haemarthrosis — bleeding into a joint.

Menorrhagia — excessive menstruation at normal intervals.

Metrostaxis — (metrorrhagia) — excessive irregular or continuous bleeding per vaginam between the periods.

Haemopericardium (cardiac tamponade) — bleeding into the pericardium.

Haematomyelia — bleeding into the spinal cord.

BIBLIOGRAPHY

Allison D J 1978 British Journal of Hospital Medicine 20: 707.
Machin A 1979 British Journal of Hospital Medicine 21: 294.
Weatherall D J, Pippard M J, Callender S T 1977 New England Journal of Medicine 297: 445 (Editorial).

13

Thrombosis and embolism

THROMBOSIS

Thrombosis is defined as the formation of a solid or semisolid mass from the constituents of the blood within the vascular system. It is not identical with the clotting of shed blood. Although the incidence of disease is higher in the arteries, thrombosis is commoner in veins where the more sluggish blood flow predisposes to its formation.

A thrombus may:
1. Extend and spread while still attached to the vessel wall.
2. Lyse (dissolve) spontaneously without permanent damage.
3. Organise into fibrous tissue so that the lumen of the vessel is permanently obstructed.
4. Become detached in whole or in part and be swept away into the blood stream until it lodges and blocks another blood vessel. This process is known as embolism, the detached thrombus being the embolus and the area deprived of blood is known as the infarct.

Thrombi may form in any part of the vascular system. The common sites are:

(a) *The veins of the lower limb and pelvis*, and detachment gives rise to pulmonary embolism.

(b) *The left heart chamber* in valvular disease or myocardial infarction. As the heart recovers and its action improves, an embolus may be expelled, lodge in an artery of the leg and cause acute gangrene (Ch. 23) or in the cerebral vessels and cause a hemiplegia.

(c) *On an atheromatous patch in an arteriosclerotic artery*, which results in threatened gangrene in a limb already poorly supplied with blood.

Thrombus formation in a vein is known as thrombosis. If there is concomitant inflammation of the vessel wall the condition is known as thrombophlebitis. The former is usually painless, the latter is strikingly painful.

Factors which predispose to thrombosis

Certain incidents and disease render the patient more liable to form thrombi.

1. The vessel wall may be damaged by trauma including pressure during operation. Many substances suitable for intravenous injection may cause disastrous thrombosis if injected into an artery. Before the administration of intramuscular or subcutaneous injections one should always check that the needle is not in a vein by withdrawing the piston before plunging it in, and in intravenous injections care should be taken to note that it is venous and not arterial blood that is flowing back into the syringe before administering the injection. The ampoule label should be checked to ensure that the contents are suitable for intravenous administration.

2. The prostaglandins and thrombosis. Platelets synthesize the prostaglandin TXA_2 which induces the platelets to stick to each other and to foreign surfaces including the wall of diseased blood vessels. The normal lining endothelium cells secrete a different prostaglandin PGI_2 which counteracts the action of TXA_2 and reduces the tendency of the platelets to aggregate. Imbalance may arise in a diseased blood vessel which cannot make PGI_2 and the aggregating action of TXA_2 is unopposed. This is a contributing factor in thrombus formation. The possibility that PGI_2 will be available for therapeutic anticoagulation is very real (Horton, 1979).

3. Structural changes in the vessel wall. Arteries already the site of sclerosis may be further obstructed by thrombosis.

On operating tables, particularly when amputating a leg, the popliteal artery in the opposite limb — often in a parlous state of health — must be kept free of pressure from the end of the table which may have been split.

Veins with damaged valves are more liable to form thrombi, as are heart valves which have been damaged by disease.

4. Slowing the blood flow increases the risk. Confinement to bed in conditions of hypotension and obstruction to the flow of blood by constricting bandages or bad positioning on the operating table are to be avoided.

5. Changes in the nature of the blood. Dehydration increases the viscosity of the blood. Other factors which increase its coagulability are leukaemia and splenectomy (because platelet destruction is delayed), drugs such as oestrogens (included in the contraceptive pill) and malignant disease. In many cases there is a combination of factors and thrombosis is sometimes the first clinical feature of malignant disease which even an intensive search may fail to reveal.

6. Age. The incidence increases over the age of 40.

7. Pelvic operations are more likely to be complicated by thrombosis.

CLINICAL FEATURES

Arterial thrombosis causes loss of function and usually severe pain. Common examples are coronary thrombosis or thrombosis in the main artery of a leg. In this chapter, however, we are primarily concerned with venous thrombosis. This may be present as:

1. Thrombophlebitis more usually affects the superficial veins which are already varicose. The thrombus is unlikely to become detached. It is painful. The skin over the vein is reddened and the vein itself is usually palpable as a tender, firm cord.

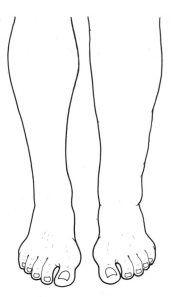

Fig. 13.1 Swelling of left leg due to thrombosis of the left iliofemoral vein.

2. *Deep vein thrombosis* which may present as:

(a) Massive thrombosis in a large vein may be relatively painless. There is swelling of the limb, which increases rapidly, and the foot particularly is usually oedematous (Fig. 13.1). The limb feels heavy and the unaffected superficial veins may be very prominent.

(b) Quiet formation is suggested by a slight rise in the patient's temperature; some aching pain in the calf of the leg; pain in the muscles of the calf on dorsiflexion of the foot (Homan's sign); slight oedema of the foot. Whatever the method of presentation, detachment of the thrombus causing pulmonary embolism is likely.

3. *Pulmonary embolism* (p. 121) may be the first sign that thrombosis has occurred.

Established thrombosis may be obvious or only suspected. In either case further investigations may be advisable to establish the diagnosis, the extent, the type and the number of thrombi, or to gauge the response to treatment.

INVESTIGATION

Radiography

Phlebography will outline the vein or show a block by a thrombus in the veins of the leg or the iliac veins.

Isotope scanning

^{125}I-labelled fibrinogen, when injected intravenously, becomes incorporated in a firm thrombus (if present) and may be detected by Geiger-counter scanning of the legs.

The ultrasonic doppler

The ultrasonic response to an increased venous flow against an obstruction has been termed the A-wave. It can be repeated as frequently as desired to assess progress without any discomfort to the patient and therefore has an advantage over radiographic and isotopic measures, but is not as accurate.

MANAGEMENT

Prevention

Large varicose veins may be temporarily controlled by crêpe bandages or ligated if the patient is undergoing a severe operation or one necessitating prolonged bed-rest.

Drugs liable to produce thrombosis such as oestrogens should be stopped four to eight weeks preoperatively. Previous venous thrombotic upsets may be an indication for prophylactic anticoagulant therapy commencing 48 to 72 hours postoperatively or even subcutaneous heparin preoperatively. The risk of bleeding has of course to be carefully considered.

Much thought has been given to the prevention of thrombosis.

Factors which diminish thrombus formation are:

1. Adequate and regular analgesia—relieves pain and makes movement easier.
2. Adequate intake of fluids prevents 'increased' viscosity of the blood.
3. No knee pillow. The patient should be operated on with the foot of the operating table elevated slightly and the heels supported by padded rings so that the calves of the legs are lifted off the table. Postoperatively the foot of the bed should be elevated and when out of bed the patient should not be allowed to sit with his legs dependent.
4. Leg and breathing exercises should be encouraged whether the patient is confined to bed or is ambulant.
5. Early mobilisation after the operation. This means walking if possible but if the patient is sitting then the legs should be elevated. The nurse should inspect the patient's ankles for swelling when bedmaking.
6. Subcutaneous heparin preoperatively is used prophylactically on high-risk patients.
7. Antiembolic stockings can be used for susceptible patients. They exert a diminishing pressure on the leg from the ankle to the thigh.

Treatment

The objects of treatment are:

1. To prevent extension of the thrombus.
2. To remove or lyse (dissolve) the thrombus.
3. To prevent detachment with embolus formation.

This is achieved in an established case by rest in bed, the foot of which is elevated, and the administration of anticoagulants until an adequate prothrombin time has been achieved.

Bed rest continues until the temperature subsides and the signs disappear—usually 5 to 8 days. Heparin 10 000 units intravenously is given at once, followed by 10 000 units 6-hourly. If it has been decided to use oral anticoagulants, which are slower in achieving their effect, these are commenced at the same time and the dose is controlled by estimation of the prothrombin time. When effective their administration is continued and heparin therapy ceases. The dosage varies with the preparation used. Warfarin has an initial dosage of 30 to 40 mg on the first day, none on the second day and a maintenance dose of 2 to 20 mg daily, depending on the level of the prothrombin time which is estimated daily. The prothrombin time should be taken at midday, and the anticoagulant given before midnight each day.

In addition to watching for signs of excessive dosage (such as haematuria, purpura, heavy periods or haematemesis), delayed haemorrhage, pyrexia, a skin rash, albuminuria and jaundice may develop because of drug sensitivity. Granulocytopenia and diarrhoea have also been noted. The fifth week is the time these symptoms may occur. The drug dosage is regulated according to the prothrombin time and steroid therapy instituted.

If at any time it is desired to reverse or diminish the effects of anticoagulants this can be achieved by 10 mg of protamine sulphate which will neutralise 1000 units (10 mg) of heparin. Warfarin is neutralised by vitamin K mg by mouth, but as it is rather slow a transfusion of fresh blood may be advisable.

Anticoagulants prevent further thrombosis and their extension, but they may not dissolve an established clot. For this reason fibrinolytic agents such as streptokinase 500 000 units may be given intravenously over 30 minutes, followed by 100 000 units hourly. Newer fibrinolysins will undoubtedly be developed. As in anticoagulant treatment, fibrinolytic treatment requires close observation, particularly for signs of haemorrhage.

The action of streptokinase may be much neutralised by the administration of tranexamic acid.

Surgical removal, thrombectomy, may be undertaken with a Fogarty venous catheter and the operation is similar to removal of an embolus from an artery (p. 211). Delaying treatment, or failure to remove the thrombus by drugs or surgery, may result in a permanent white leg by organisation of the clot. Venous bypass operations may be attempted to re-establish the blood flow.

EMBOLISM

An embolus is a foreign body momentarily free in the blood stream. The most common variety is a detached thrombus from a vein which gives rise to pulmonary embolism. Detachment of a thrombus from the left side of the heart may cause gangrene of a limb (p. 210). It used to be thought that pulmonary embolus, apart from the immediate postoperative period, was rare, but more careful observation has shown that it is not uncommon at other times. Other forms of embolus are considered and mentioned at the end of this chapter.

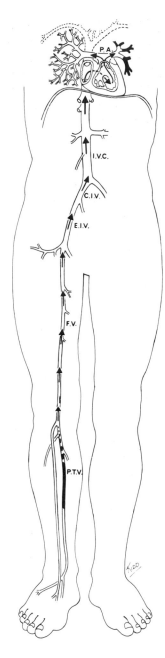

Fig. 13.2 Pulmonary embolism. The thrombus has formed in the posterior tibial veins and passes via the femoral, external iliac and common iliac veins to the inferior vena cava and thence to the right atrium of the heart. From the right atrium it passes to the right ventricle which pumps it in this case into the left pulmonary artery with infarction of the left lung.

PULMONARY EMBOLUS (Fig. 13.2).

Since embolism is a complication of thrombosis, prevention depends on avoiding thrombosis and in detecting established thrombosis as early as possible. The effect of an embolus is entirely dependent on its size. Three syndromes are recognised:

1. A relatively small embolus occludes a peripheral pulmonary artery and produces the classical picture — pleural-type pain, haemoptysis and a shadow of infarcted lung on the X-ray.

2. Repeated embolism without pain initially with gradually increasing breathlessness, fatigue and a feeling of collapse on exertion.

3. A massive pulmonary embolism occluding about two-thirds of the circumference of the pulmonary artery. The onset is sudden, there are signs of right heart failure, the patient's skin is clammy and cyanosed and the veins in the neck are outstanding. The diagnosis from myocardial infarct is often difficult but vital since it is in this form that pulmonary embolectomy may be the only hope and such a procedure would be rapidly fatal in a patient with coronary thrombosis. Electrocardiography and lung scanning with radioactive xenon may be advisable. Pulmonary angiography may confirm the diagnosis with certainty — the patient may be too ill for it to be undertaken. Blood gases should be estimated — hypoxia and hypocarbia may be diagnostic of pulmonary embolism. Electrocardiography may help to confirm the diagnosis.

Treatment

Major embolism presents great difficulties in the choice and timing of treatment. The patient is kept absolutely still and oxygen is administered. If the condition is improving, treatment is conservative. Conservative treatment entails lysis of the pulmonary embolus and the prevention of further embolism by the administration of anticoagulants or fibrinolysins (p. 119).

A large loose thrombus can be removed or the vein above it ligated so that it cannot escape, e.g. the inferior vena cava may be plicated to narrow it so that the embolus cannot pass. Smaller thrombi will lyse with streptokinase given for three days, followed by anticoagulant drugs. The real anxiety is that some hours are necessary before the effects of fibrinolysis or anticoagulants become apparent. If the patient is deteriorating, pulmonary embolectomy may be undertaken as a last desperate measure.

Lesser degrees of embolism are always anxious situations since they may be the forerunner of a massive embolism. Movement is reduced to a minimum and anticoagulant treatment is instituted at once. Investigation of the state of the deep veins is undertaken by bilateral ascending and iliofemoral phlebogram by percutaneous or perosseous routes. A decision is made as to whether further measures such as thrombolytic therapy or removal of the thrombus may be advisable.

Other forms of embolism

1. Fat embolism. Fat embolism is caused as a result of fractures and in severe cases causes respiratory distress due, not to the emboli in the lungs, but to their effect on the brain which may cause death. Assisted respiration is advisable.

2. Air embolism. Air embolism is a risk of venous haemorrhage in which air is sucked into an open vein. The air causes frothing of the blood. It is avoided in intravenous injections, including transfusion, by ensuring only fluid and no air is injected.

3. Bacteria spread by emboli may be recognised by the presence of purpuric spots on the skin, tiny splinter haemorrhages under the nails, retinal haemorrhages, or from the presence of red blood cells in the urine of such patients, in cases of infective endocarditis.

4. Malignant cells. Spread by the bloodstream.

5. Foreign bodies. The most important to avoid clinically is detachment of a portion of an intravenous catheter.

BIBLIOGRAPHY

Horton E W 1979 British Journal of Hospital Medicine 22: 260

14

Shock

The supply of oxygen to the tissues is the first essential in the maintenance of life, and this can only be ensured when the circulatory system is functioning normally. Sudden collapse of the circulation known as shock is one of the commonest and most formidable conditions encountered in surgical practice. The circulation may fail from:

1. Sudden damage to the heart. This may occur because of:

(a) *Coronary arterial occlusion.*

(b) *Toxaemia*, which may be (i) bacterial (originating elsewhere in the body), (ii) chemical, including drugs and anaesthetic agents.

(c) *Trauma.*

Complete cardiac arrest is the most urgent of all conditions, and death is an inevitable sequel unless the heart can be restored within three minutes. Cardiac massage may be the only hope, and is discussed in detail at the end of this chapter. In certain arrhythmias such as ventricular fibrillation, a defibrillator is required.

2. Deficient oxygenation of the blood in the lungs. Amongst the many causes the following are the most important surgically:

(a) *Obstruction of the pulmonary artery by an embolus.* If it is complete sudden death occurs.

(b) *Thoracic injuries*, particularly 'stove in' chest, tension pneumothorax, bruising and laceration of the lungs (Ch. 30).

(c) *Postoperative atelectasis* (collapse of a large segment of lung).

The complicated issues involved in this form are discussed in the chapters on Respiratory Failure and Diseases of the Lungs and Chest Wall.

3. Reduction in the blood volume (oligaemia). This may occur from loss of:

(a) *Whole blood*—haemorrhage.

(b) *Plasma.* This is particularly significant in burns.

(c) *Water and electrolytes*, which occurs in (i) peritonitis, (ii) intestinal obstruction and paralytic ileus, (iii) acute dilatation of the stomach, and (iv) severe diarrhoea and vomiting.

4. Loss of arterial tone. This may occur in:

(a) *The common faint.* The arterioles in the muscles relax.

(b) Acute anaphylaxis (p. 55).

(c) *Acute hormone deficiency*, notably of the adrenal gland.

(d) *Absorption of metabolites or materials resulting from tissue injury.*

(e) *Overdosage of drugs, for example, analgesics like pethidine.*

(f) *Following therapy with beta-blocking agents* (for angina, hypertension, etc.).

(g) *Noxious stimuli* such as pain will, if sufficiently severe, cause vasodilatation, particularly of the splanchnic vessels with 'pooling' of blood in the area. This is the mechanism of primary or neurogenic shock. It is a condition of short duration because either the patient dies immediately, recovers spontaneously if the causal stimulus is removed or severe pain is relieved; otherwise it passes into 'secondary' oligaemic shock.

Compensatory mechanisms

Whatever the cause of sudden collapse there are certain compensatory physiological mechanisms which occur.

1. Posture. A patient in acute circulatory failure falls down. He should be left flat or, better, kept in the head-down position to an angle of 5°. This helps to supply more blood to the brain but an angle of more than 5° is harmful because it causes venous congestion.

2. Contraction of the skin vessels. Contraction of the arterioles and venules of the skin is usual so as to conserve the blood supply to the more vital centres. The application of heat dilates the skin vessels, thereby aggravating the condition, and should not be used.

3. Insensitivity. A very collapsed patient usually has little pain. Large quantities of pain-relieving drugs are unnecessary and, in any case, are ineffective because they cannot be absorbed unless given by the intravenous route. Administered subcutaneously they may result in cumulative overdosage as the circulation recovers. Because the shocked patient is insensitive his skin is more easily damaged, so he has to be handled very gently.

4. Urinary secretion is diminished to conserve fluid in the body, but it is also a sign that tissue perfusion (the circulation of blood through the kidney and other tissues) is inadequate.

5. The heart rate accelerates in most forms of circulatory failure with the important exception of the common faint. It is an attempt to ensure that the remaining fluid is circulated as rapidly as possible, thereby providing sufficient oxygen to the tissues.

6. The temperature is subnormal. This reduces the requirements of the tissues for the diminishing amount of oxygen available. The core temperature may actually be raised. The difference between the two is a measure of the degree of shock.

All these compensatory factors are temporary in their beneficial effects and, if the condition of the circulation is not restored to normal without delay, irreversible changes set in.

Clinical causes

1. Haemorrhage.
2. Severe burns.
3. Severe wounds, particularly with extensive skin or muscle laceration.
4. Multiple fractures or single fractures of a large long bone.
5. Perforation of any viscus into the peritoneal cavity.
6. Operative intervention.
7. Adrenal failure.
8. Pulmonary embolism.
9. Myocardial infarction.
10. Severe infection, particularly septicaemia.
11. Severe pain.

CLINICAL APPEARANCES OF SHOCK

The face is ashen pale and expressionless. The eyes are still and the patient takes little or no interest in his surroundings, although he may answer, slowly, questions which are asked. He makes no complaint of pain.

The skin is cold, white, and clammy and respiration is shallow. The pulse is usually rapid and thin, although sometimes it is below normal in rate, and the temperature is always subnormal.

If septicaemia is suspected, a blood culture is performed.

The most constant finding is a low systolic and diastolic blood pressure.

Clinical management

Of the many disturbances which occur in shock, oligaemia is the one best understood and most easily remedied. Its control requires observation of:

1. The central venous pressure which is the best guide to the effective circulating volume. It may be measured by passing a PVC or Teflon catheter into a peripheral vein and threading it up until it is estimated to lie within the thoracic cavity. The veins used are those on the medial side of the arm, the subclavian or the internal jugular. The cannula must be firmly fixed to the skin. Correctly sited there will always be a free rise and fall on the attached manometer.

This catheter is connected to a special venous pressure measuring drip set (Fig. 14.1).

This is distinguished by having a long side-arm. It is provided with a centimetre scale. In use, the side-arm is filled with fluid and is then connected to the patient's venous system. The level above the manubrium sternum at which the fluid in the side-arm comes to rest is a measure of the central venous pressure. In the normal subject the value will be from 0 to 2 or 3 cm of water.

In the shocked or hypovolaemic patient it will be negative while in patients who are in heart failure or who have been overtransfused it may be very high (10 to 25 cm of water).

2. A packed cell volume (PCV) of over 55 indicates the need for saline or plasma or its substitutes rather than blood.

3. Urinary output is the best guide that tissue perfusion is occurring and an indwelling catheter is inserted in all severe cases. The specific gravity of the urine should be recorded hourly, and an output of urine below 60 ml per hour is considered unsatisfactory. Urinary output above this level suggests that the blood flow to the kidney is sufficient not only to keep the organ alive but also to function, and is indirect evidence that the circulation of blood in other organs is improving and becoming adequate.

4. The heart rate is rapid and diminishes as replacement becomes adequate (Fig. 14.2).

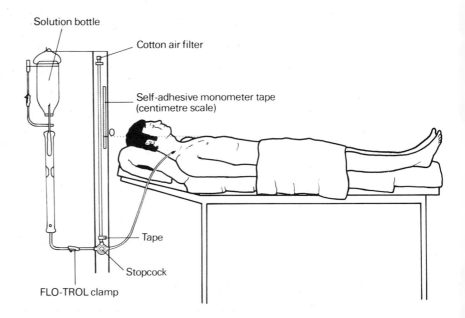

Fig. 14.1 The estimation of central venous pressure using a special Baxter drip set.

5. The blood pressure. The reversal of hypotension is in itself an unreliable sign unless accompanied by reversal of the other signs of oligaemia.

Taking the blood pressure. The patient should be at rest lying in bed, or sitting in a chair. The sleeve of the gown/jacket is rolled back or removed as necessary. The arm is extended and supported. The cuff of the sphygmomanometer is wrapped firmly and smoothly round the upper arm well above the elbow flexure. The manometer is placed level with the patient's arm, the scale being visible to the nurse. It is connected to the cuff. The nurse palpates the radial/brachial pulse, she inflates the cuff and notes the point on the manometer at which the pulse disappears. (N.B. Care should be taken to avoid discomfort to the patient by the cuff being overinflated or inflated for too long a time.) The cuff is deflated. She adjusts the ear pieces of the stethoscope, and places the other end over the brachial pulse (artery). The cuff is reinflated to above the previously noted point on the

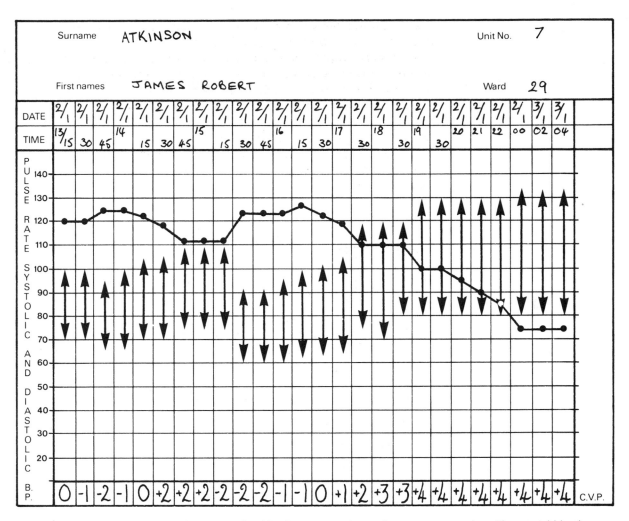

Fig. 14.2 Pulse, blood pressure and central venous pressure chart. The arterial blood pressure is measured in mm. Hg., the C.V.P. in cms. of water.

manometer. It is slowly deflated. When a tapping sound is heard, the nurse notes the point on the manometer—this gives the systolic pressure. As the cuff is deflated further, the sounds become louder, suddenly they change to a muffled sound, and then cease altogether. The point at which the sound changes from loud to muffled is noted—this gives the diastolic pressure. The manometer is disconnected. The cuff is removed and folded away into the manometer box. The patient is made comfortable.

The result is charted immediately, e.g.

BP $\frac{120}{80}$

Any significant change from previous recordings is reported to the nurse in charge. When there is difficulty in hearing the sounds or in obtaining the readings, the nurse in charge should be asked to help.

6. Temperature. Observations of differences between the peripheral skin temperature and the rectal temperature (measured by electrical thermometers) are helpful in estimating the peripheral circulation. If the temperature in the rectum and on the surface of the big toe are recorded and it is found that the big toe temperature drops or fails to rise, then all is not well. It is an even finer guide than urinary excretion to the state of tissue perfusion.

7. Expansion of the circulatory volume until it is adequate as shown by reversal of the signs of failure. This remains the most hopeful method of treatment whatever the metabolic disturbance, since restoration of normal tissue perfusion is essential.

Drugs

Vasoconstrictors are contraindicated.Drugs which may be of value if the patient fails to respond to adequate restoration of the blood volume are:

Hydrocortisone 100 mg or more in the infusion may be effective. It probably acts by stabilization of the cell membranes.

Vasodilators may be of value after the blood volume has been restored on the basis that prolonged splanchnic vasoconstriction (constriction of the arteries to the stomach and intestine) causes irreversible changes. Phenoxybenzamine has been reported to be of value as has isoprenaline which has a direct inotropic effect as well as being a vasodilator.

Correction of acidosis. A solution of 8·4 per cent sodium bicarbonate may be advisable and arterial blood-gas estimations are of value in making this decision.

Diuretics. Mannitol (a 6-carbon sugar) is an osmotic diuretic which is neither absorbed in the renal tubules nor metabolised. It may be given when acidosis and oligaemia have been corrected but if oliguria persists frusemide may also be given. If diuresis does not occur within half an hour of 40 mg of frusemide being given severe renal damage has occurred and the intake of fluid may have to be restricted on this account.

Antibiotics are essential if a bacterial element is present.

Anticoagulants may occasionally be indicated if microcirculatory thrombosis is suspected.

Electrolyte imbalance must be corrected.

Oxygen lack is corrected by administration with nasal spectacles.

Analgesics are rarely necessary until the patient's condition has been restored.

Internal haemorrhage from a ruptured organ may occur so rapidly that the risk of operating on a patient suffering from shock has to be accepted and rapid transfusion should be performed until the haemorrhage has been controlled and continued until the blood volume has been restored. The shorter the period the patient is collapsed with a low blood pressure, anoxia and loss of tissue perfusion the better, otherwise there is a risk of irreversible damage to the kidneys, the liver, and the brain, especially in the elderly.

Whatever the cause of circulatory collapse the following general principles evolve:

1. Treatment must be instituted without delay and continued until the condition has been reversed.

2. In difficult cases, where the response is slow or inadequate, the diagnosis of the cause may have to be revised.

3. Once the patient's condition has improved every precaution must be taken to see that shock does not recur. Observations on the pulse, temperature, including the colour, the state of the skin and urinary output are important. Examination of the blood and urine should be continued and the return to a sitting-up position should be instituted gradually and observantly.

Circulatory collapse should be avoided by strenuous measures if at all possible. Preoperatively the patient should be as fit as possible, and from the point of view of the circulatory system:

1. His blood should be adequate in quality and in volume.

2. His tissues should be adequately hydrated.

3. He should be mobile so that there is no stagnation in the circulatory system.

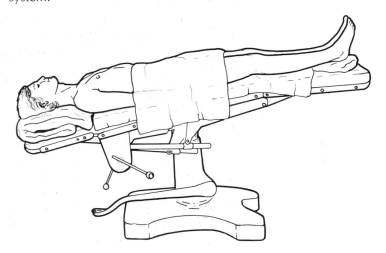

14.3 Trendelenburg position.

THE PREVENTION OF SHOCK

Every operation is an injury, but operative trauma differs from all other injuries in that the surgeon and nursing staff know its nature in advance. Further, we know the early signs of circulatory collapse.

1. The patient is kept warm on his journey from the ward to the theatre and back. Blankets should be warmed. Fear is allayed and tranquillising drugs are commonly used preoperatively.

2. The blood pressure is recorded, and in serious cases is monitored continuously, and blood replacement commenced in good time. Severe

operations are commenced only after satisfactory infusions have been established.

3. The head of the table is lowered if the blood pressure falls (the Trendelenburg position) which is shown in Figure 14.3.

4. The anaesthetist deepens the anaesthesia temporarily as specially sensitive tissues are handled. Oxygen is freely provided and cyanosis is avoided.

5. Postoperatively, fluid and electrolyte replacement (saline, 5 per cent, dextrose, Hartman's solution, plasma or blood as indicated), rest and relief from pain are continued.

6. Gentle handling of the patient by the nursing staff is very important in the prevention of shock.

There are few conditions in which a patient can improve or deteriorate so rapidly as in circulatory failure. Its treatment calls for the best organisation of the resources of a hospital and the most painstaking care from the nursing staff.

CARDIAC ARREST

The signs of cardiac arrest are:
1. Sudden collapse and the onset of unconsciousness.
2. Cessation of the heart beat—no palpable pulses.
3. Cessation of breathing—severe cyanosis.
4. Dilated pupils.

The interval between 'clinical death' which occurs with cessation of the heart beat and respiration and biological death is 3 to 5 minutes. This may be prolonged by:
1. Cardiac massage (external cardiac compression).
2. Hypothermia.
3. Extracorporeal circulation with artificial oxygenator.

Sudden stoppage of the heart requires immediate action on the part of the nursing staff, because after three minutes of cessation of blood flow to the cerebrum, cerebral damage is permanent and irreversible.

The alarm should be raised and the cardiac arrest team summoned. Ventilation of the lungs should be established at once. A free airway is ensured and the head is extended. In the absence of equipment expired air ventilation using the mouth to mouth or mouth to nose method should be employed. If available a bag and mask may be used to ventilate with air or oxygen.

Pulmonary ventilation by a bag and face mask with air or oxygen should be started immediately so that the small volume of blood which is circulating through the lungs is fully oxygenated. If no bag is available mouth to mouth or mouth to nose breathing is carried out continuously, and medical help must be summoned immediately. At the same time cardiac massage may be started. It may be more correctly called intermittent cardiac compression.

This may be performed by the nurse while another nurse continues mouth to mouth breathing simultaneously. The patient is laid flat on a firm surface (a mattress is too soft), a fracture board on a bed will do, and regular manual compression is exerted against the lower sternum at a rate of 60 times per minute (Fig. 14.4). Properly performed it can be a very exhausting effort and the rib cage may be damaged. A machine has been designed for the purpose but it is not generally available. The patient's legs should be slightly elevated to aid venous return and the head should be supported.

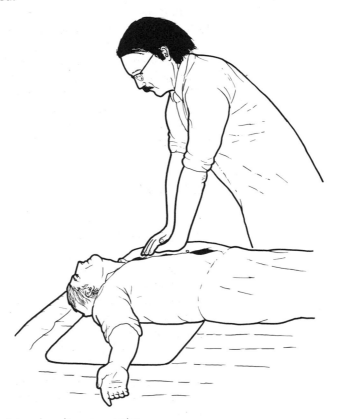

Fig. 14.4 External cardiac compression.

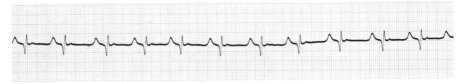

Fig. 14.5 Electrocardiograph. Normal tracing showing P Q R S and T waves.

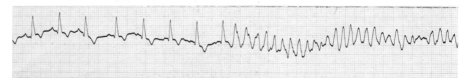

Fig. 14.6 Sinus rhythm going into ventricular fibrillation.

As soon as possible an ECG machine should be attached to the patient in order to establish which type of heart rhythm is present (Figs. 14.5 and 14.6). An intravenous infusion should be set up and a sample of heparinised arterial blood is sent for blood gas analysis. 100 mmol sodium bicarbonate should be infused.

Solutions of 1 in 10 000 adrenaline and 10 per cent calcium chloride should be immediately available for intravascular injection.

Cardiac arrest produces a severe metabolic acidosis and solutions of sodium bicarbonate will need to be infused before satisfactory cardiac action can be restored.

The provision of a cardiac arrest resuscitation trolley is now a regular feature in many blocks of wards. In addition to an oxygen cylinder with a regulator it should be furnished as follows:

Top shelf —

Ambu foot sucker	Catheter mount
Suction catheters-size 16	Ryles tube
Suction catheters-sized 14	Laryngoscope
Ambu-type bag with oxygen line	Tube KY jelly
Airway no. 3	Spencer Wells
Airway no. 2	Brook airway
7 mm endotracheal tube	Roll of Blenderm
8 mm endotracheal tube	3 in. No. 9 drain
9 mm endotracheal tube	
20 ml syringe	

Lower shelf —

Baxter intravenous set + meal hook	21 g butterfly
200 ml polyfusor sodium bic. 8·4%	19 g butterfly
500 ml dextrose 5%	Mediswabs
Cut down set	Greengauze swabs
Medicut cannulae 18g	Ethilon 320
Medicut cannulae 16g	Plain 439
Three-way taps	Ethilon 795
20 ml syringe	22 g surgical blade
5 ml syringes	15 g surgical blade
23 g needles	Roll of Blenderm
21 g needles	5 in. filling tubes
19 g needles	

Because every second is vital a 'cardiac arrest drug tray' (Fig. 14.7) should be in readiness and each compartment *boldly* labelled so that no time is wasted.

If ventricular fibrillation is present an electrical defibrillator will be required to administer an electric shock to restore normal rhythm.

Observations which should be made whilst the patient is receiving treatment are:

1. Feel for the pulse in the groin. If the circulation is maintained the pulse will be palpable.

2. Note if the pupils constrict. The pupils always dilate with circulatory arrest.

3. ECG will show activity.

4. Arterial blood gas analysis.

Aftercare. If normal cardiac function is restored these patients should be treated in an intensive care unit and be carefully monitored.

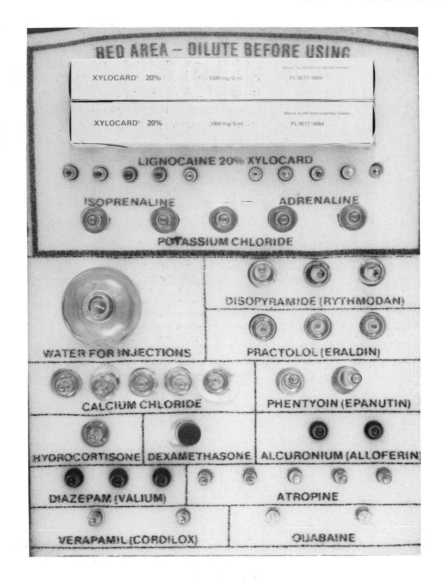

Fig. 14.7   Tray of drugs ready for rapid use in cardiac arrest.

ECG control for 24 to 48 hours is desirable. Occasionally measures for cerebral dehydration may be necessary and renal failure may follow a period of hypotension.

A useful aid to memory in the sudden emergency of the management of cardiac arrest is:

A Airway
B Breathing
C Cardiac compression
D Drugs and drip
E Electricity—ECG machine and a defibrillator.

15

Fluid and electrolyte balance and surgical nutrition

The method and forms of administration of fluid together with its complications are discussed in Chapter 16. Since fluid and electrolyte balance is a subject of great complexity and much still requires to be known, this separation is deliberate. The present discussion is a subject for the senior student.

Before abnormal states are considered an outline of the normal processes is essential.

THE FLUID

Water is the basis of all body fluids and the total quantity of body water is approximately 42 litres. This is divided into (Fig. 15.1):
1. Water inside the cells (intracellular water) and amounts to 30 l.
2. Extracellular water 12 l.
    Of which:
    (a) the plasma constitutes 3 l
    (b) the water in the tissue spaces 9 l.

The intracellular water is the fluid in which the essentials of nourishment are consumed and metabolites accumulate. The water in the tissue spaces is outside the blood stream and outside the cells. Its electrolyte composition is almost identical with that of blood plasma.

Examination of the various substances in the plasma will provide information about the composition of the fluid in the tissue spaces, but it will not tell us what the position is inside the cells.

THE ELECTROLYTES

An electrolyte is a substance which when dissolved in water splits (dissociates or ionises is the correct expression) into electrically charged particles known as ions (ion, Greek = wanderer). Each electrolyte splits into an equal number of positively (+) charged ions (known as cations) and negatively (−) charged ions (known as anions).

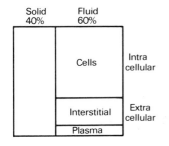

Fig. 15.1 Composition of the body.

In food an electrolyte is consumed as an independent substance, for example, common salt. To be an independent substance, which can be seen and handled, it must exist in molecular form as NaCl (its chemical formula) but in the body it exists as Na^+ (sodium ions) and Cl^- (chloride ions). Because electrolytes exist as particles, they used to be measured in terms which expressed their biological activity, namely milliequivalents per litre (mEq/l) but in the international system (SI) are now expressed in terms of their molecular weight as millimoles per litre (mmol/l).

The principal electrolytes are sodium (Na^+), potassium (K^+), chloride (Cl^-) and bicarbonate (HCO_3^-). There are many others like calcium, magnesium, phosphate, and sulphate.

Distribution of electrolytes

The extracellular and intracellular fluids show a marked difference in concentration of electrolytes. The most striking are:

1. Potassium (K^+) is the dominant cation inside the cell. Its concentration is about 144 mmol per litre against 8 mmol per litre for intracellular sodium (Na+).

2. Sodium (Na^+) is largely concentrated in the extracellular fluid and plasma with a concentration of 140 mmol per litre against 5 mmol per litre for that of potassium (K^+).

Normal metabolism tends to a production of an excess of anions over cations in the blood with the result that there is a tendency to acidosis. This state of affairs is corrected in health by the production of an acid urine. The glomeruli of the kidneys filter 170 l of fluid from the blood in 24 hours, but 168·5 l are reabsorbed by the tubules allowing 1·5 l to be passed as urine.

NORMAL CONTROL OF WATER AND ELECTROLYTES

Intake or gain is by mouth, followed by absorption from the gut.

Excretion or loss is from:

1. Extrarenal sources — the skin, respiration, and faeces. This amounts to about 1 l per day.

2. The kidneys. Five hundred millilitres of water is the minimum in which a healthy kidney can excrete the body's metabolites. The daily amount is, therefore, this quantity in addition to fluids consumed in excess of 1·5 l.

Renal control

For the kidney to function adequately it must have:

1. An intact blood supply and the blood must be supplied at adequate pressure. Its blood vessels must be intact to filter the enormous quantity of 170 l per day. In any condition of *hypo*tension the mechanism fails. In acute nephritis the glomeruli are swollen and diseased so that they allow blood to pass into the urine. In chronic nephritic conditions the glomeruli are inadequate in number and structure.

2. Normal acting tubules. To function normally and concentrate the glomerular filtrate from 170 to 1·5 l the tubules must be intact. More than this, they are under the control of hormones, viz:

(a) *The antidiuretic hormone of the pituitary*. If this is inadequate in

Fig. 15.2 Fluid and electrolyte balance and imbalance.

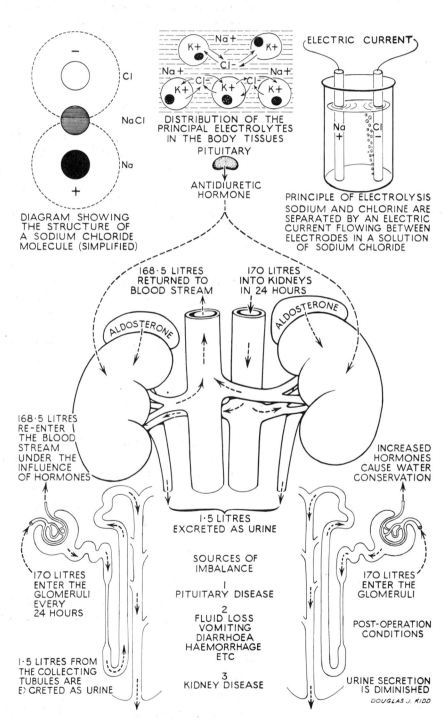

DIAGRAM SHOWING THE STRUCTURE OF A SODIUM CHLORIDE MOLECULE (SIMPLIFIED)

DISTRIBUTION OF THE PRINCIPAL ELECTROLYTES IN THE BODY TISSUES

ELECTRIC CURRENT

PRINCIPLE OF ELECTROLYSIS SODIUM AND CHLORINE ARE SEPARATED BY AN ELECTRIC CURRENT FLOWING BETWEEN ELECTRODES IN A SOLUTION OF SODIUM CHLORIDE

PITUITARY

ANTIDIURETIC HORMONE

168·5 LITRES RETURNED TO BLOOD STREAM

170 LITRES INTO KIDNEYS IN 24 HOURS

ALDOSTERONE

ALDOSTERONE

168·5 LITRES RE-ENTER THE BLOOD STREAM UNDER THE INFLUENCE OF HORMONES

INCREASED HORMONES CAUSE WATER CONSERVATION

1·5 LITRES EXCRETED AS URINE

170 LITRES ENTER THE GLOMERULI EVERY 24 HOURS

170 LITRES ENTER THE GLOMERULI

POST-OPERATION CONDITIONS

SOURCES OF IMBALANCE

1 PITUITARY DISEASE

2 FLUID LOSS VOMITING DIARRHOEA HAEMORRHAGE ETC

3 KIDNEY DISEASE

1·5 LITRES FROM THE COLLECTING TUBULES ARE EXCRETED AS URINE

URINE SECRETION IS DIMINISHED

DOUGLAS J. KIDD

amount the glomerular fluid is not concentrated and large quantities of water are lost; the condition known as diabetes insipidus in which a vast quantity of pale urine is passed is an extreme example of this failure. Pitressin by injection or by 'snuff' controls the condition.

(b) *Aldosterone*. This is a hormone which is secreted in the adrenal cortex and increases the reabsorption of sodium (Na^+) from the filtrate. This is present in large quantities in the blood and hence also in the glomerular filtrate.

THE METABOLIC RESPONSE TO INJURY

When a patient is injured, using injury in the widest sense and including bacterial infection and surgical operation, the two hormones acting on the renal tubules are excreted in excess. This is a physiological protective mechanism. The result is:

1. Water is conserved in the body. It is an everyday observation that in the first 24 to 48 hours postoperatively there is oliguria.
2. Sodium (Na^+) and chloride (Cl^-) are conserved in the body and not excreted in the urine.
3. Potassium (K^+) is lost in the urine. Potassium increases in the blood from the breakdown of cells, which is just what occurs in trauma.

The kidney allows potassium (K^+) to pass more freely, since potassium in excess is lethal, but gross lack, too, can be serious.

Once the blood volume has been restored, that is, once circulatory failure has been adequately treated, further fluid in the 24 hours postoperatively is unnecessary and may be harmful.

Estimation of electrolytes

Electrolyte estimations are determined by the laboratory on specimens of plasma from blood which has been collected in tubes containing lithium heparin. Care must be taken not to haemolyse the specimen by using a wet syringe, spirit, shaking the blood or squirting it through a fine needle. If the red cells rupture (haemolysis) they liberate enormous amounts of potassium into the plasma and render this determination valueless.

PATHOLOGICAL STATES

Depletions of fluid and electrolytes rarely occur in 'pure' forms. Sodium and water depletions, except in conditions like miner's cramp (where water has been taken without salt), usually occur together.

Sodium

Depletion occurs in:
1. Vomiting.
2. Gastric aspiration.
3. Intestinal obstruction.
4. Addison's disease.

The clinical features are those of 'dehydration', namely a dry tongue, dry wrinkled skin, sunken eyes, and a rapid, thin pulse.

It is corrected by adequate quantities of isotonic saline.

Retention is due to deficiency in the mechanism of elimination and is common in oedematous conditions. In addition, drugs such as cortisone, testosterone and stilboestrol tend to cause retention. The treatment is restriction of fluid intake and the use of diuretics.

Potassium

Depletion occurs in any illness in which there has been prolonged discharge like a fistula, paralytic ileus, or severe diarrhoea.

The clinical picture is one of apathy, drowsiness, loss of muscle power. The pulse is slow and full. The electrocardiogram shows characteristic changes.

The treatment is the administration of potassium salts.

They must always be given with caution and, if by the intravenous route, very slowly. There must be an adequate urinary output (at least 500 ml) before they are given at all.

Excess is particularly dangerous and is usually due to failure of elimination by the kidney. It occurs in conditions of:

Uraemia

Acidosis

The treatment is that of anuria (Ch. 42).

Fluid requirements

The amount of fluid the patient requires is:

Extrarenal loss	1000 ml
Add urinary loss	
Add pathological loss:	
1. Aspiration	
2. Fistula	
3. Drainage	
4. Diarrhoea	

Total fluid required in 24 hours

Fluid balance charts may be quite simple and all fluid must be measured in millilitres and totalled every 12 hours. The precise type of fluid to be given is determined by the clinical condition and the nature of the fluid lost. The state of the blood chemistry is only a rough guide in treatment and by no means helpful as a constant check. The more important normal levels are:

Serum	mmol/l
Na^+	136–144
K^+	3·4–4·5
Cl^-	95–105

Solutions

The more important solutions used in maintaining or correcting fluid and electrolyte balance are:

1. *Sodium chloride* (0·9 per cent) — Isotonic saline.
   Replaces Na^+ and Cl^-.
   150 mmol Na+ and 150 mmol Cl^- in a litre.
2. *Glucose* (5 per cent) — Isotonic.
   Replaces water.
3. *Hypertonic saline*
   Replaces Na^+ and Cl^- without water.
   Hypertonic saline (1·8 per cent) contains
   $$\left.\begin{array}{l} 154 \text{ mmol } Na^+ \\ 154 \text{ mmol } Cl^- \end{array}\right\} \text{ in 500 ml.}$$
4. *Potassium* — 5 ml 10 per cent pot. chloride w/v (13 mmol/l.)
   Added to 500 ml glucose (5 per cent).
   Replaces K^+.
5. *Compound sodium lactate solution injection BP* (formerly known as Hartman's solution) — Na^+ 131 mmol/l, Cl^- 111 mmol/l, K^+5 mmol/l and calcium lactate.
   Replaces Na^+, K^+, Cl^-, and corrects acidosis. It should be given slowly and not at all unless there is a satisfactory renal output.

THE MAINTENANCE OF NUTRITION

The maintenance of a good nutritional state presents a problem in patients who are unable to take ordinary diets by mouth. For short periods in patients who start off fit the problem is not important, as long as fluid and electrolyte balance is attended to, but the longer the inability to eat continues the more important it becomes. The patients particularly affected are long term respiratory cases, head injuries, laryngopharyngeal operations and cases of major abdominal surgery complicated by ileus, fistulae or sepsis.

The daily dietary requirements of the normal adult are:

Protein	80–100 g (provides 13–16·25 g of nitrogen)
Carbohydrates	400–500 g
Fats	80 g
Sodium	2–5 g
Potassium	2–5 g
Calcium	1 g

Trace elements — iodine, copper, manganese, zinc phosphorus and fluoride.

Calorie requirements 2500–3000 per day.

Nitrogen balance. A minimum of 40g of protein (6·59 g of nitrogen) is necessary to repair the normal breakdown of protein tissues in health. If the intake is below this level the individual is said to be in negative nitrogen balance and protein is mobilised from the body tissues which become wasted. A negative balance of 62·59 g of protein (equal to 10 g of nitrogen) causes a loss of 300 g of muscle. The estimation of the urinary nitrogen is a guide to the patient's requirements but if he has a fistula a further allowance is added for this source of protein loss.

Many diseases including burns produce a hypercatabolic state which may require up to 8000 calories per day. To ensure that protein is used to rebuild the tissues and not wasted as an energy (which fats and carbohydrates should supply) the percentage of protein to the total calorific value of the diet should be about 12·5 per cent.

Trace elements may be added when intravenous feeding is prolonged. Magnesium, which is necessary for enzyme formation may have to be given but most trace element deficiencies can be corrected by blood transfusions.

Methods of feeding

Two methods of feeding other than by mouth are available:

1. Intravenous

Until recently the only method of intravenous feeding was by the use of 5 per cent dextrose solution. In order to give enough calories excessive quantities of fluid are required and hence this was not entirely satisfactory. Emulsion of fats and solutions containing protein hydrolysates have been developed for intravenous use. These are much more satisfactory.

More recently fluids have been developed which are capable of providing a 3500 calorie diet within a fluid input of 2·5 to 3 l per day. The various solutions used include:

Aminosol 10 per cent (casein hydrolysate)

Aminosol/glucose

Aminosol/fructose/ethanol

Intralipid. Fat emulsion which is derived from the soya beans for intravenous use (10 and 20 per cent).

Aminoplex total feeding solutions.

Dextrose 50 per cent with insulin added may also be used.

It is important when patients are maintained on these solutions for long periods that vitamins and potassium (80 mmol/day) are added to the intravenous diet.

Finally the use of blood plasma as a means of restoring plasma proteins should not be forgotten. It may be used in above normal concentrations for this purpose.

Indwelling venous catheters are an important cause of hospital acquired septicaemia which is frequent after catheterisation of the large veins when this route is used for feeding. Sepsis is more frequent if blood is withdrawn through the catheter and if infection is to be kept to a minimum it must be used for no purpose other than to administer parenteral nutrition. (Ryan 1974).

2. By gastric tube

While the recent innovations in intravenous feeding have produced satisfactory methods they still involve intravenous infusions which have many hazards (upsets of fluid balance—infection—thrombosis of vessels). They are also extremely expensive. Therefore intragastric feeding has become popular for any patient who is unable to take oral food, but who has an intact and functioning gut. In this form of feeding a tube is passed via the oesophagus into the stomach and 60 ml of water are put down it hourly until it is established that the stomach is emptying normally. Then fluid diet is passed into the stomach at appropriate intervals—usually 2, 3 or 4 hourly or by a continuous drip.

Diets may be made up of eggs, milk, protein, hydrolysates and sugar, but unless great care is taken these tend to cause intractable diarrhoea.

A satisfactory method is to take the ordinary ward meals, complete with bread, butter and fish and chips not forgetting the salt and the sugar in the tea, and put it all into a liquidiser together with an appropriate amount of water. The resultant thin gruel is then passed down the intragastric tube using a funnel. Three main feeds a day (or more if required) may be given. Volumes of 300 ml per feed are acceptable to most patients. Additional in-between feeds of fluids will bring the total fluid intake up to 2·5 to 3 litres. Following severe trauma this method may fail to supply the very high calorie requirements of such patients. If this is so, intravenous feeding will have to be resorted to.

Tube feeding should proceed very cautiously until it is established that it is well tolerated. Unless the mixture is maintained at an osmolarity of 300 ml/l severe diarrhoea may result. In all forms of artificial feeding a fluid balance chart is kept and daily serum electrolyte estimation under taken.

Alternatively the longer arm of a double barrelled nasogastric tube can be threaded into the small intestine at operation and the patient fed from the first postoperation day.

Nourishment may be provided by:

1. *Elemental diet* which consists of amino acids, glucose, fats (as tri-glyceride) trace elements and vitamins. It is easily absorbed, leaves no residue and does not stimulate the secretion of gastric, pancreatic, intestinal juice or bile. It is useful in the presence of a fistula, short bowel syndromes and chronic pancreatitis. It is also useful in the preoperative preparation for intestinal surgery because it leaves no residue.

2. *Diet constituted in the hospital* is cheaper and suitable for any patient who is unable to take oral food but has an intact and functioning gut.

BIBLIOGRAPHY

Ryan J A et al 1974 New England Journal of Medicine 290: 757

16

Fluid administration

The administration of fluids is amongst the most arduous tasks the nurse can undertake. The safest and simplest route of all is by drinking. This requires:

>A cooperative conscious patient
>A normal alimentary tract
>Adequate renal function.

In these circumstances no real problem arises although occasionally gentle persuasion is required. Fluids consumed by drinking are absorbed in the lower small intestine and proximal colon, and normal excretion occurs from the kidney.

There are two main routes by which fluids may be given:

1. **Enteral** (by the gut). This includes:
   (a) Drinking.
   (b) By nasogastric tube; the lower end of the tube is in the body of the stomach.
   (c) By gastrostomy or jejunostomy.
   (d) Rectal administration.

2. **Parenteral** (by the side of the gut—which means that the fluid does not traverse the intestinal mucous membrane to reach the circulation). This includes the following methods of administration:
   (a) Subcutaneously.
   (b) Intravenously.
   (c) Intra-arterially.
   (d) Intramedullary.

ENTERAL ADMINISTRATION

Drinking

Provided the patient is conscious the nurse can do much to increase the intake if this is desirable, but she must never attempt to pour fluid into the mouth of a patient whose cough reflex is absent. It will flow into the lungs with disastrous effects.

Nasogastric tube

This may be used for a patient who has difficulty in co-operating but it is essential to ensure that the tube is in the stomach (and not coiled in the mouth or trachea) prior to feeding. This is done by aspirating a small amount before the feed and testing it with litmus paper which will turn red to indicate the presence of acid.

Gastrostomy and jejunostomy

Gastrostomy is performed in the management of infants with oesophageal atresia. A temporary jejunostomy is a little commoner. The advantage is that a wider variety of nourishment may be given than is possible by parenteral routes.

The jejunum will absorb large quantities of fluid which have been withdrawn by gastric or duodenal suction, but the extra volume of fluid which can be given should be limited to 1500 ml in 24 hours. The best method of feeding is by a continuous intrajejunal drip. Aspirated fluid should be filtered before being replaced and additional fluid which is given should be rich in carbohydrate, contain fat emulsion of small particle size, and ordinary salt is best avoided. Considerable trial and error has to be undertaken with the exact mixture of the food if severe diarrhoea, which is one of the great troubles of this type of feeding, is to be avoided.

Rectal fluids

Rectal fluids which may be administered as a single injection of 400 ml or repeated injections of 200 ml four-hourly have been largely abandoned. They may be of value in exceptional conditions where medical assistance is not available.

PARENTERAL ROUTES

The intravenous route is the usual one for parenteral administration. The intramedullary or subcutaneous ones are used only very occasionally while intra-arterial methods demand the continued presence of the doctor for the short time they are used. Their use is quite exceptional.

Blood, plasma, plasma substitute, and a wide variety of fluids for artificial feeding and the correction of electrolyte imbalance are administered by an intravenous cannula.

The type and amount of fluid required is discussed in detail in Chapter 15. This is a complex and comparatively advanced study but in this section discussion is confined to the care necessary during administration and the complications which may arise. It should be read in conjunction with the section on blood transfusion in Chapter 12.

The infusion is usually given into a vein in the forearm or hand by using the standard blood transfusion gravity set. If intravenous therapy is to be prolonged, or highly irritant solutions have to be used, a Teflon catheter is passed into one of the vena cavae. This may necessitate open infusion but more often percutaneous puncture is used.

The veins of choice are those near the hand and this has the following advantages:

(a) The patient's joints, particularly the elbow, are not immobilised.

(b) The more proximal veins are intact should further infusion be necessary.

All containers for use should be sealed and labelled with the nature and strength of the solution. If full volume is not present, then a crack must be suspected and this, as well as debris or solid matter in the flask, is an indication to abandon it. Modern practice tends to rely more on fluids supplied in flexible plastic containers. The batch and the container number should be noted in the case sheet.

The danger of plasma — that hepatitis due to a virus may be transmitted to the patient — has now been overcome by using plasma protein fraction (PPF) (Ch. 12).

To overcome the disadvantage of the danger of hepatitis from plasma, many plasma substitutes have been developed. They include:

(a) Dextran, a polysaccharide of high molecular weight.

(b) Rheomacrodex, which has the property of preventing 'sludging' of red cells and increases blood flow through the capillaries. It is a dextran of medium molecular weight.

(c) Haemaccel, a 3·5 per cent colloidal infusion solution containing gelatin.

Dextran maintains blood pressure if blood is not available, and the number of patients surviving when it is given instead of plasma closely approximates. The amount should be limited to three bags or bottles (540 ml each). Because of its anticoagulant effect, it is liable to cause some aggregation of the red cells and 10 ml of blood should be withdrawn and kept from every patient about to receive dextran. This enables blood grouping and cross-matching to be carried out with the usual technical ease should blood transfusion be called for in the next few days.

If the cause of shock is blood loss, blood has to be administered instead of plasma.

Intravenous infusion

Equipment required:

I.V.-giving set

Mediswabs

Selection of i.v. needles and cannulae

Syringe and needles

Sterile towels

Gauze swabs

Adhesive tape, Elastoplast

Appropriate fluid, e.g. normal saline

Splint

Crêpe bandage

Receiver

Fluid balance chart
Local anaesthetic, syringe and needles
Intravenous infusion stand
Tourniquet
Sphygmomanometer
Blood filters if large transfusions are contemplated.

The patient is informed of the procedure and his co-operation obtained. Privacy is ensured. He is given an opportunity to empty his bladder. The site is shaved if necessary.

The apparatus is taken to the bedside, preferably on a trolley. The site is exposed, usually the arm the patient uses least frequently. The arm is removed from the pyjama/gown sleeve. The patient is made comfortable and kept warm.

The doctor or nurse primes the giving set, fluid being caught in the receiver and air excluded. He applies the tourniquet, perhaps using the sphygmomanometer for this purpose. Using the aseptic technique, he introduces the needle and cannula into the vein. The cannula is advanced into the vein and the needle is withdrawn. He attaches the giving set to the cannula and ensures the fluid is flowing. The cannula is secured in position by adhesive tape. The limb may be lightly bandaged to a splint, taking care not to obstruct the flow.

The patient is made comfortable and the used equipment cleared away. The doctor prescribes the fluid to be given and the rate of flow. Whilst the infusion is in progress the nurse observes the rate of flow, the presence of fluid in the drip chamber/airlock, the amount of fluid remaining in the container, the giving set, the position and coverings of the cannula, the patient's arm and his general condition.

When the container is changed, two nurses check the fluid to be given. The guidelines on administration of parenteral infusion fluids are as follows:

The rate of infusion. This is determined by the doctor. The amount is determined by the size of the drops and the nurse should read the graduation of drops per millilitre on the package supplied with the set. In many sets 15 drops make 1 ml. Therefore a rate of 30 drops per minute will infuse just under 3 litres in 24 hours.

Complications

Thrombophlebitis. All solutions are mildly irritant to the wall of the vein. Its incidence is diminished by:
(a) Atraumatic vein puncture.
(b) Maintaining asepsis.
(c) Limiting the time any one vein is used, ideally not more than eight hours but in practice usually 24–48 hours.
(d) Giving specially irritant solutions by caval catheter.
(e) Changing the giving set regularly.

Extravasation of fluid into the tissue is due to the point of the cannula slipping out of the vein. The infusion usually stops and some swelling of the tissues occurs. The cannula is removed and the puncture wound dressed. Special care is required if an irritant solution is being infused. Extravasation causes necrosis of the tissues. Some antibiotic solutions such as the tetracyclines and cytotoxic agents may produce this effect.

As soon as possible fluids are taken by mouth, which is the natural and best route of all. If the patient is co-operative he takes just the right quantity. The dangers of the artificial routes are:

(a) Excess of fluid may be given, resulting in pulmonary oedema.

(b) Too little fluid is taken, causing water depletion.

(c) The wrong type of fluid may be given.

(d) Infection may be introduced or thrombosis may occur in the vein.

Contamination of intravenous fluid was extensively investigated by the Clothier Committee, and the fundamental cause of disease was found to be human failing ranging from simple carelessness to poor management of men and plant. In particular:

1. A bottle or bag which looks suspicious should not be accepted.

2. Defaced labels, loose collars, weeping from the bung, and turbidity or opalescence in the fluid render the contents suspect.

The Control of Infection Officer should be informed and stocks in the pharmacy should be immobilised pending investigation if any of the above defects is discovered in a single container.

Unit of measurement of fluid. This is expressed in the metric system. A one-thousandth part of a litre is a millilitre (ml).

17

Respiratory failure

Respiration is the process whereby the tissues are provided with oxygen (O_2) and carbon dioxide (CO_2) is eliminated. There are certain basic requirements:

1. A mechanically efficient bellows consisting of the ribs, and the muscles of respiration (i.e. the intercostals and diaphragm) with an airtight chest wall and a clear passage to the outside air through the trachea, the largnx, the mouth and the nose.

2. Enough sound lung to oxygenate the blood which passes through it and at the same time to eliminate all the carbon dioxide (CO_2) from the blood.

3. An adequate circulation of blood through the lungs and the rest of the body to carry the gases.

4. The central mechanism in the brain which controls respiratory efforts must be working and the nervous pathways from this to the muscles it controls must be intact. This centre initiates rhythmic impulses which drive the muscles of respiration and is situated in the medulla oblongata. It is sensitive to chemical changes in the blood (e.g. excess of carbon dioxide and lack of oxygen) and adjusts the rate and depth of respiration to maintain normal blood levels of those substances.

RESPIRATORY FAILURE

Respiratory failure may occur if any or all of these mechanisms are destroyed or deranged to a sufficient extent to prevent them carrying out their function.

Defects of the bellows mechanism. The bellows mechanism may be put out of action. Causes of this are:

1. Extensive fractures of the bony thoracic cage.

2. Tears in the chest wall, allowing the pleural cavity to communicate with the atmosphere and hence preventing the normal lowering of intrathoracic pressure associated with inspiration which sucks air into the lungs.

3. Paralysis of the muscles of respiration may occur due to overdosage

with muscle relaxant drugs (often used in anaesthesia), poisoning with organic phosphorus insecticides, or in myasthenia gravis.

4. Obstruction of the airway may prevent the bellows from sucking in air. This is often due to foreign bodies, sputum, secretions or trauma to the air passages or the face.

Inadequacy of lung tissue. An inadequacy of lung tissue is due either to disease, chronic bronchitis and emphysema, pneumonia, tuberculosis, carcinoma of the bronchus, pneumoconiosis, etc., or to destruction of lung tissue by surgery, irritant gases or chemicals. An example of the latter is the destruction of lung tissue caused by poisonous gases such as chlorine.

Inadequate circulation of blood. Inadequate circulation of blood may occur from heart failure or sometimes due to vascular accidents such as emboli or thrombosis within the lungs themselves.

Central failure. The central mechanism may fail from a number of causes—trauma to the skull, narcotics or toxins. The nervous pathways from the centre to the muscles may be interrupted either by injury as in cervical fractures or by disease such as poliomyelitis.

CYANOSIS

Cyanosis is a violet or sometimes a greyish colour of the skin produced by abnormally large amounts of reduced haemoglobin or less frequently by abnormal pigments such as methaemoglobin or sulphhaemoglobin.

It may be:
1. Central
(a) Arterial blood is insufficiently saturated with oxygen because the air passages are obstructed, the respiratory muscles are paralysed or a portion of the lungs is out of action from collapse or pneumonia.
(b) Blood is shunted from the pulmonary vein to the pulmonary artery without exposure to the alveoli.
2. Peripheral. The arterial blood flow in the tissues is slowed by vasoconstriction and cyanosis occurs because of the large amount of time available in the tissues for gaseous interchange. Shock and Raynaud's Disease (Chs. 14 and 23) are conditions in which this may occur.

TREATMENT

The principles underlying the treatment of all forms of respiratory failure are the same. The cardinal rule is to ensure that the lungs are ventilated efficiently by whatever means are available.

First in order to ventilate the lungs a clear airway via the mouth or nose and trachea to the lungs must be ensured. Therefore foreign bodies, secretions, etc. are removed and the tongue and jaw must be held forward in the unconscious patient. Artificial respiration is commenced. The most efficient and only really satisfactory method of doing this as a first aid measure is by mouth to mouth or mouth to nose respiration. By this method the patient's lungs are inflated by the nurse blowing through his mouth or nostrils — then they are allowed to deflate again by their own elasticity.

Mouth to mouth or mouth to nose breathing

Firstly the air passages must be cleared of any obstruction. The occiput should rest on a surface in the same plane as the patient's shoulders and buttocks and the patient's neck is extended from the normal lying position so that the tongue does not fall back and close the glottis. A special airway (Brook's), or, alternatively, a handkerchief to fit over the lips can be used if contact with the patient's mouth is undesirable.

Many favour mouth to nose instead of mouth to mouth, but for the less expert it is probably easier to nip the nose than to keep the patient's mouth closed. If a 'bag mask' type of inflating unit is available it can be used only if the operator is quite sure that she has the necessary skill.

As soon as possible this method of maintaining gaseous exchange ought to be replaced by some sort of formal artificial ventilation of the lungs.

Artificial ventilation

This may be accomplished by passing an endotracheal tube into the trachea and inflating the lungs with air or oxygen either manually, using a rubber bag, or, better, by one of the many machines available.

All mechanical lung ventilators work by intermittently blowing respirable gases into the patient's lungs. The lungs deflate by virtue of their own elasticity. Such a machine is the Manley ventilator which is driven by compressed gas. Other varieties are powered by electric motors.

The more sophisticated machines not only blow air or oxygen into the lungs but may also suck it out actively. Some of these more advanced machines, such as the Elema-Servo ventilator, have what is known as a patient-triggering device which enables them to assist the inadequate efforts of a partially paralysed patient without his attempts to breathe conflicting with the work of the machine.

All mechanical ventilators must be equipped with efficient humidifiers so that the inspired gas is saturated with water vapour. These may be devices rather like an electric kettle in which the gas is passed over hot water or may be nebulisers, either mechanical or ultrasonic. Some such as the Bennett cascade may also be heated. If the inspired gases are not rendered wet the patient's tracheal and pulmonary secretions dry up and are difficult to remove and may even crust on the tracheal mucosa.

It is essential that all equipment used in mechanical ventilation should be sterile before use. Accessories such as endotracheal and tracheostomy tubes are sterilised by steam or radiation. (Ethylene oxide should be used with care as it may become trapped between the layers of rubber — only to be liberated later when the tube is in use).

The ventilator itself should have its working parts sterilised by ultrasonically nebulised alcohol (70 per cent solution), ethylene oxide gas or suitable chemical solutions, or should be autoclaved.

Ventilators should be fitted with bacterial filters on both their inspiratory and expiratory tubes. These should be autoclaved frequently and always before the machine is used on a new patient. It is important to ensure that these filters do not become waterlogged during use as this may give rise to respiratory obstruction. Waterlogging may be avoided by siliconising the filter or by heating it.

If the use of a mechanical ventilator is expected to last for more than 48 hours it is often considered desirable to carry out a tracheostomy and inflate the patient's lungs via this route.

The reasons are:

1. Prolonged presence of an endotracheal tube in the larynx may cause sloughing with subsequent stenosis. An endotracheal Lanz tube with its overpressure safety is mandatory for prolonged use or when a cuffed tracheostomy tube is required.
2. It enables the attendant to remove secretions from the bronchial tree with great ease. This is accomplished with the aid of a suction machine and catheter (Fig. 17.1).
3. The shortening of the air passages which accompanies tracheostomy lowers their resistance to infection and helps the elimination of carbon dioxide (CO_2).
4. The patient may in fact find a tracheostomy less distressing.

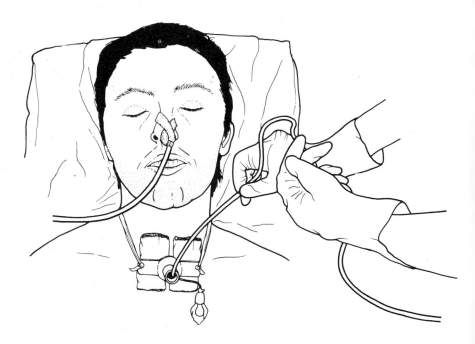

Fig. 17.1 Suction through the tracheostomy tube. The nasogastric tube is for feeding.

It is important that the nurse should understand the care of a tracheostomy. The tube which will be used for this type of patient is of plastic and has an inflatable cuff which prevents leakage of air from the trachea. The mechanical ventilator is attached to a swivel connection at the end of this tube. Whenever secretions accumulate in the tube or air passages they should be removed at once. After a suction session it is desirable to inflate the patient's lungs using a rubber bag as an inflating device.

It is impossible to overemphasise the importance of two factors in the care of a tracheostomy.

Firstly, every effort should be made to avoid introducing infection into the bronchial tree during the repeated bronchial toilets which must be carried out and, secondly, at all costs the inspired gases must be prevented from drying out the tracheal and pulmonary secretions.

Because the nose, which normally moistens the inspired air, has been bypassed patients breathing through a tracheostomy tube tend to get tenacious and viscous sputum which is hard to remove. This evil can be mitigated by humidifying all gas used in machines. Some rely on heat to saturate the gas with water vapour while others introduce an extremely finely divided spray of water into the gaseous stream. The Radcliffe humidifier is a good example of the first type. A more modern one is the Bennett cascade.

It is important to remember that whilst artificial ventilation by a machine will keep the patient alive almost indefinitely, machine failure which goes unobserved will kill him within minutes. Therefore machines should never be left unattended and manual means of inflation should always be immediately available for use in emergency.

Whilst mechanical ventilation is in progress the cause of the respiratory failure should be treated if this is possible. Infection is treated with antibiotics or the pressure on nerves caused by fractures is relieved.

Where a mechanical ventilator is in use the patient requires feeding. Some are able to take ordinary light diets, others need intragastric feeds. If they are lying very still in bed they ought to be gently rolled from one side to the other every 2 hours to prevent hypostatic pneumonia of the dependent parts of the lungs. Care of the pressure areas is important.

The services of well trained physiotherapists are essential.

TRACHEOSTOMY

Tracheostomy, or an artificial opening in the trachea, is necessary to relieve sudden laryngeal obstruction. In the very young nasotracheal intubation with a plastic Jackson-Rees tube is used rather than tracheostomy.

INDICATIONS FOR TRACHEOSTOMY

Obstructive conditions of the larynx

1. Acute oedema of the glottis. This may occur as a result of Ludwig's angina, carcinoma of the tongue, or as a result of a radium reaction inside the mouth.
2. Carcinoma of the larynx.
3. Foreign bodies impacted in the larynx.
4. Trauma.
5. Burns of the mouth or larynx.

6. Acute laryngitis particularly diphtheria; the diphtheritic membrane may block the airway completely.

Paralysis or spasm of the respiratory muscles and respiratory failure

1. Bulbar paralysis including poliomyelitis.
2. Tetanus and certain stages of coma, including some head injuries.

Some types of inability to maintain satisfactory blood gas levels during prolonged artificial ventilation

Such as respiratory failure due to lung damage — chronic bronchitis.

Haemorrhage into a cystadenoma of the thyroid gland is not an indication for tracheostomy but for laryngeal intubation followed by partial thyroidectomy.

The time for operation

The nurse must be familiar with the conditions in which a tracheostomy may be indicated, and once the possibility has arisen the instruments must be at hand and ready sterilised.

In a case of progressive respiratory obstruction a tracheostomy is usually indicated when the accessory muscles of respiration commence to be used, namely, the alae nasi and the sternomastoid. Recession of the epigastrium is also present. The patient is usually cyanosed, and the accompanying mental stress is very considerable.

Artificial respiration will not be of the slightest use should the patient collapse, because he has not a free airway, and collapse due to respiratory obstruction is an indication for lightning speed in effecting an artificial opening.

The operation

If the patient is collapsed and no instruments are at hand a penknife has, on occasion, been successfully used, and the nurse must bear in mind that of all instruments necessary in this grave emergency a knife is the most important. The patient's head must be kept well extended over a pillow or sandbag.

After the opening has been made in the trachea a tracheostomy tube, to which two tapes are attached, is inserted. The tapes must be tied immediately at the side of the patient's neck in a knot and bow. If they are tied at the back of the patient's neck they are uncomfortable to lie on, inaccessible and may be untied by mistake if the gown is also fastened by tapes. If a ventilator is to be used a cuffed plastic tube is essential.

Postoperative treatment

The patient is exhausted and dozes off to sleep. He should be laid flat in bed, rolled from side to side hourly to promote drainage and exudate should be sucked from the tracheostomy tube. When he awakens he should be propped up and kept in this position for 48 hours. If metal tracheostomy tubes have been used the inner tube will require frequent removal and a supply of autoclaved tubes should be available.

Deep breathing exercises are carried out under the direction of a physiotherapist. A suction machine must be available to enable the nurse to clear secretions from the airway, together with a supply of sterile suction

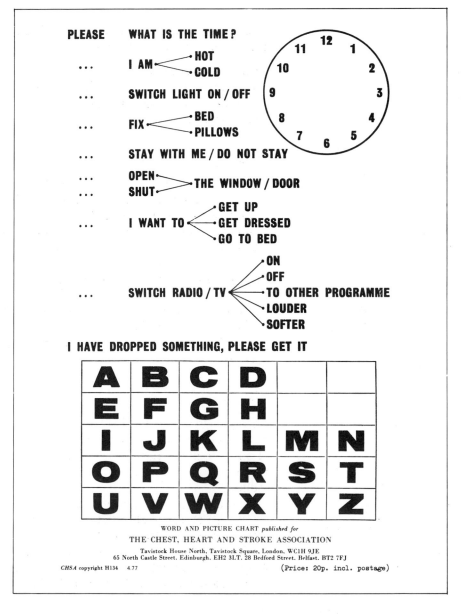

Fig. 17.2 On a table within reach of the patient is a word and picture chart, a bell, a pencil and writing pad.
(Illustration by courtesy of the Chest, Heart and Stroke Association).

catheters. Personnel should be trained in the methods used to avoid introducing infection into the trachea. Humidified oxygen may be administered via a tracheostomy mask. A pair of tracheal dilators must be always at hand in case the tube is coughed or pulled out, and a pair of scissors to cut the tapes in case the outer tube becomes blocked. A spare correctly fitting tube should be available. Gentle handling is essential as the posterior wall of the trachea is very thin and easily eroded.

All these measures are designed to prevent pneumonia, which is a very likely complication.

Swallowing may be difficult but small amounts of fluid can usually be taken. If the patient is very thirsty fluids may be given parenterally.

If the case is one of carcinoma of the larynx a tracheostomy will be permanent, but in other cases the tube is removed when the cause of the obstruction has subsided. In children, removal of the tube may be followed by considerable fright because the voice is absent *unless the wound is completely covered.*

RULES FOR TRACHEOSTOMY MANAGEMENT

The following rules are essential:
1. Scrub the hands, wear sterile disposable gloves and a mask.
2. Use prepacked sterile disposable catheters.
3. Do not allow the catheter to touch *anything* before aspirating the trachea.
4. Discard the catheter after aspiration.
5. Replace the inner tube as required. A supply of autoclaved inner tubes should be available.
6. Clean the tracheostomy wound and renew the dressing regularly. A keyhole gauze dressing is used.
7. Micro-organisms live everywhere and may kill if introduced into the bronchi. *Escherichia coli, Klebsiella bacilli* and *Pseudomonas aeruginosa* are the most common.
8. Always inflate the lungs after a suction session.
9. The use of a word chart (Fig. 17.2) to enable the patient to communicate.

CARE OF A PATIENT WITH A TRACHEOSTOMY

The following articles should be kept at the bedside:
Sterile tracheal dilators
Selection of sterile suction catheters
Sterile disposable gloves
Suction machine with half an inch of Savlon 0·5 per cent in the suction
  bottle
Bowl of Savlon 0·5 per cent
Brown wax bag
Small gallipot containing small amount of sterile normal saline to act as

a lubricant. This sterile normal saline is removed from the container using a sterile syringe and needle.

The tracheostomy tube is held in position by tapes, which are tied at the side of the patient's neck.

The tube is sucked out whenever necessary, but at least at 2-hourly intervals. Disposable gloves are put on. The packet containing the catheter is cut at the wide end of the catheter, which is connected to the pressure tubing of the suction machine. The wrapper is removed. The catheter is nipped in order to prevent suction, and dipped into the normal saline in order to lubricate it.

The tracheostomy tube is steadied and the catheter inserted not more than 4 inches. It is released to allow suction, turned, and slowly withdrawn while turning. Should it be necessary, the catheter can be reinserted once only.

When a Y-shaped connection is used, the side-arm can be opened or covered to prevent or allow suction.

After withdrawal the catheter is washed through with Savlon 0·5 per cent. It is disconnected and discarded into the brown wax bag. The pressure tubing is fixed to the handle of the suction machine using a bulldog clip. The gloves are removed and discarded into the brown wax bag.

Ideally the suction session should be attended by an anaesthetist who together with the nurse form a team and engage in what is known as 'bagging and sucking', an exercise designed to remove as much moist secretion as possible and in a way that will reduce the risk of infection and post-suction lung collapse.

Care of the tube

A cuffed tube requires attention at intervals, e.g. 2-hourly or as otherwise instructed. The pharynx is sucked out especially if the patient is not swallowing. The tracheostomy tube is sucked out using another catheter. The cuff is released for 2 minutes and then reinflated (Fig. 17.3).

The inner tube of a metal tube is removed, e.g. 2-hourly, and the outer tube sucked out. The inner tube is washed in sodium bicarbonate, and is sterilised in special Savlon or by boiling and reinserted.

The wound is cleaned as required, e.g. 4-hourly, using a suitable antiseptic aseptic technique. A gauze swab may be placed under the tube if necessary.

Emergency. If the tube becomes dislodged and the patient is having difficulty in breathing, the tapes holding the tube are cut, the tracheal dilator inserted and held open to allow entry of air. Assistance is called for. The tracheostomy may require to be sucked out.

OXYGEN THERAPY

Air contains about 20 per cent of oxygen. This is adequate to saturate the haemoglobin of the blood in a patient whose respiratory and circulatory systems are normal. In many surgical conditions the respiratory and cardiovascular systems have suffered from severe interference. The result is that the circulating haemoglobin is reduced in amount or is inadequately saturated with oxygen. For this reason the percentage of oxygen in the inspired air has to be increased.

The indication for use is hypoxia (deficient oxygen in the blood from any cause). The distress of respiratory failure is often really due to CO_2 retention, not to lack of oxygen.

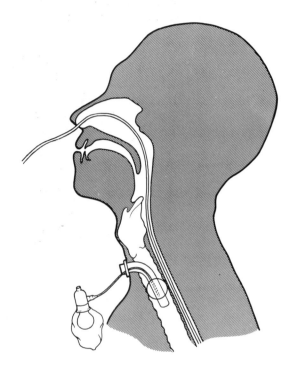

Fig. 17.3 The cuff of the tube fills the trachea when inflated. Its deflation for two minutes two hourly relieves pressure on the softer posterior wall of the the trachea and prevents ulceration. (See also Fig. 28.10.)

CAUSES OF HYPOXIA

   1. Respiratory obstruction. This includes all conditions in which the normal exchange of gases in the lungs is impeded:
   (a) Laryngeal obstruction.
   (b) Laryngeal spasm.
   (c) Pneumonia.
   (d) Collapse of the lungs.
   (e) Pneumothorax.
   2. Shock and heart failure. Stagnant anoxia.
   3. Diminished oxygen-carrying capacity. Anaemia due to haemorrhage being the most important surgically.
   4. Increased oxygen consumption, such as continuous hyperpyrexia.

It is important to stress that the decreased respiratory movements which occur postoperatively may be due to:

(a) The effects of the anaesthetic not having worn off.
(b) Bandages being too tight and impeding respiratory movement. The patient whose chest is 'crushed' should nevertheless be tightly bandaged in order to stabilise the thoracic cage.
(c) Pain.

These may be indications for assisted respiration or analgesics rather than a supply of oxygen.

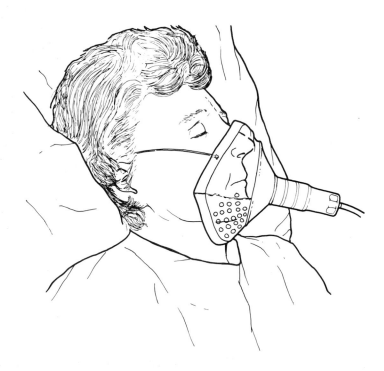

Fig. 17.4 Disposable oxygen Ventimask.

Oxygen is supplied in cylinders at a pressure of 13 800 kPa (2000 lb/in²; 6·9 kPa, or kilopascals, = 1 lb/in²) or possibly by a pipeline from a central depot. A reducing valve brings this pressure down to 34·5 kPa and a flowmeter is attached which measures the quantity of oxygen delivered in litres per minute.

Oxygen may be administered by:

1. *A face piece* — (a) the ordinary mask of an anaesthetic machine, (b) the polythene mask (Fig. 17.4).
2. *Nasal inhalation* — (a) nasal mask such as a Polymask, (b) nasal tube, nasal spectacles or a nasal catheter.
3. *Oxygen tent* — The oxygen tent has been largely abandoned. It is hot, septic and the concentration of oxygen is frequently inadequate.
4. *Incubator* for newborn hypoxic cases.

Method of administration

Pure oxygen is administered until the patient shows the maximal improvement. The oxygen is then gradually reduced and the patient's condition is satisfactory only when he can inhale air alone without any deterioration. The usual rate of administration is 4 l per minute. All oxygen should be moistened. The nose requires careful toilet if an indwelling catheter is being used and 0·1 per cent Hibitane in Xylocaine jelly is useful.

In patients such as chronic bronchitics who normally have a high blood carbon dioxide (P_{CO_2}) and low blood oxygen (P_{O_2}) care should be taken to limit oxygen flow to 4 litres of 24 per cent oxygen per min to avoid total suppression of respiration or to use one of the special masks such as the Ventimask which restricts the inspired oxygen content to 24 or 28 per cent.

Special precautions to be taken with oxygen therapy

There are no toxic changes in the fully formed tissues from a concentration of up to 70 per cent oxygen. Retrolental fibroplasia is a danger in premature infants.

The most important danger is that of fire. This is increased by:

1. Greasing the valve.
2. Smoking, the use of a naked light or electric toys.
3. The use of spirit or ether for the treatment of the patient.
4. The production of static electricity — for example by too active bed-making or nylon clothing.

Before connecting up the oxygen supply, grit should be blown out. When the oxygen cylinder is empty it should be removed and marked accordingly. If 'piped' oxygen is used the nurse must know where the cut-off valves are situated outside the room or ward in case of fire.

Details of administration of oxygen

The doctor ordering that oxygen shall be given to a patient, should indicate the means of administration and the rate of flow. Many devices are available for this purpose, e.g.:

Nasal spectacles
Ventimask
Edinburgh mask

In emergency, until the arrival of the doctor the nurse may give oxygen using the nasal spectacles with the rate of flow adjusted to 4 litres per minute.

The procedure is explained to the patient, and his co-operation obtained. The nostrils are cleaned using a wool swab held in sinus forceps and moistened in sodium bicarbonate solution. After use the swab is removed with dissecting forceps and discarded.

The nurse checks that oxygen is flowing from the piped supply. She fills the humidifier (nebuliser) with distilled water up to the level of the mark. The apparatus is connected and the flow of oxygen related to the prescribed rate. The spectacles or mask are placed in position. The patient is made comfortable. Observations are made on the effects of the oxygen on the patient's colour, breathing and general condition.

When oxygen is being administered intermittently, on the same patient, the spectacles or mask are stored in a clean paper bag attached to the locker, until next required.

The spectacles or mask and length of tubing are changed after 24 hours or more frequently as necessary. Being disposable they are discarded.

When the administration of oxygen is discontinued, the spectacles, mask and length of tubing are discarded. The humidifier is emptied, washed in Savlon 0·5 per cent, rinsed and dried, and placed back in position near the flow meter until required again.

When an oxygen cylinder is used, it is prepared and turned on outside the ward. The assembled apparatus consists of:

Cylinder with reducing valve, gauge and flow meter
Humidifier
Appropriate tubing
Appropriate means of administration.

Hyperbaric oxygen therapy

A tiny amount of oxygen is dissolved in the blood plasma. This amount can be considerably increased if the patient is placed in a chamber and oxygen is administered at a pressure of 2 atmospheres. (Oxygen at a greater pressure than that of the atmosphere is described as hyperbaric.) This may be of value in saving a threatened limb. There is a specially devised bed which avoids the necessity of a pressure chamber. It has been used before megavoltage radiotherapy to increase the response to treatment. It is also used for patients in severe shock, for enhancing the chances of 'take' in extensive skin graft, in the treatment of gas gangrene and in combating carbon monoxide poisoning. Paradoxically the development of North Sea gas, which contains no carbon monoxide, has reduced the need for hyperbaric oxygen as a treatment for gas poisoning but increased the demand for hyperbaric facilities in hospitals close to off-shore rigs because of the conditions of pressure in which divers work.

INTENSIVE CARE UNITS

An intensive care unit is one where there is the concentration of skill, equipment and staff required for the treatment or resuscitation of a seriously ill patient. The object is to maintain the highest level of medical and nursing care by day and by night. The essential features are:

1. Structure

Extensive floor space per patient is necessary and easy access all around the patient's bed should be provided. There should be good observation of the patient from a centrally placed panel. Exceptionally extensive electrical provisions are made for portable X-rays as well as for respirators, suction machines and monitoring apparatus. At the nurse's station are telephones and light indicators for night use, switches for the control of lighting and indicators relating to piped oxygen, suction and emergency electricity generation.

2. Equipment

This is necessarily on a lavish scale. The nurse cannot be expected to know how everything works but she should know what she may or may not do with it, whether it is working and what measures to take if it ceases to function. The most efficient suction machine will not function if the top of the reservoir is not fitted in an airtight manner! All the equipment necessary and already discussed in the sections on acute circulatory and respiratory failure must be available. A small laboratory near by is an essential.

Because of the ever-present danger of cross-infection, facilities for the total isolation of very clean from 'very dirty' patients are an essential feature of all modern intensive care units.

3. Staff

To afford complete 24-hour coverage a three-shift system of duty is required with an average of five trained nurses and supporting nursing auxiliaries or ward orderly staff for each patient.

The types of condition for which patients are admitted vary enormously. They may be postoperative conditions, severe road accidents, coal-gas poisoning, frost-bite, myocardial infarction or cerebral thrombosis. Most will have some degree of respiratory, circulatory or metabolic disturbance. In addition to specialised procedures to counteract these conditions all patients require good basic nursing care. Careful records, attention to general and oral hygiene are as important as elsewhere in the hospital.

CONTROL OF RESUSCITATIVE THERAPY

The control of resuscitative therapy, amongst which may be included oxygen, mechanical ventilation and the correction of acid base disturbances, is often achieved by reference to blood gas estimations. These are carried out on arterial blood taken into heparinised syringes. Specimens which cannot be examined at once should be refrigerated.

The normal values are:

pH   7·4

Standard bicarbonate 25 mmol per litre

P_{CO_2} 5·4 kPa
P_{O_2} 13·3 kPa

Collection of specimens

Taking blood for estimation of blood gases.
On a tray is placed:
    A receiver
    Heparin 5000 units per ml
    Syringe 5 ml
    Needle size 21 × 1½
    Wax carton of ice
    Strapping
    Red caps
    Mediswabs
    Packet of gauze swabs
A piece of strapping with the patient's name written on it is attached to the barrel of the syringe.

The doctor takes the blood from the patient's femoral artery. He removes the needle. He fixes a red cap to the nozzle of the syringe. He gently rotates the syringe. It is plunged into the wax carton of ice. It is taken immediately to the unit laboratory. The nurse maintains digital pressure on a gauze swab over the femoral artery puncture for at least 5 minutes and continues observation for several hours for signs of haemorrhage.

18

Burns and scalds

Burns are caused by dry heat and scalds by moist heat. Burns are always more serious than scalds of the same extent. The clinical features and treatment are identical, and four out of five are the result of accidents in the home.

In practice it is necessary to decide whether or not the full thickness of the skin has been destroyed; if it has, skin grafting is necessary. The degree or depth of the burn is that of its deepest part. Modern classification recognises only two degrees of burns.

1. Destruction of the epidermis (the superficial layer of the skin). Healing can occur from the epithelium in the deeper parts of the skin.

2. The whole thickness of the skin has been destroyed. Since healing can occur only from the edge of intact skin it would not only be slow but fibrosis in the open defect would cause contracture. Skin grafting is required as soon as possible. Figure 18.1 illustrates the two degrees of burns and also shows that because the cutaneous nerves are not destroyed in a superficial burn, pain is severe while a deep burn is painless. In doubtful cases the distinction may be made by using a needle point.

Causes

1. Dry heat — flame.
2. Moist heat — scalds.
3. Chemicals.
4. Electricity.
5. X-rays and radium.
6. Friction is an occasional cause.

CLINICAL FEATURES

The degree of general upset is proportional to the superficial extent of the damage rather than the depth of the burn.

1. Pain is usual, but is most marked in the more superficial burns because the sensory nerve endings in the skin are exposed. In deeper burns

they have usually been destroyed.

2. Shock is always present if the burns are moderately extensive, and in more extensive burns it is profound.

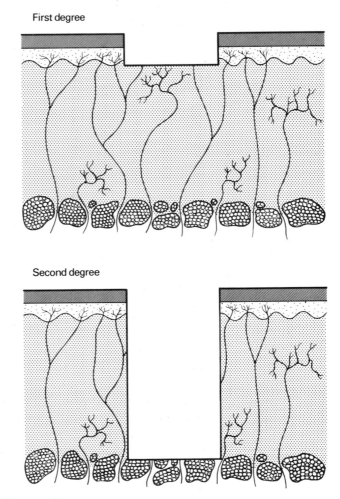

Fig. 18.1 Degrees of burns.

The treatment and nursing care of burns illness

The care of the burnt area cannot be discussed in isolation from the general and metabolic changes which result from burning. These changes are complicated and not completely understood. They vary with the extent of the burns and the general physical condition of the patient. The institution of special units for the treatment of major burns has greatly improved the end results. The advantages are a sterile air-conditioned warm atmosphere with staff wearing sterile dresses and shoes. Visitors wear gowns and overshoes — masks frighten children and are not usually worn. If a special unit is not available barrier nursing techniques are used and as in a special burns unit sterile bed linen should be provided.

The special features of burns illness are the prevention and treatment of shock, infection and other metabolic changes.

The restoration of function and the minimisation of deformity has to be borne in mind from the moment of admission.

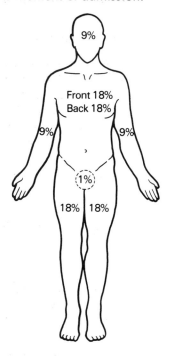

Fig. 18.2 Wallace's 'Rule of Nine' for estimating fluid requirements in the first 48 hours after burns.

1. The superficial extent of the burnt area is estimated on admission. The accompanying diagram from Wallace's 'Rules of Nine' (Fig. 18.2) is convenient. It is not often, of course, that the patient is burnt on the whole of the front of one arm or one leg so that another useful adjunct in the calculation is to assess an area covered by the surface of the patient's hand as 1 per cent. If the area exceeds 10 per cent in the child or 15 per cent in the adult the patient may die from circulatory collapse. Therefore burns of greater extent than this will require intravenous infusion.

2. Depth of the burn. Superficial and partial skin thickness burns will heal if sepsis is excluded. Deeper burns will require grafting. In the occasional areas where there has been complete charring of the limb amputation may be necessary.

3. Site. Certain additional measures may be necessary in some sites. For example, tracheostomy will be indicated where the mouth or air passages have been severely burnt, or, occasionally for a deep burn of the neck. A dorsal slit or circumcision may have to be performed for certain burns in the genital area. Large burns of the trunk or burns involving wide areas on both aspects of the leg are particularly difficult to nurse, and a special bed for nursing the patient is of value.

4. Age and general condition. The chances of a patient surviving severe burns will be greater in the previously fit and robust, than in the aged patient suffering from the chronic illness. Epileptics used to form a notable percentage of patients who are accidentally burnt, because they fall on the fire during a fit. However, this has diminished with the improvement in drugs used for the control of epileptic fits.

Management on admission

The patient should be admitted to a special resuscitation room and kept there until the danger of circulatory collapse has passed. He should be laid between sterile sheets and resuscitative measures are commenced at once by administering 500 ml of plasma (or plasma substitute) intravenously. In children an open infusion will normally be necessary and a nurse should have the necessary apparatus available. The first 500 ml may be given in a period of 5 minutes before any further observations have been made. Once the plasma is running the following records are made and repeated at quarter hourly intervals:
1. The rate of the pulse.
2. Blood pressure.
3. Temperature.
4. The central venous pressure.
Blood is taken for estimation of:
(a) The haemoglobin level.
(b) State of the electrolytes.
(c) Haematocrit reading. This reading is an indication of haemo-concentration — that is to say an estimate of the amount of plasma lost and, therefore, a guide in determining loss of blood volume.

Resuscitation

1. The amount of fluid. The total amount of fluid to be given is calculated and half this quantity is given in 8 hours and the remainder in 24 to 48 hours. The fluid loss each day may be as much as 5 litres from evaporation. If the urinary output is unsatisfactory Mannitol should be given at an early stage after initial fluid replacement. If it is effective there will be a diuresis within an hour. If there is not, then its use should not be proceeded with.

In children aged 0–9 years the percentage which each area forms of the total body surface is different from the adult. A chart of these percentages is available in all children's hospitals.

2. Type of fluid. Plasma (or plasma substitute) is of the first importance. Normal saline is also given to maintain electrolyte balance and, if there has been red blood corpuscle destruction, some whole blood is usually given. Many give one half of the saline-plasma requirements as blood.

3. The rate of infusion is determined by:
(a) Calculation of the total amount lost.
(b) Ensuring that urinary excretion is maintained (see below).
(c) Estimation of the central venous pressure.

4. Sedatives or analgesics are not always necessary, but if they are, they should be given intravenously.

5. Stopping the transfusion. This is never stopped before 24 hours and usually continued for 48 hours. The transfusion is continued until the blood tests show that stability has been achieved with very little fluid loss in the previous four hours, that is to say that the blood pressure, haematocrit and haemoglobin levels are maintained with the administration of not more than about 500 ml of fluid in this period.

Maintenance of urinary excretion

Special care is necessary to observe the volume of urinary secretion which may be diminished due to shock.

1. An indwelling catheter is inserted into the bladder and the amount of urine excreted hourly is measured. If it falls below 60 ml in the adult or 30 ml in the child the rate of the drip is increased until the central venous pressure reaches 15 cm of water.
2. If the patient is able, drinking is encouraged; if vomiting occurs nasogastric aspiration is necessary instead.
3. The urine is examined for the presence of normal and abnormal contents as well as for specific gravity.
4. The blood urea is estimated.
5. A fluid balance chart is kept.

Care of the burnt areas

The principal object is the prevention of infection and covering the burnt area with skin as soon as possible. Superficial and partial skin thickness burns will heal if infection is excluded. Deeper burns require skin grafting. Special measures to be undertaken are:

1. Bacteriological. After admission swabs are taken from all burnt areas separately as a control and at regular intervals afterwards.

2. The danger of tetanus in burns should not be overlooked and the patients immunity should be checked and brought up to date if necessary.

3. Maintenance of asepsis is very important and all in attendance must wear caps, masks, gowns and overshoes. Sterile bed linen is used. Local cleansing is not undertaken until the patient's condition is satisfactory but preferably undertaken within 12 hours under analagesia such as morphia. It consists of snipping away dead skin and cleansing with a mixture of Cetavlon and Hibitane known as Savlon 0·5 per cent. The surface is then dried with warm air or sterile towels. After this the burnt area may be treated by:

(a) *Exposure method*. The object of this method is to obtain and maintain a dry surface after cleansing with a detergent and drying with a hair drier if necessary.

Some surgeons advise that *no* antibiotic powder is used.

The sloughs are excised and grafting is performed as soon as possible in second-degree burns. The optimum time is 24 hours—if this is not possible the next time will be 10 to 21 days.

The exposure method is only really satisfactory in a sterile unit.

(b) *Closed dressing principle*. The first layer should be non-adherent and antiseptic—the antiseptic being silver sulphadiazine. Tulle gras and melolin are suitable non-adherent dressings. The second layer is cotton gauze and the third layer absorbent wool. It is not redressed for six to eight days unless the dressing is wet with serum. Hyperpyrexia is due to the absorption of toxins but it should be remembered that when skin is destroyed the skin is less effective as an organ of heat loss and heavy dressings may be aggravating this condition. If infection occurs the appropriate antibiotic is administered. For fear of producing a general- ised allergic reaction, antibiotic powders are not used locally.

Burnt hand. The fingers are bandaged separately. Early grafting is advis- able since tendons are often functioning and intact at the time of the burn, only to be destroyed by autolysis which is invariable beneath a second degree eschar. Obviously this is not possible if the patient's survival is in doubt and in such cases the hand may be enclosed in frequently changed plastic gloves soaked in a silicone.

Monafo has shown that if burns dressings were kept constantly moist with a 0·5 per cent solution of silver nitrate the heavy bacterial contamina- tion from the air, so common when burns dressings are changed, would not arise.

4. Systemic antibiotic therapy. This is usually confined to penicillin 0·5 megaunits b.d. Despite reports of penicillin sensitivity most surgeons treat- ing burns advise the use of penicillin systemically and locally and alter it only on bacteriological evidence from the laboratory.

5. Primary excision and skin grafting. Localised full thickness burns may be excised as soon as the patient has been resuscitated.

6. Secondary skin grafting is necessary in all full thickness burns and may be performed in a series of operations depending on the extent of the area to be grafted. It is a particularly difficult decision in extensively burnt patients who are not doing well, but the consensus of opinion is that if one delays until the condition is ideal and the local area bacteriologically sterile many of these patients will have died. For these extensively burnt patients the following minimal standards are necessary:

(a) A normal blood haemoglobin reading. This can be achieved by blood transfusion.

(b) The absence of haemolytic streptococci. These are almost invari- ably sensitive to penicillin and can be killed in a few days. Grafting can be undertaken in the presence of staphylococci if the appropriate anti- biotic is prescribed.

(c) A plasma protein reading of not below 55 g per 1 (5·5 g per cent).

7. Cleaning burnt area. In addition to these measures the burnt area is cleaned as much as possible:

(a) Eusol compresses followed by saline pads may be applied.

(b) Silver sulphadiazine is applied as a 1 per cent ointment to the exposed surface or it may be incorporated in a dressing in patients infected with *Pseudomonas aeruginosa*. Systemic antibiotics are of little value because of the avascularity of burns wounds, but azocillin and gentamicin are the most useful.

(c) Excision of sloughs in all deep burns is undertaken before separation occurs. The area is then covered with autografts or viable cadaveric allografts with or without tissue typing. They are preserved in a skin bag in liquid nitrogen.

Skin grafting

Skin grafting will considerably reduce the time taken for a wound or burn to heal if there has been extensive skin loss. In addition, the scar will be more supple and the degree of contracture very much diminished.

If there is doubt about the viability of the recipient area the graft can be stored in a refrigerator for up to two weeks at a temperature of 4°C. Other sources are:

1. Homografts from suitable donors provide temporary cover before rejection.
2. Cadaver homografts from a skin bank — again these provide temporary cover.
3. Pigskin — now commercially available.

Preparation of the donor area

Grafts may be taken in the form of thin sheets cut from the superficial layers of the skin (Thiersch graft), or large pedicle flaps (pedicle grafting). Pinch grafts have no place in modern plastic surgery since they leave a disfigured site and give an indifferent cosmetic result.

In cases for Thiersch grafting only the superficial cells (epidermis) of the skin are taken. In tube pedicle grafting the whole thickness of the skin is used. Antiseptics should not be applied to the donor area before grafting, since most antiseptics destroy the cells in the superficial layers of the skin. The limb or other area chosen is shaved, washed, and enclosed in a sterile towel.

Preparation of the recipient area

The wound is ready for grafting only when the granulations are healthy and sepsis has been almost eliminated. The granulating surface is healthy when it is smooth and does not bleed readily. As an additional precaution, a swab should be taken for bacteriological examination to determine the degree and nature of any infection which may be present. Antibiotics may be prescribed.

Care of the patient after skin grafting

The donor area is always painful, and this may be minimised by the application of a soothing dressing, such as petroleum jelly gauze.

The recipient area is usually covered with tulle gras and a firm pressure bandage. The nurse must take the greatest care with the grafted area to see that it is not damaged while the patient is recovering from the anaesthetic. The dressing is usually left untouched for six to seven days, and in most cases the surgeon will prefer to perform the dressing himself. At the first dressing the old applications are floated off with sterile saline. In certain areas such as the perineum or buttocks the grafts themselves can be treated by exposure instead of dressings.

When the burn has soundly healed lanoline is applied to the skin.

NURSING CARE

The care of burnt patients requires the highest nursing skills. On admission the patient has to be resuscitated immediately. There are many parameters by which this is controlled and they have to be repeated at very frequent intervals and recorded. Burnt clothing can be removed only when resuscitation has been established and forms as good a dressing as any until this has been achieved. The site of the burnt areas may pose great problems in basic nursing care; the position in bed, the treatment of pressure areas or even oral hygiene may call for great ingenuity. Feeding and the use of a bedpan require patience and perseverance. Superimposed on these problems is the anxiety and fear of a patient in discomfort with a limb immobilised by an intravenous line, severely burnt as well as the prospect of further operation procedures. The aim, the necessity and the good results which will flow from the measures should be explained and discussed as his condition improves. The importance of active movements and the purpose of special dietetic measures encourage him to help himself.

Special complications of burns in the first seven days

Additional special problems which may arise are:

1. Acute toxaemia. This condition is not unlike the crisis which occurs in hyperthyroidism. The patient becomes excitable and later increasingly drowsy; the pulse increases in rate and diminishes in volume; the temperature rises to higher levels each day. The patient suffers from vomiting and diarrhoea. If the condition is unrelieved or fails to respond to treatment coma results.

Treatment. Continuous intravenous plasma transfusion and the administration of antibiotics are continued.

2. Extensive local oedema. This complication is not unusual, and is best overcome by a change in posture of the part so that the tissue drains by gravity. In the case of the hands, it is best overcome by suspension of the hands, adequately protected with dressings, from Balkan beams.

3. Loss of morale. Morale is all-important to the immediate recovery. The physical weight of the dressings and the severe distress of the accident weigh heavily on many patients. Their dread of disfigurement is very great. The hair should be brushed and the patient should be encouraged to use cosmetics or anything which increases morale. This produces a sense of well-being and restores confidence.

It should not be forgotten that there may be deep psychological aspects in the relationship between parent and child following burns. Parents may feel a sense of guilt that their child has been burnt through some neglect on their part. In other patients the parents are aggrieved that the child has been burnt from its own fault.

4. Metabolic changes. There is a great loss of nitrogen and the patient is in a hypercatabolic state. Once fluid and electrolyte balance has been stabilised a high protein high calorie diet with generous supplements of vitamin C has to be provided.

5. Renal failure. This may occur and the urine should be tested for albumin, which is a nitrogen loss and the volume measured each day, no matter how well the patient is progressing. A fluid balance chart should be kept.

6. Pulmonary complications. For example, pneumonia and bronchitis frequently occur, particularly in elderly patients. Pulmonary oedema, believed to be caused by unidentified toxins, may develop although the burning has not involved the respiratory tract.

7. Liver failure and jaundice may occur quite suddenly from toxaemia from tissue destruction or sepsis.

8. Bone marrow suppression may develop as a result of infection and cause anaemia.

9. Contractures and deformities. These are best overcome by early light splintage, active movements and early skin grafting.

10. Gastrointestinal bleeding from acute ulceration, the classical but rarest form being an acute duodenal ulcer (Curling's ulcer).

Chemical burns

Chemical burns are treated on lines similar to those described above, but those due to acid should be irrigated with sodium bicarbonate solution and those due to alkalis with 1 per cent acetic acid as soon as possible after infliction. With acid or alkaline burns of the mouth the following buffer solution may be used:

Potassium dihydrogen phosphate (30 g)
Disodium hydrogen phosphate (200 g)
Aqua ad. 1 litre.

In addition to being used as a mouth wash it is suitable for irrigating the eyes.

The wide use of chemicals has led many firms to state how burns resulting from their products should be treated and burns centres throughout Great Britain can advise on treatment by telephone.

X-ray burns

X-ray burns require the application of an oily dressing. Patients who have worked as radiographers for some years are liable to develop squamous cell carcinoma (epithelioma) of the skin if the shield of the X-ray tube has been ineffective and X-rays are emitted.

On hair-bearing areas temporary depilation occurs after three weeks, or permanent alopecia (baldness) if the hair follicles have been destroyed.

19
Trauma

Trauma means injury. People may be injured singly or many at a time, e.g. train crashes, multiple pile-ups on the motorways and, regrettably, terrorist activities. When there are many injured patients the accident services of the hospital to which the casualties are taken will be severely tested and most hospitals will have a published plan to deal with such situations. Nurses should make quite sure that they are familiar with such major disaster plans as the efficient treatment of large numbers of casualties presented in a very short time depends to a large extent upon the efficient organisation of the medical and nursing staff and the ancillary staff.

MAJOR DISASTERS: SURGICAL TRIAGE

Triage is a military term used to describe the initial sorting of injured patients and this concept has been adopted to deal with major disasters in civilian hospitals. The method used to sort injured patients is to divide them into three groups. The first group of patients to identify are those whose life-threatening conditions will benefit most rapidly from the provision of basic resuscitative techniques. The second group of patients are those with serious injuries which will need hospital treatment but whose treatment can safely be deferred without threat to life until the first group of patients have been dealt with. The third group are those patients with lesser injuries who do not require urgent medical attention and many of them do not require admission to hospital.

   The critically injured patients in the first group are those in whom the air-way is at risk, or whose blood volume is seriously diminished, and those with major chest or abdominal injuries.

Patients with threats to the airway

Threats to the airway must receive absolute priority in order to re-establish a patent airway. A patient with otherwise minor injuries may very quickly die because the airway is obstructed by vomit, blood or foreign bodies. Once the airway has been re-established by removing any obstruction, by

ensuring that the tongue has not fallen back into the pharynx, by endotracheal intubation or by tracheostomy then other serious injuries can be
dealt with. Naturally occurring surgical diseases are usually confined to
natural anatomical regions, e.g. of the stomach, the peritoneum, the lung.
This is not so in the case of traumatic lesions which may transgress many
anatomical boundaries. Their treatment requires a very sound knowledge
of anatomy and a wide experience of surgery.

Blood volume

Serious external blood loss is uncommon and can in most cases be stopped
fairly easily by the application of direct pressure, but blood lost internally,
either by bleeding into the abdominal or thoracic cavities or by bleeding
into soft tissue planes from such injuries as multiple fractures is less easy to
recognise and is often underestimated. It should be suspected in all
patients who have multiple fractures, a history of high speed injury or a
penetrating injury. It is rarely necessary to transfuse such patients with
uncrossmatched blood as the blood volume can be maintained with various intravenous fluids until adequately crossmatched blood is available.

Chest injuries

All patients with major chest injuries are at risk to their life until the lungs
can be re-expanded and kept adequately ventilated. Such patients will
usually need to be kept in the resuscitation area until they are stabilised,
and may well need chest drains and intermittent positive pressure respiration. See Chapter 30, Figure 30.1.

   The second group of patients should be assessed in the resuscitation
reception area but are usually able to be passed through this area fairly
quickly and admitted to the ordinary wards for treatment when time
becomes available. The third group of patients will also need assessment in
the Casualty reception area but can often be referred for out-patient treatment or treatment by their own doctors after initial assessment.

Surgical triage: multiple casualties

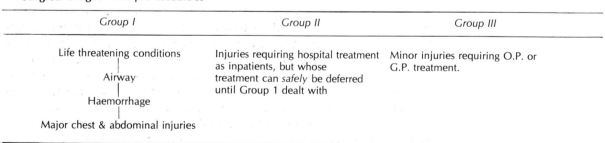

Group I	Group II	Group III
Life threatening conditions | Airway | Haemorrhage | Major chest & abdominal injuries	Injuries requiring hospital treatment as inpatients, but whose treatment can *safely* be deferred until Group 1 dealt with	Minor injuries requiring O.P. or G.P. treatment.

It is important in the treatment of large numbers of casualties that the
nursing staff should follow directions of the nursing officers in charge who
will in turn be working in close conjunction with the medical staff. The
most important member of the medical staff in such a situation is a senior

doctor who has been appointed as the triage officer and this will usually be a senior accident surgeon. He will often ask the nursing officers to allocate a nurse to a particular patient as continuous observation and re-assessment of priorities is necessary. It may be necessary to empty a ward of routine patients to use as a special reception ward for the injured and this of course will require a high level of nursing staff.

Documentation of the injured patients presents many difficulties as some of the patients may be unconscious and no names may be available. In addition the care of property of the injured patients will also have to be specially organised and continuous liaison with the police and arrangements to deal with the press and enquiries from patients relatives will have to be planned.

Shock in injured patients

This is considered in detail in Chapter 14. Shock may be caused by severe pain, by emotional factors, or by severe diminution in the blood volume. Pain can of course be relieved. Emotional factors need to be considered and a good nurse will always try and reassure a patient that he or she is in good hands and will be well looked after. The nurse should always have time to answer patients questions and to keep the patient informed as much as possible as to why various procedures are necessary. Loss of blood volume is dealt with by intravenous transfusion of blood, plasma, plasma expanders such as Dextran or other intravenous fluids as the doctor directs.

Infection

Patients with open wounds or compound fractures (remember that fractures of the base of the skull into the pharynx, the middle ear or the sinuses; fractures of the jaw into the mouth; fractures of the ribs which may penetrate the lungs; and fractures of the pelvis which may damage the bladder, the rectum or the intestines are technically compound fractures) are at risk of infection and for this reason antibiotics are usually prescribed to cover the first few days of healing. Compound wounds are often contaminated with foreign bodies (pieces of clothing, oil, metallic fragments or road debris) and the initial treatment of the compound wound should always include removing all the foreign material that can be identified in the wound. It is quite often necessary to excise the whole wound surgically in order to be sure of obtaining clean surfaces which will assist in healing. In some cases it is advisable not to close the wound immediately but to use the method known as delayed primary repair where the wound is cleaned and dressed and is not sutured for 3 or 4 days. This method is quite commonly used in crush injuries or in missile injuries and its application in war time or as a result of terrorist activities has saved many lives.

The crush syndrome

After a compressing injury of several hours duration, usually of the limbs, the patient may develop hypotension followed by acute renal failure. This is known as the crush syndrome. It is thought to be due to the release from injured tissues of substances toxic to the renal tubules.

The treatment is both to manage the renal injury by suitable dialysis and intravenous treatment, and to excise or even amputate the crushed tissue, taking special precautions to avoid infection, as this always makes the syndrome more dangerous.

Thrombosis

Thrombosis, or clotting of the blood in the large veins, is a frequent complication of injury especially in older people. Sometimes the clots break away from the walls of the vein and enter the venous circulation, passing through the heart and becoming impacted in the pulmonary arteries — pulmonary embolism. This is a serious and often fatal complication so precautions are often taken to prevent venous thrombosis by the administration of plasma expanders or occasionally by the use of anticoagulant drugs.

Other wound complications

Tissues in the depth of the wound may be deprived of their blood supply and become necrotic. This is known as sloughing and will often require excision of the dead tissue.

Secondary haemorrhage

This is haemorrhage which presents a week or 10 days after injury and is almost always due to infection which erodes the wall of the small blood vessels in the base of the wound. Such a complication may be dealt with by means of direct pressure but usually requires surgical ligation of the eroded artery and the administration of antibiotics.

Failure to heal

Persistent infection may also lead to failure of the wound to heal and the establishment of a sinus (which is a permanently discharging abscess in the wound) or a fistula (which is a connection between a hollow organ in the body and the exterior, e.g. an intestinal fistula). Wounds may burst apart after initial partial healing (e.g. a burst abdomen) or bleeding may continue deep to the skin within the wound and form a large haematoma. Occasionally a skin wound will heal with a raised pink irritable scar known as a keloid scar. These are more common in the sites where the skin is very mobile and are also more common in the darker skinned races. (Ch. 11, Fig. 11.6). The treatment of these scars is often unrewarding but radiotherapy may help as may the exhibition of local cortisone dressings. Finally the scar tissue of a wound may contract and give rise to a deformity. This is particularly so in limbs and more common in wounds close to joints.

Wound healing

Healing of the wound depends not only upon the accurate apposition and repair of wounded tissues but on the general condition of the patient, so it is important to ensure that the patients nutritional state is good and that there is an adequate haemoglobin content of the blood. Older people are often short of vitamins and plasma proteins, and the addition of vitamins and a higher proportion of proteins in the diet is sometimes necessary.

Summary

The final result achieved by an injured patient depends very largely on the adequacy of the initial treatment. In severe injuries the initial treatment is directed towards saving the patient's life particularly by attention to the airway and the replacement of any blood loss. The next important factor in the treatment is accurate repair of damaged tissues (including any fractures), the prevention of infection and the prevention of contractures. In this connection it should be stated that the aim of treatment is to return the patient to the level of function which he or she enjoyed before the injury. It must never be forgotten that re-habilitation of function is as important as the primary treatment.

BIBLIOGRAPHY

Brown A A, Nicholls R J 1977 British Journal of Surgery 64: 397
Yates DQ W 1979 British Journal of Hospital Medicine 22: 323

20

Fractures and joint injuries

Broken bones and injured or dislocated joints are very common results of trauma. There are however other conditions in which bones can be fractured and joints injured or dislocated. Fractures and joint injuries can therefore be divided into three types:
  (a) traumatic,
  (b) pathological,
  (c) stress.

Traumatic

This group is by far the most common. The injury may be "closed", i.e. the injury to the bone or joint does not communicate with the exterior or it may be compound, i.e. the broken bone or injured joint is accessible to outside pollution and is therefore much more likely to become infected. Such cases are always treated with antibiotics as well as the special treatment for the injury. Fractures may be of several anatomical types according to the severity of the injury and the direction of the force. If the bone ends are jammed together it is known as an impacted fracture. If the bone ends are splintered it is a comminuted fracture. If the bone is that of a young child it may well be only partially fractured. This is known as a greenstick fracture because it is similar to the way in which a living twig will break when a bending force is applied to it. If the fractured bone ends damage tissues close to the bones such as larger arteries or nerves, then the fracture is known as a complicated one (Fig. 20.1).

Pathological

A bone which is diseased will often fracture following a very minor trauma which would not break a normal bone. Such a fracture is known as a pathological fracture and arises in diseases such as malignant deposits in bones and in Paget's disease. Similarly a joint affected by diseases such as syphilis may dislocate spontaneously. There is a special type of pathological dislocation of the hip seen in new born babies known as congenital dislocation. This is due to abnormal joint development and is discussed in Chapter 47.

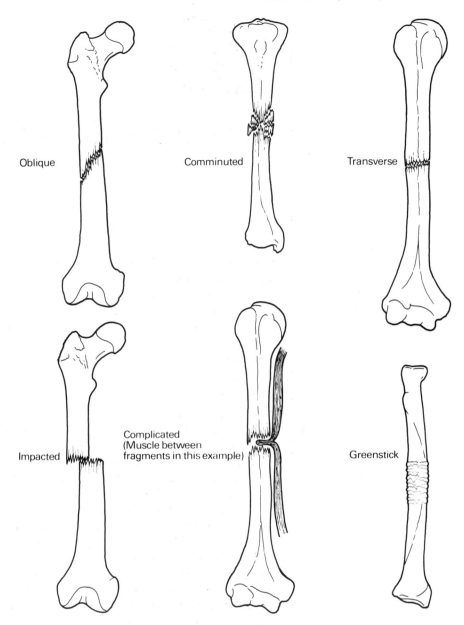

Fig. 20.1 Varieties of fractures.

Stress fractures

These arise in normal bones which have an undue and repetitive stress placed upon them. They usually start as partial fractures and as the stresses are repeated the fractures become complete, although some attempt at healing commences when the initial minor fracture appears. The most common example of this rare condition is a fracture of the neck of the second metatarsal in young recruits to the army who are required to do a great deal of marching and foot stamping in their first few weeks of training. A stress injury of a joint is best exemplified by the development of arthritic changes in the joint following undue wear and tear.

Changes resulting from fracture

In the traumatic fractures it must always be remembered that broken bones bleed and the blood loss can often be quite severe, for instance a patient with bilateral femoral fractures may well bleed six pints of blood into the muscles and soft tissues of the thighs. This accounts for the anaemia and severe pain and swelling which such an injury causes.

Fractured bones heal by the natural healing processes of the body. The blood clot between the ends of the bone becomes organized. This results in the formation of tissue known as callus in which special cells concerned with bone repair are found in plentiful amounts. One type of cell — the osteoblast — produces bone tissue whilst another cell — the osteoclast — removes and remodels excess bone so that eventually the healed bone adopts the same shape as it had prior to the fracture.

As a general rule bones take about 6 weeks to unite but the larger bones which take the full weight of the body such as the femur and the tibia will take as long again or even longer to become strong enough to take the body weight. The smaller bones and the non weight-bearing bones such as the humerus or the metacarpals may be strong enough to fulfil their normal function before the bone is fully united. It is a strange and unexplained freak of nature that those bones which can least easily be immobilised (e.g. the clavicle or the ribs) practically never fail to join whether or not they are immobilised, whereas the bones which are most easily able to be fixed (e.g. the humerus and the tibia) are the ones which most frequently fail to unite (Fig. 20.2).

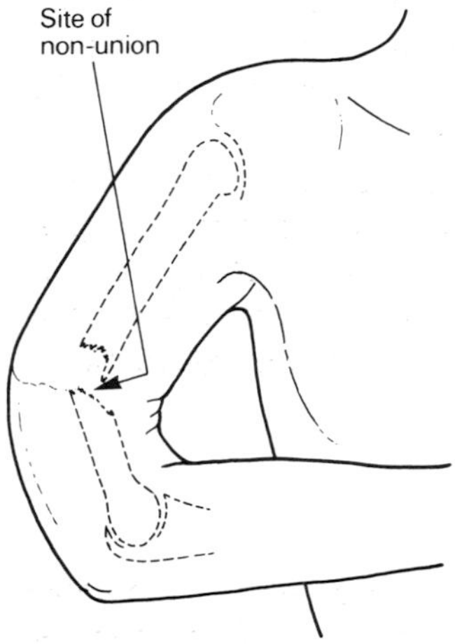

Site of
non-union

Fig. 20.2 Un-united fracture of the humerus.

Symptoms and signs of fractures

1. Pain aggravated by movement,
2. Tenderness over the fracture line,
3. Swelling,
4. Deformity,
5. Shortening of the limb,
6. Loss of function,
7. Abnormal mobility at the fracture site,
8. Occasional crepitus or grating of the bone ends as they move on each other

Sometimes all these signs and symptoms are obvious but in other cases only one or two of them may be present, depending upon the site of the fracture, the displacement and the leverage upon the fracture.

PRINCIPLES OF TREATMENT OF FRACTURES AND JOINT INJURIES

The important principles of treatment can again be classified under three headings as follows:

(a) reduce the fracture or the dislocation,
(b) rest the injury until it is healed,
(c) restore the function of the injured part.

REDUCTION

Unless a fracture is complicated (i.e. has damaged neighbouring important structures which need urgent treatment), then there is usually no urgency to reduce the displacement and the limb can often be splinted for several days if necessary until the final method of treatment is decided. On the other hand a dislocated joint must be reduced as a matter of urgency because the longer the joint remains dislocated the more likely is the articular surface to become permanently damaged.

The usual method of reduction is by manipulation either with or without anaesthesia but in certain cases it may be necessary to perform a surgical operation in order to reduce the fracture or the dislocation. This procedure technically converts the injury into a compound type. It is therefore usual to cover the postoperative period with a course of antibiotic treatment.

REST UNTIL HEALED

When considering the second principle of treatment it is important to know the various methods of splintage which are used. These vary from the most simple support such as a sling or a collar and cuff to the most complicated type of internal fixation or external splintage. A small, but important, point to note is that a sling is used to support the weight of the arm in such injuries as a fracture of the clavicle or a dislocation of the acromio-clavicular joint; whereas a collar and cuff is used to allow the weight of the arm to hang down and thus aid the realignment of the bone. The latter is used in injuries such as fractures of the surgical neck of the humerus.

The most common method of external splintage used is plaster of Paris though recently other substances have been introduced which have all the advantages of plaster of Paris as well as other advantages, such as being water-resistant, lighter and allowing X-rays to pass through more easily than plaster. It must be remembered that any rigid cast applied to a limb encircles the limb and should the tissues swell beneath the plaster then the cast can restrict the circulation, sometimes with tragic results.

The indications that a plaster is too tight are:
(a) pain which is persistent and increasing,
(b) numbness of the extremities as the blood supply to the sensory nerves is cut off,
(c) whiteness or paleness of the extremities because of circulatory interference. The nurse should draw the sister's attention to any patient in whom she notices these signs presenting.

It is much better to remove and reapply a plaster ten times than to leave on too tight a plaster which may cause loss of the limb. It must also be remembered that a poorly applied plaster cast may cause local soreness from pressure and that the sharp edges of the cast may also break the skin. The nurse must be aware of these possibilities and check plaster casts for comfort on frequent occasions.

Special splints are also used in certain circumstances and perhaps the best known of these is the Thomas splint (Fig. 20.3). This splint was first devised by Hugh Owen Thomas (p. 601), in order to rest knee joints which were infected with tuberculosis. In more recent years it has become widely used throughout the world for the treatment of fractured femoral shafts. The ring of a Thomas splint is fairly rigid and can give rise

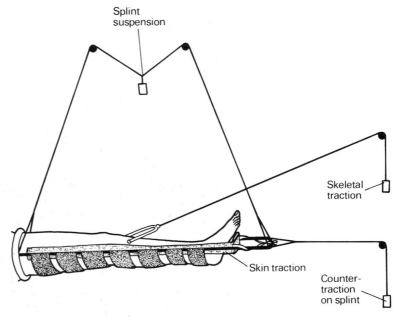

Fig. 20.3 The Thomas splint. The splint is suspended and *either* skin traction with counter-traction on the splint *or* skeletal traction is applied.

to pressure sores so it is common to apply counter traction from the bottom end of the splint over a pulley at the bottom of the bed in order to pull the ring away from the groin. A recent modification of the Thomas splint is the Povey splint which has a foam rubber ring round the upper part of the thigh which is much more comfortable than the Thomas splint. The whole splint is also much more manoeuverable for nursing purposes and the patient can easily be transported in the Povey splint. A further advantage is that the cumbersome frame needed to support a Thomas splint is unnecessary. In fractures of the femur, traction is commonly applied to the limb itself in order to keep the bone alignment in good position. Such traction can be applied through adhesive tape strapped to the sides of the lower limb (skin traction) or by means of a pin passed through the front of the upper end of the tibia (skeletal traction). Either type of traction may be fixed (i.e. fixed to the bottom end of a Thomas splint) or may be balanced (i.e. the traction is applied without fixation to the splint by means of a spring or a weight).

Any patient with fractures who is confined to bed for a long period (and this particularly applies to elderly people) is liable to pressure sores and careful nursing is essential in order to prevent these. Various types of mattress have been devised to reduce the risk of bed sores but by far the best method of preventing them is regular careful nursing care.

For a number of reasons the surgeon may decide to splint the fracture internally rather than use external splinting. Such a decision involves a surgical operation and the patient must be prepared for this in the same way as for any other major surgical operation. Particular care must be placed on preoperative shaving as an infected fracture or an infected joint

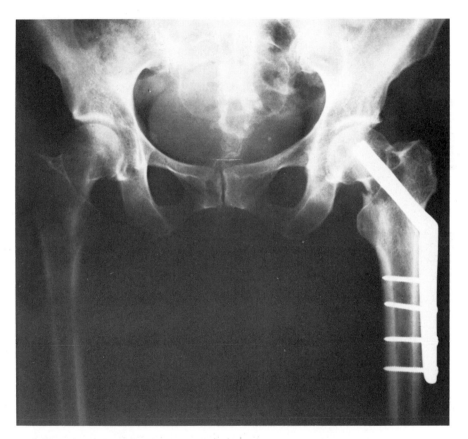

Fig. 20.4 Internal fixation. X-ray showing a fracture of the neck of the femur, fixed by a pin up the centre of the neck and a plate with screws holding it to the shaft.

as a result of unsterile surgery is a disaster for the patient. Internal fixation may be achieved by the use of bone screws, plate and screws, wire, rods within the cavity of the bone, or by a combination of one or more methods (Fig. 20.4). A useful method of fixation in dirty compound wounds is to insert threaded pins into the bone through the skin, and connect the free ends of the pins by an external bar. This fixes the fracture but allows the wound to be treated.

Usually the safest method of treatment is conservative but operative reduction and fixation is often used in elderly people, so that they may be mobilised more quickly; in cases where the fracture or dislocation is completely unstable or for ease of nursing in multiple fractures.

Compound fractures, as opposed to closed fractures, require treatment within the first few hours but it is frequently wise to spend some time in treating the patient's general condition before turning ones attention to the local treatment of the compound fracture.

During the period of resuscitation the compound wound should be covered with a thick sterile dressing and left undisturbed until the patient is taken to theatre and anaesthetised. At operation all foreign material and non-viable tissue is excised from the wound which is then closed if possible.

If plaster is applied in such cases there is always some bleeding into the plaster and staining of the plaster from the exudate. Some surgeons like to cut a window in the plaster over the wound so that it can be re-dressed without disturbing the fracture; whereas other surgeons prefer to remove the plaster, dress the wound and re-apply plaster should this become necessary. Contaminated and compound wounds will heal quite adequately beneath the plaster. Sometimes it is not possible to close the wound and in cases where there is severe tissue damage it is sometimes wise to deliberately leave the compound wound open but clean and dressed with an appropriate antiseptic dressing. The limb is therefore encased in a plaster and final closure of the wound is then delayed for several days. It must not be forgotten that fractures of the base of the skull, fractures of the ribs, fractures of the jaw and sometimes fractures of the pelvis may be compound as they all may communicate with the exterior through the various body cavities. Complicated fractures which injure important organs close to the fracture site may also need fairly immediate treatment in order to repair or lessen the chance of permanent damage to the affected structure.

The treatment of pathological fractures follows the same principles as the treatment for traumatic fractures but in addition treatment may be instituted to deal with the underlying pathology. For instance it is quite common only to discover a secondary malignant deposit in the bone by the fact that a fracture has occurred. In this case, the fracture is often fixed internally and radiotherapy treatment given locally to kill off the cancer cells in the local deposit.

The rarely occurring stress fractures also call for the same principles of treatment as in traumatic fractures, though reduction is rarely required as it is unusual to find any displacement in stress fractures.

RESTORATION OF FUNCTION

The restoration of full functional activity following a fracture of a limb or dislocation of a joint is perhaps the most important principle of the three. It is no help to the patient to obtain a perfectly healed fracture in excellent position but be unable to use the limb because of stiffness. Restoration of function begins as soon as the primary treatment has been instituted so the nurse must encourage the patient to use the muscles of the immobilised part as frequently and as actively as he can. The physiotherapist will see the patient perhaps once a day but the nurse may see the patient many times a day. A patient being nursed in a Thomas splint for a fractured femur who does not do his quadriceps exercises at least hourly and who does not exercise his calf muscles and his ankle, will find himself quite unable to walk when the splintage is finally removed, and his re-habilitation will be unduly prolonged. He may well develop a permanent limitation of movement of the joints of the limb if he has not conscientiously performed his re-habilitation exercises during the course of his treatment.

Restoration of function of course is not confined only to limbs. One of the most important aspects of treatment of fractures of the ribs is to keep the lungs fully expanded by deliberate breathing exercises. Head injuries may give rise to a certain amount of brain damage and this can affect the speech so that speech therapy becomes an important part of functional rehabilitation.

If a patient is confined to bed because of a fractured lower limb it is important not to let the muscles and joints of the other limbs become stiff, in order to achieve as early a restoration of function as possible. The patient must be continuously encouraged by the nursing staff to perform the exercises and treatment prescribed by the surgeon. There is nothing more rewarding than to see a seriously injured patient return to a full normal and active life.

IMPORTANT POINTS ABOUT PARTICULAR FRACTURES

FRACTURES OF THE SHOULDER GIRDLE AND UPPER LIMB

Shoulder girdles

Fractures of the clavicle are treated by 2 to 3 weeks rest in a broad arm sling followed by mobilisation. There is rarely any difficulty in achieving union and full movement. Fractures of the scapula require rest in a sling until the pain and swelling subsides. No particular treatment other than this is necessary.

Fractures of the humerus

A fracture of the greater tuberosity of the humerus is commonly associated with a dislocation of the shoulder joint. The treatment for this is reduction of the dislocation as early as possible and this usually achieves a satisfactory position of the fracture of the greater tuberosity. Rest in a sling for 10 days followed by mobilisation of the arm is an acceptable form of treatment. Fractures of the surgical neck of the humerus are common in the elderly and are almost always impacted. Fractures of the mid shaft of the humerus are common and usually unite well. These usually require immobilisation in a plaster slab from the point of the shoulder round the elbow together with a collar and cuff so that the weight of the arm keeps the humerus well aligned. An important point to check in all these fractures is that the radial nerve has not been damaged (Ch. 46). This is tested by asking the patient to dorsiflex the wrist.

Fractures around the elbow

These are common in children and as a result of high velocity injuries such as car crashes. A supracondylar fracture of the humerus in children should be reduced by manipulation under general anaesthesia and supported in a collar and cuff with the elbow flexed beyond the right angle. One of the complications is compression of the brachial artery by swelling in front of the elbow and the nurse must check the radial pulse at hourly intervals as, if the pulse disappears, the flexion at the elbow must be lessened. As a general rule fractures around the elbow joint do not need to be immobilised in plaster but some complicated fractures do need open reduction and internal fixation.

FRACTURES OF THE FOREARM BONES

It is essential to obtain an accurate reduction in these cases as, if there is angulation or residual displacement after manipulation, the important function of rotation of the forearm will be limited. It is therefore quite common for fractures of the forearm bones to require open operation and internal fixation in order to get an absolutely accurate reduction.

Fractures of the distal forearm

The so-called Colles' fracture—an impacted fracture of the lower end of the radius with dorsal and radial angulation and displacement is one of the commonest fractures seen. It is particularly common in elderly people with frail bones and requires manipulative reduction followed by a plaster slab for 4 to 5 weeks.

Fractures of the wrist and hand

Because of the poor blood supply of this bone, fractures of the scaphoid may take many weeks to achieve full union and until union is achieved a scaphoid plaster cast is necessary. Fractures of the metacarpals usually do not present any difficulty and rarely require immobilisation but fractures of the fingers are most important and if badly treated will give rise to permanent deformities and limitation of movement.

FRACTURES OF THE SKULL

These are dealt with in the chapter on head injuries. The important features of these injuries is whether there has been underlying brain damage or damage to the blood vessels which supply the brain. Occasionally one sees a depressed fracture when the skull has been struck with a hard round object which has the effect of depressing a circular portion of the skull below the general level of the skull, causing local injury to the underlying brain.

FRACTURES OF THE SPINAL COLUMN

Such injuries are becoming more and more common and, as with fractures of the skull, it is important to decide whether or not the fracture of the spinal column is associated with damage to the spinal cord.

Compression fractures of the vertebral bodies are the most common types of spinal fracture and are usually not associated with any spinal cord injury. They are treated by bed rest until the pain settles down. Extension exercises of the spine should be started as soon as the patient can comfortably perform them. Once the pain has diminished then the patient is allowed up and about.

Dislocations of the spine however frequently give rise to neurological complications and from the point of view of treatment and nursing it is important to decide whether such dislocations are stable or unstable. A stable dislocation without neurological damage is treated by reduction of the dislocation if possible followed by treatment in the same way as for a compression fracture. An unstable dislocation without spinal cord damage is uncommon but requires urgent reduction and operative fixation in order to prevent spinal cord injury during the various nursing procedures necessary whilst the patient is in hospital. Dislocations, whether stable or unstable, with neurological damage should be reduced although the amount of recovery to be expected is variable. As a general rule patients who are completely paralysed and have an unstable dislocation make no recovery of their spinal cord function distal to the level of the lesion (Fig. 20.5).

In these cases nursing care becomes most important as the patient will be confined to bed or a wheelchair for a long period and pressure sores develop very easily in skin without sensation. Two hourly turning is necessary and for this reason some surgeons will fix the dislocated spine by surgical means after reduction purely in order to facilitate the nursing care. Other important requirements are care of the bladder, breathing exercises and the prevention of fixed deformities in the paralysed part of the body. The most difficult cases to manage of course are those with the dislocation in the cervical spine where the legs, the intercostal muscles, and a variable proportion of the upper limb muscles are paralysed. However, it is surprising how well these people manage their ordinary lives if they receive skilled medical treatment and nursing in the first few weeks after injuries.

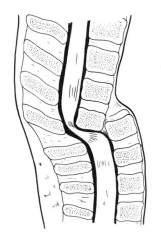

Fig. 20.5 Dislocation of the cervical spine. Note the displacement of the bones and the severe angulation of the spinal cord.

FRACTURES OF THE RIBS (See also Chapter 30)

The fractures of the ribs themselves are of little significance and no particular local treatment is performed for the fractures themselves. The major consideration is what damage has been done to underlying structures. The fractured ends of the ribs may pierce the lungs giving rise to a haemothorax and pneumothorax. If the hole in the lung exerts a valvular effect so that air can escape from it but cannot be sucked back into the lungs then a particularly dangerous situation exists as a tension pneumothorax will develop. This requires urgent treatment otherwise the patient will die.

If a large segment of the chest becomes flail because of double fractures of several ribs then the mechanism of respiration is damaged and the flail piece of chest sinks in with inspiration and moves outwards on expiration. This is known as paradoxical respiration and is best treated by means of intermittent positive pressure respiration on a ventilator. Fractured ribs may also damage the spleen, the kidney, the stomach and the liver and laparotomy is often necessary in this case.

FRACTURES OF THE PELVIS

The pelvis surrounds internal organs which may be damaged by fractures of the pelvis. These organs include the urethra, the bladder and the bowel and urgent surgical treatment is necessary for these damaged organs.

Fractures of the pelvis which do not pass through the weight bearing area of the pelvis are treated merely by rest until the painful symptoms subside. Fractures of the pelvis involving the acetabulum or the sacroiliac joints require much longer periods of bed rest and sometimes need open reduction and fixation.

FRACTURES OF THE LOWER LIMBS

Fracture of the neck of the femur is one of the most common reasons for admission to hospital of elderly people. Because this is an injury of the aged it is almost always treated surgically in order to allow them to be up and about as soon as possible. Those fractures close to the femoral head are usually treated by removal of the femoral head and the insertion of a metallic prosthesis. This is because the head of the femur is likely to die as a result of damage to its blood supply and subsequent avascular necrosis. Fractures lower down the femoral neck are usually treated by means of a pin, which passes up the neck into the femoral head, attached to a plate which is screwed to the upper shaft of the femur (Fig. 20.4). It must be remembered that because patients with fractures of the femoral neck are usually old, they may well have other concurrent diseases. In addition the patient may be in a poor state of nutrition (often these old people live at home alone and eat poorly — in fact many of them are not found for some hours after the fall which has broken their femoral neck). They may be diabetic, in some degree of heart failure, myxoedematous or suffering from malignant disease. Many of them are anaemic and all these various problems must be considered preoperatively so that the patient's general condition is as good as possible before surgical treatment is undertaken.

Postoperatively, as much attention must be given to the patient's general condition as to the fractured femoral neck. It is usual to mobilise these patients as soon as possible after their operation taking partial weight on the injured limb, progressing to full weight-bearing as soon as they are comfortable.

Dislocation of the hip

Although dislocation of the hip is not common it is occurring with increasing frequency. The treatment is to reduce it as soon as possible and to make quite sure that the sciatic nerve has not been injured. A patient with a dislocated hip who cannot dorsiflex the foot on that side has very likely contused the sciatic nerve.

Fractures of the shaft of the femur

The safest way in which to treat these fractures is by immobilisation on a Thomas splint or other similar splint. The leg must rest snugly in the splint and must not lie on top of tightly stretched slings around the splint. Half the thickness of the limb must sit comfortably in suitably shaped slings under the splint whilst the other half should be visible above the splint. If skin traction is applied it is as well to shave the leg before application of the skin traction and to cover the skin with a Tinct. Benz. spray. This helps to prevent soreness of the skin and adds to the adhesiveness of the extension strapping. The care of a leg splint for the three months it takes until the fracture is solid requires regular attention and inspection by the nursing staff to check that the groin ring is not too tight, that the slings supporting the leg are at the right tension, and that the traction cords are kept taut.

Occasionally however a fractured shaft of femur is treated by surgical fixation either with a Kuntscher nail down the medullary cavity or by means of a heavy duty plate and screws.

Fractures of the patella

Crack fracture of the patella without separation of the fragments means that the extensor apparatus of the knee is still intact. The treatment required is aspiration of the knee joint to remove the blood and rest in a plaster of Paris cylinder for 3 to 4 weeks. However if the patellar fragments are widely separated then the extensor mechanism has been badly torn and requires surgical repair together with repair or excision of the patella. Once again plaster immobilisation is necessary for some 5 to 6 weeks after this.

Fractures into the knee joint

These fractures should be treated by aspiration of the blood from the knee joint, manipulative reduction if possible or open reduction if indicated followed by immobilisation in a plaster cylinder for several weeks depending upon the age of the patient.

Fractures of the tibia

These are best dealt with by means of plaster of Paris immobilisation but the plaster needs to extend from the upper thigh down to the toes in order to immobilise the tibia adequately. These fractures may take up to 4 or 5 months before solid union occurs. Fractures of the lower tibial shaft occasionally fail to unite for no very obvious reason. In this case bone grafting or internal fixation may become necessary. Some surgical centres treat fractures of the tibia initially by internal fixation although this increases the risk of infection. However this risk is acceptable in some circumstances.

Fractures around the ankle joint

The ankle joint is a hinge joint but there is also an element of gliding movement. The bony walls containing the talus are often fractured by forced rotation movement and, according to the force applied, one or more bones will fracture. These fractures are commonly known as Potts fractures. They are usually treated by manipulative reduction and immobilisation in a plaster cast from the toes to just below the knee. The plaster is left in place for 6 to 12 weeks depending on the nature of the fracture. Occasionally they require open reduction and fixation with screws or wire.

Fractures of the heel bone

Fractures of the os calcis can be quite crippling injuries particularly if the fracture passes into the joint between the talus and the os calcis. This joint is responsible for accommodating the position of the foot to rough ground and a fracture which interferes with the movement of this joint will give rise to a permanent painful limp. Fractures of the os calcis are not therefore immobilised in plaster but the patient is kept from weight bearing until the fracture is united. During this period exercises to increase the mobility of the joint are performed regularly. Occasionally it is necessary to arthrodese the joint if it is badly damaged. Fractures of the mid foot and forefoot require immobilisation until united usually for 5 or 6 weeks but fractures of the toes can be treated without immobilisation.

21
Diseases of the skin

PRESSURE SORES

Pressure sores are an important complication which may develop from confining the patient to bed. In many cases they are preventable by skilled nursing, but in some cases no effort or skill can avoid their development, and the condition is frequently a terminal one.

Causes and predisposing factors

The cause is long-continued pressure, and the pressure required need only be high enough to compress the blood vessels in conditions of hypotension resulting from shock or blood loss. Then otherwise tolerable pressure on the skin may cause a sore. Pressure causes discomfort, but in the debilitated and in paraplegics with a sensory loss, such discomfort may not be appreciated by the patient. The surface appearance of a pressure sore gives little indication of what may be its ultimate size.

General

    (a) Emaciation due to malnutrition or disease.
    (b) Senility.
    (c) Diabetes, anaemia, and other severe constitutional disturbances.
    (d) Immobility — paralysed patients.

Local

    (a) Pressure. The patient's body weight renders movement difficult if he is obese. In a thin subject the bony prominences are exposed to greater pressure.
    (b) Loss of skin sensation. This is usually due to a lesion of the spinal cord or the peripheral nerves.
    (c) Incontinence is a potent source of pressure sore formation, since the skin becomes moist and septic. Incontinence increases the risk of pressure sores five-fold.

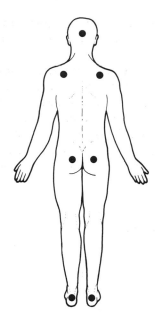

Fig. 21.1 The pressure areas.

(d) Excessive sweating causes a moist skin.
(e) Friction such as too vigorous rubbing and the presence of foreign bodies — wrinkled sheets, breadcrumbs, etc.
(f) Impaired circulation, e.g. patients suffering from heart disease.
(g) Oedema.

The pressure areas

The pressure areas are those portions of the body on which the greatest weight is borne when the patient is recumbent, and it is at these sites that sores are liable to occur. They include the heels, buttocks, sacrum, scapular areas, elbows, the spinous processes of the verterbrae, and the occiput (Fig. 21.1).

The prevention of pressure sores

1. Pressure must be relieved by frequent change of posture, and the circulation revived by stimulation of the skin.
2. A carefully made bed, in which the sheets are pulled tight, smooth and freed from crumbs and wrinkles.
3. Sorbo or air rings and cushions are used if necessary, and the nurse should ensure that pressure is evenly distributed and that the patient is moved about in bed. Although frowned on by some authorities rubber rings are useful in the correct position.
4. The skin must be kept clean and dry.

All these objects are ensured by:

(a) Attention to the skin. The skin should be washed with soap and water, rinsed and carefully dried. Massage which was carried out with apparent success is now very much frowned upon since research has shown that careful washing and drying alone is more effective. Silicone preparations are only of use as a barrier against incontinence.

(b) There are a number of sophisticated beds which are very effective but are extremely expensive. They include the Egerton net suspension bed in which the patient lies in a hammock, water beds and the Mediscus air bed.

The ripple bed was a considerable advance in the treatment and prevention of pressure sores. It has an alternating pressure-point pad used over the patient's ordinary mattress under the bottom sheet to provide regular, frequent automatic redistribution of the pressure areas. The pad consists of a vinyl plastic pad with alternating sets of air cells running transversely across the width of the regular mattress, with an air pump which automatically controls the cycle. Single pads are now available and a new twin pulsator will operate two pads.

(c) Immediately incontinence occurs, the patient must be washed from the waist to the knees and dried thoroughly. All soiled bedclothes are changed and zinc and castor oil ointment or silicones form a waterproof covering for the skin. An indwelling catheter is essential to prevent bed-wetting in the persistently incontinent patient. 'Inco pads' may be used. These are made of several thicknesses of soft paper which can be easily changed and are disposable. They are useful only in as much as they protect bed linen. If left in position too long they can also aggravate the skin by causing friction.

(d) Seventy-eight per cent of all pressure sores occur in the ischial region and are consistently more common in chair-bound than in bed-fast patients with the same degree of helplessness. Bowker and Davidson have designed a cushion (Fig. 21.2) that is effective in relieving high pressure points by distributing body weight uniformly over a large area of the buttocks and thighs. It consists of a foam outer cushion fitted with a waterproof vinyl cover on a polyvinyl chloride bag containing five litres of the thixotropic gel.

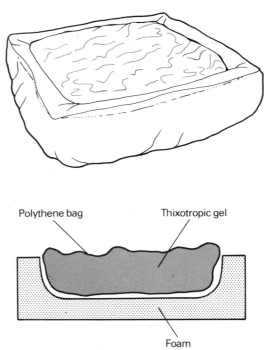

Polythene bag   Thixotropic gel

Foam

Fig. 21.2 Cushion containing thixotropic gell.
(By courtesy of Bowker and Davidson).

Established pressure sores

The first decision to be made is whether the sore is superficial or deep. Superficial sores which are painful, account for about 75 per cent of the total and will usually heal. A deep sore is painless, life-threatening and will not heal until the slough has been removed. Organisms colonise rather than invade the tissues so that antibiotics have no place in treatment.

When the lesion is still limited to an area of erythema of the skin, relief of pressure is most important. The patient's posture must be changed at least 2-hourly, and on occasions the patient may be allowed to sit out of bed with considerable benefit. The doctor in charge of the case should always be asked if this is possible in a case of threatened sores. Sitting out of bed may be substituting one form of immobility for another so frequent care is still necessary

In some patients, particularly those in whom there has been complete transection of the spinal cord, the development of an ulcerated sore would appear to be inevitable, yet they almost never develop a pressure sore when they are cared for in special spinal injury units.

If some part of the sore is healing by granulation, 1 per cent gentian violet or red lotion is of value. In the young subject who shows every sign of recovery from a long illness, and who has been unfortunate enough to develop a large pressure sore as a complication, a further skin graft may be necessary to accelerate recovery. When ulceration has developed the same aseptic precautions should be followed as when dealing with a wound.

ULCERATION

An ulcer is a breach of the epithelial surface. Important in maintaining the discontinuity of the epithelium and preventing healing are pathogenic bacteria, defective oxygenation as a result of venous or arterial disease, oedema from circulatory defects or infection, a defective nerve supply, and continued trauma.

Types of ulcers

1. Inflammatory:
   (a) Non-specific, e.g. carbuncle which has pointed.
   (b) Specific — tuberculosis, syphilis.
2. Varicose (Ch. 23).
3. Bed sores (p. 189).
4. Trophic.
5. Malignant.
6. Rodent ulcer (Ch. 27).

The parts of an ulcer are:

The floor — the portion which can be seen.

The edge — side walls.

The base, i.e. the portion that can be felt.

COMPLICATIONS OF A SCAR

Wounds, ulcers, and burns which have involved the dermis leave a scar. Complications which may arise are:

1. Keloid formation. This is very common after operations performed during pregnancy, following burns and after wounds in the Negro races.
2. Ulceration (from defective blood supply).
3. Contracture.
4. Neuroma (gives rise to pain).
5. Adherence to deep tissues.

6. Neoplastic changes.
7. Latent tetanus.

OTHER SURGICAL LESIONS OF THE SKIN AND SUBCUTANEOUS TISSUES

Injuries

Bee and wasp stings. The sting causes considerable pain. After removal of the sting by squeezing a compress of ammonia for a bee and vinegar for a wasp sting is applied. Bee and wasp stings cause 4 or 5 deaths a year in Great Britain due to anaphylaxis. A vaccine has been developed to nullify the effect of future stings in the estimated 60 000 people allergic to the stings.

Dog bites are treated with surgical toilet to the wound and the administration of tetanus toxoid and antibiotics. If the animal is suffering from hydrophobia (rabies), which is extremely rare in this country, the appropriate antitoxin must be obtained and administered as soon as possible to prevent the condition arising in the patient. The animal is isolated and kept alive to observe its behaviour before killing it when its central nervous system is examined for rabies.

Foreign bodies. Needles, splinters of metal and wood, and fragments of glass frequently become embedded in the tissues. If the end of the foreign body is protruding an X-ray is taken and the surgeon will advise if its removal is necessary. Most types of glass because of their lead content, are opaque to X-rays and therefore cast a shadow on the film because the component materials have a high atomic weight.

If it has been decided to remove the foreign body, the part is kept splinted and at rest and a further X-ray is taken immediately before the operation.

Removal of a foreign body in certain sites may cause greater damage than if it is left alone. Many foreign bodies cause no trouble and become surrounded by and embedded in fibrous tissue.

The Burman metal detector is an electromagnetic detecting device which will locate quickly and accurately metallic foreign bodies. Location is based on the indications of a meter and of a small loudspeaker operating simultaneously. The instrument, which is set to give sound of uniform pitch, remains unchanged until the probe approaches close to the metallic foreign body when the sound and meter reading both rise sharply. When used following an incision the probe is covered with a specially designed rubber jacket which can be sterilised by autoclaving or can be boiled. Non-responsive retractors supplied with the instrument are used for retraction.

Localised infection of the skin

1. Boils. A boil is caused by infection of a hair follicle by the *Staphylococcus pyogenes*. The first symptom is a localised itching pimple which increases in size, and the surrounding area becomes indurated and painful. As pus forms on the surface a yellow discharge occurs. Later there is sloughing, which is replaced by granulation tissue as healing commences. Should resolution occur without suppuration, the condition is known as a 'blind boil'.

2. Carbuncles. A carbuncle is a gangrenous process of the subcutaneous tissues. It is due to infection of multiple hair follicles, and the commonest site is the back of the neck. Diabetics are particularly liable to develop carbuncles.

Treatment. The urine is tested for the presence of sugar. If the patient is a diabetic the dosage of insulin will usually have to be increased and the co-operation of the physician sought. The best method of treatment of a boil or carbuncle is by administration of the appropriate antibiotic; resolution is usual and the acute stage is greatly shortened. If pus forms drainage will be necessary.

3. Subcutaneous abscess is a common condition. It is a frequent termination of cellulitis. The classical signs of acute inflammation are present.

Treatment. When pus is present drainage is necessary.

Tumours of the skin

Papillomas and haemangiomas are fairly common.

Malignant tumours are:
1. Rodent ulcer.
2. Squamous-celled carcinoma. } See Chapter 22.
3. Melanoma.

Septic fingers

Infection of a tendon sheath is responsible for the crippling disability which may be seen in many cases as the end result of a septic finger.

Cause

Septic pinpricks and cuts from glass are the usual causes.

Symptoms

1. Pain in the finger which is aggravated by movement.
2. The finger is swollen and throbbing.
3. Extension of the metacarpo-phalangeal joint is extremely painful.
4. Red lines on the arm (lymphangitis) and enlarged axillary lymphatic nodes (lymphadenitis).

General constitutional signs, flushed face, pyrexia, and loss of appetite, are present.

Treatment

1. Absolute rest. The arm should be kept supported in a sling.

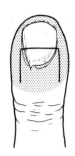

Fig. 21.3 Nail base removed for paronychia.

2. Antibacterial therapy.

3. Incision and drainage followed by hypertonic sodium sulphate baths and active movement. Splinters or foreign bodies present will be removed at the same time. In addition, the general treatment of an acute infection is undertaken. Active movements of the fingers as soon as they are painless are very important.

Paronychia is the occurrence of infection around the nail bed. As soon as pus forms the bed is incised and the proximal half of the nail is removed to effect drainage (Fig. 21.3). The distal half is left covering the sensitive tissues. A new nail grows when the infection subsides and the portion of the old nail which has been left drops off. In a neglected case infection of the bone (the distal phalanx) develops.

Pulp space infection. The dense tissue of the finger tip is often infected by needle pricks. Unless early treatment is sought, necrosis of the underlying bone occurs.

Diffuse infection of the spaces in the palm may occur as a result of a tendon sheath infection or a subcutaneous abscess which has not been drained adequately.

BIBLIOGRAPHY

Bailey B N 1970 British Journal of Hospital Medicine 3: 223
Bowker P, Davidson L M 1979 British Medical Journal 2: 958
Gibbs J R 1977 Lancet 1: 174
Scales J T In: Bedsore biomechanics, Macmillan, London, p 259.

22

Oncology

The science of new growth or tumour formation is known as oncology. A tumour, or new growth, is a mass of cells similar to those of a body tissue, growing at the expense of the body and fulfilling no useful purpose. It is not true that tumour cells proliferate faster than normal cells. Further, it has become clear that a tumour is not a relatively stable mass of cells which increase in size and number as a result of a steady rate of cell division. It increases in size only when the rate of proliferation is higher than the rate of cell loss.

A new growth may be simple or malignant, and the difference is that unchecked a malignant growth will invariably kill the patient. Simple tumours are nonetheless important because, untreated, they may cause death by interfering with some vital function. A simple tumour of the meninges, for example, will cause cerebral compression and, unrelieved, the patient will die in a coma. A malignant growth is commonly known as a cancer.

THE CAUSE OF CANCER

The cause, or causes, of cancer are unknown, but there is, nonetheless, a vast amount of valuable information about the factors predisposing to its occurrence. Not all malignant growths are incurable, the number of cures is increasing. In some sites cancer is invariably fatal, but in others the results of treatment are highly successful.

Predisposing factors

1. *Heredity*. Notable examples are the development of carcinoma of the colon in patients with familial polyposis and carcinoma of the oesophagus in the skin disease known as tylosis.

2. *Chronic irritation*. Chronic irritation has long been recognised as a predisposing factor. Constant irritation from coal-tar products or excessive exposure to sunlight may result in growths of the skin. Excessive cigarette smoking in bronchial carcinoma and β-naphthylamine in carcinoma of the

bladder are well recognised carcinogens.

Many pioneers of radiology lost their lives from skin cancer, the result of exposure to unprotected X-ray tubes.

3. Chronic sepsis. Carcinoma of the tongue is very frequently associated with long-standing syphilitic infection, and the condition hardly ever develops in a clean mouth.

In the pages which follow are described growths as they appear to the naked eye or under the microscope — that is, their morphological character. Malignant growths may well be due to the loss of essential cellular constituents or to faulty synthesis and logical treatment would lie in substitution or replacement therapy. A biochemical characterisation of cancer rather than a morphological one would then be logical. There is evidence that with some tumours syndromes occur as a result of circulating hormones secreted by the primary tumour.

4. Immunological aspects. Tumours are not autonomous — that is to say they are not independent of all the normal constraints which contain tissue metabolism. It is known that spontaneous regression can occur and yet sudden reappearance may be made after a period of complete quiescence. It is of interest to note that circulating tumour cells often fail to establish metastases.

5. Viruses and alterations in the hormonal balance are other factors which predispose to malignant new growth. In experimental animals a condition indistinguishable from carcinoma of the breast can be produced by a virus.

THE DEVELOPMENT OF A MALIGNANT NEW GROWTH.

It is now believed that carcinogenesis occurs in two stages. The first stage (tumour initiation) is a gene mutation in individual body cells. The second stage (tumour promotion) enables the genetically altered cell to proliferate to form a tumour. The factors which cause tumour promotion may ultimately be more amenable to intervention than the initial change in the cell.

SCREENING FOR THE EARLY DETECTION OF CANCER

This may take the form of:

Clinical examination

Exfoliative cytology. Examples are:
1. Cervical smear for detection of carcinoma cervix (p. 585).
2. Screening of urine in rubber and dye workers who are liable to car cinoma of the bladder (p. 465).

Radiography has been used for carcinoma of the breast but is not of proven value. More important in breast carcinoma is clinical examination of the breasts when smear screening for cervical cancer is undertaken. The opportunity should be taken at the same time to examine the breasts for the presence of lumps. Mammography may reveal patches of calcification in the breast which were clinically not palpable (Ch. 29).

SIMPLE NEW GROWTHS

Much confusion has arisen in following the terminology of tumour formation. The ending 'oma' simply means a new growth. A simple new growth is similar in substance to the tissue in which it arises and is named accordingly. Malignant new growths are named after the cells from which they arise.

Here are considered only the main types of simple new growths and the way in which they differ from malignant growths. Under the appropriate regions their clinical features are considered in detail.

Type of growth	Tissue of origin
Lipoma	Fat
Neuroma	Nerve tissue
Chondroma	Cartilage
Myoma	Muscle
Osteoma	Bone
Fibroma	Fibrous tissue
Angioma (naevus)	Blood vessels
Myeloma	Bone marrow
Odontoma	Teeth
Adenoma	Gland

A papilloma is a pedunculated tumour of the skin or of an epithelial lining. Some new growths are multiple. They have arisen separately and not from

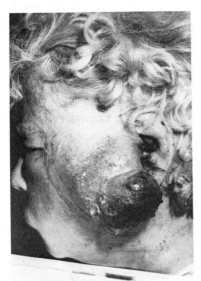

Fig. 22.1 Carcinoma of the parotid gland (fungating).

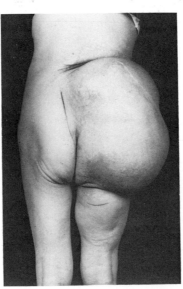

Fig. 22.2 Sarcoma of the right buttock.

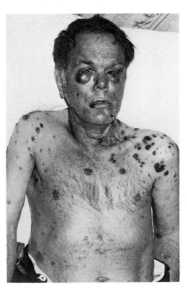

Fig. 22.3 Disseminated malignant melanoma.

metastasis. Common multiple simple new growths are:
    Lipomas
    Neurofibromas
    Naevi

Characteristics of simple new growths

1. The increase in size is slow. The tumour is limited by a capsule.
2. Spread into the neighbouring tissues does not occur. The tissue is pushed aside but not invaded.
3. They do not spread by the blood stream or by the lymphatic system.
4. They may cause symptoms as a result of their size or by pressure on the neighbouring tissues.
5. There is no tendency to recur after excision.

The usual treatment is excision or in suitable cases treatment by cryosurgery (p. 202).

MALIGNANT NEW GROWTHS

The principal forms are:
1. Those arising from the epithelial lined surfaces — carcinoma.

(a) *Squamous-celled carcinoma* (syn. epithelioma), which is a squamous-celled tumour growing from tissues covered by squamous cells, e.g. the tongue and skin.

(b) *Adenocarcinoma*, which is a glandular tissue tumour, e.g. breast, stomach, large intestine, salivary (Fig. 22.1).

2. Connective tissue tumours (Fig. 22.2). Sarcoma — these arise in bone (osteogenic sarcoma) or in fibrous tissues (fibrosarcoma).

3. Pigment cells. Melanoma (Fig. 22.3) arises in the pigmented layers of the skin and in the choroid of the eye. Simple pigmented moles may develop into malignant melanomas.

In between simple and malignant growths there is a number of border-line growths, the best recognised being a rodent ulcer of the skin. They are locally malignant in that they destroy tissue, but rarely spread to remote sites or into the lymphatic system.

Papillomas of the urinary tract, which were always known to become malignant if untreated, are now believed to be the first manifestation of carcinoma of the bladder.

The spread of malignant new growths

Malignant new growths may spread:

1. Locally. The growth increases in size and invades the neighbouring tissues eroding blood vessels, the skin and bony tissues if adjacent.

2. By metastasis (i.e. by secondary growth formation). The word metastasis means a mirror image.

(a) *By the lymphatic stream*. Carcinomas almost invariably metastasise or spread first by this route. The local lymphatic glands enlarge as spread progresses. Sarcomas invade the glands very late in their course.

(b) *By the blood stream*. The tumour may be widely disseminated to other tissues, and the deposit is also known as a metastasis or secondary new growth. This is a common method of spread of sarcomas, and this characteristic renders them rapidly fatal. Carcinomas have a lesser tendency to invade the blood stream in their earlier stages.

Secondary growths in bone are commonly the result of a primary growth in the breast, lung, prostate, kidney and thyroid.

3. By contact. Tumours of the bladder have an evil reputation in this connection but the true explanation is probably that they are multicentric in origin.

4. Transperitoneal implantation. Cells shed from a growth of the stomach may fall on to the structures in the pelvis and give rise to secondary growths. The ovaries are the organs most frequently invaded by secondary growths in this way.

5. Surgical implantation. This is not a frequent occurrence, but is seen occasionally in the scar of an operation wound through which a new growth has been excised.

Characteristics of malignant new growths

1. Untreated, the patient usually dies from the disease.
2. Increase in size is progressive. They have no limiting capsule.
3. Spread occurs to the other tissues as described above and gives rise to secondary growths.
4. Ulceration and infection are common, and many of the symptoms and signs are due to infection of the growth. Infection is particularly liable to result in secondary haemorrhage.

Symptoms and signs of malignant new growths

The symptoms and signs described in this book, as we follow the course of new growths in each organ, are those of moderately advanced tumours. The early symptoms and signs are:

1. *A lump* — this should invariably be a cause for seeking medical advice.
2. *Bleeding* — from any part of the body. A few drops of blood lost even on only one occasion are important.
3. *Slight alteration in normal habits or functions* — to mention only a few: (a) increasing constipation; (b) difficulty with swallowing, walking, talking, or eating.
4. *Changes in metabolism*. Since some tumours such as those of the pancreas, the pituitary or the adrenal add to the function of these organs, a change in metabolism may be the first indication of tumour formation.

New growths in the early stages will be diagnosed only by careful clinical examination and painstaking investigation. When symptoms are marked the growth is usually well advanced.

Biopsy. In cases of doubt, a small portion of the growth is removed and examined under the microscope. This procedure is often of great value in diagnosis, but is not without danger because more rapid spread of the growth may result. The recovery of malignant cells from the interior of organs or in secretion or excretion is sometimes of great value in diagnosis.

Exfoliative cytology is the process by which cells recovered from natural secretions like the gastric juice or the urine are centrifuged, sectioned in a paraffin block and examined under a microscope. Scrapings from organs like the cervix of the uterus may be treated similarly, and the opinion of an experienced pathologist is invaluable in the detection of cancer at a very early stage.

Biopsy and exfoliative cytology material will be examined by the pathologist. When a growth is malignant certain terms are used. Anaplastic means that cell division has been rapid. Another term used in this connection is undifferentiated which means that cells are very poorly formed and bear little or no resemblance to the cells from which they arose. They are more malignant than a growth in which the cells are well differentiated and more like the cells of origin. It can be compared to drawing a square with a pencil on paper. The normal accurate square is drawn with a ruler — normal cells — it takes time. Drawn more hurriedly without a ruler but joined together it will still resemble a square — well differentiated but not an accurate square. Drawn still more rapidly it may have only two sides and be unjoined — poorly differentiated and anaplastic — rapid and bad.

TREATMENT

Unfortunately neoplasia is all too often a generalised disease with many subclinical foci and it is these undetectable micro-metastases which later become manifest. For many years surgery and radiotherapy were the main forms of therapy for most solid tumours with chemotherapy used as a last resort in disseminated cancer. Over the last decade considerable advances have been made in the treatment of a few types of solid tumours — Burkitt's lymphoma, chorion carcinoma, acute lymphoblastic leukaemia and Hodgkin's disease.

In many cases the results of multicentre trials must be awaited before the value of a chemotherapeutic drug can be evaluated in the treatment of a particular tumour. The chance of cure from chemotherapy is at its highest when the tumour mass is small, for at this stage the proportion of cells in division is highest. This is immediately after the apparently successful excision of a tumour or when there is only minimal residual tumour.

Immunotherapy which builds up lost resistance is also becoming increasingly important in the treatment of cancer.

The best method of treatment of an individual tumour is a matter of multidisciplinary consultation.

The treatment of childhood cancer by surgery, radiotherapy or chemotherapy has already resulted in the cure of several thousands of children in Britain. With a long life span there is a proportionately greater chance of long-term damage to normal tissues and organs to emerge. The mutagenic effects of radiotherapy and chemotherapy on the gonads are an obvious hazard to any offspring. The results of studies so far are reassuring but are incomplete.

Radical treatment

Surgical excision consists of removal of the growth and the whole of the area between it and the lymphatic glands, together with the glands themselves. The results are best when the glands are not invaded. Occasionally, and particularly in tumours resistant to other forms of treatment, a 'second look' operation is undertaken for recurrent disease. In some patients further progress is achieved in controlling or eradicating the disease.

Radiotherapy. In certain sites, such as the tongue, where the mutilation of surgical excision is very great, this method is usually employed. In this particular growth it is as effective as operation. Radiations act by destruction of the cancer cells.

Cryotherapy is the destruction of living tissue by cold. The fundamental premise of cryodestructive surgery is that the living cells are first injured and later die from the results of freezing. A machine circulates liquid nitrogen through a partially insulated probe. A cryolesion is produced around a central freezing point.

The majority of skin tumours, benign and malignant, are best treated in this way. Postoperatively a slight haemorrhagic ooze may accompany the thawing process but ceases within a few hours. This may be followed by blister formation and subsequently by an eschar. This separates after several weeks and epithelialises.

Adjuvent chemotherapy implies the use of systemic agents in the destruction of disseminated microfoci of malignancy at a time when there is no clinical or investigative evidence of residual disease. In England and Wales 150 000 people die of malignant disease each year and it is estimated that 70 to 80 per cent die of metastatic disease. In the U.S.A. 700 000 new cases of malignant disease are registered each year and 50 per cent are estimated to have metastatic disease at the time of diagnosis or a high risk of recurrence following the presently available surgical or radiotherapeutic primary treatment (De Vita et al 1975).

The size of the total body burden of tumour has long been recognised as a factor influencing the response to chemotherapy. When the burden is reduced by surgical excision of the primary growth or shrunk by radiotherapy, chemotherapy is theoretically likely to be most effective in the destruction of micrometastases. The selection of patients will be determined only after the results of clinical trials now in operation. But already it is clear that for Wilms tumour and osteogenic sarcoma the results have been substantially improved with adjuvant chemotherapy.

Palliative treatment

Radiotherapy is frequently of value in causing retrogression and, in the advanced case, may delay deterioration. In the presence of gross sepsis, however, it is not satisfactory, because the tumour is more resistant and infection may flare up. Radiotherapy is also a satisfactory method of relieving pain from secondary deposits in bone.

Surgery. Palliative operations are frequently undertaken to relieve symptoms such as obstruction.

The duty of a doctor or nurse is to relieve suffering, and, although not able to cure the patient of his disease, the treatment of his symptoms is all-important to him.

Adrenalectomy and gonadectomy for carcinoma of the breast or prostate.

Hormonal antidotes are still in the process of development. Prostatic cancer may be treated with stilboestrol (5 mg t.d.s.) taken orally, and carcinoma of the breast in the male or elderly women by ethinyl oestradiol 1 mg t.d.s.

Cytotoxic agents (chemotherapy) also destroy bone marrow — an effect which is put to therapeutic use in the treatment of the leukaemias. The concentration of the drug at the tumour site is increased by:

(a) Injection into a malignant effusion.
(b) Injection into an artery supplying the tumour (regional perfusion).
(c) Intravenous injection (depending on the blood count).

Side-effects include leucopenia, diminution in platelets, alopecia, haematuria and nausea. The principal cytotoxic agents used clinically are methotrexate, cyclophosphamide and thiotepa.

Cytotoxic agents act by interfering with the metabolism of the cancer cell. In conditions such as Hodgkin's disease, some leukaemias and chorion carcinoma, the results of single or combined drug therapy are very encouraging. Some of the many groups of drugs used in combination are:

Vinblastin
Prednisolone
Nitrogen mustard
Procarbazine
5 Fluorouracil.

Local perfusion. Local intra-arterial perfusion with cytotoxic agents will increase the concentration of the drug at the site of the disease. As a method of treatment for secondary disease within the liver local perfusion with 5-Fluorouracil via the hepatic artery offers some hope of controlling what is otherwise a hopeless condition.

Antiviral agents. (Ch. 6) Interferon has been used but no conclusive results are yet available.

Anabolic synthetic chemicals increase resistance by increasing metabolism in the tissues. Durabolin or decadurabolin given by injection are examples of the type of preparation used — others are the corticosteroids.

RADIOTHERAPY

As the name implies, treatment by radiation includes radium, 'X-irradiation', and radioactive isotopes.

The aim of radiotherapy is either:
1. Radical to cure the disease.
2. Palliative to relieve a symptom such as the pain of a bony metastasis, dysphagia in carcinoma of the oesophagus or bleeding from a carcinoma of the uterus.

Radium

Radium emits several rays—alpha and beta particles, and gamma rays. Only gamma rays are used in the treatment of cancer.

The radium salt is enclosed in a platinum needle, the platinum absorbing the alpha and beta particles, which are highly damaging to the tissues.

Radon is a gaseous emanation of radium. The seeds are radioactive for about nine days. This form of application is particularly suitable for sites such as the bladder, the parotid gland, the skin, and pharynx. The seeds do not require removal.

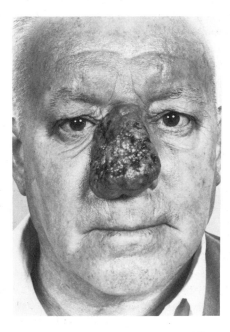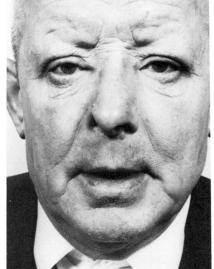

Fig. 22.4 Effect of radium.
A. Squamous-celled carcinoma of the nose before treatment.

B. Same patient after treatment.

Some growths are more sensitive to irradiation in a hyperbaric oxygen chamber.

The forms of radiotherapy have been classified by Paine (1980) as:

1. External beam irradiation

(a) Conventional X-ray therapy delivered from a superficial or deep

X-ray set similar to diagnostic X-ray equipment. The energy output is relatively low (40–140 RV).

   (b) Megavoltage radiation supplied by:

      (i) X-ray sources from a linear accelerater with an output of 4–25 MeV.

      (ii) Gamma ray sources, either Cobalt (^{60}Co) or Caesium (^{137}Cs). The energy output is 1·2 MeV.

2. Bradytherapy

The delivery of the radiation is relatively slow — the source being placed within or near the growth. It may be:

   (a) Intracavitary. This is the usual treatment of malignant uterine tumours. Originally carried out with radium the treatment is now delivered with ^{137}Cs and can be afterloaded into a tube placed in the patient previously or by the Cathetron technique. In this technique the whole irradiation is carried out under general anaesthesia in a few minutes. The source holders are carefully placed by the operator and when all attendants have moved to an adjoining room from where the patient can be safely monitored then ^{60}Co sources are afterloaded mechanically.

   (b) Interstitial therapy. Radium needles have been largely superseded by ^{192}Ir wires or ^{137}Cs needles (Paine 1972).

Radioactive isotopes

The radioactive isotope is a form of an element which behaves chemically in the same way as its normal form, but because of a different combination of particles within its nucleus, it is unstable and changes into a different element, releasing energy in the form of X-rays, gamma-rays, alpha and beta particles. The energy released enables them to be used in amounts small enough not to interfere with normal physiology and this is also the reason for their use in radiotherapy. They are used in three ways.

   1. Research.

   2. Diagnosis. Radio isotope imaging of bone with ^{99m}Tc-labelled phosphates is the most frequently performed scan in departments of nuclear medicine for pre-treatment assessment, staging and follow up. One quarter of clinically early cases of carcinoma of the breast have a positive bone scan. Unnecessary surgery is avoided and early palliative treatment is commenced.

   Radioactive iodine, which is concentrated in thyroid tissue, outlines the thyroid gland and will show if any gland tissue lies retrosternally. Scans using special isotopes are now common to outline the kidney, the lungs, the bones, the liver and the pancreas.

   3. Treatment.

   (a) Carcinoma of the thyroid — this sometimes takes up radioactive iodine and the radioactivity concentrated in the thyroid kills the carcinoma cells. Metastases from this tumour sometimes take up radioactive iodine. Radioactive iodine is also used to treat thyrotoxicosis.

   (b) Multiple myelomatosis — radioactive phosphorus (^{32}P) is injected intravenously and concentrates in bones.

(c) Caesium or cobalt is used as a beam in place of deep X-rays.

(d) Gold, injected into pleural and peritoneal fluid, commonly abolishes the fluid, but does not cure the disease. It is a palliative treatment.

(e) Yttrium or preferably radioactive gold is implanted into the pituitary—this procedure has the same effect in breast carcinoma as adrenalectomy, but can be used after adrenalectomy has failed.

All the substances actually injected into the body have a short life and the patient is not 'radioactive' for long. Also they are very local in their effects and other people can be in contact with them in safety.

Faeces and urine may need to be stored in protected containers until any radioactivity in them has diminished to a minimal quantity. This usually takes only a few days; then the excreta can be emptied into the drains in the usual way.

The mode of action of radiations

The gamma rays or X-rays destroy cells which are about to divide. Cancer cells divide frequently, hence the more rapidly growing the tumour the more radiosensitive it is likely to be. Some damage to the skin and tissues is inevitable with radical radiotherapy, and this is known as a 'radiation reaction'.

The care of the patient undergoing radium treatment

Care of the radium application locally

The nurse must see that the radium does not slip out of place and must report any mishap at once. Loss of radium is prevented by keeping the patient in bed with a special sign, such as a large red 'R' hung over the bed to indicate that radium is being used. All dressings, etc. should be kept in a special bucket until the radium has been removed from the patient and the needles counted and found correct. All excreta are preserved while there is radium in the patient's body and inspected before disposal.

Preparation of the skin

Only pure surgical spirit should be used for the preparation of the skin before the application or insertion of radium. Metallic substances which give off secondary radiations should not be used. These include pins, strapping, metallic chains, metallic lotions and ointments.

Radiotherapy reactions

Radiotherapy may give rise to general and local reactions.

General reaction

This may consist of nausea and general malaise. From its effect on the blood system anaemia and leucopaenia may develop.

Local reaction (radiation reaction)

On the intact skin radium produces a painful erythema which, if severe, may lead to an indurated area of cellulitis. The stages are:
1. Erythema.
2. Dry desquamation.
3. Moist desquamation.

On the skin zinc (in strapping) and mercurial lotions are avoided. The skin is kept dry with minimal cleansing and if it weeps only light sterile gauze is applied. Chafing is avoided and hypnotics are prescribed.

In the mouth and throat sloughing and infection are inevitable. A careful watch should be kept for secondary haemorrhage and blood cross matched if it is suspected. Antibiotics may be necessary to control sepsis and particular attention is paid to feeding. Peanut butter is helpful and dry food like biscuits are avoided. A spray of 10 per cent lignocaine enables fluids to be taken in less discomfort. Smoking in the room and any source of fumes increase irritation of the mucous membrane.

The bladder. Increased frequency of micturition and infected urine are common symptoms. Bladder wash-outs (Ch. 43) may be necessary.

The rectum. Irritation and diarrhoea may develop.

Local disabilities induced by radiotherapy

Damage which may occur from radiation includes:
1. Renal damage may develop following abdominal radiation and may induce acute or chronic nephritis followed about a year later by hypertension.
2. Osteoporosis may result in fracture after radiation of the cervical spine.
3. Radiation pneumonitis is a possible complication of radiotherapy to the breast.
4. Myelitis of the cervical spinal cord may arise from radiotherapy in the neck.
5. Damage to the rectum and sigmoid colon may occur after radiation to the cervix.
6. Fistula and perforation may occur from radiation necrosis.

All these local complications are diminished by improved techniques.

Occupational therapy and rehabilitation. The patient must be kept occupied while in hospital. Light work like rug making helps to pass away the time and take the patient's mind off his illness. The follow-up of patients suffering from cancer is important to the patient because recurrences are frequently treatable. It is also important to the hospital, so that the end results of treatment may be studied and correlated.

Protection of the nursing staff

Radium and X-rays are powerful poisons and sources of danger to the health of the nursing staff if adequate precautions are not taken. The nurse must not handle radium with the fingers. The nurse should not expose herself unnecessarily to radium, and the staff attending radium cases should be changed frequently and should wear small badges to indicate the level of radiation to which they have been exposed and should be tested regularly. A blood count should be performed every three months to detect early damage to the nurse's health.

NURSING CARE

In this chapter the nature, the diagnosis and technical aspects of treatment have been considered and in many of the pages which follow the management of malignancy in various regional sites is described. There is always a danger that the anxieties and fears of the patient are overlooked in our desire to effect a cure.

Many patients are investigated for symptoms which may be due to a malignant growth and while some are aware of the possibility others are quite oblivious. At this stage the nurse has every reason to be cheerful to the anxious patient. In many instances the patient suspects the worst, fears the consequences and loses all hope when there is a possibility of cure. At this stage and at all stages in the management of the patient the nurse must be a good listener and however hurried she may be the patient must be given every opportunity to speak his thoughts. It is at this time that the staff can give the patient what is most needed, a sense of companionship and trust.

Once the diagnosis has been established a decision has to be made on the best method of treatment and the patient may be confronted by an increasing number of consultants as the decision is often a multidisciplinary one. All methods of treatment are almost always unpleasant either alone or in combination. Surgery is rarely of a minor nature and often radical and mutilating. Radiotherapy and chemotherapy to be effective have to be given in doses bordering on the toxic. A knowledge of the type of operation, the effects of irradiation at various sites as well as the toxic manifestations of chemotherapy with cytotoxic drugs is an essential background for the nurse. She can prepare the patient for the onset of unpleasant symptoms which may arise from treatment and if they occur he will feel reassured that they are transitory and not as he may otherwise presume due to extension of the disease.

The decision of how and to what extent a patient is informed is a medical one and the nurse must be aware of the decision of the doctor in charge of the patient. She should answer questions from the patient unhesitatingly within the general policy of the unit. Relatives should normally be taken into the picture but on occasions the patient wants to know the whole truth and insistent that his relatives should not be distressed. On many occasions the patient almost certainly knows the diagnosis but obviously prefers no serious discussion.

The patient and his relatives need information and if possible reassurance on many aspects of his condition. The possibility of returning to a normal life or occupation is the first consideration and this varies with the site and extent of the lesion. All are anxious that pain be controlled and in the majority of patients this reassurance can be given (Ch. 5).

The maintenance of health is the first priority in a patient afflicted with malignant disease. The maintenance of nutrition, the correction of anaemia and the control of infection are essential. Nor should it be forgotten that the patient may develop nonmalignant disease which if not diagnosed and treated correctly may be lethal.

Quite as important with these patients as the length of life is the quality of life and good nursing care can do much to improve it. A check on body weight is a good general guide.

BIBLIOGRAPHY

Bush H 1978 British Journal of Hospital Medicine 20: 260
De Vita V T 1977. In: Salmon S E, Jones S E (ed) Adjuvant therapy of cancer, Elsever North Holland, Amsterdam, p. 640.
Paine C H 1972 Clinical Radiology 23: 263
Paine C H 1980 British Journal of Hospital Medicine 23: 544

23
Diseases of arteries and veins

ARTERIES

Arteries (apart from the pulmonary artery) carry oxygenated blood to the tissues and therefore any impairment to the normal flow will lead to anoxia of the tissues. The blood flow within a vessel is governed by several factors including its diameter, the cardiac output and the viscosity of the blood itself. The increased viscosity which may develop in some forms of blood disease such as leukaemia may lead to thrombosis. The flow in small vessels is much less than in larger ones and a critical closing pressure exists below which flow ceases, a point of importance in the development of thrombosis following vascular spasm and generalised hypotension.

Muscular activity plays an important part in the regulation of blood flow. When a muscle such as the calf muscle is exercised its demands for oxygen and glucose are increased. The waste products of metabolism act locally by producing vasodilation but if insufficient arterial blood is reaching the leg muscles these products accumulate in the tissues and lead to troublesome cramp-like pain felt within the calf. The pain, which is referred to as intermittent claudication, disappears with rest only to return with resumption of activity. As the degree of arterial obstruction increases, the claudication distance will diminish. Eventually the patient may complain of pain at rest which is sufficiently severe to keep him awake at night.

OCCLUSIVE ARTERIAL DISEASE

Arterial occlusion may occur suddenly, following an embolus or thrombosis, or gradually as in atherosclerosis (Fig 23.1) and thromboangiitis obliterans. These conditions principally involve the lower limbs.

Embolism

This is due to the transmission of an organised thrombus from one part of the circulation to another where it becomes lodged, generally at the point of division of an artery. The embolus usually orginates either within the left atrium, as in mitral stenosis, within the left ventricle as following myocardial infarction, or indeed within an atheromatous aorta.

Impaction takes place at the site of division of peripheral vessels, the majority occurring within the common femoral artery at the origin of the profunda femoris.

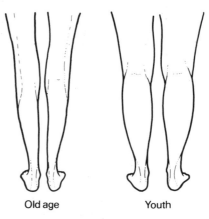

Old age   Youth

Fig. 23.1 Legs of old age showing absorption of the muscle mass due to the diminishing blood supply. Legs of youth showing good muscles.

While cerebral embolism is common and often fatal, embolism within the upper limb is less common and rarely produces any problem. Obstruction of the circulation produces sudden ischaemia of the affected part which if not relieved may proceed to actual gangrene.

Clinical features

Pain of sudden onset.
Pallor of the limb giving way eventually to a blotchy blue discoloration.
Paralysis of the affected limb.
Loss of cutaneous sensation.
Feeling of coldness.
Loss of pulsation within the artery distal to the point of occlusion.

Treatment

Early diagnosis and treatment are both important in saving limb and life. Whilst a small peripheral embolus may be treated conservatively with intravenous heparin to prevent propagation of the clot distal to the site of occlusion, an embolus which occludes a major artery such as the femoral is a surgical emergency. The operative management of arterial emboli has been revolutionised by the introduction of the Fogarty balloon catheter. The catheter may be introduced into the artery through a small arteriotomy and the thrombus retrieved in a 'chimney sweep' fashion from its site of impaction.

Anticoagulant therapy with intravenous heparin is commenced as soon as possible and continued postoperatively but because of the risk of bleeding it has to be carefully controlled (Ch. 13). The nurse should observe the colour and temperature of the toes as well as palpate the pulses in the arteries distal to the operation site to ensure that the blood supply is satisfactory. Absent pulsation or pallor and coldness of the toes should be reported without delay.

Atherosclerosis

The aetiology of this condition is unknown but it is characterised by the deposition of fatty material within the wall of the artery and predominantly within the subintimal layers. This deposition, together with the subsequent thrombus formation, leads to a narrowing of the lumen. The disease appears to be widespread throughout the circulatory system but tends to be concentrated at sites of bifurcation such as the aortoiliac region.

Clinical features

It is only when the blood flow is reduced to critical levels that the disease produces symptoms and these are gradual in onset. When it involves the main vessels to the leg the commonest symptom is that of intermittent claudication. In this condition, a cramp-like pain appears with exercise. It is generally felt within the calf but it may also be experienced within the thigh and gluteal region. The walking distance required to produce the pain gradually becomes shorter and within time proves to be incapacitating. Rest pain may become a distressing factor. It indicates marked ischaemia and as it is often worse at night, causing loss of sleep, leads to a rapid deterioration of morale.

Management

Patient must learn to live with it.
Reducing weight will lead to relief.
Stop smoking.
Avoid injury to the area of ischaemia. Nail trimming (Fig. 23.2) should be done with great care the nails being kept long to avoid injury. As most sufferers have poor eyesight and tremulous hands they are advised not to attempt to cut their toenails.
Correct any anaemia.
Careful control of diabetes.
Reconstructive arterial surgery should be considered only if the symptoms are severe and do not respond to conservative measures. The feasibility of such surgery will depend on arteriographic evaluation of the affected vessel. This involves the injection of radio-opaque material under general anaesthesia into the arterial tree proximal to the site of obstruction. In the case of the lower limb the femoral artery may be punctured directly within the groin or the aorta may be punctured through the back, the needle passing to the left of the vertebral bodies.
Two types of operative procedures may be carried out.

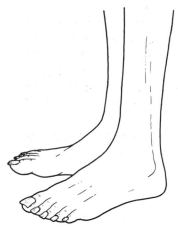

Fig. 23.2 Toe nails must not be cut short. Note the thin wasted limbs so characteristic of arterial insufficiency.

1. Thromboendarterectomy. The inner lining of the diseased artery together with its contained thrombus is cored out either through a long incision or through several small incisions using a special ring stripper. The arterial incisions are then closed either by direct suturing or by incorporating a vein patch graft (Fig. 23.3).

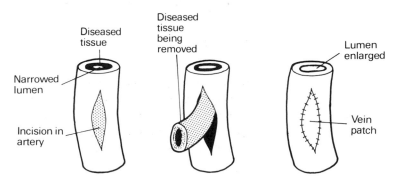

Fig. 23.3 Thromboendarterectomy through an incision made over the blocked segment. The inner core consisting of the diseased tissue is removed and the incision repaired by means of a vein patch graft.

2. Bypass grafts The diseased segment may be left in situ and the region by-passed using the patient's own saphenous vein anastomosed to the femoral artery above and to the popliteal below (Fig. 23.4).

If it is technically impossible to perform any kind of reconstructive surgery it may be possible to relieve the rest pain by means of a lumbar sympathectomy.

Aneurysms

An aneurysm is a localised dilatation of an artery resulting from weakness of its wall, atherosclerosis being the commonest cause.

Degeneration of the whole of the arterial wall may give rise to a spindle-shaped enlargement of fusiform type whereas localised weakness of part of the wall may produce a saccular form. The weakness within the arterial wall may also be of a congenital nature such as the so-called berry aneurysm of the intracranial vessels (Ch. 44). Inflammatory changes in the arterial wall such as are found in syphilis may also lead to aneurysmal formation.

A traumatic aneurysm is really a false aneurysm with the development of an aneurysmal sac in a haematoma surrounding a damaged artery.

Clinical features

Presence of an expansile swelling which may be painful or painless.
Palpable thrill and audible bruit.
Left untreated an aneurysm may rupture into the surrounding tissues or may thrombose with impairment of the peripheral arterial circulation.
Rupture of an abdominal aortic aneurysm is preceded by severe back

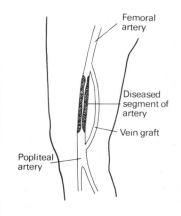

Fig. 23.4 A saphenous vein bypass graft.

pain. Profuse haemorrhage into the retroperitoneal tissues leads to severe shock and a tender abdominal mass is usually palpable.

Treatment

Complete excision of the aneurysm and its replacement by an arterial Dacron graft is the ideal procedure (Fig. 23.5).

The condition of a patient suffering from an aortic aneurysm is assessed before operation and prepared in the usual manner for an abdominal operation. A nasogastric tube has been found to be unnecessary and omission has reduced postoperative pulmonary complications from 16 to 7·5 per cent.

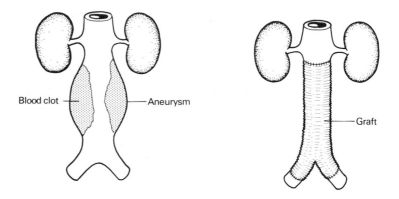

Fig. 23.5 An abdominal aortic aneurysm containing a thrombus and its replacement by a Dacron arterial graft.

A ruptured abdominal aneurysm is a very different situation. Some patients die before reaching an operating table and amongst those who do undergo surgery there is a mortality of 45 per cent compared to 8·5 per cent when the aneurysm is unruptured. What the patient requires above all else is that the bleeding is controlled by placing a clamp across the aorta above the aneurysm.

A pressurised suit advocated by Lewis may be life-saving. On arrival at the hospital the patient is taken straight to the theatre. As rapidly as possible a nasogastric tube is passed (essential as the contents of his stomach are unknown), and the skin of the abdomen is prepared. An intravenous line (preferably two) is set up. Twelve units of blood are ordered.

If the patient's condition permits resuscitation is commenced but the systolic blood pressure is not raised above 100 mm Hg in case further bleeding occurs. The anaesthetist only induces the anaesthetic when the surgeon is ready to open the abdomen. Within 2 minutes of induction the surgeon opens the abdomen and immediately puts a clamp across the aorta. Effective resuscitation is now possible and when the hypotension has been corrected by blood transfusion the patient is heparinised and the operation proceeds.

Postoperatively the patient is treated in an intensive care unit, where the blood pressure, the blood gases, serum electrolytes and all the other para-meters which guide treatment are monitored. Paralytic ileus is a common complication.

The pulses in both lower limbs should be palpated half-hourly for the first 24 hours and any deficiency reported.

Thromboangiitis obliterans

Although this condition is regarded by some to be simply an early form of atherosclerosis it is described here as a separate entity.

The disease tends to affect young men and is characterised by an inflammatory reaction which involves the arterial wall together with the adjoining vein and nerve. Remissions and relapses are often encountered with gangrenous changes appearing later in one or more toes and remaining localised for some time.

Treatment

Smoking should be stopped completely but although vasodilator drugs are often prescribed their efficacy is doubtful. The results of lumbar sympathectomy are variable but if pain is severe it is worthy of trial. Limited amputation of the toes is successful in this condition and major amputation should be withheld for as long as possible.

Raynaud's disease

This is an uncommon condition which affects the hands of young women. There appears to be an exaggerated vasospastic response to cold, the attacks being characterised by blanching of the digits followed by blueness and pain and later by redness. Patches of gangrene may appear on the

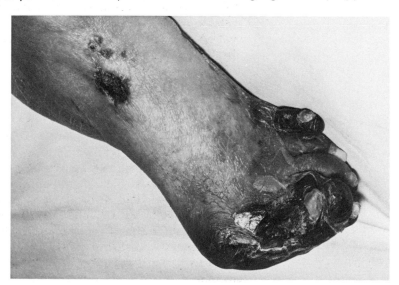

Fig. 23.6 Gangrene of the foot.

fingertips, and treatment is primarily directed towards protection from the cold and the administration of vasodilator drugs. Cervical sympathectomy may lead to relief of symptoms.

Gangrene

This means death of tissue and may be massive in type as in the death of a whole limb (Fig. 23.6) or it may be localised in form as for example involving the fingertip.

Causes

Loss of blood supply as in atherosclerosis.
Physical or chemical violence as in burns.
Infection such as gas gangrene.
Gangrene in general, apart from gas gangrene, may be of two types.
1. Moist gangrene. The tissues are moist and infection spreads rapidly. Toxic products are absorbed in the tissues near to the gangrenous area. If the gangrene is moist the area must be treated as a septic wound and amputation is undertaken as soon as possible.
2. Dry gangrene. This form is usually vascular in origin and the spread is slow. So long as the part is kept dry the gangrenous portion may separate at a line of demarcation, the tissues proximal to this being healthy and viable.

Treatment of the gangrenous limb

(a) Keep the limb cool so that its metabolism is reduced.
(b) Keep the affected part dry. This is best accomplished by complete exposure and the toes involved may be kept separated by dental rolls.
(c) The limb should be protected from the weight of the bedclothes by a bed-cage and the heel supported on a foam pad.
(d) Adequate relief of pain.
(e) Lumbar sympathectomy may result in vasodilatation of the collateral blood vessels and an improvement in the cutaneous blood flow.
(f) When gangrene threatens the patient's life amputation should be considered.

Gangrene of digits is a definite indication for direct arterial surgery because if successful a major amputation is avoided. If unsuccessful then some form of amputation is inevitable. Obviously this is a serious undertaking in an elderly feeble patient and the nursing care of such cases is of paramount importance. A constant anxiety is the healing of the amputation flaps in tissues which are obviously depleted of blood supply. A compromise has to be made. The higher the level of the amputation such as mid-thigh the better the chances of healing but against this must be placed the fact that amputation above the knee joint means that rehabilitation of the patient is going to be much more difficult. All amputations require vigorous skin preparation in the theatre and all should have intramuscular penicillin commencing on the day before surgery and continuing for seven days after operation. These measures are essential to prevent gas gangrene in the amputation stump.

Postoperative management

Avoid injury to the stump.

The stump must be wrapped in crêpe bandage (Fig. 23.7) and then left exposed.

No pillow is placed behind the stump as a flexion deformity may develop.

Remove drainage tube in 48 hours.

Exercise the limb from the second day.

Early mobilisation on crutches and fitting of the artificial limb.

Removal of skin sutures on the 10th day.

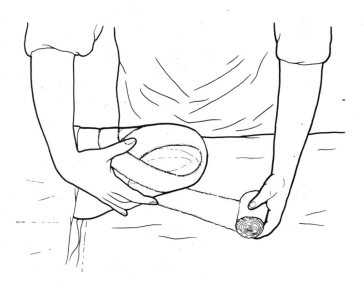

Fig. 23.7 Bandaging an amputation stump.

Complications

Reactionary haemorrhage within the first 12 hours.

Secondary haemorrhage at 7–10 days.

Infection. This may be associated with disease in the bone.

Phantom pains. The patient may still complain of pain in the foot or hand which has been amputated.

Amputation stump neuroma.

Seventy per cent of all amputations performed are on patients over 70 years of age and half of all unilateral amputees who survive 3 years will lose the other leg.

VEINS

Anatomy

The internal saphenous vein runs in front of the medial malleolus, ascends the leg within the subcutaneous tissue just behind the medial border of the tibia, passes behind the posterolateral aspect of the knee and then continues along the medial aspect of the thigh to perforate the deep fascia at the saphenous opening to join the femoral vein. The main vein has many tributaries, the principal one being the posterior arch vein. Both the internal saphenous and the posterior tributary communicate with the deep intramuscular veins via communicating channels which perforate the deep fascia. The natural flow of blood is from the superficial veins via the perforating channels into the deep veins, the valves present within directing the flow and preventing any tendency to back-flow.

Varicose veins

Destruction of these valves allows for back-flow into the superficial veins and as a result elevation of the pressure (especially during exercise) within the superficial veins. This eventually leads to the varicosities (Fig. 23.8).

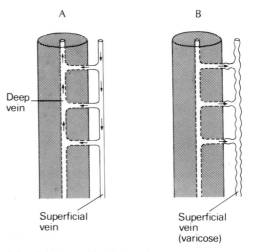

Fig. 23.8   A. Normal flow of venous blood through competent communicating veins from the superficial system to the deep system.
B. Reversal of flow following incompetence of the communicating veins with the development of varicosities within the superficial system.

Clinical features

Small varicose veins give rise to no symptoms. The principal symptom in the more prominent veins is a dull aching pain within the calf towards the end of the day. Women often complain of the unsightly appearance (Fig. 23.9) and enlargement of the vein at the saphenous opening may produce a soft swelling often 2 cm in diameter which has a well-marked cough impulse and empties on lying down. This is known as a saphena varix.

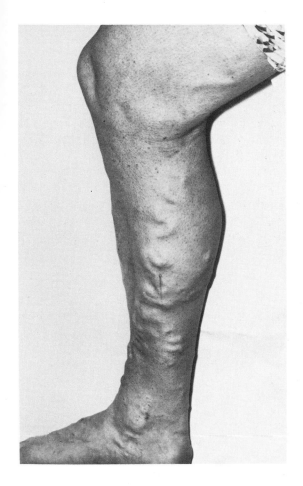

Fig. 23.9 Varicose veins.

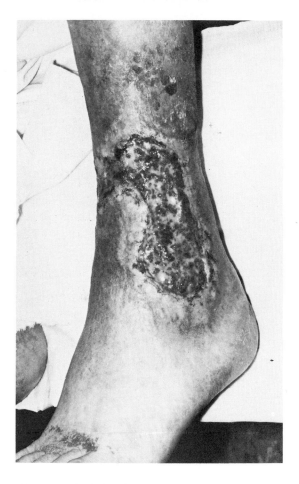

Fig. 23.10 Varicose ulcer.

Treatment

1. Elastic crêpe support stockings may be used to provide relief in patients unfit or unwilling to undergo surgery.

2. Injection sclerotherapy. This is suitable for the milder varicosities, the aim being to induce a thrombophlebitis within the vein which is then transformed into a thick fibrous cord. The agent used is sodium tetradecyl sulphate and it is injected at three or four sites into the vein, which is emptied by elevation of the leg. Pressure pads over crêpe bandages are then applied from the foot to the thigh; a full-length elastic stocking is worn for support for 6 weeks. The patient is encouraged to walk 2 miles per day.

3. Surgery. This approach is the most successful and consists of completely stripping the whole vein from the ankle to the groin where it is tied flush with the femoral vein. The patient wears a supporting stocking for 4 weeks.

The popular use of the saphenous vein as a bypass vascular graft may influence the surgeon in his decision to resort to surgery.

Complications

1. Phlebitis-treated by rest, lead and opium dressings and antibiotics.
2. Haemorrhage-treated by elevation of the leg.
3. Ulceration. Varicose ulceration (Fig. 23.10) may be treated conservatively initially with bed rest and occlusive dressings. If this is unsuccessful a direct attack on the incompetent perforating veins may be carried out surgically.

BIBLIOGRAPHY

Lewis D G, McKenzie A, McNeil I F 1973 Annals of the Royal College of Surgeons of England 52: 53–58

24

The nature of disease

In the preceding pages the various processes of disease have been covered. For the remainder of the book, disease as it affects specific systems and organs of the body will be described. This chapter serves as a link between the two sections, and provides an opportunity to take a slightly broader view of the nature of disease before proceeding to a more detailed description of its site.

The causes of disease are of fundamental importance. The clinical picture as revealed by signs and symptoms has to be known if it is to be recognised and the correct treatment undertaken. Changes which result from disease have one or more of the following effects:

1. *Tissue destruction*. When it is gross it is known as gangrene or putrefaction; lesser degrees of destruction are termed necrosis.
2. *Obstruction* is a common cause or result of disease. Lesions occur in far dispersed sites in the body which have little or nothing in common aetiologically yet they share an identical, simple mechanical process. It is more likely to occur in the narrowest part of an organ or duct. Some of these sites are illustrated in Figure 24.1.

Loss or diminution of blood supply is due to obstructive changes in the blood vessel walls or the valves of the heart. Solidification of normal contents in other channels results in stone formation in the biliary or urinary tract whilst the same process in the blood is called thrombosis. In addition to disease of the wall and obstruction of the lumen the whole organ may be compressed by pressure from without.

3. *Fluid leakage*. Fluid loss may be in a gross clinically perceptible form such as occurs in haemorrhage, perforation, ascites, burns, diarrhoea, vomiting or only in a more delicate physicochemical sense of change between the extracellular spaces and the blood.
4. *Degeneration*. The tissues wear out.
5. *Hormonal excess or inadequacy*.

In any illness an assessment has to be made of the nature of the changes produced.

ANATOMICAL NARROWS

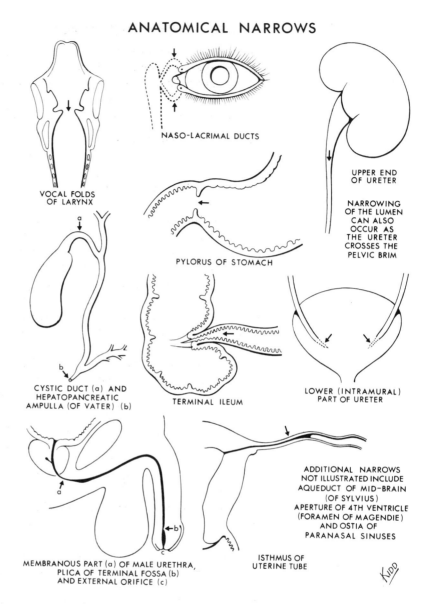

Fig. 24.1 Obstruction is more likely to occur where the lumen is narrowest.

THE NATURE OF THE CHANGES PRODUCED

The following are a few examples of these processes:

(a) A small wound causes fluid leakage due to haemorrhage and fluid leakage occurs from the inflammatory reaction in healing;

(b) a 30 per cent burn causes fluid leakage and tissue destruction;

(c) in a strangulated hernia containing a loop of small intestine the blood vessels to the bowel are obstructed and the flow of intestinal contents along the lumen of the intestine is prevented.

The degree or severity of the change

Taking the above examples —
(a) is usually completely trivial;
(b) requires immediate and urgent treatment of the extensive fluid loss if the patient is to survive;
(c) unless there is immediate surgical relief the patient will die.

If the normal vital reactions of the body can restore health no special treatment is required. If these reactions are overwhelmed treatment is necessary.

Health is the preservation of a constant internal environment in the body. Small changes in this environment — the 'milieu intérieur' of Claude Bernard — produce reactions which restore this state. Living cells apart from those on the surface of the skin are provided with a fluid environment, with a constant hydrogen ion concentration, osmotic pressure and temperature. Oxygen and food are carried to the cells by the arterial blood which is oxygenated in the lungs and waste products including carbon dioxide removed by the venous blood and the lymphatic system to be eliminated by the lungs and the kidneys. The whole process is regulated by the activities of the hormones and the nervous system. Cannon named this restoration of a constant environment 'homeostasis'.

Many diseases produce a state in which these reactions are strained or severely threatened and unless efforts are successful in re-creating conditions in which it is possible for the body to readjust the patient will lose his life. Treatment must be based on measures which logically assist these reactions and it is very easy to aggravate the patient's condition by well meaning but thoughtless action. For example, it is not so very long ago that heat in the form of hot water bottles and radiant heat cradles which appear so comforting in the management of the shocked patient were used routinely. They forced dilatation of the skin vessels which the physiological reaction was trying to constrict to maintain the blood pressure as well as to retain fluid in the body and provide as much blood as possible to the vital centres within the brain.

The measurement of the pulse, temperature and respiration are routine checks on the physiological state of the patient, but in serious conditions many more parameters of the body's activities have to be checked — the arterial blood pressure, the central venous pressure, the blood gases, the serum electrolytes, to mention only a few examples. Since the patient's condition is changing rapidly many tests have to be repeated at frequent intervals. In many cases a continuous check — monitoring — is essential. It is for this reason that a patient who requires such observation is nursed in an intensive care unit.

Man has survived much injury and disease from Adam to the present day without the help of antibiotics, extensive resuscitative measures and all the other facilities of modern medicine, including the social services. It is but a few years ago that the pulse, arterial blood pressure, temperature, blood haemoglobin and the blood urea were the only physical and chemical measurements of his well-being. To understand what we are really trying to do to help the patient it is worth considering very briefly what vital reactions occur in the patient's body, all of which are designed for his survival. It is the study of these in depth that has enabled considerable progress to be made in the care of the patient.

VITAL REACTIONS

1. Haemostasis has been considered in detail in Chapter 12. It is a natural reaction and, however large or small the haemorrhage, it is essential in controlling bleeding. Detailed study of its mechanism has enabled us to make good deficiencies of clotting factors as well as to prevent or disperse undersirable thrombus formation. Blood transfusion has saved lives of patients whose blood loss has been too rapid and too great to be overcome by the body.

2. The reaction to injury explains how the body takes special precautions to conserve vital fluids and electrolytes when it is assaulted by injury, using the term 'injury' in the widest sense of physical trauma or bacterial invasion. The immediate changes are:

(a) Increased secretion of antidiuretic hormone by the pituitary. The result is that water is conserved in the body. The kidney secretes a highly concentrated urine of high specific gravity. The volume is small so that what fluid is lost as urine is used to the greatest advantage to remove the maximal quantity of waste products.

(b) *The adrenal glands* secrete large quantities of aldosterone which has the effect of retaining Na^+ in the body; K^+ is increased in quantity from the breakdown of protein tissue and an excess which is very toxic is freely excreted by the kidneys in larger quantities than normal. These changes are reversed when the body commences to rebuild — Na^+ is freely excreted and K^+ necessary for the building up of cells is retained.

There are many other reactions but the above are examples of the types of changes which occur.

3. The inflammatory reaction has already been discussed and its failure to occur may be fatal (Ch. 8).

4. Physiological changes in fluid loss whether of whole blood, water, plasma, or electrolytes (Ch. 15.).

5. Immunological reactions are generally beneficial but a fuller understanding is necessary to treat and prevent organ rejection.

6. Psychological reactions to disease are important to the surgical nurse and the surgeon in the management of the patient and his disease.

All these vital reactions occur in and around a living cell in a fluid medium. The one essential is an adequate supply of blood and efficient venous drainage. Figure 24.2 illustrates in simplified diagrammatic form how the normal mechanism operates at the level of a single cell. For the purposes of illustration a single cell in the upper part of the small intestine secreting intestinal juice (succus entericus) is taken as an example and for the purposes of illustration only we shall assume that the adjoining cell secretes the hormone secretin which warns the pancreas that pancreatic juice should be secreted.

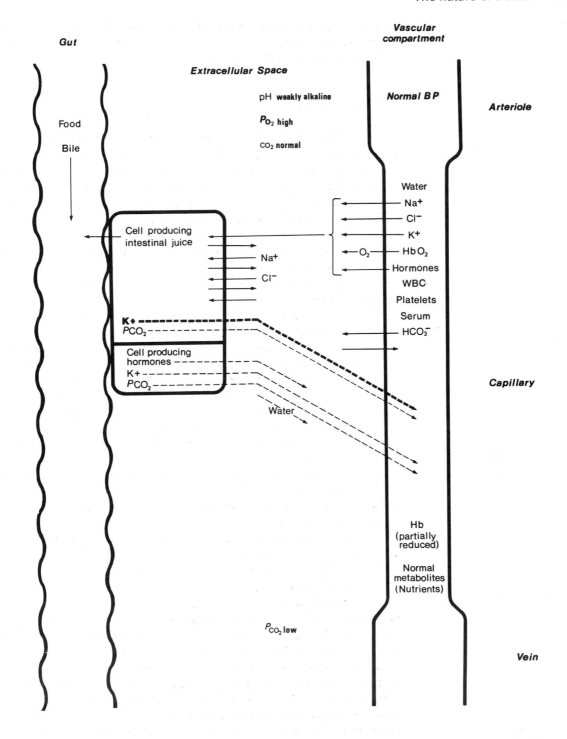

Fig. 24.2 Some of the normal exchanges at cell level in the small intestine in health (see text). K$^+$ and Na$^+$ pass freely across the cell membrane, CO$_2$ is excreted. Intestinal juice is produced and intestinal hormones are secreted and carried away in the venous blood.

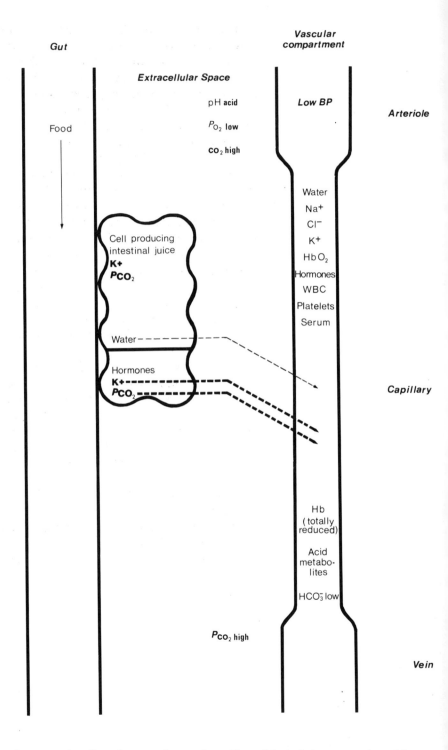

Fig. 24.3 The effect of a severe haemorrhage. The cell is denied oxygen and nourishment. Water is withdrawn from the extracellular space and ultimately from the cell. CO₂ first accumulates in excess in the cell then in the extracellular space and in the venous blood.

Figure 24.3 shows the changes which occur in the cell as a result of depletion of blood volume from haemorrhage anywhere in the body.

The junior nurse may well think — this is all very interesting, but has it any relevance to what she does at the bedside? Indeed it has. For example, it determines many nursing procedures.

1. The position of the patient. It explains why pressure sores may develop and are kept active. The blood supply is compressed and the cell dies. If there is an excess of fluid in a limb from deficient venous drainage raising the limb will help increase the flow of fluid from the leg. When the femoral artery is blocked by an embolus the patient is nursed on the opposite side and not resting on his buttock, so compressing the little blood which could flow in from this area to the leg.

2. The prevention of thrombosis. It is obvious that the more dehydrated the patient the greater is the viscosity of the blood (Fig. 24.3) and the more likely thrombi are to form. The risk of thrombosis is increased if the patient is immobilised or the blood platelets are increased as after splenectomy.

3. Corticosteroid therapy by interfering with fluid exchange and causing water retention interferes with normal reactions. It also prevents the adrenal glands from functioning normally and in stress more corticosteroids have to be supplied or the patient will collapse since he is unable to react to injury.

4. The poorer reaction of the older patient is in large measure due to inadequate blood supply because the vessels are arteriosclerotic. Hormones, immune bodies, white blood corpuscles, and antibiotics are not so easily concentrated where they are required as they are in the younger patient with a better cardiovascular system.

5. Abnormal white cells are ineffective in infection and the leukaemic patient is unable to deal with invading organisms. Shortage of white cells has a similar effect.

6. Inadequate renal or pulmonary function results in a build-up of waste products.

The outstanding lesson that emerges from a study of the changes in disease at the cell level is that the shorter the time that elapses from deprivation of blood and all the bad things it brings the better it is for health.

25

The lymphatic system and the spleen

Lymph is a tissue fluid which collects within the prelymphatic extracellular spaces from where it is conveyed to the larger lymphatic channels and by these eventually to the blood stream. It passes to the lymph nodes which are structurally adapted to filter and sample the lymph passing through them. This enables the system to isolate infection and when necessary triggers off host defence mechanisms. This response is mediated through lymphoid follicles contained within each node.

The principal sites of lymph nodes are indicated in Figure 25.1. Individual areas of the body drain to regional or primary groups of nodes. Efferent vessels from these lead to secondary groups of lymph nodes and may communicate with channels leading to the larger main ducts which join the venous system at the root of the neck.

Both the lymphatic channels and the nodes may be displayed by radiographic techniques following the injection of contrast media into a small subcutaneous lymphatic, a technique known as lymphangiography. Lymphatic structures can also be examined by radioisotope scanning and open excision biopsy of the node.

These techniques are now applied to the clinical investigation of oedema and malignant disease.

THE LYMPHATIC GLANDS

INFLAMMATORY CONDITIONS

Acute lymphadenitis. This is commonly due to an acute septic focus, such as a boil, tonsillitis, or a septic wound.

The primary cause must be treated. Locally, a counter-irritant relieves pain, and in many cases the infection subsides without very much trouble. Occasionally suppuration occurs and incision and drainage may be necessary.

Chronic lymphadenitis. *Tuberculous*. This is now a comparatively rare condition. Resolution usually occurs with rest and antituberculous chemotherapy. If the glandular mass enlarges, excision of the glands is

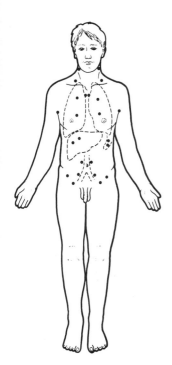

Fig. 25.1 The principal sites of the lymphatic glands.

performed. A cold abscess may be aspirated or drainage may be performed and the gland removed by curettage. In the abdomen, tuberculous glands usually heal by calcification, and may give rise to symptoms on account of mechanical interference with the functions of the intestine.

Other causes of chronic lymphadenitis include sarcoidosis, infectious mononucleosis and syphilis.

MALIGNANT TUMOURS OF LYMPH NODES

These may be primary or secondary.

1. Secondary malignancy is by far the commonest, the lymph node being the first 'port of call' of most malignancies once it moves outside its primary site.

2. Primary malignancy i.e. Lymphoma (Fig. 25.2). This is less common, Hodgkin's disease being the commonest variety. Once a definite diagnosis has been made by open lymph node biopsy the patient is thoroughly investigated to determine the extent of the disease before treatment is planned. Lymphoma may be found wherever there is lymphoid tissue e.g. the liver, the spleen, the gastrointestinal tract as well as the lymph node areas. The extent of involvement determines to a large extent the choice of therapy and has a direct relationship to the prognosis. This is determined by clinical examination of all the lymphatic drainage areas, a chest radiograph, an exploratory 'staging', laparotomy and more recently lymphangiography.

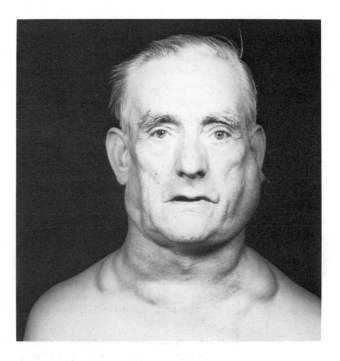

Fig. 25.2 Lymphoma. The glands of the neck are visibly enlarged.

Many patients with Hodgkin's disease and other malignant lymphomas can look forward to a normal span of life following radiotherapy or chemotherapy.

Lymphatics

Several clinical syndromes associated with oedema of unknown aetiology affecting infants, children and young adults are related to congenital developmental abnormalities demonstrated by lymphangiography. These conditions are usually difficult to treat and only the most severe cases should be subjected to surgery. This consists of excision of the oedematous subcutaneous tissue with the construction of skin graft procedures.

Lymphoedema from lymphatic obstruction also occurs as a result of:
(a) invasion of the lymphatics by cancer cells,
(b) surgical removal of the lymph nodes,
(c) parasitic infestation of the lymph channels e.g. Filariasis.

THE SPLEEN

The spleen is closely allied to the lymphatic system and it is frequently enlarged in lymphatic disorders, e.g. Hodgkin's disease and infective mononucleosis. It may also be enlarged in conditions unrelated to the lymphatic system such as portal hypertension, thrombocytopenic purpura and myelofibrosis.

INDICATIONS FOR SPLENECTOMY

1. Rupture is the commonest indication. The spleen is torn in a crush injury of the left hypochondrium. The patient complains of left sided abdominal pain and exhibits all the signs of internal bleeding.

2. Hereditary spherocytosis is a condition in which the red blood cells are fragile and are broken down by the spleen leading to anaemia and jaundice.

3. As part of a staging laparotomy for lymphomas.

4. In certain cases of portal hypertension.

5. Thrombocytopenic purpura is a bleeding disorder caused by a reduction of circulating platelets and the site of platelet consumption (the spleen) is removed.

Preparation for splenectomy

The preparation is similar to that for any major abdominal operation. A blood platelet count is almost always performed before operation.

The spleen is situated in the left hypochondrium, and access is difficult if the stomach is distended. For this reason a nasogastric tube is passed before the patient leaves the ward and left in position during the operation and for 24 hours afterwards.

Postoperative care

Thrombosis is the only special complication to be feared, and the measures described to prevent it should be energetically pursued.

Collapse or pneumonia of the lower lobe of the left lung is an occasional complication and may be prevented by deep-breathing exercises. Acute dilatation of the stomach is prevented by leaving the nasogastric tube in position and aspirating the stomach until it is emptying normally.

26

Organ transplantation

When an organ ceases to function owing to disease it can occasionally be replaced by artificial materials or by an organ taken from another individual.

Artificial materials introduced into the human body encounter a hostile environment and no material has yet been devised which combines ideal mechanical properties with perfect compatibility with human tissues. Having said this, many prostheses enjoy a considerable measure of success, good examples being the hip joint prostheses in joint replacement surgery and Dacron arterial grafts in vascular surgery.

The replacement of a diseased organ by one removed from another individual has, in recent years, become a reality although the potential rejection by the body of the transplanted organ remains a major obstacle.

Types of transplant

1. Autograft. (Fig. 26.1). Tissue taken from one area of the body and placed in another. A good example of this is skin grafts.

2. Allograft. Tissue taken from one individual in a species and placed in another of the same species. Examples are renal and hepatic transplants.

3. Xenograft. Tissue from one species transplanted into a member of another species.

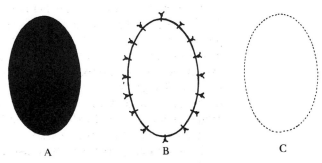

Fig. 26.1 Autograft. Skin defect (A) is closed by autograft of skin (B) and remains healed when the graft has 'taken' (C).

TISSUE REJECTION

The process is essentially an immunological one. When skin of guinea pig A is grafted on to guinea pig B the grafted tissue is initially accepted but at about the 10th day thrombosis occurs within the blood vessels which have grown into the grafted tissue, and the skin dies (Fig. 26.2). This phenomenon is known as tissue rejection. If a second piece of skin is grafted on to guinea pig B rejection is more rapid, occurring in 3–5 days.

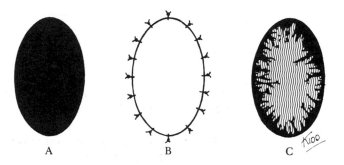

A   B   C

Fig. 26.2 Homograft reaction. Skin defect (A) is closed by homograft of skin (B) and gradually withers away (C) owing to the homograft reaction.

The process of rejection is accompanied by the features of an inflammatory response with infiltration of the area with leucocytes and exudation of fluid into the intercellular space. Within the cell membranes of the grafted organs are a number of factors called transplantation antigens. These antigens are recognised as foreign by the recipient lymphocytes. A generation of lymphocytes is produced which are specifically committed to the destruction of the grafts. The lymphocytes enter the blood stream and infiltrate the graft. This reaction on the part of the lymphocyte represents the cellular component of the immune response. In addition there is a humoral component in which the lymphocytes produce and release into the circulation antibodies which act upon the foreign antigens on the cell membranes of the graft.

In order that any allograft procedure may succeed, the process of rejection must be modified. At present this may be accomplished in two ways.

(a) Donor matching. Transplantation antigens are inherited characteristics. If donor and recipient are of the same genetic make-up, as in identical twins, no rejection will occur and the graft may survive indefinitely. Attempts have therefore been made to determine compatibility between the antigens of the donor and recipient, an assessment called tissue matching. The first part of the matching process is to ensure that the blood groups of the donor and recipient are the same. Following this the HLA system is matched for each individual. A good tissue match is compatible with a long survival of the grafted tissue.

(b) Immunosuppression. It is also possible to modify the production of antibodies by suppressing their manufacture. The drugs that are used to suppress the immune response are azothioprine and prednisolone. Whilst the former interferes with the metabolism of the lymphocyte the latter works by modifying the inflammatory response.

Antilymphocytic globulin, when injected into a recipient, reduces the number of circulating lymphocytes and thus modifies the process of rejection.

Clinical applications

Renal transplantation is now clinically acceptable. The good results achieved by transplantation are better than by any form of dialysis. Most donor material is obtained from car accidents, and as it must be removed from the donor's body not more than 30 minutes after death considerable ethical procedures are raised with respect to the definition of death and there are obvious difficulties in obtaining permission from the relatives for this to be done.

The donor kidney is transplanted into the right iliac fossa (Fig. 26.3) of the recipient, the renal vessels being anastomosed to the iliac vessels, whilst the ureter is implanted into the dome of the bladder.

Although both liver and heart transplants have been carried out at many centres the results do not compare favourably with those of renal transplantation. The consensus of opinion, therefore, is that until the rejection problem has been finally conquered both liver and heart transplantation should be confined to one or two international centres.

The results of liver transplantation are showing improvement as a result of better surgical technique. Rejection episodes are easily controlled with immunosuppressive drugs and hypothermic preservation will keep the donor liver in good condition for 10 hours.

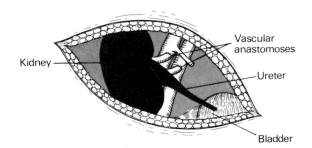

Fig. 26.3 A transplanted kidney in position.

27

The face, the mouth and the tongue

A patient suffering from a surgical lesion of the face or lip usually seeks medical advice in the early stages of the disability. The mildest lesion of the face is usually of some concern even to the most self-effacing individual, and facial disease or deformity can depress the morale of a patient out of all proportion to the size or severity of the lesion. Unsightly scars or naevi will effect profound changes in the attitude and outlook of the patient. They may affect his whole life, and the importance of the work of the plastic surgeon lies in reducing his disabilities.

Wounds

Wounds of the face, because of the abundant blood supply to the part, heal rapidly. Thorough cleansing and the removal of grit is important, as failure to do this results in an ugly discoloured scar. The fine stitches inserted should be removed on the third or fourth day to avoid permanent stitch marks. Sepsis is rare, dressings are unnecessary and the wound may be left exposed.

A depressed fracture of the malar bone is not uncommon, and early elevation is undertaken so that the cheek prominence is restored.

Inflammatory conditions and cysts

Cellulitis and carbuncle. The lips may be affected. Infection of the upper lip, once regarded as a most dangerous condition, is now easily resolved by the use of antibiotics.

Chancre of the lip. A primary syphilitic lesion (chancre) may appear on the lip. The glands in the neck are enlarged.

Chronic inflammatory conditions. Chronic inflammatory conditions are not common. The rhagades of congenital syphilis may be seen as healed scars in the adult.

Cysts of the face. Sebaceous cysts (Fig. 27.1) are common, particularly on the nose and around the ears. They are due to blockage of the duct of a sebaceous gland. The pent-up secretion of sebum is responsible for the swelling, and the lining of the cyst is the stretched sebaceous gland. The treatment is excision.

Dermoid cysts may form at the line of fusion of the skull and face and may be found at the root of the nose or over the external angular process of the orbit (Fig. 27.2).

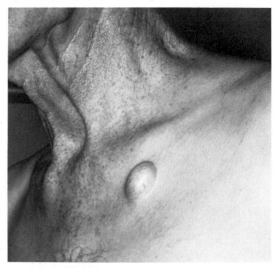

Fig. 27.1   Sebaceous cyst below the left clavicle.

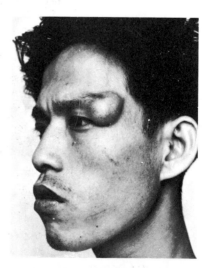

Fig. 27.2   External angular dermoid cyst. The overlying skin is freely movable.

NEW GROWTHS OF THE FACE AND LIPS

Simple tumours

Simple tumours, particularly naevi, may be disfiguring. They are usually treated by destruction with carbon dioxide snow, by surgical excision or by radiotherapy if they do not regress spontaneously. The best method is probably by cryosurgery.

Basal cell carcinoma (Syn. Rodent ulcer)

A rodent ulcer (Fig. 27.3) usually occurs on the upper part of the face, and is frequently situated dangerously near to the eye. It is locally malignant and, untreated, will erode the bones of the face and skull until a septic meningitis kills the patient. Its progress is very slow at first.

Radium to the surface, excision or cryodestruction are effective. In late cases the eyeball may have to be removed.

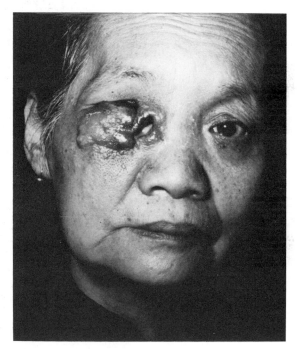

Fig. 27.3 Rodent ulcer.

Squamous-cell carcinoma

Cancer is commoner on the lower than on the upper lip, and used to be frequently associated with a long-standing habit of smoking a hot clay pipe.

Clinical features. The growth appears as a hard nodule which later becomes either papilliferous and warty in appearance, or it assumes the characteristics of a typical malignant ulcer. The base is fixed and the edge is hard and everted. The lymphatic glands underneath the chin and the lower jaw enlarge as spread occurs. Untreated, the tumour erodes the lower jaw.

Treatment. Surgical excision, radiotherapy or, better, cryosurgery may be used. The glands are treated by subsequent block dissection.

Cleft lip and cleft palate

Cleft lip and cleft palate are congenital deformities due to the failure of fusion of the various tissues forming the lips and the palate. Cortisone intoxication, virus infections such as rubella, oxygen and vitamin deficiency, as well as radiation damage during foetal life, are now known to be causal factors. Cleft lip almost invariably affects the upper lip, and may involve one or both sides. It may occur alone or in association with a cleft palate. In all cases there is some deformity of the face and nose. A cleft palate may involve the hard and the soft palate or only a portion of the soft palate. The disability of these lesions may be summarised as follows:

    1. The obvious cosmetic deformity.

    2. Feeding is difficult with a cleft palate but a cleft lip causes no interference.

    3. Nasal catarrh and respiratory infections are common because the mouth and the nose communicate.

    4. The speech is seriously impaired.

Treatment

A cleft lip is repaired as soon as possible. The edges are freshened and sutured together under a general anaesthetic.

The orthodontist by making a plate (Fig. 27.4) for the newborn baby with the cleft palate can aid the baby to suck. Furthermore modification of the plate can mould the cleft into correct alignment before surgical closure is undertaken. This has given vastly superior cosmetic results; in particular, deformity of the nose is very much reduced.

The repair of a cleft palate is undertaken in the first year or two of life. The soft palate must be repaired if good speech is to be attained. The hard palate may be united by suture, or the cleft may be blocked with an obturator (a dental plate similar to that on which artificial teeth are set).

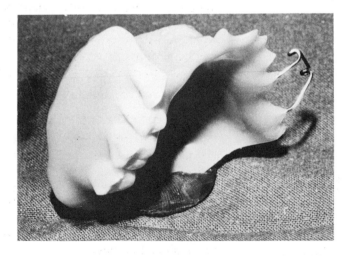

Fig. 27.4 Dental obturator to repair palatal defect.

Preoperative care of a case of cleft lip

The infant must be trained to take food from a special spoon (Fig. 27.5) or dropper, and his reaction to this form of feeding must be satisfactory before operation is contemplated. Sucking with a soft teat is preferable if a dental plate can be fitted. He should be gaining weight. The blood haemoglobin should be not less than 12 g/dl. The mouth must be gently rinsed or swabbed very carefully with glycothymolin or other suitable mouthwash, and swabbed with sodium bicarbonate solution to remove mucus. Preoperatively, systemic antibiotics will usually be prescribed to counteract any infection which may develop.

Swabs of the nose and throat should be taken before operation and the child should be in hospital for at least a week.

Postoperative care of cleft lip

1. Antibiotics will be continued postoperatively. The wound is left exposed. The mouth and nose are frequently cleansed so as to avoid infection. The sutures are removed on the fifth day after operation or earlier as the surgeon directs.

A Logan's bow may be applied for 14 days to keep the lip in the normal pouting position.

2. The arms are splinted lightly to prevent the infant 'picking' the dressing.

3. Feeding must be as careful as before operation.

4. Rest is essential. Crying must be reduced to a minimum, since it tends to stretch the suture line. Sedatives, such as chloral hydrate, are prescribed at frequent intervals for 4 or 5 days after the operation.

Preoperative care of cleft palate

The child's general condition must be satisfactory before operation is performed and sepsis must be eliminated. The mother can be assured of a good cosmetic result. Removal of the tonsils may be advised but this practice is avoided if possible as removal of the tonsils and adenoids tends to impair effective palatopharyngeal closure.

Postoperative care of cleft palate

1. The arms are splinted to prevent the child injuring the suture line in the mouth. The patient is propped upright in bed. Atropine (0·3 mg) is administered to diminish salivation for 2 or 3 days.

2. Feeding is carefully carried out. Since the mouth is now smaller than previously, and also very tender, there may be considerable difficulty in feeding. The diet should consist of milk, jelly, blancmange, fruit juice, and soup. Rusks, vegetables, and toast are avoided lest the suture line in the mouth should be injured.

3. The mouth is cleansed with several spoonfuls of sterile water before and after every feed.

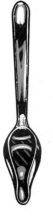

Fig. 27.5 Spoon adapted for feeding infant with cleft lip or cleft palate.

4. The stitches do not require removal, since catgut is usually employed and will dissolve spontaneously. Wire sutures, if inserted, will be removed by the surgeon.

5. Rest is secured, as described in the postoperative care of a cleft lip.

Continual supervision and further operations to correct associated deformity are necessary until adult life.

A long convalescence is necessary, and the child must be under the care of a speech therapist as soon as possible after operation.

THE MOUTH AND THE TONGUE

The most serious disease inside the mouth is a carcinoma originating in the buccal mucosa or in the mucous membrane of the tongue. The condition is frequently associated with chronic irritation, and is rarely seen inside a clean mouth.

Glossitis

The commonest cause of inflammation of the tongue is antibiotics causing vitamin B_2 deficiency. Cytotoxic drugs are an occasional cause.

Chronic glossitis in which the tongue is firm, fissured and later white and cracked on the surface (leukoplakia) is a pre-cancerous condition. Excisional biopsy and cryosurgical excision of the affected area is undertaken.

Cysts in the mouth

1. Simple mucous retention cysts are not uncommon.
2. A ranula is a cystic swelling of the floor of the mouth.
3. A dermoid cyst may protrude into the floor of the mouth.
Excision is the usual treatment.

Ulceration of the tongue

Ulceration of the tongue may be:

A dental ulcer. A dental ulcer is always situated on the side of the tongue in the neighbourhood of a jagged tooth.

Syphilitic ulceration is painless, and the ulcer has a typical punched out appearance.

Malignant ulceration is discussed below.

Aphthous ulcers. Aphthous ulcers are characterised by the development of single or multiple erosive lesions in the oral mucosa surrounded by an area of oedema and hyperaemia. They vary in size from 2 to 10 mm and may be episodic. In women, characteristically they occur premenstrually. The cause is unknown, but oestrogen therapy is effective in healing most patients with premenstrual aphthous ulcer as well as in some in whom the ulcer is not related to the menstrual cycle. Stilboestrol 3 mg daily is a suitable dosage.

NEW GROWTHS OF THE TONGUE

Simple new growths

1. Papilloma.
2. Angioma.

The patient feels the nodule. In the case of angiomas slight haemorrhage is usually present. These growths are excised with a diathermy knife.

Malignant new growths

The incidence of carcinoma of the tongue has been greatly reduced by routine dental care and the effective treatment of syphilis.

Symptoms and signs

Pain may be present in the tongue or referred to the ear.

Haemorrhage. Small haemorrhages are common once ulceration has occurred. A massive fatal secondary haemorrhage is a not unusual termination.

Ulceration. Ulceration has usually occurred by the time the patient seeks advice. It takes the form of a sloughing ulcer with a firm, indurated base and a large everted edge (Fig. 27.6). As the disease advances the patient may be unable to protrude the tongue from his mouth. Salivation is excessive as a result of irritation, and the exudation of pus which results from secondary infection of the growth. Secondary deposits may occur in the lymphatic glands in the neck.

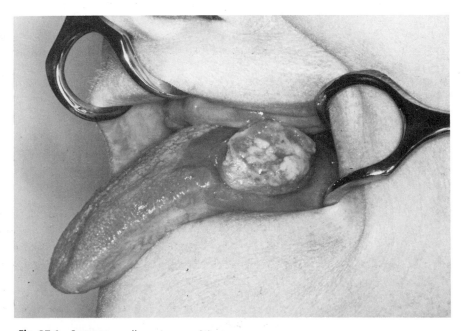

Fig. 27.6 Squamous-cell carcinoma of the tongue.

Course of the disease

Untreated, death occurs from:
1. Broncho-pneumonia, which results from the inhalation of the infection in the growth.
2. Secondary haemorrhage.
3. Starvation and exhaustion as a result of pain, and extension of the growth into the tissues of the neck and mouth.

Treatment

Dental treatment is undertaken before any surgical treatment can be attempted. The teeth and gums are invariably septic.

Radiotherapy. Interstitial radium is the treatment of choice usually applied to the primary growth, but radiotherapy has given disappointing results in the treatment of the glandular field.

If the glands are invaded they are treated by what is known as a 'block dissection' of the neck. This is usually undertaken after the primary growth has been treated by radium. For this operation the skin is prepared from about 15 cm below the clavicle up to the hair-line.

If the glands are not invaded a careful watch is kept on their condition.

Nursing care. The patient with radium in the mouth requires very special care. *The threads of the needles* must be securely fixed on the face with strapping and regularly inspected and counted to ensure that a radium needle has not been swallowed. All excreta are inspected before disposal. Frequent bland mouthwashes must be given, and a fluid diet, as rich as possible in protein and other nutrients, must be provided. Meat soups, eggs, milk, jellies and fruit juice to which glucose has been added can all be taken. Peanut butter is very useful to keep the mouth moist.

The mouth is septic and irrigation with hydrogen peroxide or eusol diminishes foetor.

He should be nursed upright in bed and provided with:
1. A bowl into which saliva can drain.
2. Gauze swabs or disposable tissues to wipe his lips. The bowl for salivation and the swabs should be checked in case they contain a radium needle.
3. A pencil and paper to communicate his wishes.

Pain is usually severe, and morphia may be necessary for its relief. Earache, although not due to an organic cause in the ear, may be treated by the instillation of phenol drops (5 per cent) into the ear and a cotton-wool plug. They act as a counter-irritant at the site to which pain is referred.

The radium reaction is frequently severe, and secondary haemorrhage is most liable to occur 2 or 3 days after the radium has been removed. Its risk is minimised by frequent cleansing of the mouth and encouraging the patient to wash out the mouth as often as possible. Chemotherapy may be prescribed to control infection. Should bleeding occur, the nurse must pull the patient's tongue well forward with the tongue forceps. This frequently controls the haemorrhage temporarily. If this is not successful, the common carotid artery pressure point at the root of the neck must be compressed at once and medical aid summoned without delay.

THE SALIVARY GLANDS

The normal healthy mouth, apart from cleansing of the teeth, does not require mouthwashes. The mouth of the patient who is toxic, dehydrated or forbidden to take fluid becomes dry and more septic than usual. He has little stimulus to excite salivation. The result is that infection creeps up the ducts down which saliva normally flows profusely, and an inflammatory condition develops in the gland. It is for this reason that moistening of the mouth, and mouthwashes, are so important in preventing infection in the conditions just mentioned. Even better than moistening the mouth is to stimulate the flow of saliva, and this can be achieved by giving the patient chewing gum or barley sugar.

Acute sialadenitis (acute inflammation of a salivary gland)

This is due to the conditions which we have mentioned above, and is common only in the parotid glands.

The face is tender and swollen over the affected parotid gland. The patient complains of difficulty in opening his mouth.

The prevention and treatment have already been indicated, namely, mouthwashes, chewing gum and drinking plenty of fluids, if they are allowed. Should suppuration develop, incision will be necessary.

Acute non-suppurative parotitis (mumps)

This is a virus infection and an entirely separate condition. Both parotid glands are usually swollen. Orchitis and very rarely pancreatitis may occur as complications.

Chronic sialadenitis and salivary calculi

The secretion from the parotid gland is thin and serous; that from the submandibular gland is thick and mucoid. As a result of obstruction or stricture of the duct, a low-grade chronic inflammation may arise in a gland. In some cases a calculus forms and blocks the duct. Because of the thicker secretion, 95 per cent of calculi are formed in the submandibular gland.

Symptoms and signs

The patient complains of a swelling in the submandibular region which increases in size at meal times and diminishes in the periods between meals. The enlarged gland can be palpated. A radiograph is taken to prove the presence of a calculus.

Treatment

Treatment may consist of:
1. Removal of the calculus.
2. Dilatation of Wharton's duct with lacrimal probes.
3. Excision of the gland.

A calculus in Wharton's duct is removed from inside the mouth. No special local preoperative preparation is necessary. Postoperatively, these patients may be sent from the theatre with a small swab in the mouth, which is attached outside to a pair of Spencer Wells forceps. The patient is usually coughing by the time he leaves the theatre, and the swab can be removed shortly afterwards. It is unusual for severe haemorrhage to develop. Stitches in the mouth are usually of catgut and do not require removal.

Dilatation of Wharton's duct is usually undertaken for strictures; dabbing the surface with local anaesthetic may suffice, or no anaesthetic may be necessary. The preparation for an excision of the gland is similar to that for excision of the lymphatic glands of the neck.

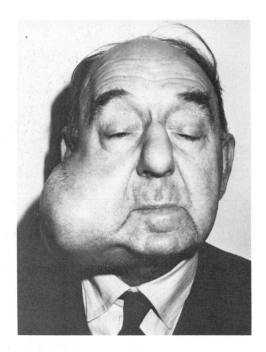

Fig. 27.7 Mixed parotid tumour.

Parotid tumours

1. Mixed parotid tumour (Fig. 27.7)—75 per cent are benign. The superficial lobe of the parotid gland is excised.
2. Carcinoma—the facial nerve is invaded. It is treated by total removal of the parotid.
3. Some rarer tumours, such as adenolymphoma, may occur.

THE TEETH AND THE JAWS

In the first or deciduous dentition there are 20 teeth which erupt at intervals from about 6 months to 2 years of age. The permanent teeth, which number 32, follow the deciduous teeth and commence to erupt at the age of 6 years. They continue their eruption until the age of 12, when only the third molar (wisdom) teeth are unerupted. Their eruption occurs in the late teens. The roots take three years to develop completely after the teeth have commenced to erupt. Failure to erupt may result in impaction (Fig. 27.8).

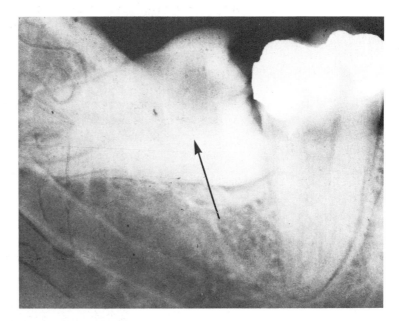

Fig. 27.8 Impacted third molar (wisdom tooth).

Each tooth forms a firm joint with the jaw, being held in its socket in the alveolar bone by a fibrous ligament, the periodontal ligament, which is attached to the tooth root and to the bone.

ABSCESSES ARISING FROM THE TEETH

An abscess arising from a tooth may be the cause of infection at remote sites in the body. Infection arising from teeth may be of two types:

1. Open sepsis. Open sepsis occurs almost invariably from infection of the gum margins and from decayed teeth and roots. It is commonly caused initially by the deposits of calculus (tartar) which irritate and inflame the gum margins. It is known as open sepsis because the infected material drains into the mouth. The pus forms in the pocket between the gum margin and the root of the tooth and drains into the mouth producing halitosis (bad breath). Infection may spread to the sinuses, tonsils and stomach. Open oral sepsis predisposes to chest infections after general anaesthesia.

2. Closed sepsis. Closed sepsis is considerably more important than the open type. Infection almost invariably commences as dental caries (decay) and if this is untreated it spreads and infects the pulp of the tooth, from which it is but a short step to the jaw and the venous blood stream, through which it is passed around the body. Such bacterial spread (bacteraemia) is dangerous in patients suffering from congenital or rheumatic heart disease because it can lead to bacterial endocarditis.

Dental abscess

1. Acute. An acute dental abscess (alveolar abscess) arises from an infected tooth. The onset is heralded by acute pain, increasing in severity. Swelling is not marked at this stage.

About the third day there is characteristically a sudden remission of the pain as the inflamed, congested tooth pulp dies. Soon the infected material escapes through the root end and produces inflammation of the periodontal ligament. This makes the tooth tender to touch and to bite on, and pain returns in the jaw. With the pus tracking through the periosteum into the soft tissues, a generalised swelling occurs. The patient feels unwell, looks ill and the temperature, which should not be taken in the mouth, is elevated.

Treatment consists of extraction of the offending tooth. This will usually provide sufficient drainage, but in the presence of extensive facial swelling with pus, external drainage may be necessary in addition. Antibiotics will be used in severe cases. Nursing treatment, apart from vigorous hot mouth-washes, is on the general lines of an acute toxic condition.

2. Chronic. A chronic abscess may follow an acute abscess which has

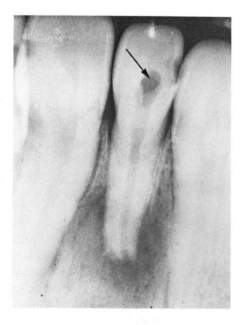

Fig. 27.9 Apical abscess.

pointed in the mouth, leaving a sinus which has failed to heal. More commonly they are chronic from the beginning, caused by low grade infection from the dead pulp of a tooth over a prolonged period (Fig. 27.9.).

Odontomes

Odontomes are cysts or tumours arising from the cells from which teeth are formed. Excision and removal of the epithelial elements is undertaken, together with malformed dental hard tissues — i.e. masses composed of enamel, dentine and cementum in differing proportions.

Dental caries

Dental caries is a very common disease in civilised peoples and its treatment is a matter for the dental surgeon. It is the progressive destruction of the enamel and dentine of a tooth by acids produced by oral bacteria. The bacteria (which are part of the normal flora of the mouth) convert carbohydrates such as sugar and starch to acid — e.g. lactic acid, which can slowly dissolve the hard tooth tissues. The dental plaque, a film lying on uncleaned teeth, is the site where bacteria act to produce the acid. It follows that in simple terms, caries can be controlled by (a) reduction of the amount of sugar in the diet, and particularly by cutting down the duration of time it is present in the mouth; (b) removal of the dental plaque by brushing between the teeth conscientiously; (c) making tooth structure more resistant to acid attack by applying fluoride gels to the teeth or, better still, incorporating fluoride in the developing tooth through the intake of fluoridated drinking water. The addition of minute quantities of fluorine (as sodium fluoride) to water supplies where this element is naturally lacking significantly reduces the incidence of dental caries.

A nurse should never advise a patient to have his teeth extracted, however bad they may appear — only to seek dental advice. Conservative treatment may well be possible.

Haemorrhage following the extraction of teeth

As we would expect, this may be primary, reactionary or secondary. Reactionary, or intermediate haemorrhage, occurring a few hours after extraction is by far the most common and is probably caused by excessive vigorous rinsing of the mouth or by licking the clot and dislodging it.

Treatment

The head is raised on pillows and the mouth cleaned and examined with a good light. A pressure pack is placed over the bleeding socket. A gauze swab soaked in hot water and wrung out is placed over the socket and the patient is instructed to bite on it. 'Surgicel' gauze may be packed into the socket before applying the pressure pack. If this fails, the gum will probably have to be sutured, usually after giving a local anaesthetic. Make sure the patient does not suffer from a constitutional bleeding disorder — e.g.

purpura, haemophilia or is on anticoagulants. Morphia 15 mg may be useful to reduce apprehension and agitation.

FRACTURES OF THE JAW

Almost all fractures of the jaw are caused by violence — e.g. the car accident victim or the boxer. Pathological fractures occasionally occur as a complication of osteomyelitis or as a complication of a large dental cyst or neoplasm.

The immediate treatment is to ensure a free airway. The muscular control of the tongue, because of its dependence on an intact lower jaw, may be lost in a fracture and if the patient is laid flat on his back there is a considerable risk of the tongue falling back, causing asphyxia. This may be prevented by placing a suture through the tongue, by tongue forceps, or by nursing the patient lying on the face until either the mandible has been immobilised in a forward position or the patient's control of the tongue has returned.

All patients suffering from a fracture of the jaw are transported in the prone position.

Treatment of fractures of the mandible

The aims of treatment are reduction of the fracture, its immobilisation and the prevention of infection. It may be immobilised by:

1. Gunning splints (in the edentulous patient).
2. Eyelet wiring.
3. Cast metal splints.

The teeth are fixed together either by wires or metal cap/splints to ensure correct relationship upper to lower. If they occlude correctly then the bone, of necessity, must be in correct alignment. Maintaining the teeth in occlusion may be necessary for 5 to 6 weeks. The mouth is syringed with sodium bicarbonate 1·60 using a 20 ml plastic syringe, and as soon as possible, the patient is encouraged to clean his teeth with a small toothbrush and paste. Corsodyl mouth wash (containing 0·2% chlorhexidine gluconate) 10 ml twice daily, is a useful antiseptic and cleansing agent which reduces dental plaque and helps good oral hygiene. Food, which has to be in liquid form, may be given by a catheter and plastic funnel, or by flexible straw. Meals should be small and given frequently.

Actinomycosis

This is an example of chronic infection due to a fungus which may occur in the jaw. Classically, an extensive brawny swelling develops and in the later stages multiple sinuses which discharge sulphur granules are present. An alternative form simulates an acute dental abscess, but healing is delayed. Infection usually arises following a dental extraction or any lesion involving a breach of the oral mucous membrane. The organisms are present in normal mouths, but can occasionally enter the tissues and produce a persistent infection.

Treatment consists of the administration of penicillin or tetracycline for 6 weeks. Surgery is confined to providing free drainage from the abscess.

TUMOURS OF THE JAW

Simple tumours

Simple tumours are usually osteomata. They are not very common. Simple tumours of the mouth such as fibromas are often seen, particularly if an irritant factor such as an ill-fitting denture is present.

Malignant tumours

These may be:

1. Sarcoma. A sarcoma may develop in the upper or lower jaw but is much less frequent than a carcinoma.

2. Carcinoma. A carcinomatous growth may arise in the lining of the maxillary antrum which extends in all directions—upwards towards the eye, inwards to block the nostril, downwards eroding the hard palate and forwards into the muscles and skin of the face. Carcinoma may arise in the oral epithelium, for example in the floor of the mouth or cheek, and spread to involve the jaw bones. When well established it presents as a large ulcerated lesion which is painful and bleeds easily.

Treatment

Radiotherapy and surgery are usually combined in the treatment, the affected half of the jaw being removed in the case of carcinoma rising from the maxillary antrum. The dental surgeon will make an appliance to repair the loss of tissue.

THE NECK

Wounds

Wounds in this area bleed freely, and deep wounds may open massive blood vessels, like the carotid artery or internal jugular vein. A further danger of a wound in this area is damage to the larynx or trachea with resulting respiratory obstruction. Tracheostomy may be necessary.

Swellings in the neck

Swellings in the neck are common. They are:
1. Lymphatic glandular swellings.
2. Goitre (Ch. 28).
3. Sebaceous cyst.
4. Thyroglossal cyst, which arises in the midline above the prominence

of the thyroid cartilage. It arises on a vestigial tract running from the tongue to the thyroid. Excision is the usual treatment.

5. A branchial cyst, which arises high in the neck near the angle of the lower jaw. It is a developmental abnormality. Excision is usually performed and it may be quite an extensive operation.

6. Cystic hygroma is a condition of dilatation of the lymphatic vessels. It occurs in children and frequently becomes mildly infected. Infection sometimes results in recession. Excision is the usual treatment.

7. Ludwig's angina, which is a dangerous condition of cellulitis of the floor of the mouth. Rapid swelling appears even before pyrexia. Tracheostomy instruments should always be ready in case of respiratory obstruction. The patient should be kept very still as heart failure may cause sudden death.

28

The endocrine glands

Apart from the thyroid gland the majority of the endocrine glands are small in size and deeply situated in the body. Their vital role in all disease processes as well as in sustaining the patient during and after operation is well recognised although an enormous amount of research has still to be done to unravel their complex functions.

In addition to clinical manifestations resulting from excessive or diminished function, investigations are undertaken where appropriate in an attempt to:

1. Outline the gland anatomically and functionally by X-rays including angiography and by scanning.

2. Measure the level of a hormone in the blood directly or by radiological immuno-assay.

3. Assess the target organ response where one hormone stimulates the secretion of another. The administration of adrenocorticotrophic hormone (ACTH) stimulates the normal adrenal cortex to secrete cortisone. Failure of secretion is indicative of adrenal insufficiency.

4. Detect the level of substances in the blood or urine which may be in excess or diminished as a result of hormonal dysfunction. The electrolytes, glucose, calcium and the 17 ketosteroids are examples.

Endocrinology is a rapidly expanding science and, as a result of many sophisticated tests, some of which are mentioned in outline above, disease is diagnosed much earlier and in many cases the diagnosis is made when the patient has very few symptoms and no physical signs. This is particularly fortunate since the physical appearance of some of these patients is a cause of great distress to the patient and his relatives. In the more florid stages of some endocrine diseases the signs are not easy to conceal. We should treat these patients as human beings, which they are, and with the special sympathy which they deserve. Many of the conditions are controlable or curable and, as far as possible, this hope should be conveyed to them in our conversation and attitude. Patients with thyrotoxicosis may be irritable, moody and demanding, while the patient with acromegaly is usually embarrassed.

THE PITUITARY

The pituitary gland, weighs about 0·6 g and lies in the sella tursica (pituitary fossa) in the sphenoid bone. The roof of the fossa, formed of dense dura mater, is pierced by a stalk which connects the gland to the hypothalamus. The optic chiasma lies above the roof and upward extension of a growth of the gland may press on the nerve fibres causing defects in the visual field. There are two active lobes, an anterior and a posterior.

The secretions of the two lobes and their function are shown in Figure 28.1. The page cross references in the table after each hormone are to the pages in this book where their action is relevant to the topic under discussion in that place. Perhaps in a small measure this stresses the importance of a knowledge of their action in the general surgical management where the gland itself is not the site of disease or dysfunction.

Fig. 28.1 The pituitary hormones and their action

Hormone	Physiological action.
From the Anterior Lobe	
1. Growth hormone (GH) (Somatotrophin)	Skeletal and connective tissue growth-antagonises the action of insulin.
2. Thyrotrophic hormones (TSH) (p. 256)	Regulates secretion of thyroxine.
3. Adrenocorticotrophic hormones (ACTH) (p. 268)	Controls adrenocortical activity and secretion of cortisol.
4. Gonadotrophic hormones	Essential in development of the sexual organs in both sexes.
(i) Follicle stimulating hormone (FSH) (p. 570)	Stimulatus ripening of the ovarian follicle in the female and spermatogenesis in the male.
(ii) Leutinising hormone (LH) (p. 570)	Maintains the corpus leuteum which secretes progesterone. In the male stimulates testosterone.
5. Prolactin (p. 272)	Stimulates milk production.
From the Posterior Lobe	
1. Pitressin (antidiuretic hormone)	Antidiuretic (The action on smooth muscle contraction is pharmological rather than physiological).
2. Oxytocin (p. 272)	Contracts uterine muscle. Propulsive action on milk ducts in the breasts.

SURGERY OF THE PITUITARY GLAND

Pituitary dysfunction arises from oversecretion or undersecretion of one or more hormones. This may arise from tumour formation, vascular diseases, trauma, or be a sequal of an infective process. It also follows surgical removal or destruction of the gland by irradiation. The lesions in which surgical intervention may be advised are:

1. Chromophobe adenoma which, by pressure on the cells which secrete thyrotrophic and gonadotrophic hormones, produce widespread effects. The patient is over weight, sluggish and the metabolic rate is depressed. Amemorrhoea is usual. The tumours are radioresistant and surgery is undertaken.

2. Acidophil adenoma results in gigantism in the young or acromegaly (Fig. 28.2) in the adult from excess of growth hormone. Radiotherapy to destroy the gland is the usual treatment.

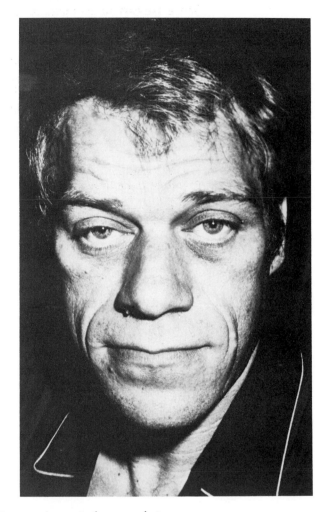

Fig. 28.2 Acromegaly — note the coarse features.

Hypophysectomy (Removal of the pituitary)

Preparation

The patient is admitted a week before operation and the urinary excretion of 17-ketosteroids estimated. The uptake of radioactive iodine is estimated for subsequent assessment of thyroid function.

Six days before operation cortisone, 50 mg by mouth, rising to 400 mg on the day of operation, is administered. Half of this is given by mouth and the other half by intramuscular injection.

Pleural or ascitic collections are aspirated.

The usual preparation for craniotomy (Ch. 44) is undertaken for a transfrontal approach. An alternative approach either for excision or for the implant of yttrium-90 is transphenoidally.

Postoperative care

The pituitary controls all the other ductless glands so that removal causes widespread effects and the postoperative care reflects some of the methods of dealing with this upset. Consciousness is quickly regained: 350 mg of cortisone is given and gradually reduced to 50 mg daily.

The wound heals uneventfully: 300 mg of DOCA may be implanted beneath the sheath of the rectus muscle in the abdominal wall before discharge from hospital.

Special dangers
1. Lassitude.
2. Anorexia.
3. Low blood pressure.
4. Danger of infection.
5. Electrolyte imbalance—salt depletion, retention of potassium and a rise in blood urea.

Salt capsules, 4 g daily, may be given if the blood pressure is low. If the blood pressure is raised salt is forbidden.

Occasional complications
1. *Fits*. The risk may be diminished by administering antiepileptic drugs.
2. *Diabetes insipidus*. 40 mg of post-pituitary snuff, once to three times daily, may be advised.
3. *Hypothyroidism*. Thyroxine may be given but is to be avoided if possible on account of the danger of stimulating the neoplasm.

After adrenalectomy or hypophysectomy vomiting is a most important symptom and is usually due to lack of cortisone.

DISEASES OF THE THYROID GLAND

A goitre is an enlargement of the thyroid gland. The thyroid gland is an endocrine gland situated at the root of the neck in front of and at the sides of the trachea and oesophagus (Fig. 28.3.) The diseases to which it is subject are unusual in that they do not conform to the pattern of those to which we are accustomed elsewhere.

The thyroid secretes three hormones:

Thyroxine
Tri-iodothyronine
Calcitonin.

The first two hormones, of which thyroxine accounts for 90 per cent, are essential for normal growth in infancy and for the maintenance of a bal-

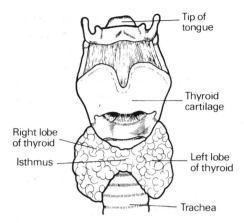

Fig. 28.3 The thyroid gland consists of two lobes joined in front of the trachea by an isthmus.

anced metabolism in adult life. If iodine is deficient in the diet, or if the demands of the body for thyroxine are temporarily in excess of the gland's capacity to produce it, the gland substance may enlarge in an attempt to compensate. Later, the enlargement may subside evenly and smoothly, but frequently it is so large or retrogression so patchy that the patient is left with an irregular nodular goitre. The absence of the gland, or the failure to produce sufficient thyroxine, results in cretinism in infants (Fig. 28.4) and myxoedema in adults (Fig. 28.5). The whole tempo of the activities of the body is depressed in these conditions. On the other hand, an excessive amount of secretion results in the condition known as thyrotoxicosis, with the result that the whole pace of the patient's activities is accelerated.

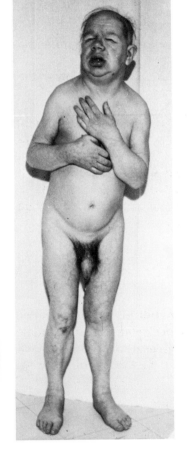

Fig. 28.4 An untreated cretin in adult life.

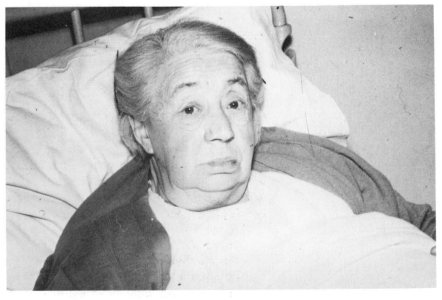

Fig. 28.5 Myxoedema showing thin hair and dry skin.

A thyrotropic hormone (thyroid stimulating) in the pituitary regulates the production of thyroxine which is manufactured in the secretory cells of the vesicles of the thyroid. Iodine is taken up from the blood and when the hormone is released into the blood stream it combines with the plasma proteins. This is known as the protein-bound iodine (PBI). An increase is a manifestation of excessive thyroid secretion and a diminution occurs in myxoedema but it is now more usual to estimate the level of thyroxine in the serum, the normal level being $3.0-7.5$ μg per 100 ml.

Secondarily, as a result of enlargement, symptoms due to pressure on the neighbouring organs may occur.

Calcitonin—a serum calcium-lowering hormone which inhibits bone destruction is now known to be secreted in the thyroid—in addition to thyroxine.

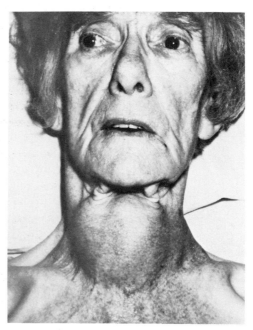

Fig. 28.6 Simple nontoxic goitre.

SIMPLE ENLARGEMENTS OF THE THYROID

Simple or non-toxic enlargement of the thyroid is fairly common (Fig. 28.6). The gland usually enlarges in the neck, but occasionally the enlargement occurs behind the upper portion of the sternum (retrosternal goitre).

Causes

During periods of special stress, such as puberty, the calls for thyroxine are greater, and a diffuse enlargement of the gland may occur. It is physiological in origin, and the colloid goitre of puberty requires no special surgical intervention.

Since iodinised salt has been used, endemic goitres with a definite geographical distribution have almost disappeared.

The simple enlargement may subside if not excessive, or subsidence may occur in one portion of the gland and not in another. This process results in the production of nodules in the gland. They may be single (adenoma) or multiple, known as nodular goitre.

Symptoms and signs

The most obvious and frequently the only complaint is the goitre itself. A goitre always moves on swallowing because it is attached to the larynx. Surgical interference is indicated if the patient complains of:
1. Pressure symptoms which may be:
    (a) Dysphagia (difficulty in swallowing).
    (b) Dyspnoea (difficulty in breathing—the trachea, which is normally C shaped and thinner posteriorly because there is no cartilage, is so compressed on both sides that it may be 'scabbard' in shape).
    (c) Hoarseness due to pressure on the recurrent laryngeal nerves.
2. Cosmetic disfigurement.
3. Symptoms suggestive of toxic or malignant changes.

Radiography of the trachea and chest is usually ordered to determine the degree (if any) of the deformity of the trachea resulting from pressure.

Treatment

Surgical operation consists of partial thyroidectomy. The after-care is similar to that of toxic goitre, but antithyroid drugs are unnecessary.

Complications of a simple goitre

1. The onset of toxic symptoms.
2. The occurrence of haemorrhage into an adenoma with the sudden onset of severe dyspnoea.
3. Malignancy.

THYROTOXICOSIS

Toxic goitre is a condition in which the secretion of thyroxine is excessive in quantity. The disease is more common in women.

The disease may commence in a gland which was previously normal, or it may develop in a thyroid already subject to simple enlargement. The former is described as primary thyrotoxicosis or Graves' disease and the latter as secondary thyrotoxicosis. The main distinction is that the patient is usually older in the secondary type and the heart muscle is less fit to withstand being driven so much faster. The other clinical distinction is that the eye signs, particularly exophthalmos, are nearly always present in Graves' disease.

Symptoms and signs

The onset of toxic symptoms may follow a severe mental shock or anxiety. The thyroid gland may be very large, or there may be almost no enlargement at all. The severity of the symptoms bears no relationship to the size of the goitre. The symptoms are those of an accelerated metabolism. The body is being driven ever faster.

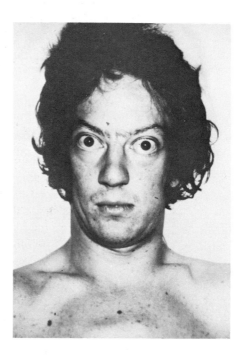

Fig. 28.7   Thyrotoxicosis.

General symptoms and signs

1. The skin is moist and vascular. Sweating may be profuse, and cold weather is preferred to a warm sunny day.

2. The eyes are protruding (exophthalmos), staring, and have a frightened look. This is common in Graves' disease (Fig. 28.7) but unusual in secondary thyrotoxicosis in the older patient.

3. Loss of weight is marked but the appetite is good.

4. Tremors of the fingers are present.

5. Mentally, the patient is hyperexcitable, nervous, and difficult to get on with. Frequently the patient with a toxic goitre will insist on leaving hospital in the midst of treatment.

6. Diarrhoea and vomiting may be present, and are due to overactivity of the intestinal tract.

Laryngoscopy is undertaken to inspect movement of the vocal cords and to detect paralysis if present.

Cardiovascular symptoms

The heart rate is always increased and palpitation is a common complaint. The systolic blood pressure is raised and the diastolic pressure lowered, with the result that the pulse pressure is increased and the pulse is full and bounding.

Later, irregularity of the heart beat occurs, usually in the form of atrial fibrillation, and unrelieved, the patient dies of cardiac failure, which is usually associated with acute mania.

Radioiodine tracer studies may be necessary to reveal thyroid overactivity in atypical cases. The blood serum thyroxine level is raised and the blood cholesterol level lowered.

Treatment

1. Mild cases may be treated medically by sedatives and prolonged rest which will include rearrangement of the patient's life. Carbimazole (Neo-Mercazole) (10 mg t.d.s.) or other antithyroid drug may be given until the patient's weight is rising and then reduced to smaller doses. Agranulocytosis is now comparatively rare but should always be considered as a possible complication of this drug. The disadvantage of all antithyroid drugs is that in the presence of moderate enlargement they increase the size of the gland. Radioactive iodine is being used with increasing frequency.

2. For severe cases and for moderate cases where the patient must lead his normal life and earn his living, subtotal thyroidectomy or radioactive iodine therapy gives the best chance of permanent cure.

Radioactive iodine is contraindicated in:

(a) Patients under 40 years of age for fear of causing carcinomatous change in the thyroid.

(b) Pregnancy.

It is specially indicated in:

(a) Recurrent thyrotoxicosis where a second operation carries a much higher risk of damage to the recurrent laryngeal nerves.

(b) In patients with concurrent medical disease which precludes safe operative intervention.

THE NURSING CARE OF A CASE OF THYROIDECTOMY FOR THYROTOXICOSIS

All patients require a period of medical treatment before operation can be undertaken.

The operation is performed when the patient is in a euthyroid state, that is a condition of normal thyroid function. The patient is now feeling better, less excitable (the heart rate is about 80 per minute) and gaining weight. This is confirmed by a normal serum thyroxine reading.

Drugs which are used in the preoperative stage are:

(a) Carbimazole (Neo-Mercazole) is given for several weeks before admission but its administration is stopped 10 days before the operation. Some surgeons continue antithyroid drugs up to the day of operation.

(b) Lugol's iodine (0·3 to 0·9 ml t.d.s.) in milk may be given for the 10 days before operation but many surgeons now omit it.

(c) Propanolol (120/160 mg daily in divided doses) may be used as the only preoperative preparation for thyroidectomy. As it acts on the heart and target organs the serum thyroxine is not lowered. Therefore it must be continued on the day of operation and for the subsequent 5 to 7 days.

(d) Valium 5 mg b.d. quietens the patient and ensures sound sleep.

(e) Digitalis is given if atrial fibrillation is present. This is given in the form of digoxin (0·25 mg) sufficiently frequently to control the fibrillation.

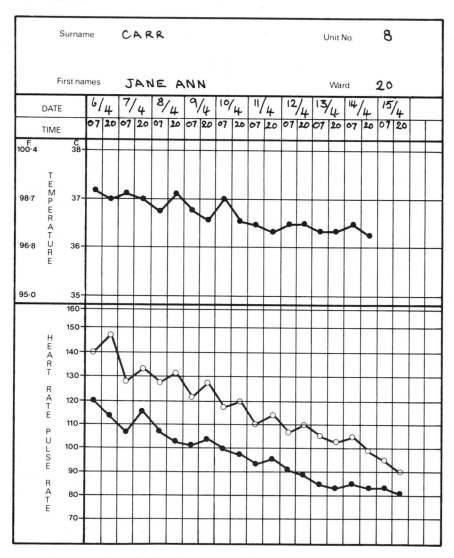

Fig. 28.8 The pulse and heart rate must be recorded in atrial fibrillation. (The upper-most graph is the heart rate).

Observations:

    (a) The sleeping pulse rate is the most important guide of progress.

    (b) The *heart rate* must be counted if the patient is fibrillating (Fig. 28.8).

Immediate preoperative care

The skin of the neck, the upper half of the chest area, the axillae and the upper arms are shaved and washed with 2 per cent hexachlorophane soap.

The operation

Up to nine-tenths of the gland is removed at operation which is usually performed under general anaesthesia. The wound is closed and drained through a tube brought out through a separate stab incision.

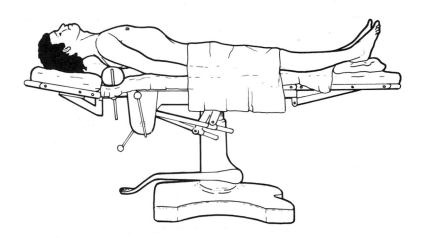

Fig. 28.9 Position for thyroid operation. Note shoulder support.

The postoperative care

Position in bed

If a general anaesthetic has been administered, the patient is laid in the lateral position until recovery takes place and is then propped up as soon as possible supported by a back rest. This relieves venous congestion. In all movements the head is supported and extension of the neck is avoided.

Treatment immediately on return from the theatre

    (a) Digoxin (0·25 mg) may be given subcutaneously, especially if the patient was fibrillating before the operation.

    (b) The respirations are frequently shallow and slow. A careful watch is necessary, and oxygen administered if required.

Difficulty with breathing may be caused by haemorrhage. An excess of blood in the Redivac bottle or swelling of the neck should be reported at once. Respiratory obstruction may develop some hours postoperatively due to oedema in the subglottic area of the larynx, i.e. just below the vocal cords and intubation may be necessary to avoid brain damage from hypoxia.

(c) The patient should swallow a little fluid as soon as possible, as it serves to clean the mouth. She should speak only in a whisper so as to decrease the pain in the neck.

(d) The bedclothing should not be too heavy, and frequent cold sponging is important as sweating is invariable. A room which is too warm must be cooled by a fan.

During the night

(a) *Haemorrhage.* A careful watch must be kept for excessive bleeding. It is important to remember that the site to look for haemorrhage is at the *back* of the dressing, if an open drain has been used.

(b) *Drugs* to encourage sleep are prescribed and given before the patient is too lively.

Care of the tube

The tube is removed not later than 48 hours after the operation and the stitches should be removed on the fourth or fifth day. If Michel's clips have been used, alternate clips should be removed on the third day and the remainder on the fourth day. After the fifth day a nobecutane spray is all that is necessary. If serum collects in the wound aspiration may be necessary.

Complications and their treatment

Haemorrhage. Some bleeding is usual, but excessive haemorrhage must be notified at once. Severe haemorrhage will cause bulging of the wound and severe dyspnoea due to formation of a haematoma. Reopening of the wound may be necessary.

Tetany. Removal of trauma to the parathyroid glands may result in tetany. The patient complains of a tingling and numbness of the face, lips and hands, and twitching of the muscles. Most cases subside spontaneously, but calcium gluconate usually gives rapid relief. The blood calcium is estimated. More remotely a high dosage of vitamin D and oral calcium supplements are used.

Apart from tetany, it is advisable to estimate the blood calcium three months after thyroidectomy. It has been shown that latent parathyroid deficiency may give rise to such distressing conditions as bilateral cataracts.

Respiratory complications. Soreness of the throat and neck are almost invariable complaints, and are soothed by giving the patient blackcurrant pastilles to suck. Chest infections are unusual.

Hoarseness is usually due to the trauma of the operation, and clears up rapidly. Occasionally it is caused by damage to the recurrent laryngeal nerve and this will be seen when a laryngoscope is passed and the vocal cords are not moving. In cases where both nerves have been damaged, the paralysed vocal cords lie almost in apposition so that the space between them is negligible. The result is that the patient has acute respiratory distress and tracheostomy must be performed without delay.

Myxoedema may occur as a remote complication in about 10 per cent of patients but not all show deposition of mucopolysaccharide substance which gives the typical 'solid' appearance in this condition.

Recurrent thyrotoxicosis.

Instructions to the patient on leaving hospital

Two or 3 months are necessary to gain the full benefit from the operation. Weight increases and, 3 months later, most patients are fit to lead a normal life. The patient can be reassured that a necklace will adequately conceal the scar. Many patients now feel the cold and must wear warmer clothing.

At a follow-up 3 months later the serum calcium and thyroxine are estimated and larygoscopic examination undertaken. An assessment is made to detect early myxoedema or recurrent thyrotoxicosis.

RADIOACTIVE ISOTOPES

Radioactive iodine is now used in the diagnosis and treatment of thyroid gland diseases. This material disintegrates with the emission of energy in the form of gamma rays which can be detected by Geiger counters. In diagnosis, a small (tracer) dose is given orally or intravenously and the amount in the thyroid and in the urine measured. A high thyroid uptake with low urinary excretion is indicative of hyperthyroidism, whilst a low thyroid uptake and high urinary excretion suggests hypothyroidism. Treatment by this means can be given by a large dose and is used at present for those in whom surgery is contraindicated and medical treatment not suitable. In thyroid cancer about 10 per cent of patients take up sufficient radioactive iodine in the gland and its metastases to be treatable by this method.

Certain thyroid carcinomas are under the influence of the anterior pituitary gland and by the administration of thyroid hormone the growth may be suppressed.

NEW GROWTHS OF THE THYROID

An adenoma is the commonest new growth. Many malignant neoplasms arise in a pre-existing adenoma and have a particular tendency to metastasise in bone. The local spread is into the trachea, oesophagus, skin and veins of the neck. In only a few cases are radioactive isotopes of value. Radical surgery may be performed if the disease is not too extensive and some types of tumour are slow growing and have a good prognosis.

INFLAMMATIONS

A diffuse iron hardness of the gland sometimes occurs and is known as Riedel's thyroiditis. Its main importance lies in its tendency to resemble carcinoma.

A rare but interesting type of chronic inflammation of the thyroid gland is Hashimoto's thyroiditis which is thought to be an auto-immune disease. In this condition the body reacts to some of its constituent proteins.

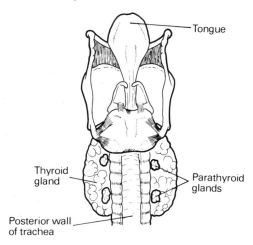

Fig. 28.10   The four parathyroid glands are situated on the posterior border of the thyroid. Also illustrates that the posterior wall of the trachea is weak because it has no cartilage.

THE PARATHYROIDS

The parathyroids are two pairs of tiny glands situated behind the posterior border of the thyroid gland (Fig. 28.10). The upper parathyroids are fairly constant in position but the lower two are much more variable in position and may even be situated in the mediastinum. Their secretion, parathormone, acts by:

1. Mobilising calcium and phosphate from bone;
2. Increasing calcium absorption from the gut;
3. Increasing the reabsorption of calcium from the renal tubules.

HYPERPARATHYROIDISM

Excessive secretion of parathormone may be due to an adenoma or hyperplasia and may present as:

1. *Bone disease* varying from decalcification to cystic formation (osteitis fibrosa cystica).

2. *Urinary stone* formation. All patients with urinary stones are investigated for overactivity of the parathyroids.

3. Dyspeptic symptoms.

4. Mental agitation.

Investigations

These include:
1. **Estimation** of the
    (a) serum calcium level (normal 2·25−2·62 mmols/l).
    (b) serum alkaline phosphatase.
    (c) Calcium excretion in the urine.
    (d) Renal function including a urogram.
2. **Radiography** of the skeleton.

Treatment

An adenoma is removed. In hyperplasia three whole parathyroid glands and one half of the remaining one are removed. The operative approach is the same as for a thyroidectomy. A parathyroid is a minute gland and even a tumour is tiny in size and soft in consistency. Not only is a parathyroid not palpable clinically, it is rarely palpable at operation. To add to the surgeon's difficulties the lower glands are variable in position and may be situated in the mediastinum so that exploration of the chest may be necessary to find the tumour. Even in the most experienced hands there is sometimes failure to find the tumour. The possibility should be discussed with the patient before he consents to the operation.

The nursing care is similar to that of a thyroidectomy in the care of the wound and gentleness in not extending the neck.

Special observations

The sudden withdrawal of excess parathormone from the blood in the immediate postoperative period may cause tetany. The serum calcium level is monitored at frequent intervals but the nurse should be specially alert to note any symptoms suggestive of tetany and test clinically for the classical signs discussed below. Intravenous calcium gluconate may be prescribed. When the condition is stabilised the patient is given a high calcium diet or calcium supplements as ordered by the surgeon after further studies of the patient's calcium metabolism.

HYPOPARATHYROIDISM

Lack of sufficient parathormone causes a fall in the serum calcium with great irritability of the nerves. This is manifested by spasm and twitching of the muscles. Known as tetany, it may be caused by conditions other than lack of parathormone such as excessive vomiting or hyperventilation (usually of hysterical origin).

The common surgical cause is removal or damage to the parathyroid glands. The clinical features are:
1. **Paraesthesia**. The commonest site is around the side of the neck, the fingers and toes.
2. **Muscle twitching** which may affect all muscles but particularly those

of the forearm and hand as well as those of the leg and foot (carpopedal spasm). Two signs may be elicited by the nurse:

(a) *Chvostek's sign* — tapping over the skin at the angle of the jaw will stimulate the branches of the facial nerve to produce twitching of the eyelids and the angle of the mouth.

(b) A sphygmomanometer cuff applied to the arm and inflated above the systolic pressure for not more than 2 minutes will cause carpal spasm.

In most severe cases the respiratory muscles are involved with stridor and fear of suffocation. Generalised twitching may be mistaken for epilepsy but there is no loss of consciousness. *Investigations* of parathyroid function are undertaken. *Treatment* is as outlined for tetany complicating thyroidectomy.

THE ADRENAL GLAND

The adrenal glands are two flat, canary yellow, structures lying above the upper pole of each kidney (Fig. 28.11). Each gland consists of a cortical and a medullary portion which, although anatomically joined, are physiologically separate. Blood containing the secreted hormones drains into the adrenal veins — the right draining directly into the inferior vena cava, the left into the left renal vein which, in turn, joins the inferior vena cava.

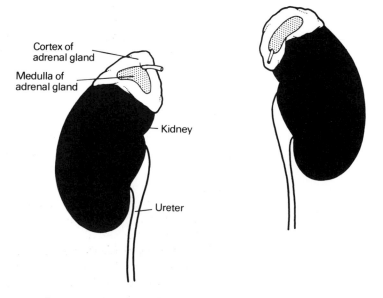

Fig. 28.11 The adrenal glands.

THE CORTICAL HORMONES

These are very numerous, at least 50 have been discovered. The principal groups are:

1. The mineralocorticoids which regulate water and electrolyte balance, the most important being aldosterone which conserves sodium in the body.

2. The glucocorticoids which convert body protein to carbohydrate. In addition hydrocortisone (which is converted in the body from cortisone) enables the body to respond to stress, inhibits the action of insulin and is important in maintaining blood pressure. In excess it inhibits the inflammatory reaction and also the rejection reaction in tissue transplantation.

3. The sex hormones. Androgens and oestrogens are secreted. ACTH stimulates the adrenal cortex to secrete glucocorticoids and the sex hormones and excess of hydrocortisone in the blood inhibits the secretion of ACTH. The secretion of the mineralocorticoids is independent of the pituitary.

THE MEDULLARY HORMONES

These are:

1. Noradrenalin

2. Adrenalin

Both hormones stimulate the sympathetic nervous system including the blood vessels causing vasoconstriction. Noradrenalin which is shorter acting than adrenalin accounts for 20 per cent of the secretion but in phaeochromocytoma the proportion is reversed.

Disease of the adrenal glands may cause over or under activity of the cortex or of the medulla. Under activity from disease or surgical excision for therapeutic reasons will require replacement therapy.

HYPOCORTICISM

Acute adrenal failure is most commonly a sequence of bilateral adrenalectomy where the patient has failed to take the prescribed amount of cortisone or has been vomiting. Sudden and unexpected postoperative collapse due to an adrenal haemorrhage is a rare occurrence.

The clinical picture is one of muscular weakness, severe shock, hypotension and vomiting. The immediate administration of hydrocortisone intraveneously is essential.

Chronic adrenal insufficiency (**Addison's disease**) is caused by tuberculous infection of the adrenal or atrophy of the tissues of the gland. Muscular weakness, a persistent low blood pressure and skin pigmentation occur. Replacement therapy and antituberculous drugs are indicated if necessary.

HYPERCORTISM

Hypercortism is due to a tumour or hyperplasia of the cortex. The clinical features are similar to those resulting from the administration of excessive doses of cortisone or excessive secretion of ACTH and is known as Cushing's Syndrome (Fig. 28.12). The moon shaped face, obesity from water and salt retention, hypertension, muscular wasting and hirsutes are all characteristics. The treatment is removal of the tumour if present or, in cases of hyperplasia, subtotal adrenalectomy.

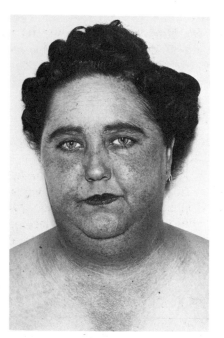
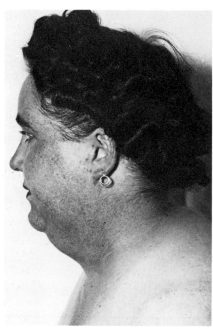

Fig. 28.12 Cushing's syndrome in the adult, showing buffalo hump (side view), acne, hirsutes, plethoric appearance.

MEDULLARY OVER-ACTIVITY

This is almost always due to a tumour—a phaeochromocytoma, and the symptoms and signs are those of excessive secretion of adrenalin and noradrenalin. They arise from hypertension and are headache, palpitation, dyspnoea and weakness. The treatment is excision but special care is necessary to neutralise the effects of increased adrenalin secretion before and during the operation as well as to counter hypotension postoperatively. The nursing care and postoperative checks are similar to that described below for adrenalectomy with the following additional precautions, the details of which will be prescribed by the surgeon. Preoperatively phentolamine is administered by mouth for some days to suppress the secretion and immediately preoperatively it is given intravenously. During the operation it is given when the gland is handled by the surgeon as this results in flooding the circulation with adrenalines. Following excision, dangerous hypotension may occur and noradrenalin should always be available to counteract the fall in blood pressure. These patients should be handled with the greatest gentleness, particularly when being positioned on the operating table since any pressure on the loin or abdomen is liable to cause a further increase in adrenalin secretion.

ADRENALECTOMY

Bilateral removal of the adrenals may be indicated in disseminated carcinoma of the breast or prostate when it is beyond other methods of control. Other indications for bilateral removal of the adrenals are selected cases of Cushing's syndrome.

Preoperative management

Patients selected for adrenalectomy for disseminated carcinoma of the breast are always at an advanced stage of the disease. The extent of the malignancy must also be mapped out carefully. A low blood count must be corrected by transfusions. Hydrocortisone is given by intramuscular injection of 100 mg one hour before operation. Both adrenal glands are usually excised at one operation but if it is decided to remove one at a time the opposite one is removed 10 days later. Because of danger of delay in healing and trauma on the table to a healing wound, the stitches from the first wound are not removed until the second operation has been completed. Pethidine, 50 to 100 mg, is preferable to morphia because of the danger of liver damage from secondary deposits.

The striking benefit of adrenalectomy is immediate relief of pain in most cases of secondary deposits in bone. After 18 months to 2 years most patients relapse.

Postoperative care

Following operation hydrocortisone is given in 100 mg doses, intramuscularly 6-hourly, for one day. Close observation of the blood pressure is essential, and if the patient becomes hypotensive the dosage and/or frequency of hydrocortisone must be increased. This is reduced to two doses of 100 mg on the next day after operation and continued orally as cortisone acetate in 25 mg doses 6-hourly for 2 days. On the fourth day cortisone is reduced to 75 mg and from the sixth day most patients are maintained on a dose of 50 mg a day. It is explained to the patient that the adrenal glands, which produce a substance called cortisone, essential to life, have been removed. Cortisone must be taken in tablet form for the rest of the patient's life. The patient should take a normal diet with plenty of salt. A few patients require in addition fludrocortisone (a mineralocorticoid) 0·1 mg daily. If she is not feeling well or gets tired, she should return at once. If she vomits, cortisone can be given by injection. If she goes abroad, she must make sure that she can get a maintenance dose of cortisone or she will die. It is essential that patients should carry 'steroid cards' to the effect that they are on maintenance cortisone therapy.

When adrenalectomy is performed for carcinoma of the breast the ovaries are also removed so that no oestrin-producing tissue remains in the body. The patient who has had only one adrenal removed requires replacement therapy — the other adrenal may be functionless from secondary deposits.

THE SURGICAL SIGNIFICANCE OF CORTICOSTEROIDS

Patients who have been on corticosteroids for any length of time usually have a medically induced adrenal insufficiency due to the suppressive action of the administered steroids on the pituitary gland.

The dose of cortisone should be increased before, during and immediately after operation to cover the increased demands made by anaesthesia and surgical intervention. Failure to observe this principle may lead to death of the patient from acute adrenal insufficiency.

Corticosteroids may be used as:

1. Replacement therapy, e.g. Addison's disease, hypopituitarism, and after bilateral adrenalectomy.

2. Therapeutically. Apart from adrenal insufficiency, cortisone is widely used in the group of diseases known as the collagenoses: notably rheumatoid arthritis, scleroderma, periarteritis nodosa, and lupus erythematosus. In addition it may be used in such diseases as iritis, thrombocytopenic purpura, and status asthmaticus.

Corticosteroids given in a dose beyond what is normally required for the maintenance of life cause the body to: (1) retain sodium salts, (2) excrete potassium salts. If more than 50 mg is used potassium chloride (3 g daily) should be given to make good the increased excretion of potassium salts. In addition a low salt diet is necessary. The patient who has undergone bilateral adrenalectomy, on the other hand, should take a normal salt diet because her replacement dosage of cortisone is equal to the normal secretion of the hormone.

Many patients receiving corticosteroid therapy may come for urgent surgical intervention and the dosage of steroids has to be increased before and after operation.

There are many complications of cortisone which may be of surgical importance. The commonest are:

1. Reactivation of a latent pulmonary tuberculous focus.

2. Bleeding from a peptic ulcer.

3. Development of silent fulminating infections, for example, appendicitis.

4. Rapid development of cardiac failure.

5. Oedema including 'moon'-shaped face usually due to overdosage.

Other complications include thrombosis, osteoporosis, psychosis, and skin reactions such as acne and mild hirsutism.

BIBLIOGRAPHY

Wade J S H 1978 British Journal of Hospital Medicine 20: 456.

29
Diseases of the breast

The protuberant portion of the breast lies on the anterior chest wall but breast tissue extends towards the midline, to the lateral chest wall and towards the axilla (the axillary tail). The alveoli which produce milk ultimately empty by lactiferous ducts whose orifices are situated in the apex of the nipple. The areola which surrounds the nipple contains sweat glands, sebaceous glands and accessory mammary glands. The lymphatic drainage of the breast is to glands situated in the axilla and along the internal mammary artery which runs down behind the costal cartilages in the anterior mediastinum.

The breast has a rich blood supply and this increases in pregnancy. After delivery the anterior pituitary releases the hormone prolactin which stimulates the alveoli of the breast to produce milk. The sucking stimulus of the child initiates the release from the posterior pituitary of oxytocin which causes contraction of the alveoli and results in the flow of milk along the ducts.

The breast differs from other exocrine glands in experiencing full physiological activity only periodically during reproductive life, i.e. when lactation is established.

Breast disease usually presents itself in three ways:

1. A palpable lump is frequently the only complaint. The general physical upset is slight but the mental anguish may be overwhelming.

When a patient confides to a nurse that she has discovered a lump in her breast the only advice she can be given is to consult her doctor without delay. The nurse can add the small consolation that four out of five lumps felt by patients are simple and non-malignant.

2. Discomfort within the breast

3. A discharge from the nipple. This may be bloodstained as in the case of a duct papilloma or carcinoma, milky following lactation, or a clear brown or greenish fluid in the case of fibroadenosis.

A discharge from the breast should be tested for the presence of haemoglobin.

BENIGN CONDITIONS OF THE BREAST

CONGENITAL ABNORMALITIES

These are uncommon apart from retraction of the nipple. One occasionally encounters an accessory nipple situated in the same plane as the normal nipple and even more rarely an accessory breast.

INFECTION OF THE BREAST — ACUTE MASTITIS

This is not uncommon during lactation, when cracks or fissures are likely to develop in the nipple and areolar regions. Acute lactational mastitis also develops in an area of milk engorgement due to a blocked lactiferous duct. A breast engorged with milk is an excellent medium for the proliferation of organisms, usually *staphloccocus pyogenes*.

Symptoms and signs

The affected portion of the breast is painful, tender, warm and indurated. The patient feels ill and the general signs of inflammation may be present. As pus develops, throbbing pain occurs and the patient is pale and tired from lack of rest and toxic absorption.

Treatment and nursing care

Prevention

Breast abscess is best prevented by careful preparation of the nipple in the last 2 months of pregnancy and the institution of scrupulous hygiene during lactation. The nipples should be massaged with a good toilet soap and water. Rolling the nipples between the fingers may get them accustomed to the friction of sucking. Any suitable ointment may be applied twice weekly but is not really necessary.

Treatment of established infection

   1. In the early stages the administration of flucloxacillin may control the inflammatory reaction. The infant should be weaned from the affected breast, which should be elevated and supported. A sedative is usually prescribed to promote sleep. The infant, of course, is fed at the other breast. The practice of manual expression of milk from the breast if excessive milk production occurs whilst breast feeding avoids galactocoele formation.
   2. Drainage is necessary as soon as pus forms, and a tube is usually inserted. At this stage weaning is inevitable from both breasts.
   Lactation is best suppressed by a tight binder. The nurse must show that she understands that the engorged breast will be initially uncomfortable and that an occasional sedative may be required. Without the stimulation of suckling the high prolactin concentrations in the blood fall to normal and lactation ceases within a week. Fluid restriction is unnecessary, causes further discomfort and has little effect on milk secretion. Oestrogens so

long used for suppression have been abandoned because of the risk of thrombo-embolism. In the occasional patient in whom stronger measures are necessary bromcriptine may be prescribed. To overcome the occasional nausea which it may cause it is advisable that it be taken with meals.

Antibioma

Occasionally an acute mastitis treated with antibiotics forms an encysted abscess, the pus is buried beneath a thick firm wall and a month later the patient is worried because she has a large lump in her breast. Simple incision and drainage are all that is necessary.

Drugs and breast feeding. Whether a drug prescribed for the mother will conflict with breast feeding is not a question that can be answered reliably and what information there is is often conflicting. In general prescribing is avoided and, if not, advice from the nearest drug information centre may be sought.

FIBROADENOSIS

The breasts enlarge and develop their adult characteristics at puberty, due to hormonal influences generated in the pituitary, the ovary, and possibly in the thyroid gland. During each menstrual cycle, some slight enlargement of the breasts occurs, to be followed by retrogression until the next cycle. Normally this periodic enlargement and retrogression occurs evenly throughout the whole of both breasts. Occasionally, however, due either to the excessive enlargement of one segment or the failure of another to subside evenly, irregularity may occur in the breast substance, with the result that the patient complains of a lump, which is usually painful in the days immediately before menstruation. These lumps, or masses, are known as fibroadenosis. They may take several different forms,

1. Generalised. The whole of one or both breasts may be hard and irregular. There may be a discharge of clear or greenish coloured fluid from the nipple.

2. Segmental. May be limited to one segment or a quadrant of one or both breasts.

3. Cystic type. Cyst formation is a predominant feature.

Treatment

The local mass is usually excised and examined under the microscope so that the diagnosis can be confirmed with certainty, and nothing reassures the patient more. The cavity in the breast is almost obliterated, but a small drain may be brought out through a separate stab incision, and the main wound in the skin is closed. The drain is removed in 24 to 48 hours. To prevent separation of the wound and consequent broadening of the skin scar the sides of the incision must be supported by gauze and strapping or Elastoplast drawn up from the sides so that the wound is not flattened (Fig. 29.1).

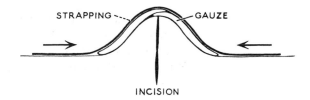

STRAPPING GAUZE

INCISION

Fig. 29.1 Diagrammatic cross-section of wound (incision) showing correct method of applying strapping over gauze to pull edges together as indicated by arrows.

Aspiration of a cyst may be undertaken with caution because there is a danger of missing an intracystic neoplasm. Any fluid aspirated is sent for examination for cancer cells.

SIMPLE TUMOURS OF THE BREAST

These are always best excised so that the diagnosis can be confirmed by pathological examination and the patient's anxieties arrested. They are:

1. Fibroadenoma.
2. Duct papilloma. This is a benign tumour which arises in one of the terminal lactiferous ducts. It causes a blood-stained discharge from the nipple. As these tumours are liable to develop into duct carcinoma, excision is advisable.

TRAUMA

Injuries to the breast may result in:

1. A haematoma which may organise to form a swelling and exploration may be necessary to settle the diagnosis.
2. Fat necrosis. A hard, craggy mass which is frequently adherent to the skin appears. The diagnosis may be suspected clinically but excision is mandatory so that a scirrhous carcinoma is excluded.

CARCINOMA OF THE BREAST

Every woman who discovers a lump in her breast has a not unnatural dread that it is a carcinoma. Unfortunately, this dread too often results in concealment of her condition until it is too late, yet the breast remains one of the most favourable sites for the treatment of a new growth. The earlier treatment is instituted, the greater the chances of cure.

One in seventeen of all women acquire the disease and more than 50 per cent eventually die from it irrespective of the form of treatment. There is an overall mortality of 8 per cent per year with a higher rate in the first three years. One half are dead in five years and three-quarters succumb eventually even as long as 20 years from diagnosis.

Carcinoma of the breast should be regarded as a systemic disease until it is proved otherwise. No big improvement can be expected until a method is found to combat micrometastases at the time of diagnosis of the lesion in the breast. Hence the potential importance of scanning clinics.

It used to be believed that cancer of the breast in old women was a fairly benign condition and for that reason labelled as an atrophic scirrhous growth. Mullen has shown that most women in the age group 71–100 are likely to die of their cancer and that this justifies a more aggressive approach to treatment.

Evidence to date suggests that the use of oral contraceptives is unrelated to the risk of breast cancer. Nonetheless it should be remembered that it must be many years before the possible relationship between oral contraceptives and breast cancer is finally settled. Oral contraceptives do increase the incidence of non-malignant lumps in the breast.

Screening for carcinoma of the breast

The effectiveness of screening has still to be evaluated. Clinical examination will discover a palpable lump but the mass may be too small to be felt with the hand. Mammography will show an area of calcification if present but repeated mammograms expose the patient to radiation hazards. Screening requires back up services for biopsy.

Varieties of carcinoma of the breast

1. Scirrhous carcinoma. This is the commonest form. It is hard in consistency.

2. Encephaloid carcinoma is a softer growth and spreads more rapidly than the scirrhous type.

3. Duct carcinoma. The rarest growth is characterised by bleeding from the nipple and is occasionally associated with an eczematous-like condition of the nipple and areola (Paget's disease). It is a favourable growth to treat.

4. Acute carcinomatosis of lactation is fortunately rare. The patient develops a growth while lactating, and the great vascularity of the breast at this time causes rapid spread.

The spread of carcinoma of the breast

1. Locally spread occurs by invasion of the skin overlying the growth and invasion of the pectoral muscles of the chest wall.

2. Lymphatic spread occurs to the axillary lymphatic glands and later to the supraclavicular group. Spread to the lymphatic glands in the chest may occur early in growths of the inner segments of the breast.

3. Spread by the blood stream may result in invasion of the bones (particularly the vertebrae) the liver and the lungs.

Clinical staging of carcinoma of the breast

Stage 1. A small growth with no localised spread.

Stage 2. Evidence of local extension such as a skin attachment and enlarged mobile lymph glands.

Stage 3. Fixed lymph glands and pectoral fascia or skin involvement.

Stage 4. Disseminated spread.

Although clinically a growth may be stage 1, undetected secondary deposits may already be well established and the disease is already well advanced.

Symptoms and signs

1. A painless, hard, irregular mass in the breast is the usual complaint. It has been noticed while washing, or as a result of a trivial knock. It is easily felt with the flat of the hand. There is usually some elevation of the breast. With a lump in the breast, as in vaginal bleeding, the greatest service a nurse can do is to refer the patient immediately to her doctor.

2. Attachment to the skin and the deeper structures, namely, the pectoral muscles and the ribs, occurs as the growth extends.

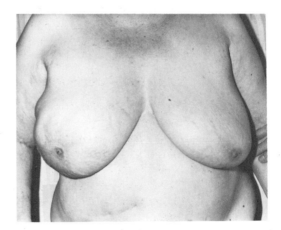

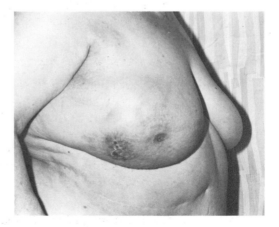

Fig. 29.2 Carcinoma of breast showing elevation and retraction of the nipple (*top*) and peau d'orange (*below*).

3. Recent retraction of the nipple may be present. This sign is diagnostic.

4. A coarsening of the skin, known as *peau d'orange*, may be present, due to blockage of the subcutaneous lymphatic vessels (Fig. 29.2).

5. Ulceration and fungation occur in late and untreated cases (Fig. 29.3).

6. The lymphatic glands in the axilla may be enlarged and hard.

7. Frozen microscopic section as soon as the lump has been removed is the only certain method of diagnosis in the very earliest cases.

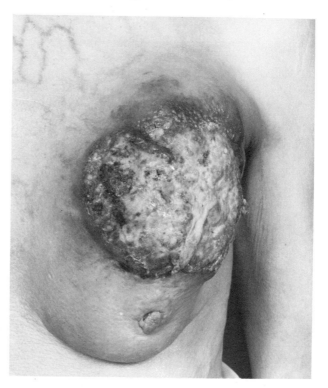

Fig. 29.3 Advanced fungating carcinoma of the breast.

Investigations

1. Radiography of the chest. Total skeletal X-ray is not of great value.
2. Bone scanning may be undertaken before deciding the appropriate method of treatment but the most careful scanning may fail to reveal micrometastases.
3. Estimation of urinary hydroxy-proline which is raised if bone metastases are present.
4. Full blood count.

A truly accurate diagnosis can only come from histological analysis of the tissue. This may be obtained by Tru-cut needle biopsy, open excision biopsy or preferably by a high speed drill biopsy preceeding any elective surgery.

MANAGEMENT

The subsequent management of the patient will depend on the local extent of the primary disease and the presence or absence of metastases.

If the disease is apparently localised to the breast the following avenues of treatment are available:

(a) Radical mastectomy i.e. removal of the breast, the overlying skin, the pectoral muscles and the axillary lymphatic glands. This procedure is not as popular as it was in the past.

(b) Patey mastectomy (Fig. 29.4) is the same as a radical mastectomy with the exception that the pectoralis major muscle is preserved. It provides adequate tumour clearance without the obvious deformity that results from removal of the muscles.

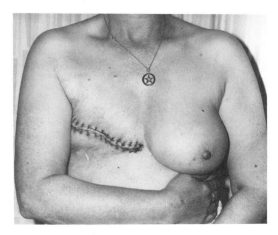

Fig. 29.4 External rotation of the shoulder joint is the only movement which it is important to recover in the first week following mastectomy. If this is full, abduction will also be full. This patient has had a Patey mastectomy performed.

(c) Simple mastectomy followed by radiotherapy if the axillary nodes are found to be involved.

(d) Wide excision of the lump followed by radiotherapy.

(e) Radiotherapy may be used alone for those cases with inoperable primary disease.

(f) Immunotherapy, using B.C.G. vaccine as a non-specific stimulus of the immune defence mechanisms may be prescribed.

Care of the mastectomy patient

Preparation of the skin

1. Local. Both axillae are shaved, the affected one because it comes into the incision, and the opposite one because the bandages pass around it. The area of both breasts, the arms to the wrists, and the abdomen to below the umbilicus, are washed with 2 per cent hexachlorophane soap.

2. The thigh. The ipsilateral thigh should be shaved and washed so that it is ready as a donor area should a skin graft be required.

The operation

The prepared area is generously towelled off.

The care of the arm during the operation. The arm is held by a nurse until the patient is towelled for operation. It is held abducted, one of the nurse's hands holding the patient's wrist and the other hand resting on the table to protect the patient's radial nerve on the lower third of the humerus. The nurse must be careful not to over-abduct the arm for fear of causing damage to the large nerve-trunks. It is then fixed on a suitably padded side arm of the operating table (Fig. 29.5).

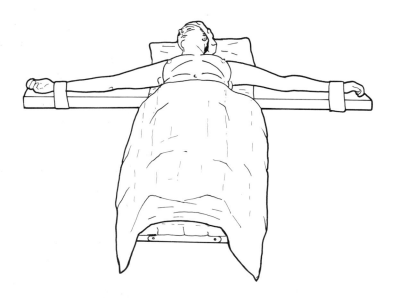

Fig. 29.5 Position for operations on the breast.

Postoperative care

When recovery from the anaesthetic has taken place, the patient is propped up and a pillow is placed at the bottom of the bed, so that she can push against it with her feet. She is mobilised the next day.

Haemorrhage and care of the drainage tube. A tube is invariably inserted, and in the first 24 hours oozing of blood and serum always occurs. A careful watch must be kept for haemorrhage, and the dressing can be repacked if it becomes saturated. The bandage must be firmly secured. Any excessive haemorrhage should, of course, be reported at once. The tube is rotated and eased a little after 24 hours and removed after 48 to 72 hours. Some surgeons prefer suction drainage of the axilla and the tube is attached to a suction machine or Redivac drain. Some surgeons insert two drainage tubes.

Pain is relieved by morphia (15 mg), which is usually prescribed on the night following the operation.

Care of the wound. The edges of the wound should be inspected for undue tension during dressing, and stitches are released if necessary. Ballooning of the flaps may occur, and air and serum are evacuated by aspiration or by the gentle insertion of sinus forceps. The flaps themselves must be observed for sloughing, and, should it occur, eusol compresses are applied.

The sutures are removed as follows: alternate sutures are removed on the tenth day and the remainder on the 12th day.

If a bare area has been grafted great care must be taken to 'float off' with sterile saline the innermost dressing, which is usually a small flap of tulle gras.

Care of the arm. It is important to commence arm movements on the second day after operation, but it is unwise to insist on much abduction for 4 or 5 days. The wound is disturbed and serum oozing increases. The patient must be encouraged to externally rotate the shoulder joint gently, and by the tenth day should have no trouble in touching the back of her head with her hand. If she has full external rotation at once she will have no difficulty in achieving full abduction. This is important, since her greatest disability will be in fastening her clothes at the back and doing her hair.

The nurse must remember that in the early days the patient will require some assistance with drinks and food because of the disability of the arm. Her locker or bed-table should be placed on the side opposite to that on which the operation was performed.

Complications

1. Respiratory complications. Respiration may be impaired by the trauma of the operation and the restriction of chest movements caused by the firm bandaging. Deep-breathing exercises although difficult in this situation must be encouraged.

2. Sloughing of the flaps. Should extensive sloughing occur, skin grafting must be undertaken later, when the area has granulated cleanly. Sloughs must be removed and sepsis reduced to a minimum as soon as possible. Eusol compresses are valuable before and just after the sloughs have separated.

3. Oedema of the arm may occur immediately if ligation of the axillary vein has had to be performed. More remotely, it may be due to lymphatic obstruction, constriction of the axillary vein from fibrosis or to recurrence of the growth and is a most distressing symptom. Elevation of the arm at night may control moderate swelling.

4. Thrombosis of the axillary vein may occur occasionally.

Cosmetic deformity

This is easily concealed by a TruLife prosthesis attached to the patient's clothing.

The management of advanced carcinoma of the breast.

The main priority of treatment is to improve the quality of life. Questions which face us are which form of treatment to give, when it should be used and what are the chances of success. These are still largely unanswered and the usual practice is to use an increasingly aggressive form of therapy in sequence.

Local therapy still has a part to play in the management of advanced disease. Whereas radiotherapy can control pain from bone metastases and heal ulcerating tumour masses, surgery can relieve functional upsets usually from tumour compression, e.g. the spinal cord.

However, most patients require systemic treatment. This may be either endocrine therapy or chemotherapy. Endocrine therapy is by ablative or additive methods. Surgical removal of the ovaries, the adrenals and the pituitary or destruction of the pituitary by the implantation of radioactive substances are standard procedures (Ch. 28).

They are either oestrogenic, androgenic or progestogenic in their action. A new compound Tamoxifen has specific antioestrogenic properties and is generally regarded as the best agent available. Many still regard oophorectomy as the treatment of choice for pre-menopausal women with advanced disease. If a response occurs then further endocrine ablation by adrenalectomy or hypophysectomy is worth while.

An alternative is to use chemotherapy with several combinations of multiple agents (Ch. 22) on a cyclical basis — remembering of course the need for regular white blood cell counts since all these agents cause leucopenia.

Mastectomy and the patient

The surgeon is well aware of the psychological insult that may arise from mastectomy. Subcutaneous mastectomy followed by a silicone implant has been undertaken in the belief that patients delay seeking advice because of fear of mastectomy. But surveys show that healthy women, should they develop carcinoma of the breast, would be more concerned about the adequacy of the clearance than resultant deformity. Self confidence is more likely to be restored by faith in their treatment and the provision of a prosthesis.

DISEASES OF THE MALE BREAST

Since the male breast is a vestigial organ, disease is uncommon.

Fibroadenosis is the most common simple lesion and is frequently due to pressure from braces. The treatment is excision. Gynaecomastia, which may be very painful, is sometimes seen as a complication of stilboestrol therapy for carcinoma of the prostate. At puberty, and sometimes in the newborn infant, enlargement of the breast occurs.

Carcinoma of the male breast occurs occasionally, accounting for 1 per cent of all breast cancer. The symptoms and signs are the same as in women, but because there is almost no breast tissue for the growth to invade, fixation to and invasion of the underlying muscle and ribs occur very early.

BIBLIOGRAPHY.

Baum, M. British Medical Journal. 1976. 1439.
Mueller C.B et al Surgery 1978 83 123
Rolland and Schellens L.J. Obst. and Gyn. 1973 80 945.
Williams E.M., Baum M. and Hughes L.E. Clinical Oncology. 1976. 327.

30

Lungs, chest wall and pleura

PNEUMOTHORAX

There are two types of pneumothorax — (a) spontaneous and (b) traumatic. Either kind can develop into a 'tension' pneumothorax.

Spontaneous pneumothorax

This is the more common variety and is seen more frequently in males than females, often between the ages of 20 and 40 years. Air escapes into the pleural cavity as a result of rupture of a small emphysematous bulla on the surface of the lung, usually at the apex. The bulla ruptures quite spontaneously and there is not usually any associated history of straining or sudden exertion. The patient complains of pain in the chest and dyspnoea, the severity depending on the size of the pneumothorax. The lung is separated from the chest wall by the air in the pleural cavity and the underlying lung is progressively reduced in size. If adhesions are present, or if the air leak stops, the underlying lung may only partially collapse.

Treatment

A small pneumothorax probably requires no active treatment and the patient is advised to remain quiet and to restrict his activities. The air is gradually absorbed over the following 7 to 10 days and the underlying lung re-expands. If the lung should fail to re-expand, or if the pneumothorax occupies more than 20 per cent of the thoracic cavity, an intercostal drainage tube is inserted through the second intercostal space anteriorly, and connected to an underwater-seal drainage bottle (Fig. 30.1). With each expiration, air bubbles will be seen to escape down the tube and through the water. Air cannot re-enter the tube and pleural cavity because of the water seal. So long as the air leak in the lung persists, bubbles of air will escape. However, if the lung can be made to expand fully, and this may require applying suction to the drainage system, the lung will begin to stick to the pleural lining of the chest wall and the hole will be gradually sealed off. When this happens, the escape of air ceases

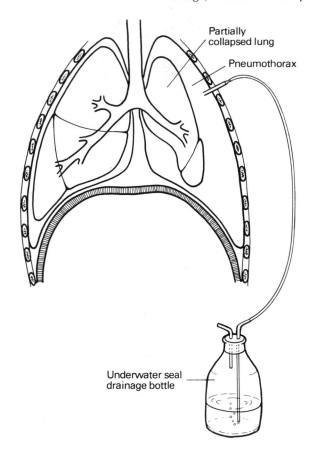

Partially
collapsed lung

Pneumothorax

Underwater seal
drainage bottle

Fig. 30.1   Pneumothorax. Intercostal tube in situ.

and the intercostal tube is normally removed 24 hours later. Many patients
will develop a second pneumothorax weeks, months or even years after
the first. These patients are very likely to go on and develop further recurrent pneumothoraces on the same side and, therefore, more active treatment than simple intubation is normally recommended after the second
pneumothorax. There is some debate as to which is the best method of
treating recurrent pneumothorax. The instillation of various irritant solutions into the pleural cavity has been recommended, e.g. Tetracycline
solution and iodized talc powder. The aim of these is to promote adhesions
between the lung and the chest wall, thus preventing further collapse of the
lung. A more certain way of achieving the same effect is to submit the
patient to parietal pleurectomy. Through a standard thoracotomy, the
parietal pleura is stripped off the chest wall leaving the raw surface of ribs
and muscles exposed. The lung sticks to this surface extensively and recurrent pneumothorax is most uncommon after this procedure. However, it is
a major operation. It does, though, have the advantage that any emphysematous bullae on the surface of the lung can be ligated or plicated
and thus further reduce the risk of future pneumothoraces. Occasionally,
thoracotomy, pleurectomy and ligation of bulla is essential for a persistent

air leak that is not responding to conservative treatment.

Traumatic pneumothorax

This is most commonly associated with fractured ribs when the surface of the lung is punctured by the sharp edge of a broken rib. It can, however, result from an external blow with no apparent rib injury. Traumatic pneumothorax is frequently associated with bleeding into the pleural cavity resulting in a haemopneumothorax. Tension pneumothorax is more likely to develop after trauma because the air leak is usually larger and may, indeed, be from a tear in the trachea or major bronchus.

Treatment

Treatment is similar to that for spontaneous pneumothorax except that active intervention is usually more frequently necessary. An intercostal tube is inserted and suction applied to draw the lung out against the chest wall in the hope that it will stick and the air leak becomes sealed. A large air leak suggests fracture of the trachea or bronchus. This can be confirmed at bronchoscopy and thoracotomy and repair of the tear is indicated. Similarly, a large tear in the lung substance will produce a large air leak and thoracotomy may be required to suture the lung. If a haemothorax is also present, two tubes will usually be necessary—one at the apex to evacuate air and the other at the base of the pleural cavity to evacuate blood.

Tension pneumothorax

Normally when air escapes into the pleural cavity, a balance of pressures is achieved with the lung either partially or fully collapsed. Some times, however, when the air leak is large, air continues to escape into the pleural cavity, even after the lung is fully deflated. With each inspiration more air is sucked into the cavity and gradually the heart and mediastinum are pushed to the opposite side. As the mediastinum moves over to the good side, the underlying good lung becomes compressed so that eventually the lung on the pneumothorax side is completely collapsed and the good lung is seriously compressed. The patient is intensely cyanotic and the circulation is grossly embarrassed. Death ensues unless urgent measures are taken.

Treatment

The tension can be easily and quickly relieved by insertion of an open needle through the chest wall into the pneumothorax. Air whistles out, the heart begins to return to the midline and the compression of the good lung is reduced. An intercostal tube should be inserted as soon as possible and connected to an underwater sealed drainage bottle. Subsequent treatment is as described above.

Tension pneumothorax presents a serious, life-threatening emergency which responds to simple urgent measures.

CHEST INJURIES

A patient with a major chest injury can present a frightening situation to an inexperienced nurse or doctor. However, many of the injuries though serious can be simply and effectively treated. A cool head and a knowledge of the structures within the chest which are liable to injury and the types of injury which can occur to each, can be of considerable help to those who have to deal with this type of patient.

Structures which may be injured

1. Chest wall, ribs, sternum, costal cartilages and soft tissues.
2. Lungs, bronchi, trachea
3. Oesophagus
4. Diaphragm
5. Heart and great vessels
6. Abdominal viscera
7. Other injuries (head, limbs, spine etc.)

Types of injuries

(a) **Bruising and lacerations** are dealt with as in any other part of the body. A penetrating injury through the soft tissues into the pleural cavity can result in a sucking wound, so that on each inspiration air is drawn into the pleural cavity through the chest wall. The air is not able to escape because on expiration the soft tissues fall together again. A pneumothorax develops which can progress to a tension pneumothorax. The hole can be sealed in an emergency situation by application of a finger, or preferably a wad of jellynet gauze. An intercostal tube can then be inserted and the wound in the chest wall later repaired.

(b) **Fractured ribs**. Simple fractures of the ribs can be very painful and treatment consists in relieving the pain until they heal. However, in the elderly patient or chronic bronchitic, serious complications can develop following simple fractured ribs. These patients are reluctant to cough because of the associated pain and do not, therefore, clear their bronchial secretions adequately. Patchy collapse develops in the lungs which can progress to pneumonia. It is essential in this type of patient that pain is adequately relieved so that vigorous chest therapy can be applied. Regular analgesia is given, particularly before physiotherapy. Fractured ribs may be complicated by pneumothorax or haemothorax and these are dealt with on their merits.

If several ribs are fractured in two places, a flail segment can develop. An area of chest wall loses its rigidity and fixation to the remainder of the chest wall and begins to move paradoxically with respiration (Fig. 30.2). Normally, on inspiration the chest wall expands but the loose flail segment moves inwards, sucked in by the negative pressure within the thorax. On expiration, the flail segment moves out again as the remainder of the chest wall moves in. The portion of lung underlying the flail segment cannot expand with inspiration. This is not important if the flail segment is small, but a large flail segment will result in collapse of a wide area of underlying lung. This lung is not properly ventilated and the patient becomes cyanosed with a falling arterial blood pO_2. If this reaches critical levels, active intervention is essential. This will normally consist in passing an endotracheal tube and putting the patient on positive pressure ventilation. The lungs are then expanded by positive pressue and the flail segment moves synchronously in and out with the remainder of the chest wall. This is continued for between 10 and 20 days, by which time the fractures have begun to heal, the chest wall moves as one piece again and the patient can be weaned off the ventilator. If thoracotomy is necessary to deal with internal injuries, the fractured ribs can be wired together so that the period of ventilation required is considerably shortened.

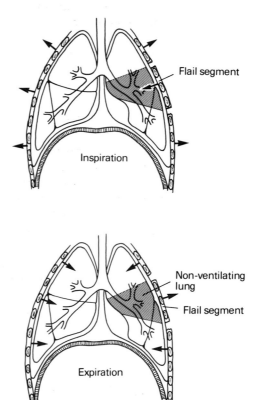

Fig. 30.2 Flail segment. Paradoxical movement on respiration.

Fractures of the costal cartilages and a stove-in sternum can behave like a flail segment and the treatment is similar.

(c) **Pneumothorax**. This has already been dealt with earlier in this chapter.

(d) **Haemothorax**. Bleeding can occur into the pleural cavity following injury from three common sources. An intercostal artery can be ruptured in association with a fractured rib, a tear of the lung may be associated with bleeding therefrom and injuries to the aorta may also occur. Aspiration of the blood from the pleural space is usually indicated. If the bleeding continues an intercostal tube should be inserted and the bleeding monitored. Thoracotomy is indicated for persistent or profuse bleeding.

INFECTIONS OF THE CHEST

Lung abscess

A lung abscess is formed by the development within the lung tissue of a cavity filled with pus. Abscesses may be single, or multiple, large or small, and involve one or two lungs. The condition is much less common nowadays since the advent of antibiotics, with improved anaesthesia and dental care. It may be due to specific infections of the lung such as staphylococcal pneumonia and tuberculosis, or to occlusion of the bronchus supplying the affected portion of lung, e.g. by carcinoma or foreign body. Aspiration of vomit following anaesthesia or intoxication with alcohol is another common cause of lung abscess. An abscess can also develop in the lung following pulmonary embolus, or lung trauma.

Patients complain of cough, fever and malaise and may have pleuritic pain. Weight loss is common and patients may be very ill. If the abscess communicates with the bronchial tree, purulent sputum will be expectorated. Chest X-ray shows one or more cavities in the lung field, often with a fluid level and tomograms can be helpful in distinguishing between a breaking-down carcinoma and a simple lung abscess. Treatment consists of bronchoscopy to exclude bronchial occlusion by carcinoma or foreign body and, if possible, to obtain secretions for culture. Antibiotics are given on the basis of culture sensitivities and these should be continued so long as the condition appears to respond. Lung resection is indicated if the lesion fails to respond to medical treatment, if a neoplasm is suspected, if haemoptysis is troublesome or if a broncho-pleural fistula develops. Occasionally patients are too ill for major chest surgery and the abscess is then simply drained externally.

Bronchiectasis

Bronchiectasis, like lung abscess, is much less frequently seen since the advent of antibiotics. The condition is caused by a combination of bronchial obstruction and pulmonary infection. A common cause is enlargement of hilar lymph glands during an infection in childhood. The infection which occurs distal to the obstruction damages the walls of the smaller bronchi which lose their elasticity and become dilated. The mucosa of the bronchial wall is damaged and secretions collect in the dilated bronchi. These secretions are prone to infection, giving rise to the symptoms and complications of bronchiectasis.

Patients complain of a chronic cough productive of purulent sputum. The amount and degree of infection of the sputum varies. Haemoptysis is common, as are acute exacerbations of infection in the surrounding lung tissue. Infection of the pleural space can lead to empyema and embolism of infected material can reach the brain causing cerebral abscess. Clubbing of the fingers is often seen in patients with bronchiectasis. Chest X-ray may appear normal, or show increased vascular markings with a honeycomb-like appearance in the affected areas. Bronchoscopy should be carried out to exclude bronchial obstruction and a bronchogram is essential to define the extent of the disease.

Medical treatment consists of postural drainage with short courses of antibiotics for bouts of acute infection. Surgery is indicated if the bronchiectasis is localised to one area of the lung. Removal of this part of lung results in complete cure. Surgery is not indicated, however, when the disease is extensive in both lungs.

Empyema

An empyema is a collection of pus within the pleural cavity. It may be secondary to an infective condition in the lung, e.g. simple abscess, bronchiectasis, pneumonia or tuberculosis. It may also be seen after thoracotomy, or following perforation of the oesophagus. Chest wall injuries may also give rise to empyema and a secondary empyema may develop in relation to a sub-phrenic abscess.

Patients may complain of cough and chest pain and are usually toxic with a fever. Chest X-ray reveals a pleural effusion and aspiration of this confirms the presence of pus. Because the abscess is usually walled off by a thick layer of fibrous tissue, systemic antibiotics are not usually effective, though they may be indicated to control toxicity.

Treatment consists initially in aspiration of the pus and injection of appropriate antibiotics into the pleural space. Many will resolve in this way, but if the pus becomes too thick for aspiration, surgical drainage by rib resection and insertion of a large drain is essential. Excision of the empyema and decortication of the underlying lung may be necessary for chronic empyema. Occasionally, when the underlying lung is grossly diseased, pleuropneumonectomy is indicated.

Tuberculosis

Most patients with pulmonary tuberculosis respond to medical treatment and do not require surgery. However, there are still a few indications for lung resection and these include the following:

1. When the sputum is still positive for tubercle bacilli 3 to 6 months after starting treatment, especially if the organism is resistant to one of the major drugs.

2. When the affected lobe or lung is destroyed by the disease.
3. Persistent haemoptysis, or troublesome bronchiectasis.
4. A persistent cavity, in spite of treatment.
5. When a neoplasm is suspected in addition to the tuberculosis.
6. When a patient proves very unreliable in taking drugs, or attending follow-up.

Surgery will usually consist of lobectomy but occasionally a totally destroyed bronchiectatic lung will be removed by pneumonectomy.

TUMOURS OF THE BRONCHI AND LUNGS

Bronchial adenoma

Bronchial adenomata are rare tumours which may occur in either sex, commonly between the ages of 20 and 40 years. They are of low grade malignancy and grow slowly but may metastasize. They usually occur in the central air passages and cause their effects either by bleeding and causing haemoptysis, or by occluding one major bronchus with collapse of a lobe. Most bronchial adenomata are usually visible at bronchoscopy and treatment is surgical. The tumour is removed together with the portion of lung supplied by the affected bronchus. The reported survival rates vary between 50 and 95 per cent at 5 years.

Hamartoma

A hamartoma is a benign tumour consisting of several different elements normally found in lung tissue, e.g. cartilage, fibrous tissue, epithelium. This type of tumour does not give rise to symptoms and is usually found by chance on a routine chest X-ray. However, it may be difficult to differentiate a hamartoma from a carcinoma and thoracotomy and surgical removal is usually indicated.

Carcinoma

At least 30 000 people die every year in England and Wales from carcinoma of the lung. The disease affects men more commonly than women but the ratio between the two is narrowing. The cause of lung cancer is not known, but there is a strong relationship to the number of cigarettes smoked. There may also be an increased incidence among people who work in arsenic and cobalt mines, or in the chromate and nickel industry.

Pathology

The three main pathological types are squamous carcinoma (50 per cent), undifferentiated carcinoma (30 per cent) and adeno-carcinoma (20 per cent). There is another type of lung cancer which is only infrequently seen and this is the alveolar cell carcinoma.

Squamous growths grow more slowly than the other varieties and metastasize later. Tumour tissue in the centre of the growth may break down and the appearances on chest X-ray then resemble a lung abscess. Undifferentiated growths, particularly the oat cell variety, metastasize early and carry a poor prognosis. Adenocarcinomata tend to occur in the periphery of the lung and their growth rate is intermediate between the other types.

Spread of lung cancer occurs either directly to the surrounding structures, e.g. mediastinum or chest wall, or along lymphatic channels to central lymph nodes or directly via the blood stream to distant organs. The most common sites of metastases are brain, bone and liver, though secondary deposits may occur anywhere.

Symptoms

One of the difficulties in the successful treatment of lung cancer is that there is an initial latent period during which a tumour may grow for a long time before producing any symptoms. When symptoms do occur the condition is already frequently inoperable. Symptoms will depend on the location of the tumour (Fig. 30.3). Involvement of the bronchus may cause cough, haemoptysis, wheezing and dyspnoea. Occlusion of a bronchus may produce pneumonia with fever and toxicity. Weight loss is common and involvement of the chest wall causes pain. Dysphagia results from obstruction of the oesophagus either by the tumour itself or by glands which may also compress the superior vena cava, resulting in superior mediastinal obstruction with swelling and cyanosis of the head and neck and dilatation of the veins over the upper chest wall. Hoarseness may develop from involvement of the recurrent laryngeal nerve supplying the vocal cord, and involvement of the pericardium may produce cardiac symptoms. Tumours of the lung can secrete hormones into the circulation producing an endocrine disorder or peripheral neuropathies. Headaches and vomiting may result from cerebral secondaries, pathological fractures from involvement of bone and abdominal pain and swelling from liver metastases.

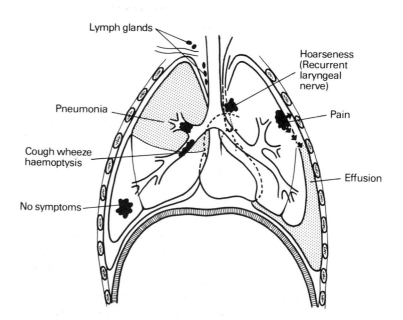

Fig. 30.3 Symptoms and signs of lung carcinoma in relation to location of tumour.

Investigation

Examination of the sputum for malignant cells will give a high incidence of reliable results if a good specimen of bronchial secretions is presented to an expert pathologist. Chest X-ray, including a lateral film, will frequently allow a confident diagnosis, but tomograms of the suspicious area will give clearer definition and will help to differentiate a simple pneumonia or abscess from a neoplasm. Bronchoscopy should be carried out in all suspected cases and if the lesion is within range of the instrument, a biopsy should be taken. If a pleural effusion is present, this should be aspirated and a specimen sent for cytological examination. A blood stained effusion invariably implies malignant involvement of the pleura. If cytology of the fluid is negative and neoplasm is still suspected, thoracoscopy can be a useful method of obtaining a biopsy from the surface of the lung or pleura. Mediastinoscopy may also be indicated in order to obtain a mediastinal gland for examination if it is suspected that these are involved by growth.

Surgery

At least 75 per cent of patients with carcinoma of the lung are already inoperable by the time they first present to the doctor either because they have distant metastases, or the tumour has spread locally to involve the chest wall or mediastinum. Sometimes the lesion is still resectable, but the patient's respiratory function is so poor that lung resection is contraindicated. About 20 per cent of patients, however, will be considered suitable for operation when all investigations have been completed.

Preoperative preparation is most important. Since most patients have been smokers and many of them have bronchitis, it is essential to start chest physiotherapy before operation. They must also stop smoking and if the sputum grows pathological organisms on culture, this is treated with appropriate antibiotics. The operation is explained to the patient and his relatives and every effort made to gain the patient's confidence for the difficult postoperative period. Operation is performed through a thoracotomy on the side of the lesion. The tumour is assessed for position, size and evidence of spread. Approximately one fifth of patients who are operated on will prove to be inoperable at operation. If the tumour is removable, a decision is made as to whether it can be completely removed together with any involved glands by lobectomy or pneumonectomy. The pulmonary arteries and veins are ligated and divided individually and the bronchus is then dealt with. This is divided close to the trachea for a pneumonectomy, and near the origin of the lobar bronchus for a lobectomy (Fig. 30.4). The open end is closed with either interrupted nonabsorbable sutures, or with a stapling clamp. If possible, the bronchial stump is covered with a flap of parietal pleura to reduce the risk of postoperative bronchopleural fistula.

Following lobectomy, two tubes are left in the chest (Fig. 30.5) one at the apex to evacuate air and to allow the remaining lobe to expand to fill the space and one at the base of the thorax to evacuate any blood drainage. The basal drain can usually be removed within 48 hours, but the apical drain is left until all air leak has ceased, and this may take several days. Following pneumonectomy, a single tube is left in the pleural space to evacuate blood drainage and to equalise pressures on both sides of the chest. This tube can usually be removed within twenty four to forty eight hours.

In the immediate postoperative period it is most important to observe the

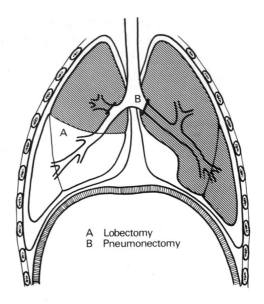

A Lobectomy
B Pneumonectomy

Fig. 30.4 A. Line of resection for lobectomy. B. Line of resection for pneumonectomy.

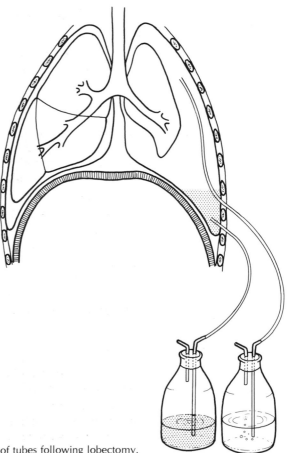

Fig. 30.5 Arrangement of tubes following lobectomy.

behaviour of the chest tubes. Excessive blood drainage should immediately be reported and the decision to remove an apical tube will often depend on the observations of a nurse regarding air leakage. Tubes should be removed quickly and cleanly to prevent entry of air or infection into the thoracic cavity.

After operation, the patient's colour, respiratory rate, blood pressure and pulse rate and rhythm are carefully monitored and any abnormalities reported. A thoracotomy wound is painful and regular analgesia is essential. Because of the pain, patients often have difficulty in coughing and clearing their secretions, and although chest physiotherapy will regularly be given by a trained physiotherapist, it will always be necessary for the nurse taking care of the patient to encourage and help him to clear his secretions between the visits of the physiotherapist. This is particularly important at night. Retained secretions can lead to serious complications with collapse and infection in the residual lobe or lung. Occasionally bronchoscopy is necessary to clear the secretions when chest physiotherapy cannot cope, and tracheostomy may even be required if bronchoscopy is insufficient to keep the airways clear.

Without operation, 99 per cent of patients with lung cancer are dead within 2 years. Even with surgery, the 5 years survival is limited. Prognosis depends on several factors but mainly the histological type of the carcinoma, the size of the lesion and the degree of involvement of the lymph glands. Approximately 40 per cent of patients undergoing resection for squamous cell carcinoma, 15 per cent of patients with adenocarcinoma and 10 per cent of patients with oat cell tumours will live 5 years or more.

Radiotherapy

Radiotherapy seldom cures a patient with carcinoma of the lung. It can also cause unpleasant side effects and patients are usually quickly aware of their diagnosis when referred for this treatment. It should, therefore, on the whole, be reserved for specific indications and not offered to every patient with carcinoma of the lung who is unsuitable for surgery. Radiotherapy can be very effective in controlling certain symptoms such as pain, dyspnoea, haemoptysis, dysphagia and superior mediastinal obstruction so that, if these symptoms are significant, it is often worthwhile referring them for radiotherapy. There are also some patients with an operable lesion who, for some other reason, are not suitable for surgery and these may also be treated. Generally speaking, however, long term survival is not improved by radiotherapy and patients should be carefully selected.

Chemotherapy

The use of drugs in the treatment of lung cancer is continually progressing and for the future this perhaps holds the best hope of improvements in prognosis. However, at the present time, survival is not significantly affected by chemotherapy and the use of drugs, like radiotherapy, should be for selected patients only.

31

Surgery of the heart

...The blood is passed through the lungs and the heart by the pulsation of the ventricles, is forcibly ejected to all parts of the body, therein steals into the veins and porosities of the flesh, flows back everywhere through those very veins from the circumference to the centre, from small veins into larger ones and hence comes at last into the vena cava, and to the auricles of the heart...

Harvey 1628

STRUCTURE

The heart consists of a connective tissue framework of four fibrous rings (Fig. 31.1). The atria, ventricles, valves and roots of the pulmonary artery and aorta are attached to this framework. It is enveloped in a serofibrinous sac called the pericardium.

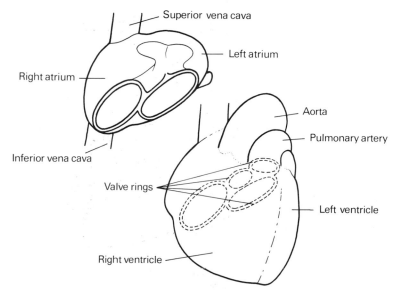

Fig. 31.1 The relationships of the cardiac chambers to the arterial roots and fibrous skeleton of the heart.

The ventricles are the pumps which provide most of the energy for the circulation of the blood. The right ventricle is like a bellows useful for propelling a large volume against a low resistance. The left ventricle is spherical and thus efficient at pumping against a high resistance.

Each atrium lies behind and to the right of its corresponding ventricle. The atria transfer blood from the veins (pulmonary and systemic) into the ventricular pumps. They may be likened to booster pumps.

Cardiac valve movements are passive. The atrioventricular valves (mitral and tricuspid) are funnel shaped. The chordae tendineae extend like guy ropes from the valve cusps into the papillary muscles. The semilunar valves (aortic and pulmonary) consist of three symmetrical cusps attached to the roots of the great vessels.

The pericardium with its fluid lubricates the heart, holds it in a fixed anatomical position and separates it from the other mediastinal structures.

The heart's blood supply is provided by two coronary arteries which arise from the sinuses of Valsalva of the aortic root. The left main coronary artery (Fig. 31.2A) divides 2 cm from its ostium into two main divisions, the anterior descending and the circumflex. The anterior descending branch runs down the anterior interventricular groove, round the apex and ascends for a short distance in the posterior interventricular groove. The circumflex branch courses around the base of the left ventricle. The right coronary artery (Fig. 31.2B) passes beneath the left atrial appendage to the atrioventricular groove to reach the posterior interventricular groove. The venous drainage of the myocardium consists of a superficial and deep system. The very extensive superficial system of veins converge to form the coronary sinus which terminates in the right atrium. The deep system of veins communicates directly with the atria and ventricles through the thebesian veins.

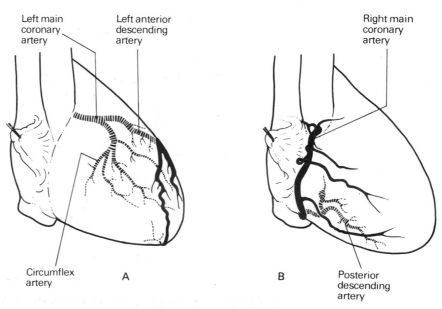

Fig. 31.2 A and B The superficial coronary arteries.

FUNCTION

The delivery of blood to all organs of the body is accomplished by the pumping action of the heart.

Systemic circulation

The systemic circulation consists of three functional divisions — the arterial pressure reservoir, the capillaries and the venous volume reservoir.

The left ventricle ejects blood into the aorta and other elastic arteries. When the ventricles relax the flow of blood from the ventricles ceases but the elastic wall tension in the arteries continues to drive the blood through the capillaries (Fig. 31.3).

The velocity (speed) of blood flow through the capillaries is less than elsewhere in the circulation because of the very great cross section area of the capillary bed. Thus the blood comes into close contact with the

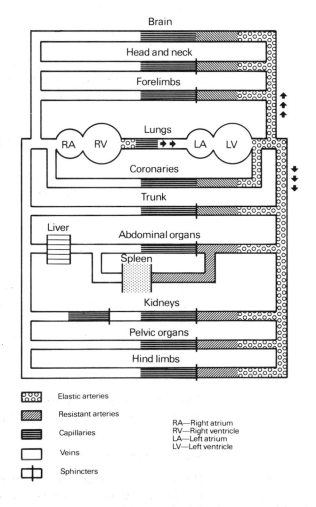

Fig. 31.3 Schematic representation of functionally defined segments of the circulation.

extravascular tissues. These features of capillary flow provide ideal conditions for the rapid transfer of substances by diffusion.

The systemic veins provide a mechanism whereby the volume can be varied over wide limits with only slight changes in pressure. The venous return is a most important regulator of cardiac output. If the pumping action (contractility) of the heart is unimpaired an increased venous return will increase cardiac output; conversely a decreased venous return will decrease cardiac output.

The systemic circulation may be described as a high pressure, high resistance system which supplies the variable requirements of many different tissues, thus it requires many controls. 'Central' control is mediated through the sympathetic nervous system and governed largely by the vasomotor centre of the medulla oblongata. In addition blood flow through various tissues may be adjusted locally in response to their metabolism and oxygen requirements.

Pulmonary circulation

The right ventricle pumps mixed venous blood through the pulmonary arteries and arterioles into the pulmonary capillary bed where gas exchange takes place. The pulmonary circulation in contrast to systemic circulation may be seen as a low pressure, low resistance circuit supplying a single function to one organ.

THE SCOPE OF CARDIAC SURGERY

Surgical correction of most of the serious congenital and acquired heart lesions is now possible. The patient is usually returned to a useful and active life.

CARDIAC CATHETERISATION

This special investigation is necessary to provide the surgeon with precise anatomical information. The catheter is a flexible tube about 100 cm long. It is connected to a continuous infusion drip containing heparin to prevent intravascular clotting. It is usually passed under local anaesthesia.

Right heart catheterisation

The catheter is passed through the antecubital vein to enter in succession the right atrium, right ventricle and pulmonary artery.

Left heart catheterisation

The left heart chambers may be entered in an antegrade fashion by passing a catheter into the right atrium, and then penetrating the atrial septum, the catheter enters the left atrium and may be advanced into the left ventricle.

A catheter may be introduced into the brachial or femoral artery and passed retrogradely up the aorta and into the left ventricle.

The pressures in all the chambers of the heart may be measured. The maximum normal pressures are:

Right atrium	6 mmHg
Right ventricle	30 mmHg
Pulmonary artery	30 mmHg
Left atrium	12 mmHg
Left ventricle	120 mmHg
Aorta	120 mmHg

Changes in pressures show the presence of disease, e.g. a high left ventricular pressure with a simultaneous low aortic pressure shows a pressure drop (gradient) across the aortic valve, thus revealing the presence and severity of aortic stenosis.

Blood samples can be withdrawn from the different chambers. Measurements of the oxygen saturation and tension may show the presence of abnormal communications between the systemic and pulmonary circulations.

Angiocardiography

Radio-opaque dye is injected through a catheter into a selected cardiac chamber. This will show the shape and size of the chamber and helps to detect any abnormality of cardiac contraction. The presence of a thrombus or a tumour within the chamber will be revealed. Regurgitation of the dye from one chamber to another confirms the presence of a valve leak or abnormal communication and is helpful in assessing the severity of the leak.

Coronary arteriography

Specially shaped catheters are inserted into the brachial or femoral artery and passed up the aorta, and then directly into the orifice of the coronary arteries. Dye injected through these catheters outlines the coronary arteries and this is essential for the precise localisation of coronary artery disease.

Preoperative care of the patient

Particular attention is given to the elimination of infection which may be the cause of postoperative bacterial endocarditis. Careful dental inspection and radiographic studies will reveal any septic foci and these are eradicated. Cultures of throat, nose, skin, hair and urine are obtained and any infection found is treated appropriately.

A history of dyspepsia should be carefully evaluated and if necessary barium studies and fibreoptic gastroscopy should be performed.

The patient will be admitted a few days prior to surgery. Very ill patients will require a longer period of intensive medical and nursing care before surgery. Digoxin will usually be stopped 48 hours before open-heart surgery.

Cardiac disease is a source of great anxiety to the patient and the family. It is essential that the surgeon should explain the nature of the disease, the proposed surgical procedure and the likely outcome of treatment to both patient and family.

All members of the caring team should likewise ensure that they understand the nature of the patient's disease and the operation to be performed. They can then make it easy for the patient and family to ask questions which will be answered in simple nontechnical language. This gives the patient confidence in those who are caring for him and a knowledge that his welfare is their primary objective.

Cardiopulmonary bypass

Most heart operations are performed with the assistance of a heart-lung machine. The heart is exposed through a median sternotomy incision, in which the sternum is split down the middle and spread widely by a mechanical retractor.

Intravenous heparin is given to prevent the blood clotting as it passes through the heart-lung machine. Tubes are inserted into the superior and inferior vena cava and the patient's venous blood is drained into an artificial oxygenator. The oxygenated blood is pumped back into the patient usually through a tube placed in the ascending aorta, but occasionally into the femoral artery. Thus the patient's heart and lungs are bypassed and the surgeon is able to operate inside the cavities of the heart. When the surgeon has closed the cardiac chambers the heart and lungs resume their normal function, and the tubes are removed from the vena cava and aorta. Any excess heparin is neutralised by the appropriate dose of protamine sulphate.

CONGENITAL HEART DISEASE

Congenital abnormalities of the heart result from an arrested or defective embryonic development. The eight most frequently encountered anomalies which account for 85 per cent of all congenital cardiac lesions will be described.

It may be useful for the student to group congenital heart defects as follows:

1. Abnormal communication between the pulmonary and systemic circuits which permits the passage of blood from the systemic to the pulmonary circulation, i.e. left to right shunt. This leads to overloading of the pulmonary circulation. Examples of this are patent ductus arteriosus, atrial septal defect and ventricular septal defect.

2. Abnormal communication between the pulmonary and systemic circuits which allows passage of blood from systemic veins to systemic arteries without first traversing the lungs. This leads to arterial hypoxaemia and cyanosis. Examples are the tetralogy of Fallot and transposition of the great vessels.

3. Lesions which do not cause shunts. Examples are coarctation of the aorta, pulmonary stenosis and aortic stenosis.

Patent ductus arteriosus

The ductus arteriosus connects the pulmonary and systemic circulations in foetal life, so that blood is short-circuited away from the lungs where it is not required. At birth spontaneous closure usually takes place, but occasionally the ductus remains open and the blood flows from the systemic to the pulmonary circulation. Congestive cardiac failure and bacterial endocarditis are the commonest complications. The operation to close the patent ductus is performed through a left thoracotomy. The ductus may be ligated, but some surgeons prefer to divide it and suture the ends to avoid the possibility of recanalisation.

Atrial septal defect

There is a communication between the two atria resulting in a large flow of blood from the left to the right atrium. There is a high pulmonary blood flow which may result in pulmonary hypertension and right ventricular failure.

The defect is closed by direct suture with the assistance of cardio-pulmonary bypass.

Ventricular septal defect

A communication between the left and right ventricles results in a large flow of blood passing from left to right ventricle, and then through the lungs. Cardiac failure and pulmonary hypertension supervene.

The defect is closed by inserting a patch of Dacron with the assistance of cardiopulmonary bypass.

Tetralogy of Fallot

The tetralogy of Fallot is a combination of:

  (a) Pulmonary stenosis
  (b) Ventricular septal defect
  (c) Dextroposition of the aorta
  (d) Right ventricular hypertrophy.

The obstruction caused by the pulmonary stenosis reduces the blood flow to the lungs, and thus the blood is shunted from the right ventricle through the ventricular septal defect to the left ventricle and into the aorta. The ingress of 'venous' blood to the aorta causes hypoxaemia and cyanosis.

Complete correction of the defect may not be possible in infants; temporary improvement may be produced, by increasing the blood flow to the lungs. This is achieved by creating a shunt between the aorta or subclavian artery and the pulmonary artery.

Correction of the defect is performed using the heart-lung machine. The pulmonary stenosis is relieved and the ventricular septal defect is closed by a patch.

Transposition of the great vessels

The great arteries arise from the anatomically inappropriate ventricles; the aorta from the right ventricle and the pulmonary artery from the left ventricle. Thus venous blood enters the right ventricle and is then pumped into the aorta and systemic arteries causing hypoxaemia and cyanosis.

Treatment

The operation is performed with the assistance of cardiopulmonary bypass. The right atrium is opened and the atrial septum excised. A large patch of pericardium or dacron is inserted so that oxygenated blood from the pulmonary veins is directed to the right ventricle and then pumped to the aorta; and the systemic venous blood directed into the left ventricle and pumped into the pulmonary artery (Mustards' technique).

Coarctation of the aorta

This is a narrowing of the aorta just distal to the origin of the left subclavian artery, which causes a high blood pressure in the cerebral circulation and the arms. The blood to the lower two-thirds of the body reaches it by way of a series of anastomotic channels, which run back into the aorta via the intercostal vessels.

Treatment

The coarctation is exposed through a left thoracotomy incision. The narrowed segment is excised and the cut ends of the aorta are sutured together. A tube graft of Dacron is inserted if the ends will not come together.

Pulmonary stenosis

There is a dome-like fusion of the cusps of the pulmonary valve with a central perforation often only 2–4 mm in diameter. The pressure in the right ventricle is increased and the pressure in the pulmonary artery is reduced. This leads to right ventricular hypertrophy, and eventually to right ventricular failure.

Treatment

The operation to relieve the stenosis is performed with the aid of cardiopulmonary bypass. The pulmonary artery is opened and the valve is divided with the scissors.

Aortic stenosis

The valve tissue is thickened and there is fusion of the commissures. In the most extreme cases the valve is dome-shaped with a central pin-hole opening. Frequently the valve has only two cusps instead of the usual three.

Surgery is indicated if the degree of obstruction is severe enough to result in symptoms.

Treatment

The operation is performed with the assistance of cardiopulmonary bypass. The valve is exposed and the fused commissures are carefully opened. It is likely that most of these patients will require valve replacement in later life.

ACQUIRED HEART DISEASE

Mitral valve disease

Rheumatic endocarditis is the most frequent cause of mitral valve disease; other causes include bacterial endocarditis, rupture or dysfunction of papillary muscle secondary to myocardial infarction, and spontaneous rupture of chordae tendineae.

Mitral stenosis. The rheumatic valvulitis leads to scarring, thickening and deformity of the cusps. There may be scarring, thickening and fusion of the chordae tendineae. Eventually calcification may occur.

The pressure in the left atrium rises as the orifice of the valve becomes smaller. This results in pulmonary congestion. Atrial fibrillation is a frequent complication.

Treatment

Mitral valvotomy is performed when the valve cusps are pliable and there is no significant regurgitation. Exposure of the heart is by left thoracotomy. A finger is inserted into the left atrium through a small incision in the auricular appendage (Fig. 31.4). A Tubbs' dilator is inserted into the left ventricle through a small incision in the left ventricular apex. The finger in the left atrium guides the tip of the dilator into the valve orifice and the fused cusps are separated by opening the dilator (Fig. 31.4).

Mitral valve replacement. When the principal lesion is mitral regurgitation or if the mitral stenosis is not suitable for valvotomy, then the valve is excised and a new valve is inserted. Cardiopulmonary bypass is necessary for this operation.

Valve substitutes. The most commonly used valve substitutes are:

(a) Prosthetic valve—this is a man-made mechanical valve. Most frequently used are the tilting disc valve (Bjork Shiley valve; Fig. 31.5A) and the caged-ball valve (Starr Edwards valve; Fig. 31.5B).

(b) Homograft—a human aortic valve removed as soon as possible after death, sterilised, and stored in a preservative solution.

(c) Heterograft—an animal (usually pig) aortic valve which is sterilised and stored in a preservative solution.

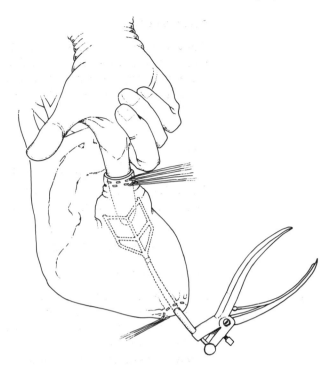

Fig. 31.4 Transventricular mitral valvotomy. The surgeon's index finger is in the left auricle—the Tubbs' dilator through the apex of the left ventricle.

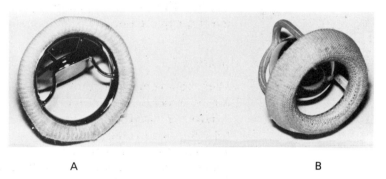

A   B

Fig. 31.5 Prosthetic heart valves. A. Tilting disc valve (Bjork Shiley). B. Caged ball valve (Starr Edwards).

Aortic valve disease

The principal causes are rheumatic fever, congenital bicuspid aortic valve, bacterial endocarditis and syphilis.

Aortic stenosis. Narrowing of the aortic valve orifice, frequently with calcification of the valve leaflets. This results in a raised left ventricular pressure and a reduced aortic pressure. It is a very serious disease, and when angina pectoris, blackouts, or left ventricular failure occur valve replacement should not be delayed.

Aortic regurgitation. The cusps become thickened, rigid, and deformed, allowing blood to leak from the aorta into the left ventricle. The volume of blood in the ventricle is greatly increased, which may lead to left ventricular failure.

Treatment

Excision of the diseased valve and insertion of a new valve. Cardiopulmonary bypass is required.

Angina pectoris (coronary artery disease)

Angina pectoris is a condition in which chest pain with 'a sense of strangling and anxiety' is produced by exercise or emotion, and relieved rapidly by rest. It is most frequently associated with disease of the coronary arteries.

The site of narrowing or obstruction of the coronary arteries is demonstrated by coronary arteriography.

Treatment

Surgery is indicated when severe angina is not relieved by medical therapy. The operation is performed with the assistance of cardiopulmonary bypass. A length of saphenous vein is removed from the leg. The vein is reversed and anastomosed proximally to the aorta and distally to the coronary artery beyond the site of narrowing or obstruction—aorto coronary saphenous vein bypass graft. This bypass restores the blood supply to the ischaemic area of myocardium and relieves the angina.

ANEURYSMS OF THE THORACIC AORTA

Aneurysms of the thoracic aorta may be fusiform or saccular. They may be located in the ascending, transverse arch or descending thoracic aorta. Arteriosclerosis is the most common cause but they may be due to cystic medionecrosis or syphilis. Chest X-ray will reveal the aneurysm as a mediastinal mass but aortography is essential for precise definition of site and size.

Treatment

The aneurysm is excised and a Dacron tube graft is inserted. The surgical approach would be dictated by the site of the aneurysm.

Dissecting aneurysm

A tear in the intimal layer permits the force of the blood stream to cause the separation of the intramural layers of the aorta. The dissection usually begins just beyond the origin of the left subclavian artery or in the ascending aorta a few centimetres above the aortic valve. Almost all the patients suffer from hypertension. The patient will present with sudden onset of severe pain in the chest, back, or epigastrium.

Treatment

Rest, sedation and antihypertensive agents are usually an effective form of therapy. Surgical intervention is indicated by failure to control hypertension, persistence of pain, or life threatening complications.

Chronic constrictive pericarditis

Almost any form of acute pericarditis may result in chronic pericarditis. Despite the most careful investigation the aetiological agent is not identified in over 50 per cent of patients. The thickened pericardium and its inflammatory exudate encase the heart and impede the relaxation of the ventricles.

The patient presents with signs of right heart failure, i.e. raised venous pressure, ascites, hepatomegaly and oedema.

Treatment

Pericardiectomy is the only definitive treatment. The thickened pericardium and exudate which prevent ventricular relaxation must be completely excised.

CARDIAC PACEMAKERS

Types of pacemakers

Pacemakers are either fixed rate or non-competitive/Demand.

The fixed rate pacemaker stimulates the heart at a pre-set rate regardless of the heart's own activity. There is, therefore, a possibility of a stimulus occurring during the vulnerable period and thus triggering ventricular fibrillation. This type of device is now used less frequently because of the greater availability of non-competitive systems.

Non-competitive/Demand. The two most commonly used are:

(a) The Demand R synchronous which synchronises its output with the R wave providing a stimulus which falls in the absolute refractory period.

(b) The Demand R inhibited which is inhibited by ventricular depolarisation and stimulates only when the ventricular rate is below its preset rate.

Pacing may be a temporary measure or a permanent form of therapy.

Indications

Temporary

1. Complete heart block or other marked bradycardia. Used as an emergency measure pacing may be life saving in a patient with Adams-

Stokes attacks. The temporary system is left in place until a reliable permanent system is functioning.

2. Acute myocardial infarction. Pacing is required in only a small percentage of patients who have had an acute myocardial infarction.

3. Certain intractable arrhythmias.

Temporary pacing is achieved by inserting an electrode through a vein and passing it into the right ventricle until the tip of the electrode is in contact with the endocardium. The electrode is attached to an external pacing device (Fig. 31.6).

Permanent pacing

Permanent pacing may be used for any chronic disorder of rhythm or conduction that produces symptomatic bradycardia. These include complete heart block, sinus arrest and complete AV block. Permanent pacing may be carried out by the transvenous route or by attaching an electrode to the epicardial surface of the heart. A thoracotomy is required for the insertion of an epicardial lead. The pacemaker (Fig. 31.7) is implanted into a suitable site in the patient's abdominal or chest wall. The transvenous route is preferred because of its lower operative mortality and morbidity.

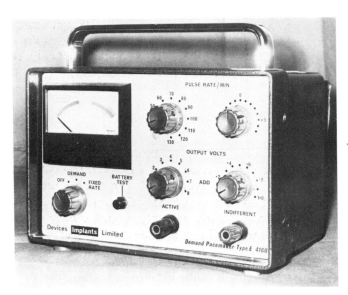

Fig. 31.6 External pacemaking device.

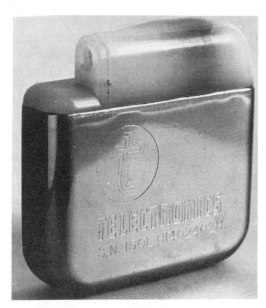

Fig. 31.7 Implantable pacemaker.

Complications

Epicardial. Early postoperative complications are usually those associated with a thoracotomy.

Transvenous (Endocardial). Infection, phlebitis or haematoma may occur at the site of the venous cut-down. The electrode may perforate the myocardium causing tamponade, or allow stimulation of extra-cardiac structures such as the diaphragm. Thrombosis associated with the electrode may give rise to pulmonary emboli.

A wide variety of arrhythmias may complicate the insertion of any type of pacemaker.

Failure may present as a cessation of pacing, aberrant stimulation, or change in timing characteristics. Failure may be due to:

  (a) Failure of the battery
  (b) Fracture of an electrode
  (c) Displacement of an electrode
  (d) Increase in pacing threshold

Pacemaker Clinic

Regular checks for the patient and the electronic device are essential. This is best achieved by a special Pacemaker Clinic which is fully equipped to assess pacemaker function. In such a setting the goals of maximum pacemaker longevity, minimum surgical procedures and maximum patient safety can be achieved.

POSTOPERATIVE CARE

The care of the patient who has had a mitral valvotomy, resection of coarctation, insertion of pacemaker or closure of patent ductus arteriosus is similar to that previously described for the patient who has had a lobectomy (p. 293). Usually only one drainage tube will have been inserted.

Intensive care

The patient whose cardiac surgery has been performed with the aid of cardiopulmonary bypass will return to the intensive care unit. The patient's ECG, blood pressure, central venous pressure and skin temperature are constantly monitored and electronically displayed. Urine flow is measured hourly and frequent estimations of blood electrolytes and arterial blood gases are performed. Some patients will require intermittent positive pressure ventilation.

32

Diseases of the oesophagus

ANATOMY

The oesophagus is a hollow, muscular tube which extends from the cricopharyngeus muscle in the neck, at the level of the sixth cervical vertebra, through the posterior mediastinum and oesophageal hiatus in the diaphragm to the stomach. (There is, therefore, a short length of cervical oesophagus and a short length of intra-abdominal oesophagus.) Most of the organ, however, lies within the thoracic cavity, running down behind the trachea, heart and pericardium. The aortic arch crosses it to the left in the mid-thoracic region. Behind the oesophagus lie the thoracic vertebrae in the upper part and the descending aorta in its lower part (Fig. 32.1).

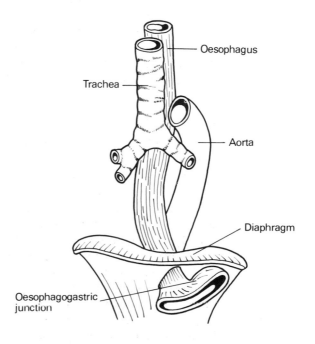

Fig. 32.1 Anatomy of the oesophagus.

The oesophagus receives its arterial blood supply from branches of the inferior thyroid artery in the neck, from branches of the aorta in the thorax and from branches of the left gastric artery below the diaphragm. Venous drainage mirrors the arterial supply to a large extent. There are, however, numerous communications between the venous plexuses throughout the oesophagus and these are important in the development of oesophageal varices (Ch. 36). The veins draining the thoracic part of the oesophagus to the azygos veins communicate freely with those draining the intra-abdominal oesophagus to the portal system. Lymphatic drainage is to the glands in the neck, the central glands in the mediastinum and the coeliac glands below the diaphragm. Again, there are extensive communications between the lymphatic channels.

PHYSIOLOGY

The oesophagus is not an inert tube, but is a physiological organ and disturbances in the nervous mechanism controlling it can result in distressing symptoms. Parasympathetic control is through the vagus nerves and sympathetic from the thoracic sympathetic chain. The oesophagus has a physiological sphincter at both upper and lower ends which are under nervous control. Their relaxation is controlled during the act of swallowing and after the bolus of food has passed they regain their tone, preventing reflux and regurgitation of the swallowed food. As the muscles of the pharynx contract on swallowing, the upper sphincter relaxes to allow the food through and then contracts again. A peristaltic wave passes down the oesophagus, taking the bolus with it. Immediately prior to the arrival of the peristaltic wave at the lower oesophageal sphincter, the sphincter relaxes and opens the way for the food to enter the stomach. It then closes again, preventing reflux of gastric contents in to the oesophagus. Disturbances of this finely coordinated mechanism, as occurs in, for example, achalasia and hiatus hernia, can result in serious difficulties of swallowing (dysphagia).

Investigation

1. Radiology. Screening of the oesophagus on swallowing barium suspension can give much information on the movements of the oesophagus and will also demonstrate the presence of tumours, strictures and foreign bodies. If a perforation is suspected, a water soluble contrast medium (e.g. Gastrografin) is normally used since this is absorbed from the tissues into which the medium might escape.

2. Oesophagoscopy. This can be done under either general or local anaesthesia depending on the preference of the patient and the endoscopist. It can also be done with the larger rigid metal oesophagoscope or the flexible fibre-optic instrument. The rigid oesophagoscope allows for better suction, removal of food debris and larger biopsy. The flexible instrument (Fig. 35.1) is less bulky to pass and probably gives better views of the intra-abdominal oesophagus and the junction with the stomach. In addition, it can be passed on in to the stomach and duodenum for examination of these areas if this is indicated.

3. Manometry. If a soft, fine bore catheter is passed into the oeso- phagus and connected to a pressure transducer, the pressure within the lumen of the oesophagus at different levels can be measured and a pressure trace produced on paper. There is a normal 'pressure profile' for the oesophagus which demonstrates the presence and position of the upper and lower sphincters and which records the contraction and relaxation in these sphincters and in the remainder of the oesophagus as the peristaltic wave passes down in response to swallowing. Certain abnormalities in this pressure profile have been recognised in different disease states and these characteristic abnormalities are sometimes diagnostic in difficult cases when radiology and oesophagoscopy are negative.

HIATUS HERNIA

A hiatus hernia is a hernia of the stomach through the oesophageal open- ing (hiatus) in the diaphragm. There are two main types of hiatus hernia: a) sliding (Fig. 32.2), b) rolling (or para-oesophageal Fig. 32.4). A combina- tion of the two can occur. Many people have a hiatus hernia and are either unaware of it or have few or no symptoms.

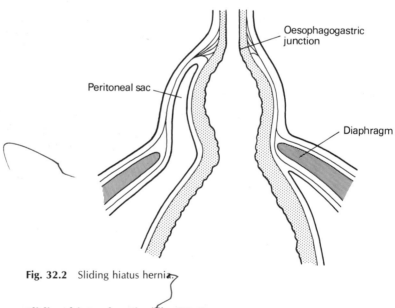

Oesophagogastric junction

Peritoneal sac

Diaphragm

Fig. 32.2   Sliding hiatus hernia

Sliding hiatus hernia (Fig. 32.2)

This is by far the commonest type comprising 85 per cent to 90 per cent of all hiatus herniae. The essential problem in sliding hiatus hernia is that the mechanism preventing reflux of gastric contents into the oesophagus breaks down (Fig. 32.3). Food can be regurgitated into the mouth and the oesophageal mucosa is bathed in acid secretions. The symptoms of sliding hiatus hernia result either from this gastro-oesophageal reflux, or from

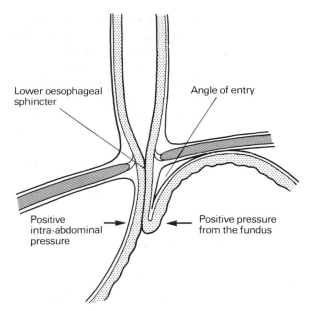

Fig. 32.3   Control of gastro-oesophageal reflux.

impaction of the hernia in the oesophageal hiatus. Inflammation of the oesophageal mucosa gives rise to the pain of heartburn or oesophageal spasm. Healing of the inflammation can result in scarring of the oesophagus which may eventually produce a stricture. Dysphagia may be due to either oesophageal spasm, stricture formation or impaction of the hernia.

Investigation

A barium swallow and meal will, in most cases, demonstrate the presence of the hernia and of any gastro-oesophageal reflux, although small hernias can be difficult to demonstrate. The location and severity of any associated stricture will also be shown.

Oesophagoscopy is necessary to determine the degree of inflammation of the oesophageal mucosa (oesophagitis) and to assess any stricture present.

Manometry can be helpful in patients with persistent symptoms and negative barium studies and oesophagoscopy.

Treatment

Many patients will require no treatment because they have few or no symptoms. If symptoms are present, medical treatment should normally be tried in the first place. Medical treatment consists of three basic components:
  1. Weight reduction
  2. Posture
  3. Drugs
Many patients will find that their symptoms are completely relieved sim-

ply by losing weight. This takes the pressure off the abdomen and allows the herniated stomach to fall back into place. Since the symptoms of reflux are frequently made worse by lying down or bending over, patients should be advised to avoid sleeping flat and stooping. The head of the bed should be raised on blocks or at least the patient should be supported with several pillows. Numerous drugs have been used to alleviate the symptoms of reflux and these fall into three broad categories: (a) antacids which neutralise the gastric acid, (b) drugs which form a bland neutral layer on top of the gastric contents so that when reflux occurs it is this bland, non-irritating fluid which is refluxed and (c) drugs which reduce the acid-secretion of the stomach. None of these drugs will do anything to relieve symptoms of regurgitation or impaction of the hernia, but they do help to relieve acid heartburn and may reduce the degree of oesophagitis. They do, of course, have to be continued indefinitely.

Other measures which are of value are to stop smoking, to avoid wearing tight garments, to eat smaller meals and to avoid eating and drinking before going to bed.

Surgery

Surgery is indicated in the following circumstances:

1. Patients in whom the above medical treatment has failed to relieve distressing symptoms.

2. Patients who either cannot or will not accept medical treatment indefinitely and who have significant symptoms.

3. Patients who have developed complications of hiatus hernia, e.g. stricture.

The hiatus can be approached either from below the diaphragm through an abdominal incision, or from above the diaphragm by thoracotomy. The advantages of the thoracic approach are better exposure of the region of the hiatus and, more importantly, it is possible by this approach to mobilise the oesophagus, to free it from its adhesions and thus to carry out a repair which is devoid of tension. As oesophagitis develops, the oesophagus usually becomes thicker and shorter and mobilisation, therefore, becomes increasingly important to obtain a tension-free repair. A number of operations have been described for the repair of hiatus hernia and all the successful ones have the aim of reducing the hernia, restoring the intra-abdominal segment of the oesophagus and the lower oesophageal sphincter to their normal positions below the diaphragm, and to recreate the angle of entry of the oesophagus into the stomach. When these have been achieved, the margins of the hiatus are narrowed down around the oesophagus.

Postoperative care

Following thoracotomy, the patient will have an intercostal drain which should be connected to an underwater seal drainage bottle and left unclamped on open drainage. This is usually removed after 24 to 48 hours. A nasogastric tube is usually unnecessary and the patient is allowed small amounts of fluid the day after operation, progressing over the next few days to free fluids, semi-solids and a normal diet. Chest physiotherapy is important to prevent respiratory infections and early mobilisation is encouraged. Pain should be relieved by analgesics initially by intra-muscular injections and later by oral administration. The patient is normally discharged from hospital between 10 and 14 days after operation.

Management of peptic stricture

Peptic stricture is a late complication of reflux oesophagitis. Persistent inflammation leads to the formation of scar tissue in the oesophageal mucosa and wall. The patient usually gives a history of hiatus hernia for several years with the onset of slowly progressive dysphagia. The condition has to be distinguished from carcinoma of the oesophagus and this is done on the basis of the clinical history, barium examination and oesophagoscopy. There are three ways of dealing with the problem:-

1. Repeated oesophagoscopy and dilatation. This is usually reserved for elderly and infirm patients who are not considered suitable for major surgery.

2. Repair of the hiatus hernia with one or two dilatations. This method of treatment is only suitable if the stricture is still relatively soft and easily dilated. In this situation, repairing the hernia and stopping the acid reflux can prevent the stricture progressing and one or two dilatations are sufficient to open up the way through.

3. Resection of the stricture and replacement of the removed oesophagus with a segment of colon. Alternatively, the whole oesophagus can be removed and the stomach brought up through the chest to the neck and anastomosed to the cervical oesophagus. Both these operations give good relief of dysphagia.

Rolling (para-oesophageal) hiatus hernia (Fig. 32.4)

Although this type of hiatus hernia occurs through the same opening in the diaphragm as the sliding variety, the symptoms and complications of the two conditions are completely different. The intra-abdominal segment of the oesophagus retains its proper position below the diaphragm and gastro-oesophageal reflux does not occur. The hernial sac is present in front of the oesophagus and through this the fundus of the stomach enters the chest. As the hernia enlarges, the greater curvature of the stomach also rolls up into the chest and may take with it the greater omentum and the transverse colon.

Symptoms

Because gastro-oesophageal reflux does not occur, the symptoms are not those of reflux oesophagitis. In fact, there may be few symptoms associated with this type of hernia though if they do occur they may consist of vague indigestion and discomfort in the epigastrium after meals. Patients may also complain of retrosternal or chest pain, and nausea and vomiting. The com-

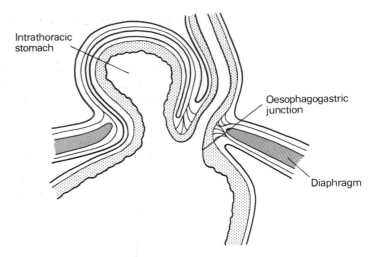

Fig. 32.4   Para-oesophageal (rolling) hiatus hernia.

plications of this type of hernia are serious and can be life threatening. Bleeding is common and may take the form either of chronic blood loss, leading to an iron deficiency anaemia, or haematemesis of sufficient severity to require blood transfusion. The contents of the hernia are liable to the same complications as, for instance, an inguinal hernia. The stomach may become twisted (volvulus) and this can lead to strangulation. Other abdominal viscera pulled up into the chest may become incarcerated and obstructed.

Treatment

There is no useful medical treatment for rolling hiatus hernia. Since gastro-oesophageal reflux does not occur, the medical measures advocated for sliding hiatus hernia are ineffective. Elderly or infirm patients with few symptoms are usually left alone without treatment. However, because of the risk of serious complications, the patient with a rolling type of hernia is normally recommended to have a surgical repair. The preparation of these patients for operation and their post-operative care is similar to that for a sliding hernia. The actual operative technique differs only a little.

ACHALASIA

The word achalasia means 'failure to relax' and the disease is so called because the main problem is a failure of the lower oesophageal sphincter to relax on swallowing. This normally relaxes to meet a peristaltic wave carrying a bolus of food down the oesophagus. In achalasia, the sphincter remains in tone so that when the bolus of food reaches it, it remains closed and forms a functional obstruction to the passage of food. The condition can occur at any age and its cause is not known for certain. Examination of the oesophagus shows degeneration of the nerve cells and plexuses in the wall of the oesophagus which coordinate the movements of the oesophagus. The muscular wall of the oesophagus usually becomes hypertrophied and thickened in an attempt to overcome the obstruction at the lower end, but the wall gradually becomes weaker and weaker and the oesophagus dilates until it is no more than an inert, thin-walled tube containing a great deal of fluid and food residue (Fig. 32.5).

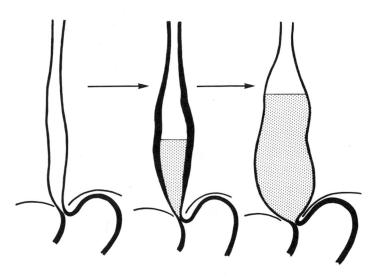

Fig. 32.5 Achalasia. Progression of changes in oesophagus.

Symptoms

The principal symptom is dysphagia which usually comes on slowly but the patient may complain of a sudden onset of symptoms after an emotional shock. The food tends to stick behind the lower sternum and the patient has trouble with both fluids and solids. The patient may experience retrosternal pain after eating caused by incoordinated spasms of the oesophagus. As the oesophagus dilates and fills with fluid and food, the patient may complain of regurgitation particularly on lying flat or bending over. Sometimes the oesophageal contents are aspirated into the trachea causing respiratory symptoms. Weight loss is common and may be severe.

Investigation

The X-ray appearances on barium examination are typical with a dilated oesophagus narrowing down to a taper point at its lower end. Even air has difficulty in passing into the stomach and the gastric bubble is frequently absent.

Oesophagoscopy is not usually necessary to establish the diagnosis, but is usually done to exclude other diseases such as carcinoma and to clean out the oesophagus before operation.

The muscular disorder in the oesophagus in achalasia can be clearly demonstrated by oesophageal manometry and this is a useful method of confirming the diagnosis.

Treatment

There are no drugs of value in the treatment of achalasia and patients are usually managed either by intra-luminal dilatation of the lower oesophageal sphincter, or by operation. Dilatation is frequently followed by recurrence of the achalasia and is accompanied by a certain risk of perforation. Surgery is, therefore, generally preferred.

Operation

Prior to operation, the patient should be kept on a liquid diet for 48 hours and the oesophagus emptied by a large bore nasogastric tube the night before and morning of surgery. Surgery is carried out through a left thoracotomy and the operation of choice is a Heller's myotomy. This consists of a vertical incision dividing the circular muscle at the lower end of the oesophagus rather like a Ramstedt's operation for pyloric stenosis (Fig. 32.6). The muscle is divided down to the mucosa which is allowed to pout through. The encircling fibres are thereby divided and the efficiency of the lower oesophageal sphincter is destroyed. This interference with the lower oesophageal sphincter will usually result in postoperative reflux of gastric secretions into the oesophagus unless an anti-reflux operation is carried out at the same time, and a repair of the hiatus hernia is usually combined with the Heller's myotomy.

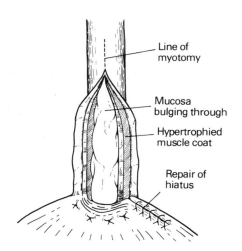

Line of
myotomy

Mucosa
bulging through

Hypertrophied
muscle coat

Repair of
hiatus

Fig. 32.6 Heller's myotomy for achalasia with repair of hiatus hernia.

Postoperative care

An intercostal tube will be in place and this should be connected to an underwater seal drainage bottle. The tube can usually be removed 24 to 48 hours after operation. Oral fluids can often be commenced the day after operation with progression to semi-solids and a solid diet over the following 5 to 7 days. Dysphagia is usually markedly improved but may never be quite normal again due to the generalised muscular incoordination and weakness of the remainder of the oesophagus.

CARCINOMA OF THE OESOPHAGUS

Carcinoma of the oesophagus is a condition more common in men than women, which presents more frequently in later life. Its cause is unknown. The incidence and sex distribution of the disease varies considerably in different parts of the world, and dietary factors have been implicated. Certain disorders, such as achalasia, the Plummer-Vinson syndrome and caustic burns of the oesophagus, are associated with a higher incidence of the disease.

Pathology

Most of the tumours are squamous cell carcinomas, but some of those arising near the oesophago-gastric junction are adeno-carcinomas. Tumours can occur in any part of the oesophagus but are most common in the lower third. Tumours spread by direct invasion of surrounding structures, to the lymph glands in the neck, the mediastinum and along the course of the left gastric artery to the coeliac axis. Widespread dissemination of the disease can occur through the blood stream, particularly to the liver.

Symptoms

A carcinoma is usually present in the oesophagus for some time before it produces symptoms and it is this early latent period which hinders successful treatment. The main symptom is dysphagia which is experienced at first with certain types of solid food, but is steadily progressive until the patient has difficulty even with liquids. The poor dietary intake is associated with weight loss and bleeding may also occur.

Investigation

A barium swallow will demonstrate the presence of an obstructive carcinoma. The lesion can then be visualised at oesophagoscopy and a biopsy taken. A liver scan is sometimes helpful in determining whether spread has occurred to the liver. Oesophageal manometry has no place in the diagnosis of malignant tumours of the oesophagus.

Surgery

Surgical resection offers the only real prospect for cure in the present state of treatment. In addition, removal of the tumour is often the best form of palliative treatment and the patients are able to eat and swallow their own saliva until they die. If the tumour is not removable or if widespread metastases are present and the patient is not expected to live for more than a few weeks, palliation is obtained by the insertion of an indwelling tube through the growth (Fig. 32.7).

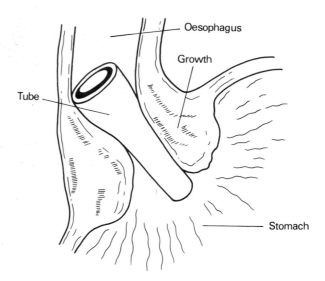

Fig. 32.7 Indwelling tube for inoperable carcinoma of the oesophago-gastric junction.

Preoperative preparation

Many patients with carcinoma of the oesophagus are in a poor nutritional state with disturbances of fluid and electrolyte balance. These should be corrected with a nourishing fluid diet, or, if necessary, with intravenous fluids. Anaemia, if present, should be corrected and vigorous chest physiotherapy commenced, since many patients have poor respiratory function and may even have developed areas of aspiration pneumonitis due to tipping over of fluid from the obstructed oesophagus into the bronchial tree.

Operation

The amount of oesophagus and stomach removed will depend on the location of the tumour. For tumours in the lower third of the oesophagus, the whole of the oesophagus below the tumour plus approximately 5 cm above the upper limit of the tumour together with the upper third of the stomach, the spleen and the associated lymph glands will be removed (Fig. 32.8). A similar amount of oesophagus, but less stomach is removed for tumours of the middle third. Almost the entire oesophagus is removed for tumours of the upper third of the oesophagus within the chest. Continuity is restored by anastomosing the cut end of the oesophagus to the remaining portion of the stomach which is brought up through the hiatus into the chest. For tumours of the upper third of the oesophagus, this anastomosis will usually be in the neck to the cervical oesophagus.

The incision used will vary with the preference of the surgeon. For

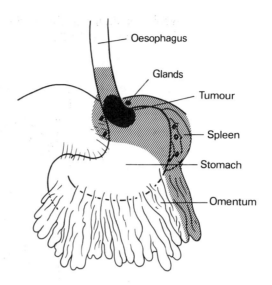

Fig. 32.8 Oesophagogastrectomy for carcinoma. Extent of resection.

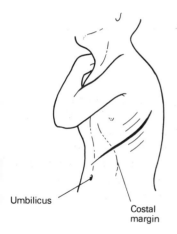

Fig. 32.9 Thoraco-abdominal incision for oesophagogastrectomy.

tumours at the lower end of the oesophagus, most surgeons will use a left thoraco-abdominal incision extending from the chest across the costal margin on to the left upper abdomen (Fig. 32.9). When the ribs are spread and the costal margin and diaphragm divided, an excellent exposure is obtained of the whole region. For tumours higher in the oesophagus, resection can be carried out through an extension of this incision on the left side together with a separate cervical incision if necessary. However many surgeons prefer the Ivor Lewis procedure in which an incision is first made in the abdomen to mobilise the stomach and when this has been closed the patient is turned on the left side and an incision is made in the right chest for resection of the tumour and construction of the anastomosis. Since the vagus nerves are necessarily divided during the resection, a drainage procedure is frequently carried out on the pylorus to prevent gastric stasis. A formal pyloroplasty may be done or a more simple pyloromyotomy with division of the encircling muscle layer.

Postoperative care

An intercostal drain will be present and this should be connected to an underwater seal drainage bottle. A nasogastric tube will be left in the stomach and this is aspirated at hourly intervals. The nasogastric tube should be treated with great care; it will have been carefully placed in position at operation and if it becomes dislodged will need to be passed again blindly with the risk of pushing it through the newly constructed anastomosis. The tube should therefore be securely taped to the patient's nose and great care exercised in handling it. The amount of aspirate usually diminishes over the first 3 to 4 days after which the tube can be removed. The incision is a painful one and regular analgesia is required postoperatively. Chest physiotherapy is of considerable importance, particularly since many of the patients are elderly and have poor respiratory function.

The patient is allowed nothing by mouth for several days after operation. The normal period is 4 days, after which the patient is allowed small amounts of clear fluid and if this is tolerated he will progress to free fluids, a sloppy diet and solid food over the next 5 or 6 days. During the period of nothing by mouth, fluid and electrolyte balance is maintained by an intravenous drip.

Sutures are removed after 10 days and the patient is usually able to return home 2 weeks after operation by which time he should be able to manage a reasonable diet. However, because of the reduction in the size of the stomach, many patients find that they cannot eat normal quantities of food and they should be encouraged instead to eat smaller amounts more frequently. The mechanisms which normally prevent reflux of gastric contents into the oesophagus have been removed at operation, and patients are likely, therefore, to complain of regurgitation or vomiting on lying flat. These symptoms can usually be controlled if the patient sleeps propped up on several pillows.

Results of surgery

Patients with adeno-carcinoma do less well than those with squamous cell carcinoma, and patients with squamous growths in the upper and mid-oesophagus do less well than patients with squamous growths at the lower end. In the majority of patients, surgery is purely palliative and allows them to eat and swallow their own saliva. Only 10 per cent to 15 per cent of patients live for 5 years or more after resection. These results are poor and are not likely to improve until either earlier diagnosis can be made, or alternative forms of treatment are discovered. Irradiation is sometimes combined with surgery but generally speaking irradiation is ineffective in the treatment of oesophageal carcinoma. However, tumours of the upper oesophagus, particularly the cervical oesophagus, do very poorly with surgery and many people consider that irradiation should be the first line of treatment for tumours situated in this region. Chemotherapy has little place at the moment in management of carcinoma of the oesophagus, but drugs and different combinations of drugs are being developed all the time and it is likely that improvements in this form of treatment will be made in the next few years.

Palliative intubation

Several different kinds of tubes have been manufactured for the palliative treatment of carcinoma of the oesophagus in patients considered unsuitable for resection. Some of these can be inserted from above through an oesophagoscope, but others require a laparotomy and opening of the stomach to pull the tube through and fix it in position.

The most commonly used tubes which are inserted through a laparotomy are the Mousseau-Barbin tube and the Celestin tube. The stomach is opened through a short incision and the tube is fed down from above by the anaesthetist and pulled through the growth by the surgeon, so that its upper wide mouth lies above the tumour. The lower end is cut short by the surgeon and fixed to the side wall of the stomach. The stomach is then closed and the wound repaired.

Patients are normally able to take fluids 48 hours after such a procedure and progress quite quickly to a sloppy type of diet. More solid food can be taken provided the patient chews it well and washes it down frequently with a fizzy drink. The tube can become blocked by food or by growth growing up and around the orifice. Displacement can also occur as well as ulceration of the lining of the oesophagus or stomach by the edge of the tube. Generally speaking, however, these type of tubes provide a reasonable palliation for the short length of time the patient survives.

FOREIGN BODIES

Foreign bodies can become lodged in the oesophagus at any age, but are more common in children and in elderly people with either no teeth or poorly fitting dentures. The object may lodge in the oesophagus, either because of its bulk or because of a pathological narrowing of the oesophagus itself. In the normal oesophagus there are three narrowed areas: at the cricopharyngeus, the arch of the aorta and the diaphragm. Pathological narrowing is usually due to a peptic stricture but may be due to a carcinoma.

The patient will often complain of pain in the chest and an inability to swallow either solids or fluid. Perforation of the oesophagus may occur with all the serious complications associated with this. Plain P.A. and lateral films should be done together with a gastrographin swallow to localise the foreign body and identify any leak from the oesophagus.

Management

If a foreign body has lodged in the region of the cricopharyngeus there may be associated respiratory obstruction. A child should be tipped head down and given a sharp blow between the shoulder blades. In the adult, a similar blow may dislodge the foreign body but failing this the patient should be grasped from behind with the arms encircling the lower chest and the hands gripped together in the epigastrium. A sudden bearhug in this situation is often effective in dislodging the foreign body. There is no urgency usually about removing foreign bodies further down the oesophagus and this is done at oesophagoscopy under general anaesthesia.

Perforation of the oesophagus by a foreign body is a serious complication. After removal of the foreign body, the patient is turned on the side and through a thoracotomy the hole in the oesophagus is repaired. Mediastinitis and infection of the pleural space develop very rapidly after perforation of the oesophagus and treatment is urgent. Without treatment, the patient invariably dies and if treatment is delayed recovery is, at the best, prolonged and complicated.

PERFORATION OF THE OESOPHAGUS

Aetiology

1. Instrumental. Perforation of the oesophagus is not uncommon after oesophagoscopy, particularly if this is done inexpertly or with undue force. A tear may occur in the cervical oesophagus in trying to pass the instrument through the cricopharyngeus muscle. Lower down the oesophagus, perforation is usually due to either inexpert dilatation of a stricture or carcinoma, or to an unduly generous biopsy.

2. Foreign body. A sharp foreign body can perforate the oesophagus at any level but is more likely to do so at the three narrowed regions of the oesophagus, as described under 'Foreign bodies'.

3. Spontaneous. Perforation of the oesophagus can occur spontaneously during violent vomiting, particularly after a heavy meal or excessive alcohol intake. A tear develops usually in the lower third of the oesophagus on the left hand side, but may occur in the mid oesophagus on the right side.

Consequences of perforation

(a) **Cervical perforation**. Air escapes into the tissues of the neck giving rise to surgical emphysema. If the condition is untreated, an abscess will subsequently develop in the neck.

(b) **Intra-thoracic perforation**. Air escapes into the mediastinum and pleural space. The air can track up the mediastinum into the neck and again produce surgical emphysema. Air in the pleural space results in a pneumothorax. The communication between the oesophagus and the mediastinum and pleural space allows infection to develop and mediastinitis and empyema ensue (Fig. 32.10). If the patient has vomited on a full stomach, part of the vomit will find its way into the pleural cavity and the

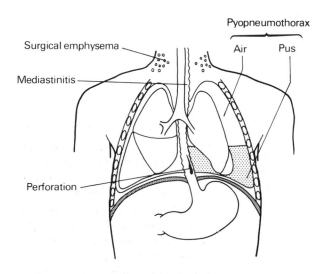

Fig. 32.10 Complications — perforated or ruptured oesophagus.

infection is particularly severe and rapidly developing. Untreated, the patient will die and the chances of the patient surviving are poor if the diagnosis is delayed for more than a few hours.

Management

(a) **Cervical perforation**. If recognised early, this type of perforation can usually be managed quite simply with antibiotics and nil by mouth for several days. Infection of the cervical spaces does not occur and the tear usually heals. If this condition is not recognised and an abscess develops, this will have to be drained.

(b) **Intra-thoracic perforation**. It is important that the condition is recognised quickly. Chest X-ray will show a pneumothorax and perhaps also a fluid level in the pleural cavity. A gastrografin swallow will demonstrate the site of the perforation.

An intercostal tube is inserted to relieve the pneumothorax and oesophagoscopy performed to carry out toilet of the oesophagus, to remove any foreign body and to verify the position of the perforation. Thoracotomy is performed immediately to drain the mediastinitis and empyema and to repair, if possible, the tear in the oesophagus. If surgery has been delayed by more than a few hours, the tissues of the oesophagus around the tear become very soft and will not hold sutures, in which case the best that can be done is to place a large drainage tube to the site of the perforation.

Postoperative recovery can be quick if surgery is carried out soon after the perforation, otherwise recovery is prolonged and it is several weeks before the perforation closes and the empyema settles down. Until the fistula is closed the patient is allowed nothing by mouth and is fed either intravenously or by gastrostomy or jejunostomy. If the perforation is associated with a stricture or tumour of the oesophagus, it is unlikely to close unless the obstruction is removed and this is usually done at the first operation if the patient's general condition permits.

OESOPHAGEAL ATRESIA

The oesophagus ends blindly in the upper chest. Usually the lower end communicates normally with the stomach and has a proximal fistula into the trachea (Fig. 32.11). The baby is often born to a mother who has had hydramnios. The child is unable to swallow normally, continually dribbles mucus from its mouth and may have cyanotic attacks. If atresia is suspected no feed should be given to prevent inhalation into the lungs. A soft radio-opaque catheter should be passed into the pharynx and if it will pass no further than 4 inches it is likely that the baby has an atresia. An X-ray, with the catheter in position, confirms the diagnosis. Until operation can be performed the baby should be nursed on its abdomen in the head-down position, but some believe that in order to prevent gastric juice entering the trachea the body should be propped up and the mucus extractor should be taken on the journey to the hospital. The nasopharynx is aspirated and no feed of any kind given. An intravenous infusion is set up and blood cross-

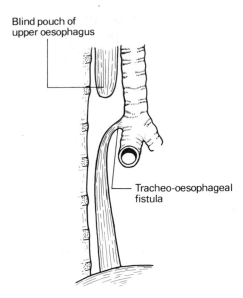

Blind pouch of
upper oesophagus

Tracheo-oesophageal
fistula

Fig. 32.11   Oesophageal atresia.

matched. At early operation, usually through a right thoracotomy, the fistula is closed. It may be possible to join the two ends of the oesophagus. If they are too far apart primary anastomosis may not be possible. The upper pouch is brought out into the neck to allow saliva to dribble away and the baby is nourished through a gastrostomy tube. Later, when the baby is stronger (perhaps several months old) an isolated length of colon with its blood supply intact is passed up through the anterior mediastinum and is anastomosed to the oesophageal pouch above and to the stomach below.

33

Pathophysiology of the gastrointestinal tract

The surgical anatomy of the gastrointestinal tract is outlined in Figure 33.1. The liver and biliary apparatus on the one hand and the pancreas on the other develop as diverticula of the gastrointestinal tract to which they remain connected by the common bile duct and the pancreatic duct. Their external (exocrine) secretions are discharged into the second part of the duodenum, usually through a common opening guarded by the muscular sphincter of Oddi into the biliary papilla.

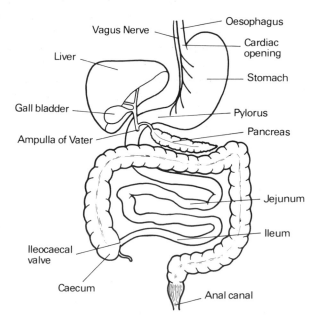

Fig. 33.1 Normal anatomy of the gastrointestinal tract.

The remainder of the gastrointestinal tract runs in continuity (apart from the appendix) from the cardiac sphincter of the stomach to the anal canal. The stomach with its thick muscular walls and deep mucous lining is in continuity with the oesophagus. The cardiac sphincter prevents the reflux into the oesophagus of acid and pepsin which are secreted in the cells of the fundus and body of the stomach. The pyloric antrum which is not acid-secreting leads to the pyloric canal which is guarded by the pyloric sphincter — the distal opening being the pylorus. The rich blood supply comes from the coeliac axis and the venous drainage is ultimately to the portal vein. The nerve supply is from the vagus nerves and the sympathetic plexus.

The small intestine consists of the C-shaped duodenum, the jejunum and lower small intestine known as the ileum, which is the narrowest portion of the bowel and enters the caecum through the ileo caecal valve. The total length of the small intestine is about 3·6 to 3·9 m (10 to 11 feet); the older estimates of 23 feet which were made on postmortem specimens are now thought to be erroneous. The jejunum accounts for about 60 per cent of the total length, the ileum about 40 per cent. The duodenum receives chyme, acid and pepsin from the stomach, bile and pancreatic juice through the biliary papilla. Digestion and absorption take place predominantly in the jejunum and the products absorbed ultimately enter the portal circulation.

The large intestine from the caecum to the rectum is about 121 cms (4·5 feet) in length, the rectum 11·25 cm (5 inches) and the anal canal 4·75 cm (1·5 inches).

The functioning of the gastrointestinal tract is under nervous and hormonal control. The complex churning movements of the stomach mix the food and prepare the mixture for the duodenal action of enzymes which are secreted in an alkaline medium which neutralises the acid chyme from the stomach. Peristalsis is the characteristic movement of the small intestine and reflex mass peristalsis once or twice daily into the large intestine.

The hormonal control of secretions is shown in Figure 33.2.

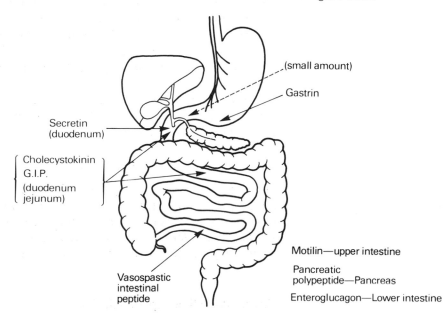

Fig. 33.2 Sites of origin of gastrointestinal hormones (G.I.P. now stands for glucose dependent insulin releasing peptide).

Acid pepsin

Acid pepsin secretion is stimulated by:

1. Vagal action. The cephalic phase of secretion in which the thought and taste of food initiate the stimulus.

2. Gastrin — a hormone secreted into the blood from the pyloric antrum which continues the second phase of the secretion of acid and enzymes; it is released by the presence of food in the stomach and intestine, some foods being more potent stimulants than others.

The stomach takes minutes to fill with food but hours (3 to 6) to empty. The trickle of chyme which occurs through the pylorus stimulates the release of hormones in the duodenum. As the pyloric sphincter relaxes a little bile enters the stomach and can be detected in gastric juice of all patients in which the pyloric canal is not obstructed.

The duodenal hormones

Those released are:

1. Secretin which stimulates the flow of pancreatic juice containing the powerful enzymes which digest protein, fat and carbohydrates. It also diminishes the secretion of gastric juice.

2. Cholecystokinin, which is secreted in response to the presence of fatty food in the duodenum. It relaxes the sphincter of Oddi and contracts the gall-bladder, which discharges its bile (concentrated 50 times) into the common bile duct and thence into the duodenum.

3. Enterogastrone, which diminishes gastric secretion and gastric emptying.

The small intestine secretes intestinal juice (succus entericus) but it is weak in enzymes and comparatively unimportant in digestion.

Digestion of food into aminoacids, glucose and fatty acid is virtually completed in the jejunum and absorption which begins in the duodenum is almost entirely completed in the jejunum. The ileal contents are almost entirely a fluid faecal residue but the terminal ileum is the area for the absorption of vitamin B_{12} and of bile salts.

The colon removes water and salts from the residue to produce semi-solid faeces but it should be noted that the majority of the body's water is *absorbed from the small intestine.*

Vasospastic intestinal peptide (V.I.P.)

This occurs in the nerve plexus of the small and large intestine. It is believed to control blood flow, secretion, and motility in the intestine. Oversecretion of the hormone may produce the clinical syndrome W.D.H.A. (Watery Diarrhorea, Hypokalaemia and Achlorhydria). Such excessive production may result from a tumour of the islet-cells of the pancreas.

Gastric inhibiting peptide (G.I.P.)

This is secreted in the mucosa of the small intestine and was originally thought to inhibit gastric acid secretion. Subsequent work has shown that its physiological action is to stimulate the release of insulin when glucose is taken by mouth. However it retains the initials G.I.P. which now stand for glucose-dependent insulin releasing peptide.

Three other peptides have been identified in the gastro intestinal tract, pancreatic polypeptide, motilin secreted in the upper small intestine and enteroglucogon secreted in the lower intestine. The action of these hormones is undecided.

PATHOPHYSIOLOGICAL CHANGES

Normal function is altered by the effects of disease or surgical intervention.

DISEASE

Mucosal damage

Lesions which result in extensive involvement of the mucous membrane result in loss of function. A carcinoma of the stomach destroys its power to secrete acid and enzymes while gastroenteritis not only prevents digestion and absorption but results in dehydration and loss of electrolytes. Extensive proctocolitis causes haemorrhage from ulceration, absorption of toxins occurs in the large areas of denuded mucosa and fluid loss may be considerable.

Perforation

This results in leakage of the contents. Outside the confines of the gastrointestinal tract all the contents are irritant and if not highly infected soon become so. The possible results are:

(a) **General peritoneal contamination** resulting in general peritonitis (Fig. 33.3). This is the usual result in peptic ulcer perforation and unless 'sealing' (described below) comes into play the same result is inevitable from perforation of the lower reaches of the gastrointestinal tract. Widespread paralysis of the bowel results and bacterial infection causes death if the condition is unrelieved.

(b) **Sealing by omentum or adjacent bowel** may occur. This gives rise to an abscess which localises the disease and may result in resolution, or it may require drainage.

(c) **Fistula formation**. A gastric ulcer may perforate into the transverse colon giving rise to a gastro-colic fistula (Fig. 33.4B). Food passes undigested into the colon but more important is that colonic contents pass into the stomach and then circulate in the duodenum and small intestine causing severe infection which is life threatening. Another very dangerous fistula is where the diseased colon forms a fistula with the bladder (Fig. 33.4C). Infected flatus causes a urinary infection and the symptom of pneumaturia (gas in the urine). The other fistula which may develop is one between the fundus of the gall bladder and the duodenum (Fig. 33.4A). This causes no trouble in itself since bile is still delivered where it is

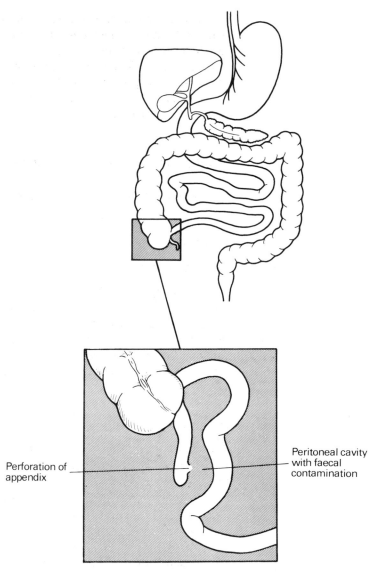

Fig. 33.3 Perforation of the appendix causes faecal peritonitis.

required, namely into the duodenum and a gallstone, if present, is passed into the gut—but if one is large then it lodges the lumen of the terminal ileum (the narrowest portion of the bowel). An acute intestinal obstruction results.

Obstruction

Figure 33.5 illustrates the effects of obstruction. Common to all obstructive lesions are:

    (a) dilatation of the segment above, accumulation of secretions, reverse flow and stagnation with resultant infection.

    (b) collapse and loss of function beyond the site of obstruction.

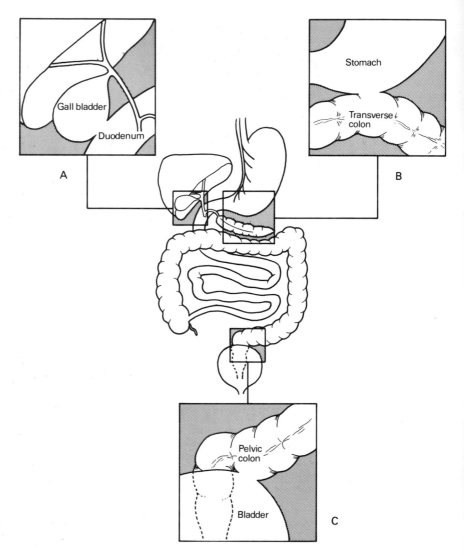

Fig. 33.4 Fistulas involving the gastrointestinal tract: A. Gall bladder to duodenum. B. Stomach to colon. C. Colon to the bladder.

The common sites of obstructions are:

(a) The pyloric end of the stomach. The stomach is dilated, filled with fluid and food (consumed perhaps days before). Bile is absent in the secretion. The patient is unable to eat, vomits copiously and, therefore, loses weight, becomes dehydrated and goes into electrolyte imbalance. Since no chyme passes to the duodenum there is weight loss from lack of nutrition.

(b) The small intestine. The great volume of material in the jejunum — chyme from the stomach, bile, pancreatic and intestinal juices well up. The bowel dilates, the contents regurgitate into the stomach and are vomited. It is important to note that because the contents are vomited abdominal distension is *minimal*. Gross dehydration and electrolyte imbalance result.

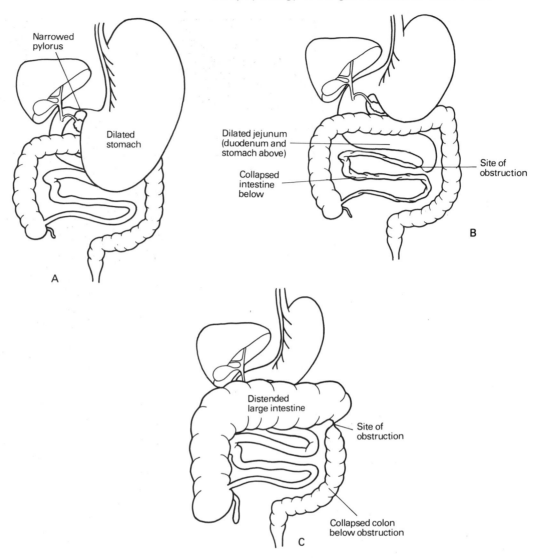

Fig. 33.5 Obstruction in the gastrointestinal tract: A. Pyloric stenosis. B. Small bowel obstruction. C. Large bowel obstruction.

(c) **The large intestine**. The large intestine contains much less fluid than the small intestine, but a large quantity of gas which, denied exit, causes enormous abdominal distension. The dominant symptom is the inability to pass this flatus as well as faeces. Regurgitation of the large bowel contents into the ileum occurs only minimally and at a very late stage. Therefore, vomiting, so marked in small bowel obstruction, is rare in obstruction of the large intestine.

(d) **The biliary tract**. Figures 36.4 and 36.5 show the sites of obstruction.

(i) *The cystic duct*. A stone impacted in the cystic duct prevents the gall bladder emptying into or filling from the common bile duct. The gall bladder, as in all obstructions, distends and the retained contents become infected. Jaundice does not develop because bile from the liver along the common bile duct can still flow into the duodenum and digestion is unaffected.

(ii) *The common bile duct* may be blocked by a stone or neoplasm. The whole duct system into the liver is dilated. Jaundice develops and if unrelieved deepens each day. Because bile is absent from the intestine the faeces are pale. Bile pigments are excreted in the urine. Retained bile salts cause pruritus of the skin. Infection (cholangitis) is heralded by the onset of rigors. Unrelieved the bile secretion by the liver ceases but mucus secretion continues (white bile).

(e) Pancreatic obstruction alone will cause steatorrhea.

SURGICAL INTERVENTION

All surgical intervention in the gastrointestinal tract, with the exception of appendicectomy, may cause physiological changes. Some are relatively mild and well within the powers of the body to compensate, others are more profound. The principal operations are:

Vagotomy

Total or truncal vagotomy diminishes:

(a) Gastric secretion — the beneficial effect.

(b) The motility of the stomach so that it distends and cannot empty adequately. A pyloroplasty or gastrojejunostomy is necessary to ensure it drains.

The effect on the intestine is variable. A significant portion of patients has more frequent bowel action but a small number suffer from attacks of uncontrollable diarrhoea.

The purpose of the more selective vagotomies (Ch. 35 and Fig. 35.4) is to cause the inhibition of gastric secretion without the undesirable side effects.

Gastrectomy

The various forms of gastrectomy are shown in Figure 35.5. The most physiological is a Billroth I in which the stomach is rejoined to the duodenum. Even in this case more rapid emptying of the stomach may occur in the absence of a pyloric sphincter.

The effects of a Polya gastrectomy are:

(a) The absence of a reservoir — 'dumping into the jejunum' en mass.

(b) Food may empty into the efferent loop before bile or pancreatic juice mix with it with the result that digestion is inadequate.

(c) Bile may rush into the stomach instead of into the efferent loop, the stomach is irritated and bile may be vomited separately from food.

(d) The efferent loop may be obstructed.

(e) Rapid passage may prevent absorption of vitamin B_{12} with resulting macrocytic anaemia. Poor absorption of iron may cause microcytic anaemia.

The results will be undernourishment, loss of weight, vitamin deficiency, and the danger of reactivation of a healed tuberculous lesion in the lung.

Enterectomy

Resection of moderate lengths of the small intestine produce very little physiological changes but loss in excess of 75 per cent may cause rapid transit, diarrhoea and malabsorption. Extensive resection of the ileum may result in megaloblastic anaemia from failure to absorb vitamin B_{12}. Bile salts are absorbed in the terminal ileum and if not absorbed may irritate the colon with resultant diarrhoea.

Colonic resection

Total colectomy results in a semi fluid continuous motion through an ileostomy but digestion and absorption are unaffected. Right hemicolectomy (Fig. 39.5) may cause more frequent bowel action partly because the faeces are less solid and partly from the reduced ability to reabsorb bile salts as the terminal ileum is resected as part of the operation.

Cholecystectomy

This causes no significant changes—bile still flows into the duodenum.

Pancreatectomy

Total pancreatectomy produces diabetes and insulin replacement is required. The absence of pancreatic secretion causes steatorrhoea as well as diminished digestion and absorption.

Shortcircuiting (by-pass) procedures

Most by-pass operations produce significant changes. A gastrojejunostomy may occasionally give rise to syndromes similar to those which occur following gastrectomy. If the upper jejunum is by-passed malabsorption may develop and by-passing the terminal ileum may cause vitamin B_{12} deficiency. One risk of all by-pass procedures is that a 'blind' loop may be left in which stasis occurs. Infection of the contents occurs, fouls the intestine and gives rise to malabsorption. Surgical correction is necessary.

34

The acute abdomen

Nowhere is surgical progress more obvious than in the management of the acute abdomen. Before the turn of the century surgical intervention was rare (although Lawson Tait performed the first successful appendicectomy in 1880). For the first half of this century it was well recognised that the progress of the primary condition had to be halted without delay before the secondary manifestations of shock, dehydration and toxaemia overwhelmed the patient and spontaneous recovery was unlikely. Operation was undertaken with the least possible delay, anaesthesia by modern standards was poor and antibacterial substances were unknown. Dehydration and electrolyte imbalance was not corrected and the value of nasogastric suction was not recognised.

The progress of the primary condition has still to be halted by operation without unnecessary delay but it is now recognised that the dangerous secondary manifestations can be largely avoided by preoperative corrective treatment. If they are, the chances of a successful outcome are greatly increased. Because of the fear that operation may be delayed even a few hours all analgesics were forbidden until the operating surgeon saw the patient. Nowadays an analgesic, the dosage of which is measured against the severity of the patient's pain, is given by the first doctor to see the patient. It enables the patient to give a coherent history, local tenderness may be even easier to detect and a mass, if present, is more easily palpable than in an abdomen with extreme rigidity.

All acute abdominal catastrophes can be resolved into three groups:

1. Peritonitis.
2. Intestinal obstruction.
3. Intra-abdominal haemorrhage. (This forms a very small group of which the symptoms and signs are those of peritonitis in addition to those of internal haemorrhage.)

These conditions almost invariably require emergency operation for their relief. The problem, however, is not as simple as that because many other conditions cause acute abdominal pain. The differentiation of those which require operation from those which do not is of vital importance.

The most important of these lesions which do not require operation are:

1. The colics

(a) Intestinal — gastroenteritis.
(b) Ureteric (p. 442)
(c) Biliary (p. 380).

} Rarely require urgent operation.

2. Extra-abdominal causes of abdominal pain

(a) Pleurisy and pneumonia
(b) Coronary thrombosis
(c) Spinal lesions
(d) Uraemia
(e) Certain blood diseases
(f) Arteriosclerosis
(g) Diabetic hyperglycaemia
(h) Herpes zoster
(i) Porphyria

} Operation harmful and unnecessary.

ACUTE PERITONITIS

The peritoneum is a continuous, thin, shiny, avascular membrane which lines the abdominal cavity. The portion behind the muscles of the anterior abdominal wall and in front of those on the posterior abdominal wall is known as the parietal peritoneum and is richly endowed with nerve endings. Irritation of this portion of the peritoneum gives rise to pain at the site at which it is stimulated.

The visceral peritoneum is the portion which is reflected to envelop most of the abdominal organs. It forms the outer or serous coat of organs like the stomach and the intestines. It has few nerve endings and is almost insensitive.

The peritoneal cavity (Fig. 34.1) which is the space between the parietal and visceral layers contains a fine film of sterile fluid. Infection of this cavity is known as peritonitis. The causes are:
1. Blood-borne (rare).
2. Penetrating wounds.
3. The escape of gastrointestinal contents.

The last is much the most frequent cause. If the gastrointestinal tract is healthy its irritant and infected contents make no contact with the peritoneal cavity, from which they are protected by the mucous, muscular and serous coats of the stomach or intestine. If a portion of these organs becomes diseased and their walls infected this infection may spread to the serous covering coat which becomes inflamed (Fig. 34.2B). The serous covering coat is part of the visceral peritoneum. If this is inflamed it irritates the adjoining parietal peritoneum and pain is felt at the spot where this is inflamed. This is known as a local peritonitis.

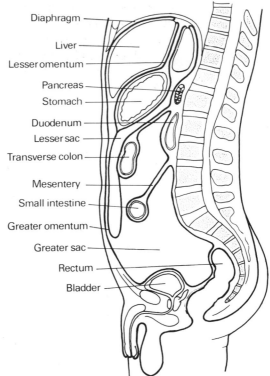

Fig. 34.1 The peritoneal cavity.

Diaphragm
Liver
Lesser omentum
Pancreas
Stomach
Duodenum
Lesser sac
Transverse colon
Mesentery
Small intestine
Greater omentum
Greater sac
Rectum
Bladder

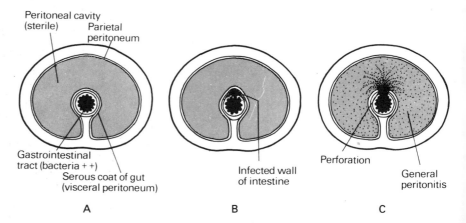

Peritoneal cavity (sterile)
Parietal peritoneum
Gastrointestinal tract (bacteria + +)
Serous coat of gut (visceral peritoneum)
Infected wall of intestine
Perforation
General peritonitis

A   B   C

Fig. 34.2 The mechanism of peritonitis.
(A) Healthy peritoneal cavity.
(B) Infected wall of bowel, bacteria spreading in the wall.
(C) Perforation of gastrointestinal contents into peritoneal cavity.

If the disease progresses and the organ ruptures the infected contents leak into the peritoneal cavity and a general peritonities has developed (Fig. 34.2C). The peritoneum responds in the ordinary way to inflammation, including an enormous outpouring of fluid. The infection can be overcome provided the supply of toxic material from the gastrointestinal tract is sealed off.

If it is not, the result is:

1. Widespread absorption of toxins.

2. Paralysis of the intestines. Nature tries to limit the out-pouring of septic contents by rest.

Treatment

The principals of treatment are:

1. To treat shock. The fluid loss is mainly plasma, water and electrolytes.

2. To rest the gastrointestinal tract—food and purgatives are forbidden and aspiration of the stomach contents is undertaken.

3. To counteract infection. All patients apart from those with recently perforated peptic ulcer are candidates for bacteraemia. Treatment with gentamicin and intravenous metronidazole should be commenced before operation.

4. To cut off the source of irritant or infection e.g. suture of a perforation or removal of a perforated appendix.

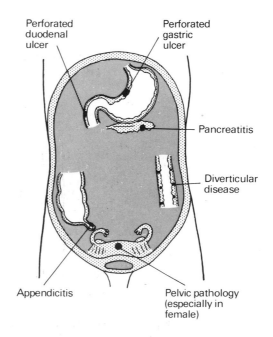

Fig. 34.3 Common sites of origin of peritonitis.

5. To cleanse or drain the peritoneum of septic contents and pus. This involves not only sucking out pus at operation but also intraperitoneal lavage with saline so that all pus, faecal material and fibrin are removed. A long vertical insision is necessary to do this.

Lesions which threaten to cause peritonitis should be terminated before peritonitis is established. The commonest causes (Fig. 34.3) of general peritonitis are:

1. Perforated acute appendicitis.
2. Perforated gastric or duodenal ulcer.
3. Perforated diverticulitis.
4. Rupture of the intestine, the rectum, or the bladder.
5. Ruptured ovarian cyst. Rupture of the uterus or Fallopian tubes.
6. Abdominal wounds penetrating the peritoneal cavity.
7. Haematogenous (blood-borne) infection.

Investigation

The nature and extent of investigation will vary with the condition of the patient, whether the underlying cause of the condition can be readily diagnosied clinically and whether they will add any information which will assist in management of the patient. Investigations considered necessary are ordered in the admission room, specimens are taken and if the patient is to be X-rayed this is done before admission to a ward bed so that unnecessary movement is avoided. Routine examination of the urine is mandatory. Other investigations which may be ordered are:

1. Radiography of the chest and abdomen. Abdominal X-rays will be inspected particularly for the presence of urinary calculi, gall stones and dilated loops of bowel and gas in the peritoneal cavity.
2. Laboratory examination of the urine for the presence of red blood cells and pus which may be positive in the presence of ureteric stones or in a urinary infection.
3. Serum amylase which is raised in acute pancreatitis.
4. Serum electrolytes which are particularly liable to be disturbed in vomiting.
5. Electrocardiograph and an estimation of the serum transaminase to exclude coronary infarction as a cause of abdominal pain.
6. A white blood cell count.
7. Blood for haemoglobin and for grouping and cross matching.
8. Peritoneal aspiration may reveal the presence of bile, pus or blood.

Clinical features of peritonitis

In the pages which follow the clinical features and management of peritonitis are discussed. Acute appendicitis is taken as an example not only because it is fairly common but the course it may follow illustrates:

1. The importance of removing a potential cause of peritonitis.
2. The nature in which the disease may be localised.
3. That diffuse peritonitis results if it perforates and contaminates the peritoneal cavity. The faecal peritonitis which results is identical to that caused by any lesion in which the bowel perforates and the basic management, complications and high mortality are the same.

ACUTE APPENDICITIS

The cause

The cause is unknown. Infection commences in the appendix, and in the more severe forms a faecolith may block the lumen of the organ, preventing the drainage of mucus and pus into the caecum. Purgatives increase peristalsis in the organ and cause perforation, i.e., bursting, with leakage of faecal material into the peritoneal cavity. In a smaller percentage of older patients the obstruction may be due to a carcinoma of the caecum. Rarer causes are a carcinoid tumour or matted worms.

The course of the disease

Without treatment the disease may take several courses:
1. Resolution may occur.
2. A localised mass or abscess may form.
3. General peritonitis may develop.

If the attack subsides, recurrence is likely. Early in the attack no one can forecast with certainty how it will progress and, for this reason, the wisest course is to remove the appendix before peritonitis has had time to develop.

Early symptoms and signs of acute appendicitis

Sudden colicky pain around the umbilicus is the first symptom (Fig. 34.4). The patient is frequently awakened with pain which comes on in attacks lasting a minute or two. It increases in severity, then passes off completely, only to recur. Vomiting may occur with considerable relief, but as the hours pass by the attacks of pain become more frequent and more severe. Later, the pain settles in the right iliac fossa, where it is no longer intermittent but constant in type. The temperature may be normal or slightly raised (37·2°C; 99°F), and the pulse rate shows a slight increase. The tongue is usually furred but moist, and no flatus is passed per rectum from the commencement of the attack.

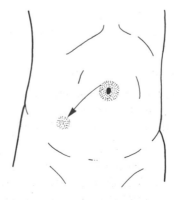

Fig. 34.4 The pain of acute appendicitis is first felt around the umbilicus and later settles over the appendix.

Should the appendix be pelvic in position, diarrhoea may be present, and if it is attached to the bladder frequency of micturition may occur.

On examination the abdomen is tender, with muscle guarding in the right iliac fossa, but elsewhere it is soft and painless. Digital examination of the rectum may reveal tenderness on the right side of the pelvis.

The clinical features of appendicitis with established peritonitis

The symptoms become more severe and the general condition of the patient deteriorates. The pain is constant and severe, but it may ease suddenly when the appendix perforates, only to return over the whole abdomen. Rigidity and tenderness are widespread, and vomiting is frequent and profuse.

As the patient becomes weaker from lack of sleep, toxaemia and fluid and electrolyte disturbances, the pain and rigidity give way to painless distension of the abdomen, and diarrhoea may be profuse.

The general appearance so typical of late peritonitis sets in. The face is shrivelled and flushed, but the eyes are glistening and bright. The mind is usually clear, but at this stage the patient is frequently too weak to give a coherent account of his illness. The result is that it may be impossible to decide with certainty the cause of his peritonitis. The temperature is always raised (38° to 39°C; 100° to 102°F) and the pulse is rapid, irregular, and of poor volume.

Appendix mass

An attack of appendicitis may terminate in the formation of a localised mass, which may form a true abscess. The surrounding coils of small intestine and omentum are bound together: they are also bound to the caecum and appendix by a fibrinous exudate. Instead of contaminating the whole of the peritoneal cavity after perforation of the organ, the infection has been limited to the area around the appendix by the great omentum. In this case, and in cases of over 48 hours' duration which appear to be subsiding, it is sometimes decided to observe their course and to operate at once should their condition deteriorate. This method of observation is known as the Ochsner-Sherren regime.

The Ochsner-Sherren regime

This method should be carried out only in the hospital, so that operation can be undertaken at once if it is considered necessary. It is a technique of observation of an acute attack and not a radical cure. The appendix will usually be removed after the attack has subsided:

1. Sedatives or analgesics are usually unnecessary at rest. The size of the swelling in the right iliac fossa should be observed and its limits marked on the skin of the abdominal wall so that increase or diminution in size can be detected.

2. The patient is nursed in whatever position he is most comfortable.

3. Vomiting or pain is reported at once.

4. Only sips of water are allowed by mouth for 48 hours. Fluid and electrolyte balance is maintained by the parenteral route.

5. The mouth is rinsed out frequently and the teeth kept clean.

6. A fluid balance chart is kept.

7. The pulse is charted hourly and the temperature two hourly for the first 12 hours. After this time a four-hourly pulse reading is substituted, so as to diminish the disturbance which hourly readings would cause to the patient.

8. The flatus tube is passed every 4 hours and left in position for at least ten minutes. No aperients are administered.

Nursing procedure for passing a flatus tube. Before this procedure, the patient is offered facilities to pass urine. A tray is prepared containing:

A small, deep bowl (or jug) of water
Kleenex wipes
Lubricant
Inco-pad
Disposable glove
Flatus tube
Paper bag (disposable)

The patient is advised of what is to happen and prepared as for rectal examination.

The Inco-pad is placed beneath the buttocks. The nurse puts on disposable gloves. The flatus tube is lubricated *around* the tip. The other end is placed in and kept below the water level in the bowl. The patient is instructed to take a breath while the nurse gently inserts the tube 2½ inches (approx.) into the rectum. She waits a few moments for air to be displaced from the tube. She then advances it, and then withdraws it slightly. The patient is asked to cough gently. This, and/or extension and flexion of the patient's legs may help to achieve the passage of flatus, seen as the escape of bubbles through the water. These manoeuvres may be repeated once or twice, but after 7 to 10 minutes, the flatus tube is removed and the anal region gently wiped clean. The patient is repositioned, and made comfortable. The used tube, gloves and tissues are discarded and the tray is cleaned. The nurse washes and dries her hands. A report is made of the result of the procedure.

Treatment

The most satisfactory case to treat is one in which the appendix is removed early in the attack. The convalescence is almost invariably smooth, and restoration of the patient to health is rapid.

If general peritonitis is present, however, removal of the appendix and drainage of the peritoneal cavity, is performed. If a large abscess is present drainage only may be undertaken and the appendix is not removed at the time. The patient is instructed to return for appendicectomy 6 months later.

Preparation of the patient with an acute abdomen for operation

This is similar to the preparation of a patient for any abdominal operation but as the time is limited the approach must be orderly so that nothing essential is omitted. Many of these patients are admitted in the small hours of the morning when the ward is relatively under-staffed.

When the patient is in bed and a final decision to operate has been made, the nature of his condition is explained and consent obtained and, if he desires it, a Minister of religion summoned. A patient may ask what will happen if he refuses operation and while this is something the medical staff must answer the nurse should bear in mind that in some conditions such as peptic perforation death is almost certain. In others, such as appendicitis which has not yet caused peritonitis, the mortality is 20 per cent if untreated so it is untruthful and foolish to say to the patient that unless he has an operation death is inevitable. The truthful answer is that at that stage no-one knows whether he is in the unfortunate 20 per cent or the 80 per cent who will recover.

An intravenous line is usually instituted and electrolyte imbalance if present is corrected. Further serum electrolyte estimations may be required.

A nasogastric tube is passed and aspirated as often as ordered. In acute intestinal obstruction the stomach may be refilled with aspirate every few minutes. The nature and quantity is recorded.

The skin preparation. The supra pubic area and the abdominal wall is shaved, washed with 2 per cent hexachlorophane soap and water and dried. The whole area from the nipples to the knees is prepared. Sometimes a second abdominal incision may be necessary. On the other hand a very ill patient in severe pain is kept still and all skin preparation, including shaving, is undesirable until he has been anaesthetised.

Premedication is given as ordered. In many cases the anaesthetist prefers to give it in the theatre.

The bladder is emptied and a further check is made that the urine has been examined and the results recorded.

Immediate preoperative ward preparation includes covering the patient's head with a disposable paper theatre cap and wrapping him in a theatre gown. The patient's identification label is written out and attached to the wrist. Dentures are removed and kept in a place of safety.

On the journey to the theatre. The patient is lifted onto a trolley protected by warm blankets. On arrival at the theatre the ward blankets are changed for theatre blankets. A small bowl and the patient's case notes and radiographs are taken to the theatre.

After the operation the ward nurse returns to the theatre and accompanies the patient back to bed, keeping a careful watch for any change in colour and his breathing. She must see that the nature of the operation and any special instructions of the surgeon or anaesthetist are recorded and understood before she leaves.

The physiology of opening the abdomen (laparotomy)

Before describing the postoperative management of the acute abdomen it should be noted that abdominal section undertaken for any condition produces certain disturbances on —

1. The gastrointestinal tract. The mobility of the stomach is diminished for 24–36 hours while that of the small intestine is relatively unimpaired. Colonic movement is more sluggish, and gas and liquid from an active small intestine pour into it and accumulate.

2. *Disordered respiratory function*. Hypoxaemia is almost uniform after upper abdominal incision. Uneven distribution of ventilation is exaggerated by a rise in the diaphragm, so producing a period at every breath in which some alveoli are closed but perfusion (i.e. blood flowing through the lungs) continues. Venous blood is inadequately oxygenated with a resultant lower pO_2. This, however, is serious only if other problems are present.

Postoperative care

If the patient is suffering from established peritonitis intravenous fluid replacement is continued and oral feeding commenced as soon as the bowel sounds recover. As soon as he recovers from the anaesthetic he should be allowed to assume whatever position he finds most comfortable. As soon as possible, and usually by the following day, he is mobilised.

The patient with faecal peritonitis has to be taken more slowly. Antibiotics and intravenous nutrition are continued. If a jejunostomy has been performed the tube is removed when ordered by the surgeon, suction is applied to the fistula and oral feeding is not commenced until the fistula has closed.

Pain. Postoperative analgesics, usually morphia (10 mg) or pethidine (50 mg), are given as soon as the patient complains of pain.

The bowel. The passage of a flatus tube twice daily prevents the usual 'distensive' pain of which many of these patients complain. About the third day a suppository is administered if the patient has not had a bowel action.

The drainage tubes are removed when ordered by the surgeon but all should be rotated and shortened a little each day to prevent one becoming adherent to a loop of intestine. Shortening is performed by withdrawing the tube slightly, cutting its external stitch and transfixing the remainder with a sterile safety pin. Removal should be recorded.

Records
1. An hourly pulse for 12 hours.
2. A four-hourly temperature reading.
3. Blood-pressure chart.
4. A fluid balance chart.

Complications

In most patients complications are few. Retention of urine (Ch. 43) or chest infection is treated as necessary. The patient with established peritonitis is more likely to develop complications.

Paralytic ileus. This is an important and not infrequent complication due to temporary loss of motor tone in the smooth muscle of the gut which is a normal response to surgery. The intestines are paralysed and dilated. Their contents regurgitate into the stomach, which may also be dilated, so that vomiting does not occur, until the stomach is overdistended with fluid.

No flatus is passed per rectum. Factors responsible for persistent ileus are:

1. Excessive handling of gut.
2. Unrelieved intestinal distension.
3. Attempts to stimulate intestinal activity by means of drugs when paralysis is still present.
4. Overdosage of drugs producing hypotension.
5. Infection (intraperitoneal).

Paralytic ileus is in large measure preventable. In cases where it is anticipated that it may develop, treatment is commenced from the end of the operation until the bowel has recovered.

Symptoms and signs. The abdomen is distended, but usually there is no pain. The distended abdomen makes breathing difficult and embarrasses the action of the heart. The pulse rate is always rapid, and in severe cases the patient is very toxic in appearance.

Treatment. Given time and rest the intestines will recover their tone. A flatus tube is passed per rectum four-hourly or, better, left in the rectum continuously. The stomach contents are aspirated continuously or every half-hour through a nasogastric tube and the volume recorded. Some surgeons use instead a Miller-Abbott tube, which is similar to a nasogastric tube and has an inflatable balloon to facilitate its passage into the intestine for a considerable distance. Some cases of paralytic ileus are due to loss of potassium. The serum electrolytes are estimated and any electrolyte deficit corrected.

Morphia (15 mg) is injected intramuscularly every 8 hours and intravenous infusions commenced so that the fluid balance is maintained.

The sign of recovery. The return of the bowel sounds and the passage of flatus per rectum, normally or by a flatus tube, are the signs that the bowel has recovered its tone. The function of the flatus tube is to overcome the resistance of the anal sphincter.

Residual abscesses. (Fig. 34.5). The commonest site for a residual abscess is in the wound and the patient improves immediately if it is drained adequately. The next most likely site is the pelvis. The onset of a pelvic abscess is heralded by pyrexia and the passage of mucus per rectum. Again drainage, which is performed through the anterior rectal wall in the male or the posterior vaginal wall in the female, leads to immediate improvement.

A subphrenic abscess is more difficult to diagnose. There may be difficulty in breathing, high temperature — evidence of general toxicity. The abscess is drained by a small incision below the subcostal margin if placed anteriorly but one sited posteriorly may require a rib resection and the post operative care is that of a pyothorax (Ch. 30).

Faecal fistula. A gangrenous appendix frequently involves a portion of the caecal wall in the inflammatory process. After operation a small portion of the wall may slough, and faecal contents contaminate the wound and excoriate the skin. The vast majority heal spontaneously in 2 or 3 weeks, but the skin must be protected from the discharge by stomadhesive or similar preparation (Ch. 38). The persistence of the fistula with 'sulphur granules' in the effluent suggests that actinomycosis may have been the underlying cause.

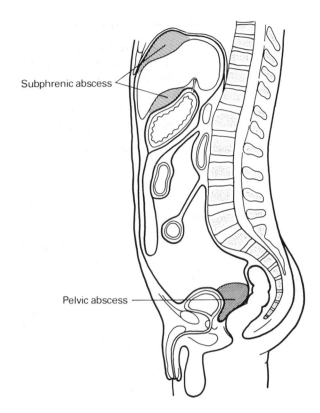

Fig. 34.5 Site of residual abscess.

Burst abdomen. This is an occasional complication of any abdominal operation. It is very rare following a gridiron incision but much commoner with longitudinal incisions. There is a sero-sanguinous discharge from the wound which separates and the intestines prolapse on to the abdominal wall. It is predisposed to by:

(a) Severe coughing.
(b) Infection of the wound.
(c) Deficiency of vitamin C, resulting in failure of the wound to heal.
(d) Removal of stitches before the wound has healed.
(e) Anaemia and malnutrition.
(f) Cortisone therapy preoperatively.

Treatment. The prolapsed intestines are wrapped in a sterile towel which has been soaked in warm saline, and the surgeon is informed at once. The patient is taken to the theatre, anaesthetised, and the wound is resutured. It is remarkable that the condition usually causes little or no circulatory failure, and the patient has an uneventful convalescence.

If a wound has not actually burst but there is a danger of this happening, a corset dressing is advisable.

Remote complications

Intestinal obstruction. This complication is more likely to occur as a result of adhesions in a patient who has recovered from extensive peritonitis. Occasionally this complication may occur a few days after the operation. The treatment is further operation to relieve the obstruction.

Incisional hernia. An incisional hernia may occur after any operation, but if it has been necessary to drain the wound the chances of it arising are greatly increased. Infection and pulmonary complications also predispose to the development of an incisional hernia because of the strain of coughing.

Intraperitoneal lavage

The value of intraperitoneal lavage in the treatment of peritonitis is now well established. It may take one of two forms after the cause has been dealt with. The first would seem to be the method of choice.

Intraoperative. In advanced peritonitis 'radical surgical debridement' is undertaken. Thorough cleansing of the whole peritoneal cavity, including every corner of the abdomen and in between loops of bowel, is undertaken with large volumes of saline to remove pus, faeces, fibrin and food. A long vertical incision is necessary. Post-operatively intestinal obstruction is a risk and in severe cases a long intestinal tube is passed through a proximal jejunostomy to the caecum to act as an internal splint. An antibiotic may be added to the fluid but this is not considered essential by Hudspeth (1978). The results are extremely good and complications are few.

Antibiotic lavage. A triple mixture of gentamicin, cephalothin and lincomycin, of which 10, 50 and 30 mg are dissolved in a litre of 1·5% Dianeal, a solution used for peritoneal dialysis. At the end of the operation at which it was sought to control the contaminating source, Portex drains (which must have a rounded cup) are inserted into the subhepatic pouch, the subsplenic area and the pelvis. Each is used in turn, the others being spigoted and through it 1 litre of solution is infused every hour, left for 30 minutes and then drained for 25 minutes. The process is continued for 72 hours. Stephen and Loewenthal claim:

(a) The maintainance of adequate antibiotic concentrations in the blood and peritoneal fluid.
(b) The dialysing fluid maintains normal serum electrolyte values.
(c) Body temperature is controlled so that the patient is rendered afebrile. The authors warn that this is a procedure only for severe peritonitis with intraperitoneal faecal leakage.

PERFORATED PEPTIC ULCER

An ulcer developing on a surface exposed to the action of acid-pepsin is known as a peptic ulcer, and includes gastric and duodenal ulcers. Perforation of a gastric ulcer is usually a more severe condition because the acid gastric juice is extremely irritant to the peritoneum and a much larger quantity of fluid leaks from a perforation in the stomach than from a similar ulcer in the duodenum. Apart from this, the clinical features and treatment are the same. Circulatory failure may be profound, and peritonitis becomes established after some hours.

A chronic ulcer may perforate but acute ulceration which is part of a widespread gastritis may also perforate. Aspirin and alcohol are recognised causes of acute ulceration. Steroid therapy is liable to reactivate a latent peptic ulcer. The most dangerous place for a patient to perforate is in hospital where an exacerbation of ulcer pain is anticipated and the patient may be sedated.

Symptoms and signs

The sudden onset of violent, constant, generalised abdominal pain is the outstanding symptom. The patient lies perfectly still where he has been smitten with pain. He feels as though he has received a powerful blow in the abdomen. Vomiting may occur. The face is pale and anxious and the skin feels cold and clammy. The temperature is invariably subnormal at first and the pulse rate is elevated. The whole abdomen is tender and extremely rigid or board-like. It does not move with respiration and there is no distension. If unrelieved the pain ceases after about 24 hours as the abdomen distends from general peritonitis. Not all patients give a history suggestive of previous indigestion.

Treatment

The tempo of deterioration is much faster in this condition than in a case of acute appendicitis. After 24 hours the patient suffering from acute appendicitis is still in a comparatively early stage because peritoneal contamination has not usually occurred. The mortality rate in patients suffering from untreated perforated peptic ulcer of 24 hours' duration is about 90 per cent.

Treatment is usually confined to closure of the perforation. If the symptoms before perforation were such that definitive surgical treatment such as vagotomy or gastrectomy was indicated this may be carried out.

Preoperative treatment

An intravenous line is set up and fluid replacement is commenced. The pain is relieved by an injection of morphia. As soon as possible the patient receives the usual preparation for an acute abdominal operation. The stomach preoperatively is aspirated, and every millilitre of gastric contents recovered lessens the damage to the peritoneal cavity.

Postoperative treatment

The general treatment is similar to that for acute appendicitis.

The hygiene of the mouth is even more important in this condition, since fluids by mouth are usually forbidden for the first 24 hours after the operation.

Diet. For the first 24 hours only parenteral fluid is given. After this a fluid diet is prescribed on return of the bowel sounds and is gradually increased to include suitable proportions of carbohydrate, fat and protein.

The immediate postoperative complications are similar to those following acute appendicectomy (p. 345), those of a case of peptic ulcer (Ch. 35) more remotely.

Instructions to the patient on discharge

It should be explained that the operation was a life-saving measure and that there is a 70 per cent chance that he will have further trouble. He can improve his chances of cure by avoiding undue stress and tobacco.

POSTOPERATIVE PERITONITIS

Postoperative peritonitis is a very important condition. It is one of the major causes of fatality following abdominal operations. It is peculiarly difficult to diagnose and in not a few cases post mortem examination reveals that deaths which have been attributed to cardiac failure and respiratory infection are, in fact, cases of true peritonitis from leakage of an anastomosis or rupture of the intestine. The real difficulty is that the severe pain and dramatic suddenness with which most peritoneal symptoms commence are clouded by:

1. Postoperative analgesics and hypnotics.
2. Some pain in the abdominal wound ⎱ which are usual
3. Some degree of pyrexia ⎰ postoperatively.

The important observations are:

1. Any complaint of undue pain should be reported.
2. Tenderness after the second day should be minimal.
3. Abdominal distension should be either responding to the usual measures or, if it is becoming worse, peritonitis should be suspected.

At an advanced stage these patients pass into acute circulatory failure and die very rapidly.

ACUTE INTESTINAL OBSTRUCTION

There are few conditions in which the real gravity of the patient's condition is more belied by his apparent well-being than in acute intestinal obstruction. The obstruction may affect the large or the small intestine; obstruction of the small intestine is always more severe than obstruction of the large intestine because of the great loss of fluid by vomiting in the former.

There are innumerable causes of intestinal obstruction, which are considered under Diseases of the Small and of the Large Intestine, but to illustrate the two main types a typical case of obstruction in each of the two portions of the intestines is discussed here.

SMALL BOWEL OBSTRUCTION

Symptoms and signs

Colicky abdominal pain commencing around the umbilicus is the first symptom. The pain waxes and wanes, is temporarily relieved by vomiting, but recurs again and again, and never moves from the centre of the abdomen.

Vomiting is constant. At first food is returned, later bile-stained gastric juice, and, in the late stages, the foul infected contents of the intestine above the obstruction. This fluid smells of faeces and is described as 'faeculent' vomit.

The loss of fluid, rich in chlorides, is considerable.

The bowels. There is usually absolute constipation, i.e. no flatus is passed after the administration of an enema or a Dulcolax suppository.

On examination the temperature is normal, but the pulse is rapid. Tenderness is unusual, unless gangrenous gut is present in the abdomen, but there is fullness of the lower abdomen. Only in very late cases is gross distension present.

Peristalsis (worm-like movements) of the bowel may be visible through a thin abdominal wall.

If an external strangulated hernia is the cause of the obstruction a tense, tender, painful irreducible swelling which has no impulse on coughing will be felt over one of the hernial sites. On the other hand, if the obstruction is due to some other cause, for example, a peritoneal band, the signs previously described will be present alone.

LARGE BOWEL OBSTRUCTION

The commonest cause is a growth narrowing the lumen of the bowel. The acute attack develops when a faecal mass blocks the already narrowed lumen.

Symptoms and signs

Obstruction in the large bowel is much better tolerated than obstruction in the small bowel. The main complaint is a feeling of abdominal distension and sometimes breathlessness, for the distension impairs the action of the heart and lungs.

Intestinal colic and vomiting appear only when a fair degree of distension has already occurred and prevents the contents of the large intestine flowing through the ileocaecal valve to the small intestine. A history of increasing constipation is almost invariable before the 'acute stoppage'.

The physical contents of the large intestine can be compared to a coal fire which consists of smoke and embers. If the chimney is blocked the real trouble arises in the room from the smoke. In the large intestine it is the gas which fills the bowel and all the striking symptoms are due to the retention of flatus and not to the presence of faeces.

The treatment of acute intestinal obstruction

The mortality rate of this condition is very high indeed, so that every care must be taken if it is to be reduced. Resuscitative measures must be instituted at once. Fluid depletion and electrolyte imbalance, which is usually severe in small bowel obstructions, has to be corrected.

A Dulcolax suppository or a disposable phosphate enema is given on admission. This serves the dual purpose of confirming the diagnosis and of clearing the bowel below the obstruction so that there is no unnecessary difficulty in the passage of the intestinal contents after the obstruction has been relieved.

A patient suffering from intestinal obstruction is given nothing by mouth before the operation.

If the obstruction is subacute, and there is no sign of gangrene an obstruction may be treated for a trial period by nasogastric suction and intravenous fluid replacement. Some patients with multiple adhesions may recover if the obstruction is due to kinking of a loop of bowel.

Very occasionally a volvulus of the pelvic colon may be reduced by passing a rectal tube through a sigmoidoscope. An intussusception (Ch. 37) may also be reduced by retrograde pressure from a barium enema given under X-ray screening control.

Immediate preoperative preparation

This is similar to the preparation for any acute abdominal operation, but special stress is laid on fluid and electrolyte replacement.

A nasogastric tube to aspirate the stomach contents is left in the stomach for 24 hours or longer after the operation. This relieves vomiting while the patient is being prepared, and prevents vomiting during the induction of anaesthesia. The aspiration of vomited material into the lungs may be fatal. If the obstruction is so severe that fluid is welling up in the stomach very rapidly, the patient is placed on the operating table in the slightly head-down position and the theatre nurse must aspirate the stomach contents even while the anaesthetist is inducing anaesthesia.

The operation

This is always confined to the simplest and quickest procedure necessary to relieve the obstruction. Division of a band or reduction of a strangulation is all that is necessary if the bowel wall is not gangrenous (Fig. 34.6). If gangrene is present, (Fig. 34.7) however, resection will be necessary, and this is a severe undertaking.

In the large intestine the most frequent method of relief is to form an artificial anus proximal to the obstruction, usually a colostomy—on rare occasions a caecostomy. The care of these fistulae is described in Chapter 38.

Postoperative treatment

Parenteral fluid replacement is continued. Continuous aspiration of the

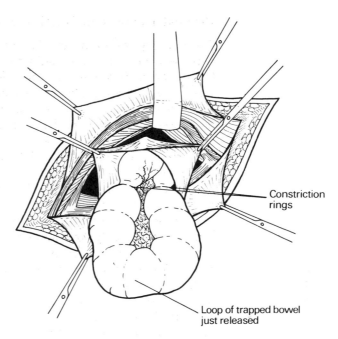

Constriction
rings

Loop of trapped bowel
just released

Fig. 34.6 Strangulated hernia. The intestine which has been released is viable. Note the released loop as well as the intestine above it is distended.

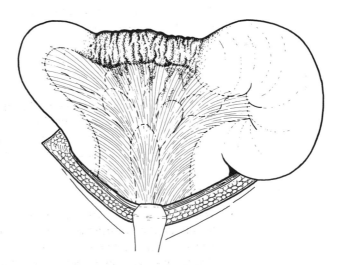

Fig. 34.7 Gangrenous small intestine. The obstruction has been relieved but as the gut is gangrenous it must be resected and continuity restored. The gut above is still distended.

stomach for 24 hours is frequently necessary, and the passage of a flatus tube per rectum is also important. These patients are sometimes very breathless from abdominal distension and are more comfortable when nursed sitting upright.

The general care of the patient and his wound is similar to that in any abdominal operation.

Postoperative complications. Particularly important in acute obstruction are:

1. Recurrence of the obstruction. The symptoms are similar to the original lesion.

2. Paralytic ileus is very common, since, although the mechanical obstruction has been relieved, the bowel wall may have developed paralysis as a result of the distension.

INTRA-ABDOMINAL HAEMORRHAGE

INTRAPERITONEAL HAEMORRHAGE

Intraperitoneal haemorrhage is not a very common cause of an acute abdomen. The only common lesion is an ectopic gestation. This is fully described in Chapter 50. Other traumatic causes include laceration of the spleen and of the liver.

The principles of treatment are:
1. Replacement of blood.
2. Control of haemorrhage by suture or removal of the affected organ.

EXTRAPERITONEAL HAEMORRHAGE

The commonest causes of *retroperitoneal* haemorrhage are:
1. A ruptured aneurysm of the abdominal aorta (Ch. 36).
2. Acute haemorrhagic pancreatitis (p. 385).

ANTEROPERITONEAL HAEMORRHAGE

The only common cause of a haemorrhage in front of the peritoneal cavity is rupture of the inferior epigastric artery which may cause sudden swelling behind the lower rectus sheath and in front of the peritoneal cavity. It is sometimes associated with severe coughing or handle-bar injuries.

CHRONIC PERITONITIS

General acute peritonitis has already been described. Chronic disease of the peritoneal cavity is described briefly to complete diseases of the peritoneal cavity.

This is usually tuberculous in origin. It may take three clinical forms:

1. Diffuse tuberculosis of the surface of the intestines and parietal peritoneum with the exudation of free clear fluid.

2. Diffuse adhesive changes which may cause intestinal obstruction. A similar condition known as sclerosing peritonitis may be caused by the drug practolol.

3. Multiple cold abscesses and fistulae usually pointing at the umbilicus.

Operation is only indicated if intestinal obstruction develops, otherwise the treatment is rest and anti-tuberculous chemotherapy.

CARCINOMA OF THE PERITONEUM

Carcinoma of the peritoneum is common, and is almost invariably secondary to growths elsewhere in the abdomen. The whole peritoneal surface may be studded with nodules of growth, and ascites is frequently abundant. No treatment of a curative nature is possible, but symptomatic relief may be given by tapping the abdomen and allowing the fluid to drain away. Radioactive gold and cytotoxic drugs are now being used in the relief of the ascites associated with this condition. A suspension of the colloidal form of the metal or drug is introduced through the aspirating needle. In 50 per cent of cases there is relief of the ascites. It does not cure the primary condition.

ASCITES

A collection of free non-purulent fluid in the peritoneal cavity is known as ascites. The term 'free' means that the fluid can move around the peritoneal cavity instead of being contained in one part of it—when it is described as encysted.

Causes

1. Carcinoma peritonei.
2. A failing heart.
3. Certain forms of renal failure.
4. Cirrhosis of the liver.
5. Some forms of tuberculous peritonitis.
6. Portal vein thrombosis.
7. Inferior venacaval obstruction.
8. Meigs' syndrome (Ovarian fibroma with ascites).
9. Escape of chyle.

Treatment

The treatment is that of the cause where possible. Locally, tapping (paracentesis) may be performed. A small trocar and disposable cannula are inserted into the peritoneal cavity after the injection of a local anaesthetic (1 per cent Lignocaine). The bladder must be emptied in preparation for the operation, and the skin of the abdominal wall is prepared in the usual way. Several pints of fluid may be withdrawn and a specimen is sent for pathological examination. A firm binder is applied after the operation to lessen further collection and assist with the drainage of fluid. If the cause is one of disseminated carcinomatosis a cytotoxic drug may be injected through the cannula.

Nursing procedure for paracentesis abdominis

A basic dressing trolley is prepared, additional items on the bottom shelf are:

Local anaesthetic and syringe	Drainage bag
Scalpel	Green' Savlon
Trocar and cannula (or other apparatus)	Iodine
Extra tubing	Green towels
Adjustable clamp	Gown, mask, gloves
Receiver	Specimen jars
Binder or many-tailed bandage	Stimulant, e.g. brandy.

The nature of the procedure is explained to the patient, and his co-operation is obtained.

The doctor prepares himself. The trolley is taken to the bedside. Privacy is ensured. The patient is made comfortable in the semi-recumbent position.

The bladder is emptied. If the patient cannot pass urine this is reported to the doctor. Catheterisation may be necessary.

The binder (or many-tailed bandage) is placed in position. The bed-clothes are turned down.

The nurse opens the outer wrappings of the basic dressing pack, opens other packets as required, and assists the doctor to assemble the apparatus. The doctor performs the procedure, assisted by the nurse. The nurse observes the patient, giving help and reassurance.

The tubing is connected to the cannula and to the drainage bag. The clamp is adjusted to allow the rate of flow ordered by the doctor. The binder is fastened in position, and readjusted as necessary.

The nurse looks after the patient whilst the drainage continues. Special observations are made on the general condition of the patient, the rate and flow of the fluid, the amount and the nature of the fluid.

The apparatus is taken down on instruction from the doctor. The wound is sealed, e.g. with Nobecutane. The trocar and cannula are rinsed in cold water, placed in the appropriate container and returned to CSSD.

PSEUDOMYXOMA PERITONEI

This is a most unpleasant condition which occurs following rupture of a pseudomucinous cyst of the ovary.

BIBLIOGRAPHY

Hudspeth A S 1975 Radical surgical debridement in the treatment of advanced peritonitis. Archives of Surgery 110: 12–33
Stephen M, Loewenthal J 1979 continuing peritoneal lavage in high risk peritonitis. Surgery 85: 603–606

35

The stomach and duodenum

The surgical anatomy and physiology of the stomach and duodenum have been considered in Chapter 33. Investigation to detect the presence of an organic lesion and to assess gastric secretory function is spread over several days. This adds to the patient's anxiety and the reason for each procedure should be explained. The passage of a nasogastric tube for investigation and in the perioperative care is a common nursing procedure.

NASOGASTRIC INTUBATION

A stomach tube is usually passed through the nose although some nurses and doctors who have undergone gastric surgery have felt that intubation was less intolerable by having it placed through the angle of the mouth. A further point to be borne in mind about passing the tube nasally is that staphylococci are often harboured in the nose and if a nasal tube is to be indwelling for some days it is advisable to take a nasal swab to make sure staphylococci are not present.

In the discussion which follows reference to the nasogastric route is equally applicable to a tube passed by mouth with two exceptions. A stomach full of retained solid foodstuff such as occurs in pyloric stenosis or one full of blood clots can be emptied only through a large bore tube and this can be passed only through the mouth.

Indications for intubation

1. Stomach wash out. Pyloric stenosis or poisoning.
2. Aspiration of excessive fluid accumulation. Pyloric stenosis, acute intestinal obstruction and acute dilation of the stomach.
3. To prevent gastric dilation in a stomach paralysed after surgery.
4. Removal/prevention of blood clots in haematemesis.
5. Gastric secretion tests.
6. Recovery of gastric juice for cytological examination.
7. Feeding where a patient who is unable to take food orally, has a functioning stomach and small intestine.

The advantages to be gained from intubation are considerable but it should not be overlooked that it is an unpleasant experience and a further discomfort following major surgery. The incidence of pulmonary complications is diminished where its use can be avoided and the danger of precipitating a hazardous staphylococcal enterocolitis should not be overlooked.

Nursing procedure for passing an intragastric tube

Equipment required:
Tube — Ryle's, oesophageal (Lenin) stomach or other
Paper towel (Kleenex roll)
Cleansing material for nose — sinus forceps
                              — cotton wool swabs
                              — sodium bicarbonate solution

Lubricant — KY jelly
Spatula and torchlight
Litmus paper
Vomit bowl, mouthwash
Medical wipes
Strapping
20 ml Syringe
Receiver
Spigot
Other apparatus, e.g. meal, suction according to reason for procedure.

The procedure is explained to a conscious patient, and his cooperation obtained. Privacy is ensured. Dentures are removed, if necessary.

When possible, the patient sits straight up, supported by pillows, with his head tilted forward. An unconscious patient lies in the semiprone position. A paper towel is placed under the chin. If he can do so, the patient is asked to blow his nose, otherwise the nurse carefully cleanses the nostrils.

The tip of the tube is lubricated. When the nasal route is used, it is gently inserted along the floor of the nose into the pharynx. When the oral route is being used, the tongue is depressed and the tube is passed over the side of the mouth and tongue into the pharynx, care being taken not to touch the uvula. When the tube is in the pharynx, the patient is asked to swallow, and the tube is gently pushed each time he does so. Sips of water may be given to assist in swallowing. In between swallows he is encouraged to take a deep breath. The nurse observes the patient for any coughing, apnoea, cyanosis or vomiting. If the tube is entering the larynx or trachea, it is removed, and the nurse passes it again when the patient has recovered from the coughing etc.

To ensure that the tube is in the stomach, the mouth is opened, the tongue depressed and the torch used to see the position of the tube in the pharynx. Using the syringe, some of the contents of the stomach are aspirated and tested with litmus paper. An acid reaction would most probably indicate that the tube is in the stomach.

A spigot is inserted into the end of the tube, and the tube is attached to the face with a piece of strapping.

When a patient has an indwelling nasogastric tube, it is necessary to attend to the cleanliness and condition of the nares and the mouth at regular intervals.

Gastric aspiration

A nasogastric tube is passed as described above.

1. Intermittent aspiration. A tray is prepared containing:

Receiver
20 ml syringe
Measure jug
Medical wipes/tissues
Disposal bag.

It is kept on the patient's locker, covered by a paper/green towel.

The patient is advised of what is to happen. The nurse holds a tissue around the junction, she removes the spigot and places it in the receiver. She ensures that there is no air in the syringe, attaches the tip to the tube and applies gentle suction. She holds the end of the tube and detaches the syringe. The aspirate is measured while still in the syringe, and then emptied into the jug. The aspiration is repeated until no fluid is aspirated. The spigot is reinserted. The total amount of aspirate is charted. The nurse leaves the tray clean, placing used tissues in the disposal bag. She reports to the nurse in charge.

2. Continuous drainage. The tube is connected to a drainage bag. The amount of drainage is measured and charted as instructed, e.g. hourly or when the bag is emptied or changed.

Removal of nasogastric tube. The patient is advised of what is to happen. The adhesive tape holding the tube is gently detached. The nurse tells the patient to take a deep breath, rapidly and smoothly withdraws the tube, and places it in a disposable bag. The patient's face is cleaned and his oral hygiene attended to. Used equipment is discarded.

Gastric washouts

Equipment required. This includes that for passing an intra-gastric tube (p. 358), with the following in addition:

Tubing 24 inches in length
Connection
Funnel
Small jug—1 litre
Large jug containing 4 litres fluid (e.g. tap water) at 100°F (37·8°C)
Bucket
2 Large polythene sheets.

The procedure is carried out very much as detailed for passing an intragastric tube (p. 358).

When the patient is unconscious, the position of the patient may be semiprone, prone or recumbent, with the head lower than the trunk. Usually, in such patients, the doctor intubates the patient and carries out the stomach lavage.

The polythene sheets are spread to protect the patient, bedding and floor. The bucket is placed on the floor. The stomach tube is passed into the stomach.

The small jug is filled with fluid. The funnel, tubing and connection are assembled. Some fluid is run through to expel air, and then stopped. The connection is attached to the stomach tube. The funnel is raised above the level of the head (or stomach if the head is low); 300 ml (half pint) of fluid is run into the stomach. Before the funnel is empty it is inverted over the bucket, and the fluid siphoned back. A specimen of the first washing is sometimes saved for analysis of gastric contents particularly drugs.

The process is repeated until the fluid returns clear, or the 4 litres of prepared fluid have been used.

Afterwards, the tube is compressed and withdrawn quickly. The patient's face is wiped, he is given a mouthwash and left comfortable in bed. An unconscious patient is kept under observation, and any alteration in the level of unconsciousness noted and reported.

Used equipment is discarded. The siphoned contents are measured and recorded, and saved for inspection.

The nurse washes and dries her hands and makes a report to the nurse in charge.

INVESTIGATIONS OF GASTRIC DISEASE

The investigations performed are:

Radiographic examination

Radiographic examination is performed after a barium meal preferably of the double contrast variety.

An aperient should be given two evenings before the barium meal examination. No food or drink is taken from midnight before the examination so that the stomach is empty of food at the time of radiological examination (say 10·00 hours).

After the barium meal is given no further solids or fluids must be given to the patient until the radiologist is satisfied with the X-rays.

Tests of gastric secretory function

In all these tests a gastric tube is passed, preferably orally, into a fasting stomach.

The patient should be as relaxed as possible. He should have been fasting for 12 hours. After spraying the throat with a local anaesthetic the tube is passed via the mouth into the stomach. An X-ray is then taken to ensure that the tube is in the body of the stomach.

The patient is now positioned in bed on his left side. A suction pump is used to withdraw the stomach contents at regular intervals, air being pumped in through a bleeder tube if the tube appears blocked.

Resting juice is aspirated and put into the first container — three quarter-hour basal specimens are then collected under continuous suction.

1. Pentagastrin. A subcutaneous injection of pentagastrin is then given (6 μg per kg body weight). Six further specimens are then collected at quarter-hour intervals. Pentagastrin has virtually no side effects.

2. Insulin. This procedure is similar to the pentagastrin test. Three quarter-hour basal specimens are collected, a blood sample being taken with the third. Intravenous injection of soluble insulin 0·25 units per kg body weight is given. Eight quarter-hour specimens are again collected and blood samples are taken half an hour and three-quarters of an hour after the insulin injection. The patient may become hypoglycaemic and sweat profusely after insulin injection. Oral or intravenous dextrose should be available but is rarely necessary.

3. Night secretion volume. After a suitable tranquiliser such as Valium, the total amount of juice secreted over a period of the 12 hours of the night is aspirated hourly or by continuous suction and the acidity is estimated. A volume in excess of 400 ml is suggestive of a duodenal ulcer while a volume of a litre suggests a gastrin-secreting pancreatic tumour.

Gastric secretion tests are particularly indicated for:
(a) X-ray negative dyspepsia.
(b) Recurrent dyspepsia after vagotomy and drainage.
(c) If the diagnosis of the Zollinger-Ellison syndrome is considered. In this condition the level of serum gastrin is greatly raised.

Four terms are used to describe the nature of gastric juice:
Hyperacidity — excess of total acid
Hyperchlorhydria — excess of hydrochloric acid
Achlorhydria — no hydrochloric acid
Achylia — no pepsin.

Tests for occult blood in the faeces

Red meat and green vegetables must be excluded from the diet for 3 days previous to the collection of the specimen. It is not necessary to submit the patient's entire stool for testing. A disposable plastic container should be used, with a tin spoon attached to the under surface of the lid.

Oesophagogastroduodeonoscopy (Fig. 35.1)

The modern fibreoptic endoscope enables the duodenum and the stomach to be viewed as well as taking specimens for biopsy. In preparation for gastroscope or flexible fibrescope is passed. No food or drink is allowed nation. It may be necessary to empty the stomach. The examination is carried out preferably between 08·00 and 09·00 hours. Before the examination the patient is given morphia (15 mg); under a local anaesthetic the gastroscope or flexible fibrescope is passed. No food or drink is allowed for half an hour afterwards, because the pharynx is anaesthetised and a little may run into the larynx.

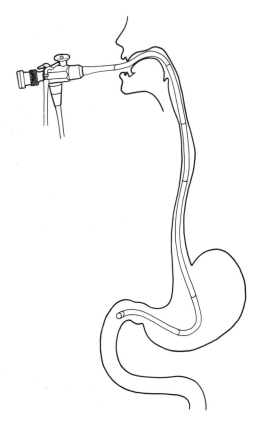

Fig. 35.1   Oesophagogastro-duodenoscopy

Gastric camera

Cytological examination

This should be performed after filtration of aspirated gastric contents.

HAEMATEMESIS AND MELAENA

When blood accumulates in the stomach the colour changes rapidly from red to black due to the action of gastric acid. It may be vomited (haematemesis) as black coffee-ground material or, if the haemorrhage is so severe that no mixing with gastric acid occurs, fresh red blood may be vomited. Alternatively the blood may pass into the duodenum and because it is irritant in the stomach and intestine it is passed very rapidly from the rectum as a tarry stool (melaena). The main causes of gastrointestinal bleeding are illustrated in Figure 35.2.

All patients with gastric bleeding require admission to hospital however mild the symptoms and signs, because no one can forecast the outcome. It may be a trivial incident or it may be the beginning of a haemorrhage that will never cease until it is controlled by surgical measures.

Corticosteroids may have activated a latent ulcer and some drugs taken

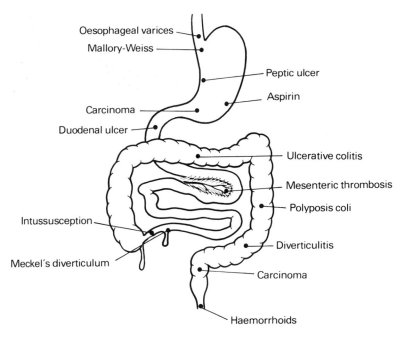

Fig. 35.2 Common causes of haemorrhage into gastrointestinal tract.

as tablets by mouth are particularly liable to erode the gastric mucous membrane. Aspirin and certain rheumatic and arthritic remedies are particularly suspect.

Management

(a) Sedation and rest.

(b) Estimation of the haemoglobin, blood grouping and cross matching of blood.

(c) Half hourly pulse and blood pressure records are kept. In more severe cases a central venous pressure line is inserted. A rising pulse rate and a falling blood pressure indicate continuing haemorrhage.

(d) The bed. Only one pillow is allowed and if the patient is very collapsed the foot of the bed is elevated.

(e) *Blood transfusion*, the rate and amount being determined by the parameter in (c).

(f) A wide bore stomach tube is passed and the stomach emptied continuously to prevent the accumulation of clot.

(g) *Antibiotics* may be prescribed because the haemorrhage is secondary in type.

(h) *Antifibrinolytic inhibitors* may be prescribed. Biggs et al have reduced the mortality from bleeding peptic ulcer using tranexamic acid.

Once the patient's condition has stabilised a barium meal and upper gastrointestinal endoscopy is carried out as a matter of some urgency to identify the cause of the bleeding. Occasionally coeliac axis angiography may be undertaken to show the site of the bleeding.

The subsequent management of the patient will depend on the radiological and endoscopic findings as well as the response to conservative measures.

PYLORIC OBSTRUCTION (STENOSIS)

The outlet of the stomach may be obstructed by:

1. Congenital hypertrophy of the muscle (congenital pyloric stenosis).

2. Simple ulceration proximal or distal to the pylorus. An ulcer may cause obstruction by its size, with considerable oedema when it is active, or by scarring when an active ulcer has healed.

3. A carcinoma in the pyloric antrum.

Whatever the cause, obstruction to the pylorus prevents food from leaving the stomach easily — solid food is retained and stagnates. As the condition becomes more severe fluid is slow to leave the stomach.

Because the stomach is nearly always full the patient has no appetite, feels distended in the epigastrium, vomits large quantities of foul material, loses weight and is constipated. Vomiting results in fluid and electrolyte depletion. On examination the patient's skin is dry and wrinkled, there is evidence of gross loss of weight and peristalsis may be visible. A hypertrophied pyloric sphincter may be palpated in the ten-day-old infant and an epigastric mass from carcinoma may be detectable in the adult suffering from carcinoma of the stomach. A barium meal will reveal delay in the emptying time of the stomach.

Management

Whatever the cause:

1. The stomach is emptied of its contents by a nasogastric tube and kept empty by frequent aspiration. If the contents are very foul a stomach washout, using a solution of sodium bicarbonate, is performed.

2. Fluid and electrolytes are replaced by intravenous infusion.

Definitive treatment depends on the cause. This may be division of the pyloric sphincter (Ramstedt's operation) in the infant, vagotomy and a drainage operation in a simple pyloric stenosis, or a partial gastrectomy for carcinoma of the stomach.

Acute dilatation of the stomach

In this condition the stomach loses its tone and may fill almost the whole abdomen. Several pints of fluid are exuded into the cavity of the organ from its own walls and from the duodenum. The condition is similar to paralytic ileus with which it is in fact often associated.

Causes

1. After operations on the stomach.

2. Occasionally it follows severe injury especially fractures of the dorsolumbar spine treated in a plaster jacket.

3. Sometimes the condition arises without any obvious cause.

Symptoms and signs

Symptoms and signs are identical with those of paralytic ileus.

Treatment

The stomach must be emptied and rested, but the fluid balance must be maintained. These objects can be achieved by:

1. Nasogastric suction for at least 24 hours or longer if necessary and intravenous fluids.

2. Elevation of the foot of the bed and turning the patient on his left side to facilitate drainage of the stomach contents.

PEPTIC ULCER

A peptic ulcer is an ulcer which occurs on a surface exposed to the action of acid pepsin. The common sites (Fig. 35.3) are:

1. The first part of the duodenum — duodenal ulcer.
2. The lesser curvature of the stomach — gastric ulcer.

Less common are:

1. The jejunum after anastomosis of the stomach to the jejunum — stomal ulcer.

2. Lower oesophagus usually associated with hiatus hernia causing a reflux oesophagitis and going on to an oesophageal ulcer.

3. An ulcer in the ileum adjoining a Meckel's diverticulum which will contain ectopic fragments of gastric mucous membrane.

All peptic ulcers are similar in pathology, basic clinical features and complications with the exception that a gastric ulcer may become, or may be mistaken for, a malignant (carcinomatous) ulcer of the stomach.

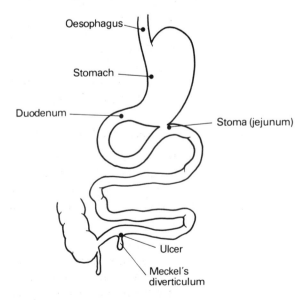

Fig. 35.3 Sites of peptic ulceration.

The cause of a peptic ulcer is unknown, but certain conditions are said to aggravate an existing ulcer or predispose to its formation in susceptible patients:

1. There is a higher incidence of duodenal ulcer amongst patients of blood group O than in the population in general.
2. Excess of acid and pepsin secretion.
3. Loss of the protective action of gastric mucus.
4. Drugs, smoking and alcohol.
5. Endocrine factors — a pancreatic gastrin secreting tumour which stimulates excessive acid secretion in the stomach is the best known.

Clinical features of an uncomplicated peptic ulcer

(a) Burning epigastric pain appearing half an hour to 2 hours after food. Food may relieve the pain of a duodenal ulcer.

(b) The appetite of a patient with a duodenal ulcer may remain good whilst the patient with a gastric ulcer is afraid to eat.

(c) Although nausea and heartburn are common features vomiting is unusual except in complicated cases.

(d) Remission and exacerbation are characteristic especially in duodenal ulcer.

The complications of a peptic ulcer

The principal ones are:
    Perforation — Chapter 33
    Haemorrhage   } discussed
    Pyloric stenosis and hour-glass contracture } above
    Carcinomatous change in a simple gastric ulcer is rare.

Penetration of adjacent organs. A chronic ulcer may invade locally the pancreas, the liver, or the intestine. The ulcer pain is usually more constant and more severe than usual, and is referred to the back.

Penetrating ulcers usually require surgical treatment. Ulceration into the colon is a serious condition, and usually results in what is known as a gastrocolic fistula (Ch. 33).

Treatment

The principles of treatment of a peptic ulcer are the same whether medical or surgical measures are employed. Basically they aim at the dilution, neutralisation or diminution of acid pepsin.

1. Dilution by frequent meals, milk drip or short circuit operation, for example, gastrojejunostomy.
2. Neutralisation:
    (a) Alkalis.
    (b) Buffers, such as milk.
3. Diminution:
    (a) Drugs inhibiting vagal action, including sedatives which diminish

anxiety. Rest in bed has a similar effect.

    (b) Drugs inhibiting acid secretion locally, e.g. cimetidine.

    (c) Vagotomy.

    (d) Gastrectomy.

    (e) Avoidance of smoking.

    4. Increasing mucosal resistance — agents such as carbenoxolone sodium stimulate protective mucorrhoea in gastric ulcer.

The prostaglandins secreted in the stomach modulate the response of the acid secreting cells to stimulants such as gastrin and histamine. This protective function is blocked by drugs such as cortisone or phenylbutazone and the administration of synthetic prostaglandins is complementary to the action of drugs like cimetidine.

The main indications for surgical treatment are:

    (a) The occurrence of complications.

    (b) The failure to respond to careful medical treatment. This requires fine judgement and the treatment of an uncomplicated ulcer requires a multidisciplinary approach including close co-operation between the physician and surgeon.

Surgical measures are either a vagotomy or a partial gastrectomy.

Investigations

    Barium Meal
    Gastric secretion tests
    Endoscopy

NEW GROWTHS OF THE STOMACH

Simple growths are rare, the commonest being a leiomyoma — a benign tumour of smooth muscle. Malignant growths are the third commonest cause of death from malignant disease and are relatively painless until far advanced. Their incidence in patients of blood group A is commoner than in the general population.

While surgery offers the only hope of cure, the survival rates, even in early cases, are extremely low. It is one of the most unfavourable sites in which to develop a neoplasm.

Symptoms and signs

The early symptoms are few and very general in type. A feeling of malaise, increasing fatigue, and slight loss of appetite are the most common. Later pain, vomiting, and anaemia may develop. Loss of weight is usually rapid, and occasionally there may be a small haematemesis. An acute onset, such as a large haematemesis or a perforation, may occur exceptionally. A growth in the pyloric antrum may cause pyloric obstruction.

On examination of the abdomen there are no physical signs in early cases, but later the malignant growth can be palpated as a hard mass in the epigastrium. The liver may be enlarged and irregular from the presence of secondary deposits.

Investigations

1. Radiographic examination after a barium meal shows the typical appearance of a filling defect.

2. Gastric secretion tests usually reveal the absence of hydrochloric acid (achlorhydria), but when the growth causes pyloric obstruction total acidity from fermentation may be increased. In all cases the amount of free hydrochloric acid is reduced. Examination of the gastric aspirate may reveal malignant cells.

3. Occult blood is usually present in the faeces.

4. Gastroscopy and the gastric camera are valuable aids to diagnosis in doubtful cases.

Treatment

Removal of the stomach (gastrectomy) is the only operation which offers any hope of cure. If the growth is inoperable but pyloric stenosis is present or impending, considerable relief may be achieved by the performance of a gastroenterostomy. Should the growth be inoperable, careful nursing can do much to render the remaining days of misery more tolerable. Analgesic and hypnotic drugs will relieve pain, and vitamins by injection will delay deterioration. Antiemetics such as perphenazine (5 mg) may be prescribed. The diet should be light and nutritious, and in particular it must be what the patient fancies from day to day.

SURGERY OF THE STOMACH

1. Vagotomy. The vagus nerves are divided within the abdomen to diminish gastric secretion (Fig. 35.4). This is known as a truncal vagotomy. If only the fibres to the stomach are divided it is known as a selective vagotomy. If only the fibres to the acid secreting parietal cell mass are divided it is called a proximal gastric vagotomy or highly selective vagotomy.

A truncal or selective vagotomy also paralyses the stomach muscle and defective gastric emptying occurs. For this reason a gastrojejunostomy or some form of drainage procedure such as a pyloroplasty is usually carried out.

2. Partial gastrectomy which may be performed for a gastric or a duodenal ulcer consists of removal of two thirds of the stomach. The stomach remnant is then sutured to the duodenum (Billroth I type, Fig. 35.5A) or to the jejunum (Billroth II or Polya Fig. 35.5B). The Billroth I reconstruction is usual in operations for gastric ulcer, the Billroth II form in cases of duodenal ulcer.

3. Total gastrectomy with anastomosis of the oesophagus to the jejunum (Fig. 35.5C) is performed in the rare case of a gastrin secreting tumour of the pancreas which may be too small to be located but persistent recurrent and often multiple peptic ulceration occurs as the stomach and duodenum are the target organs. More usually total gastrectomy is performed for carcinoma of the stomach.

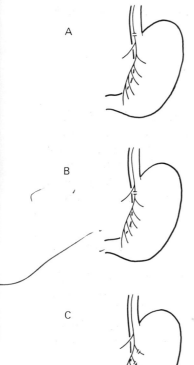

Fig. 35.4 Types of vagotomy.
A. Total truncal vagotomy.
B. Selective vagotomy.
C. Proximal gastric vagotomy.

Preoperative care

The preoperative care is similar to any major abdominal operation. Blood is crossmatched and, if necessary, anaemia is corrected. The risk of pulmonary complications is greater following surgery in the upper abdomen so pre and postoperative physiotherapy to the chest as well as the cessation of smoking is even more important. Fluid and electrolyte imbalance may require correction, especially in patients suffering from pyloric stenosis and vitamin C deficiency may have to be made good.

The stomach must be empty at the time of operation. Normally this occurs in 3 hours, and if emptying is not delayed it is unnecessary to pass a stomach tube. If pyloric stenosis is present, the stomach is emptied and washed out the evening before operation so that the patient is disturbed as little as possible the next morning. In severe pyloric stenosis gastric aspiration over several days is advisable.

A nasogastric tube is passed through the nose and left in position preoperatively. Some surgeons prefer to have the nasogastric tube passed by the anaesthetist if its use is not necessary until after the operation. The end is plugged with a tiny disposable spigot. Although the tube is usually passed through the nose some nurses and doctors who have had a gastrectomy performed have felt that intubation was rendered less intolerable by having it placed through the angle of the mouth.

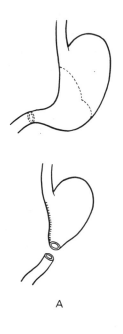

A

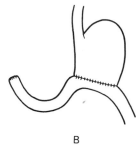

B

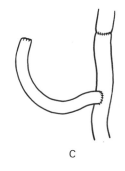

C

Fig. 35.5 Gastrectomies.
A. Billroth I partial gastrectomy.
B Polya partial gastrectomy.
C. Total gastrectomy with Roux-en-y oesophagojejunostomy.

PERIOPERATIVE USE OF THE NASOGASTRIC TUBE

Care of the nasogastric tube

This tube, which was passed before or during the operation, is left in place afterwards and the stomach contents are aspirated hourly and the amount recovered is measured and recorded. The early aspirations consist of <u>bright red blood</u> which, in a few hours, changes to dark blood and which, in 24 hours, should be bile-stained. The amount aspirated diminishes until only a few millilitres of fluid are recovered, and the bowel sounds have returned. This indicates that the gastrointestinal tract has recovered its normal activity and that it is now safe to give fluid by mouth.

Thirty ml of sterile water are given. The stomach is aspirated an hour later and, if it is emptying satisfactorily, the total amount of fluid may be increased slowly to 90 ml each hour. On the day after operation the patient is allowed up and the nasogastric tube is removed as soon as normal emptying of the stomach occurs over several days. The diet is gradually built up with citrated milk, eggs and strained soup. By the sixth day the patient is eating most foods, but he should also drink large quantities of milk.

Excessive aspirate may occur because:

1. The tube is too low and protruding through the stoma. It should be withdrawn so that it is just below the cardio-oesophageal junction. This position is attained by withdrawing the tube until no aspirate is recovered and then pushing it down again very cautiously 1 cm at a time until the stomach contents are again recovered.

2. Over-infusion of fluids in the 2 or 3 days following operation.

Report.

Alternatives and modifications of nasogastric intubation

Some believe that a nasogastric tube is unnecessary and can be dispensed with. There is no doubt that, in the majority of cases, this is correct. In a significant minority, however, dilatation of the stomach occurs quietly and sometimes disastrously and this is preventable by an indwelling tube.

Morris Lee's two-way intubation tube is a double-barrelled tube, one barrel of which is much longer than the other. The larger one is manipulated into the jejunum (or duodenum) at the end of the operation and the nasal end is connected to a reservoir of fluid. This obviates the need for intravenous fluid. The shorter barrel is in the stomach and can be aspirated in the ordinary way. The underlying principle of its use is that the jejunum is often active and functioning while the stomach is still paralysed.

Kay uses a special tube from the cavity of the stomach to the abdominal wall to obviate the need for a nasogastric tube. It is a modified gastrostomy procedure.

POSTOPERATIVE CARE

Apart from management of the nasogastric tube which has just been discussed the only special point is a special watch if a drainage tube has been used.

The drainage tube. If a corrugated tube has been inserted it should be removed on the 5th day, but if there has been a discharge of bile or intestinal contents this should be reported at once and the tube should not be removed.

The general management of fluid and electrolytes is continued until the stomach is emptying and the diet is gradually built up. In most cases the patient is mobilised on the day following operation and fit for discharge from hospital in 8 to 10 days.

Complications

1. Haemorrhage. Small quantities of blood are usually aspirated in the first 12 hours. Larger quantities of loss, however, require treatment. Morphia is administered and the foot of the bed is elevated. A nasogastric tube is usually in position and the stomach contents aspirated.

Treatment for haematemesis (p. 363) is instituted. If the bleeding persists the wound may have to be reopened and the bleeding point ligated.

2. Vomiting. Occasionally severe persistent vomiting occurs, due to the obstruction of the intestine which has been joined to the stomach. It may be necessary to reopen the wound when this complication is present. Acute dilatation of the stomach may follow gastric operations and the nasogastric tube must not be removed until the stomach has recovered its tone.

3. Staphylococcal diarrhoea, due to a pure growth of *Staphylococcus pyogenes*, may occur as a complication of any operation, but more than 50 per cent of cases are subsequent to gastrectomy. It should be stressed that:

(a) It may be epidemic.

(b) The patient is usually receiving broad-spectrum antibiotics.

(c) A nasogastric tube has been used.

Clinically the condition may simulate internal haemorrhage, coronary thrombosis or pulmonary embolism until the diarrhoea appears. There is a gross loss of fluid. In suspected cases a specimen of faeces is sent for immediate microscopic examination for Gram-positive cocci, to confirm the diagnosis. The culture is also performed for antibiotic sensitivity.

Treatment. The antibiotics in current use are discontinued. Erythromycin (0·5 g) four times daily is given intramuscularly but in severe cases 250 mg doses should be given by slow intravenous injection. Fucidin (500 mg) 6-hourly is also of value. Fluid loss is replaced by intravenous fluid. The patient is nursed in isolation.

4. Pulmonary complications may be prevented in a considerable measure by deep breathing exercises and free movement in bed. Antibiotics are administered in established disease.

5. Peritonitis may occur from leakage at the anastomosis or from rupture of the duodenal stump (Fig. 35.6). Rupture results in a duodenal fistula, which can also occur from damage to the duodenum in the operations of right hemicolectomy or nephrectomy on the right side. A small abdominal drainage tube will always discharge bile-stained fluid if the duodenum has ruptured. The commonest day for a rupture is the fourth or fifth postoperative day. It is impossible to resuture the ruptured duodenum because the ferments are already eating away its very substance. Therefore treatment consists of:

(a) Gastric aspiration.

(b) Suction drainage through the stab wound.

(c) The parenteral administration of fluid to maintain the fluid balance.

(d) The administration of antibiotics.

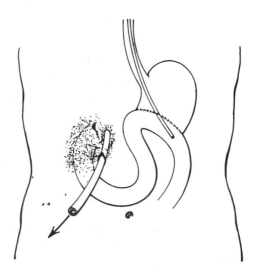

Fig. 35.6 Rupture of the duodenal stump following gastrectomy is the commonest fatal complication. The escaping enzymes destroy so much of the wall that suture is impossible and the only hope lies in removing the enzymes by nasogastric tube and suction through the fistula.

6. Stomal ulcer. A more remote complication, its onset is heralded by recurrence of the original symptoms of indigestion.

A stomal ulcer is an ulcer at the line of junction (the stoma) with the small intestine. Strict medical treatment is usually prescribed, but if this is not successful a more extensive removal of the stomach or vagotomy is performed.

A stomal ulcer may cause a gastrojejuno-colic fistula by perforation into the colon.

THE POST-GASTRECTOMY SYNDROMES

A proportion of patients develop symptoms of varying severity after the main meal. They include the 'dumping' syndrome, the symptoms of which are:

Dizziness
Sweating
Palpitation
Epigastric discomfort
Extreme weakness, and, on occasion, loss of consciousness.

These symptoms may appear half an hour to 3 hours after food, and may be relieved by lying down.

The patient is advised to avoid a large meal if any of the above symptoms appear. His diet must be revised to ensure adequate nutrition by means of smaller but more frequent meals.

Other post-gastrectomy syndromes which may appear are:
1. Bilious vomiting.
2. Malnutrition.
   (a) Anaemia.
   (b) Vitamin deficiency, particularly vitamin B.
   (c) Gross loss of weight.
   (d) Osteoporosis.

Treatment. Vitamin deficiency and anaemia can be treated medically by giving the appropriate vitamin preparation or iron. A gluten-free diet is sometimes of help.

Post-vagotomy diarrhoea. This is an occasional but very distressing sequel of vagotomy. The cause is unknown. If simple measures such as codeine phosphate fail, cholestyramine (Questran) may be advised. For intractable cases a reversed jejunal segment may be performed.

Advice on leaving hospital

It should be explained to the patient that at his operation the ulcer and a large portion of his stomach have been removed, or some other operation performed, but his tendency to form another ulcer remains.

The fundamental principles of aftertreatment must be rest, relaxation, a calm attitude to life and its incidents, plenty of soft non-irritating food, taken at frequent intervals, and not lacking in any of the essentials of a good normal diet. More important than the exact diet is the mental attitude of the patient who eats it.

The precise constitution of the diet should be varied to suit the patient's needs and tastes. The regularity and frequency of the feeds are as important as their composition. If irritants such as mustard, spices, vinegar, and alcohol are avoided, and if other food is free from gross roughage, all the common foods may be safely taken from the beginning of treatment. An elaborately graded diet is unnecessary. Meals should be served as attractively as possible and efficient mastication is essential.

BIBLIOGRAPHY

Biggs J C, Hugh T B, Dodds A J 1976 Gut 17: 729
British Medical Journal Editorial 1979 1: 642

36

Diseases of the liver, the gall bladder and the pancreas

THE LIVER

Apart from being the site of synthesis of plasma proteins, glucose metabolism and the production of essential clotting factors, the liver also conjugates the breakdown product of haemoglobin, bilirubin, into an excretable form which leaves the liver by the biliary canaliculi in conjunction with the bile acids and salts. For its various metabolic activities the liver receives an abundant blood supply from the hepatic artery and the portal vein. The blood drains into the hepatic veins which join the inferior vena cava.

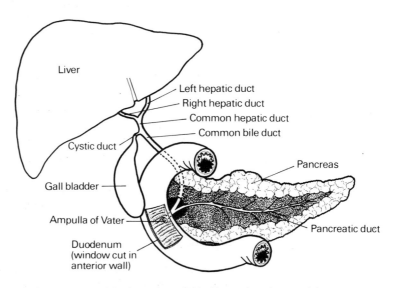

Fig. 36.1 The anatomy of the liver, the gall bladder and its ducts and the pancreas.

INJURY

Injury to the liver usually takes the form of laceration, and is due to a crush injury of the abdomen in the majority of cases. Pain in the right hypochondrium, tenderness, and the signs of internal haemorrhage will be present. It is frequently combined with multiple abdominal injuries.

Treatment

The treatment consists of an exploratory laparotomy after blood replacement. If the tear is a minor one it may be sutured or simply left undisturbed. If the tear is a severe one the situation usually calls for a formal partial hepatic resection. The liver has remarkable powers of regeneration and may indeed regain its size following right hepatic lobectomy by the end of the third postoperative week.

INFLAMMATORY CONDITIONS

Viral hepatitis

Viral hepatitis comprises two microbiologically separate diseases serologically distinguishable from each other. Infective hepatitis is epidemic and believed to be transmitted by the faecal oral route, whereas serum viral hepatitis is transmitted by physical procedures and arises from:

  (i) A pool of infected plasma or serum.
 (ii) A renal dialysis unit.
(iii) Drug addiction.

Serum hepatitis is associated with the serological entity Australian antigen (AuAg), much more commonly indicated as HB Ag, ie hepatitis B. It is acquired primarily within the walls of a hospital.

All blood and serum products are potentially infected and the following precautions must, therefore, be taken:

(a) All blood donors are tested for Hb Ag.
(b) All patients in dialysis units should be screened.
(c) The sterilisation of syringes must be adequate.
(d) Spilt blood should be disinfected with a hypochlorite solution such as Domestos or 10 per cent formalin.
(e) Specimens of blood from suspected patients should carry a distinguishing mark.
(f) All patients with liver disease, all those who have had previous blood transfusions and all drug addicts should be carefully screened.

Liver abscess

1. A solitary abscess, is usually a complication of amoebic dysentery. Surgical drainage of the abscess may be performed, but in most cases treatment consists of chloroquine or metronidazole (Flaygl) with tetracycline for the secondary infection.

2. Multiple pyaemic abscesses may occur as a complication of peritonitis. It is an extremely serious condition and chemotherapy alone offers the best prospects of cure. Multiple cholangiectatic abscesses may develop from ascending infection within the bile ducts following obstruction of the common bile duct by a calculus or a growth. Chemotherapy and surgical relief of the obstruction are necessary.

Hydatid cyst of the liver

Hydatid disease is due to an infection caused by a parasite known as the *Taenia echinococcus*. The liver is one of the commonest sites for the infection. Surgical treatment consists of excision of the lining of the cyst and drainage of the cavity.

PORTAL HYPERTENSION

Cirrhosis of the liver may be caused by excessive alcohol intake, certain toxic agents and viral hepatitis. The liver substance heals by scar tissue and this may interfere with the normal flow of blood along the portal venous pathways contained within it. As a result there is back pressure on the portal venous system, this being most marked within the veins at the cardio-oesophageal junction. In time the veins become distended and tortuous, hence the term oesophageal varices. These thin walled veins may rupture thus giving rise to a massive upper gastrointestinal haemorrhage.

Shunting of the blood from the portal system into the systemic system by anastomosis of the portal vein to the inferior vena cava may be undertaken. This leads to a fall in the portal venous pressure. If a shunt is not feasible a direct attack on the bleeding by transthoracic ligation or endoscopic sclerotherapy may be undertaken.

Carcinoma of the liver

1. Primary carcinoma is uncommon in the Western world and the treatment is resection.

2. Secondary carcinoma is almost invariably secondary to an intra-abdominal primary growth and may sometimes be controlled by intra-arterial cytotoxic agents.

LIVER FUNCTION TESTS

Although these tests are nonspecific and difficult to interpret they help to differentiate between obstructive jaundice which requires surgery and liver diseases which do not. Over three quarters of the liver may be destroyed before many of the tests show any abnormality. They attempt to provide information on:

Bile metabolism.
Plasma protein synthesis.
The liver enzymes.

Bile metabolism

Bilirubin is formed from haemoglobin in the cells of the reticuloendothelial system (spleen, bone marrow, liver) where aged red cells are broken down. The bilirubin becomes attached to albumin in the plasma and is carried by the circulating blood through the liver. The bilirubin becomes conjugated (joined) to a substance called glucuronic acid in the liver and is passed by the bile ducts into the intestine. Here bacterial action converts it into stercobilinogen most of which is excreted in the faeces where, on exposure to air, it darkens to brown and is called stercobilin. Some of the stercobilinogen is reabsorbed from the intestine into the bloodstream and excreted in the urine as urobilin.

Urobilin in the urine. In complete obstructive jaundice there is no bilirubin in the intestines for the bacteria to convert to urobilinogen. Therefore there is no uruobilin to reabsorb into the bloodstream and none to pass into the urine. Tests for urobilin therefore are negative though the urine is dark due to a high content of bilirubin glucuronide.

Urobilin (stercobilin) in the faeces. The dark colour of the faeces depends on the amount of bilirubin entering the intestine. The stools are pale in obstructive jaundice.

Bile salts also appear in the urine in obstructive jaundice as they are drained back into the blood and excreted by the kidneys. Bile salts are detected by sprinkling flowers of sulphur on the surface of the urine in a test glass. If bile salts are present the sulphur sinks due to the lowering of surface tension.

Plasma proteins

Albumin and fibrinogen are synthesised in the liver. In severe liver disease therefore their level in the blood falls. The albumin may fall as low as 25 g per litre (normal 36−50 g per litre). The globulin level, however, remains unchanged, so the normal ratio of albumin to globulin (2 : 1) may be reversed. Globulin is not a single substance but a series of similar proteins called α (alpha), β (beta) and γ (gamma) globulins. When the liver is diseased the ratio of these globulins to one another in the plasma is altered. The thymol and zinc flocculation and turbidity tests are positive when these ratios are abnormal. Prothrombin is also synthesised within the liver, a process for which vitamin K is essential. If there is no bile in the intestine vitamin K cannot be absorbed and, therefore, in obstructive jaundice the level is low. This requires correction before surgery can be carried out.

The liver enzymes

Serum alkaline phosphatase is removed from the blood by the liver and excreted in the bile. Normal values are about 2 to 10 King Armstrong units per 100 ml of serum. When the liver cells are diseased it may rise to 30 units but if the bile ducts are blocked very high levels of 100 units or more will occur. It should be noted that very high values of serum alkaline phosphatase also occur in bone diseases when osteoblastic cells are overactive, e.g. rickets, Paget's disease, hyperparathyroidism, bone tumours.

Serum glutamate pyruvate tramsaminase (SGPT) 10−35 units per ml and the serum glutamate oxalacetate tramsaminase (SGOT) 0−35 units per ml are enzymes whose levels are raised in conditions leading to damage of the liver cells such as viral hepatitis.

Liver puncture biopsy

Liver tissue may be obtained for histological examination either blindly by means of a Tru-cut needle or laparoscopically. It is helpful in the study of patients with liver disease when clinical signs and laboratory tests do not give a definite diagnosis. It is seldom indicated in jaundiced patients and is performed when sarcoidosis, Hodgkin's disease, or brucellosis are suspected.

Before the puncture is made the bleeding, clotting and prothrombin times are estimated and must be normal, liver function tests are performed, 2 units of blood are cross-matched and premedication with 15 mg morphia or 60 mg phenobarbitone instead of morphia is given if there is gross liver damage. The patient lies on her back with a pillow under her left buttock, the right hand behind the head. The skin is cleansed, a local anaesthetic infiltrated and the liver biopsy needle is plunged into the liver. The biopsy specimen is placed in normal saline, labelled and sent to the pathologist. Postoperatively a watch should be kept for signs of internal haemorrhage. **Ultrasonography and isotope scanning** provide invaluable information about the integrity of the liver substance and are, therefore, eminently suitable for the investigation of infiltrative disease of the liver, e.g. malignant secondary deposits.

JAUNDICE

Jaundice is due to the retention of bile pigments in the tissues and in the blood. When the level of bilirubin within the blood rises (normal level is less than 15·4 μmol/litre) the patient becomes clinically jaundiced. Whereas bilirubin is found in the urine in obstructive jaundice and in jaundice due to hepatitis, urobilin is absent in obstructive jaundice.

Jaundice may be classified by the site at which it is effectively caused, viz.:

Prehepatic. Haemolytic jaundice, which is a condition produced by the too rapid breaking up of the red blood corpuscles. It may be treated medically with cortisone or cured in some cases by removal of the spleen (p. 230).

Hepatic (diseases of the liver)
1. Viral jaundice has already been considered.
2. Cirrhosis.
3. Multiple secondary deposits.
4. Acute yellow atrophy.

Posthepatic (cholestatic jaundice). Due to obstruction of bile ducts:
1. Canalicular obstruction—largactil.
2. Bile ducts—stones; carcinoma of the head of the pancreas.

Jaundice is due to the retention of bile pigments in the tissues and in the blood. It is caused by a variety of diseases fully dealt with in medical textbooks. The important surgical form is due to obstruction of the common bile duct. This may result from:

(a) A stone impacted in the duct; or

(b) A carcinoma of the head of the pancreas obstructing the duct or a tumour growing in the common duct.

(c) Chronic pancreatitis (rarely).

Operative interference on a patient who is jaundiced is dangerous, because the blood has a lessened coagulability, due to the lack of vitamin K and consequently haemorrhage may be extremely difficult to control. Vitamin K is fat-soluble and therefore is not absorbed from the intestine in the absence of bile salts. For this reason vitamin K should be administered by intramuscular injection some days before and after operation. In addition, large quantities of glucose are necessary to prevent further liver damage.

After operation a jaundiced patient requires special care, since not only is internal haemorrhage more likely to occur, but it may be more easily overlooked because *pallor cannot be observed*. The pulse volume and rate should be carefully watched (Fig.36.2). As the condition improves, the colour of the stools is carefully noted each day, for they are a guide to the amount of bile reaching the intestine. When the patient is severely jaundiced the stools are almost white, and, as recovery occurs, tend to become more and more their normal colour. The urine is very dark in colour due to the presence of bile pigments.

There is an increased risk of renal failure and mannitol is used to prevent it (p. 384). Wound healing is delayed and the susceptibility to infection is greater. Intolerable itching from retention of bile salts can be very distress-

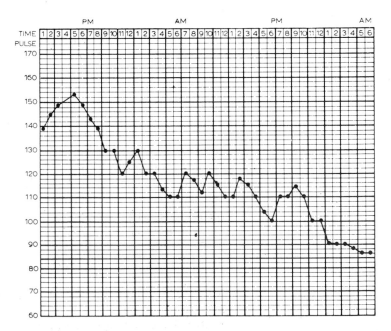

Fig. 36.2 Postoperative hourly pulse chart—always important. Vital in jaundice, as pallor from haemorrhage is unobservable.

ing in persistent jaundice. Cholestyramine, which binds bile salts, is effective in relieving this symptom.

Jaundice in any form is very depressing mentally, and the nurse must make every allowance for irritability on the part of the patient. It is part of his disease. The bleeding and coagulation times are increased. The degree of jaundice may be measured by an examination of the serum bilirubin (normal 15·4 μmol/litre).

THE GALL BLADDER

The most common disease of the gall bladder is caused by gall-stones formed by the precipitation of the constituents of bile. A gall-stone gives rise to symptoms when it moves. Movement may result in its obstructing the cystic duct with resultant acute cholecystitis, or the stone may migrate into the common bile duct causing obstruction to the main outflow of bile from the liver. There is a strong hereditary tendency in gall-stone formation. Twenty-five per cent of gall stones are pigment stones, the remaining 75 per cent being composed of cholesterol.

SYMPTOMS AND SIGNS OF GALL-STONES

It has long been said that the most typical patient is a fat parous woman about the age of 40. This, however, is far from true. Gall-stones are equally common in the thin. They are certainly more common in the female than the male but they are by no means rare in men and are occasionally seen even in children.

The patient may complain of recurrent bouts of flatulent dyspepsia precipitated by fatty foods. If a stone impacts in the neck of the gall bladder thus blocking the outflow the patient experiences severe upper abdominal pain originating in the epigastrium and then radiating around the flank to settle in the region of the right scapula (Fig. 36.3). The pain is usually colicky in type and is relieved by vomiting.

This is the classical presentation of gall bladder colic. If the pain persists and the abdomen is tender to palpation in the right hypochondrium it is very likely that the gall bladder has become acutely inflamed (acute cholecystitis), a diagnosis supported by elevated temperature and tachycardia (Fig. 36.4). Acute cholecystitis usually resolves on conservative therapy but occasionally may proceed to an empyema of the gall bladder.

Investigation of gall bladder disease

1. Direct radiographic examination of the abdomen reveals gall-stones only in 5 per cent of cases in which they are present, because the majority of gall-stones are not radio-opaque. Therefore, only a positive X-ray will be of value.

2. Cholecystogram. The cholecystographic examination varies according to the opaque medium used and the technique employed.

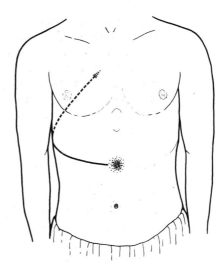

Fig. 36.3 Gall-bladder pain commences in the epigastrum and radiates to the back and shoulder.

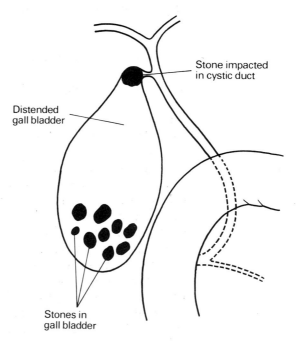

Fig. 36.4 Acute cholecystitis. A stone is impacted in the cystic duct. The gall-bladder, which contains numerous stones, is tense and distended.

The material, usually orablix, telepaque, or biloptin, is given by mouth the evening before. A radiograph is taken at 9 a.m. and if the gall bladder functions a fatty meal is then given and a further radiograph taken half an hour later. The patient will already have been prepared with the colon free from gas and faecal shadows. The material should be administered according to the makers' instructions, which should be closely followed. It is very important to be certain that the patient has not vomited the drug, as this renders the examination valueless.

A diseased gall bladder will fail to concentrate the medium. As the medium is excreted by the liver and concentrated by the gall bladder it is of little value in the presence of jaundice.

    3. Cholangiogram (outlining of the common duct). This may be done:

        (a) By the intravenous injection of biligrafin. Frequent radiographs are taken as the liver excretes the biligrafin.

        (b) When the abdomen is open at operation or before a tube is removed from the common duct.

    4. Ultrasonography. This is a valuable noninvasive investigation which is easy and quick to perform. The gall bladder and the bile ducts can be demonstrated. The presence of stones and dilation of the ducts can be seen.

    5. Percutaneous transhepatic cholangiography is a useful procedure in obstructive lesions. It is usually done as an immediate preoperative investigation in the theatre.

COMPLICATIONS OF GALL STONES

    1. Acute cholecystitis.
    2. Mucocele or empyema of the gall bladder.
    3. Common duct colic.
    4. Obstructive jaundice (Fig. 36.5).
    5. Acute pancreatitis.
    6. Fistulous communication between the gall bladder and the duodenum with the possibility of the small bowel being obstructed by a gall stone (Fig. 33.4).
    7. Carcinoma of the gall bladder.

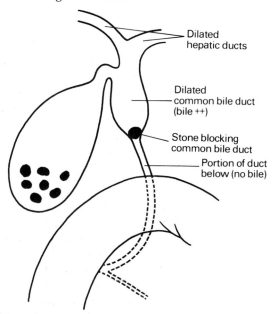

Fig. 36.5 Obstruction of the common bile duct by a stone. Note the duct above the stone and also dilatation of the hepatic ducts. This patient would be jaundiced.

Treatment

Acute cholecystitis and biliary colic. Most surgeons do not advise operation at the acute stage, and the treatment usually prescribed is:

1. Rest in bed.
2. Pethidine (100 mg) by injection. Morphia is not recommended since it is said to produce spasm of the sphincter of Oddi which guards the common bile duct and pancreatic duct at the ampulla of Vater.
3. Antibiotics.
4. Fluids (avoiding milk) by mouth. An intravenous line can usually be avoided unless vomiting is severe.

Radical cure of gall-stones. Gall-stones in a functioning gall bladder can be dissolved by the administration of chenodeoxycholic acid and although it has been used clinically it is still not acceptable for general use.

The stones must be composed of cholesterol and the gall bladder must be functioning. The treatment is protracted and the safety of the drug has not been established.

Removal of the gall bladder (cholecystectomy) removes the stones, the site of their formation, and a potential site for future problems. If excision of the organ is impossible, operation is confined to the removal of the stones and drainage of the gall bladder (cholecystostomy).

Care of the patient for gall-bladder operations

The usual preparation for any major abdominal operation is necessary. The main specific points concern the care of the drainage tubes and the nurse attending the patient in the theatre should take special care to note the exact position of each tube.

In all patients for cholecystectomy a nasogastric tube should be passed before the end of the operation. Patients after cholecystectomy tend to vomit a good deal of bile, and aspiration through a nasogastric tube for 24 hours eliminates this complication with its accompanying distress.

1. Drainage tube in the subhepatic pouch. The tube is inserted through a stab wound to drain the oozing of blood from the liver bed. It is also useful to reveal internal reactionary haemorrhage, and is usually removed after 48 hours. If there is any leakage of bile from the liver bed it also drains by this means.

2. Tube in the common duct. Bile flows along this tube, which is connected to a plastic bag. A T tube drain leading from the common duct to the outside (Fig. 36.6) will be inserted if the common bile duct has been explored. The volume of the bile excreted each day is measured and recorded and after 7 days a T tube cholangiogram is carried out. If this shows the bile duct to be patent the tube may be clamped for an hour or two. If the patient is pain free the tube may be withdrawn. The catgut sutures which previously secured it to the bile duct having by this time become friable and loose.

Operative cholangiography is now performed routinely and only after all stones in the ducts have been cleared is the gall-bladder removed. If the patient shows any of the features associated with recurrent stone

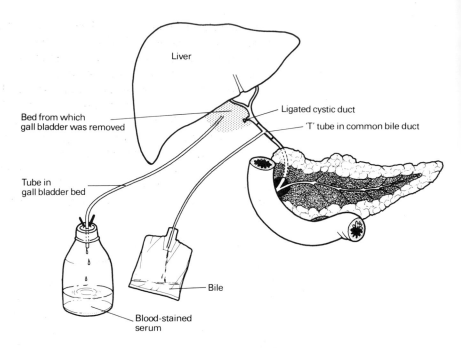

Liver

Bed from which
gall bladder was removed

Ligated cystic duct

'T' tube in common bile duct

Tube in
gall bladder bed

Bile

Blood-stained
serum

Fig. 36.6 The gall-bladder has been removed and its bed drained. The common bile duct was opened to remove a stone and closed around a 'T' tube which drains bile.

formation — the presence of biliary mud, papillary stenosis, intrahepatic stones or a grossly dilated common bile duct, an additional procedure to drain the duct may be undertaken. These include anastomosis of the duct to the duodenum or sphincteroplasty.

The intravenous line commenced in the theatre can usually be removed on the second postoperative day and a normal diet is quickly resumed. If an anastomosis of the common bile duct to the duodenum has been performed the resumption of a normal diet should be more cautious.

A specimen of bile may be sent for bacteriological examination. Where there has been severe cholangitis an antibiotic may be prescribed.

If the patient has been jaundiced or is jaundiced due to a stone in the common bile duct, vitamin K (10 mg) must be administered by injection preoperatively for three days and continued for several days after the operation. The jaundiced patient is liable to develop hepatorenal failure. This is now largely preventable by the administration of 500 ml of 10 per cent mannitol one hour before operation and this should be continued postoperatively. As mannitol produces a heavy diuresis, the fluid balance and electrolytes should be watched with great care.

Complications

1. Pulmonary complications are liable to occur especially at the base of the right lung. They may be prevented by adequate analgesia and breathing exercises.

2. Haemorrhage and bile leakage from the gall bladder bed — hence the importance of a subhepatic drainage tube.

3. Deep vein thrombosis and pulmonary embolism is more liable to occur in obese subjects. The incidence has probably decreased following the introduction of prophylactic subcutaneous heparin.

4. In the jaundiced patient there is always the danger of postoperative renal failure. This can be minimised by careful pre and postoperative intravenous fluid administration together with the administration of the osmotic diuretic mannitol during surgery.

5. Recurrent stone in the common bile duct. This will require further exploration or endoscopic division of the sphincter of Oddi may be undertaken so that the stone will pass into the duodenum.

Asiatic cholangio-hepatitis

Obstruction of the common bile duct by the liver fluke is quite common in the Far East. The smaller ducts in the liver are also involved and the patient presents with pain, Charcot's biliary fever and jaundice. As soon as he is fit the duct is emptied of stones and the liver fluke — because of similar changes in the liver a wide opening in the lower end of the duct into the duodenum is effected so that inaccessible stones and flukes as well as pus can drain. The gall bladder is also removed.

Carcinoma of the gall bladder

The new growth usually occurs in a gallbladder which contains gallstones. The rapid invasion of the liver by the growth renders most cases hopeless.

THE PANCREAS

The principal pancreatic diseases of surgical importance are acute and chronic pancreatitis and carcinoma. Rarely cysts, calculi, insulin and gastrin secreting tumours occur.

ACUTE AND RELAPSING PANCREATITIS

The great danger of this condition lies in the fact that the pancreatic juices, so potent in the digestion of fat and protein, digest the tissues with which they come in contact.

Although the exact cause remains unknown the following factors play a part in the aetiology:
(a) Gallstones.
(b) Alcohol.
(c) Viral infections such as mumps.
(d) Drugs such as steroids.
(e) Metabolic conditions — hyperparathyroidism and aminoacidurea.

Symptoms and signs

There is a sudden onset of epigastric pain and collapse, frequently after a meal. The face may be slightly cyanosed and the patient does not lie absolutely still as in the case of a perforated peptic ulcer, but tends to roll about. The temperature is subnormal in the first hours of the attack and the pulse rate is elevated. The abdomen is tender, but not rigid.

Investigation

1. The estimation of the serum amylase by the laboratory is of the greatest value. The normal is 40 to 200 Somogyi units, and in acute pancreatitis a reading of over 1000 units is usual. It should be performed in the first 24 hours.
2. A white blood count is usual.
3. The serum calcium. An estimate of the amount of calcium fixed in the formation of calcium soaps is some guide to progress.
4. Cholecystography is performed when the attack has subsided.
5. Peritoneal tap may be performed and the fluid will show the presence of pancreatic enzymes.

Complications

1. Pancreatic abscess which may require drainage.
2. Pseudocyst formation which is drained into the stomach. One in 30 patients develop a pseudocyst within the following 6 weeks.
3. Recurrence.

Treatment

There is no specific treatment for acute pancreatitis, the management of the patient being entirely supportive in type.

1. Maintenance of fluid and electrolyte balance — loss of fluid into the retroperitoneal space maybe very great. Massive transfusions of whole blood and plasma protein fraction may be vital. A careful watch is necessary to maintain an adequate urinary output. Renal failure is a very real danger.
2. Alleviation of pain — this may be very severe and intractable. Codeine phosphate by injection is the best analgesic as it relaxes the sphincter of Oddi, but pethidine may also be required.
3. Suppression of pancreatic secretion by the use of continuous gastric suction to suppress the secretion mechanism is essential.
4. Calcium gluconate 10 ml 10 per cent solution i.v. daily.

Antibiotics, and the use of anticholinergic agents to suppress pancreatic secretion are of unproven value. The use of aprotinin (Trasylol) is not only unproven but extremely expensive. Surgical interference is rarely undertaken.

CHRONIC PANCREATITIS

This is a condition in which the pancreas is slowly destroyed. It may follow acute pancreatitis but is a separate condition. Alcoholism is a prominent cause of chronic pancreatitis. It may present with:

Pain in the upper abdomen
Symptoms and signs of malabsorption
Jaundice
Diabetes

Investigations

Investigations include cholecystography, sophisticated tests to determine the secretory capacity of the pancreas and chemical examination of the stools to measure malabsorption. Duodenoscopy and cannulation of the papilla of Vater and retrograde choledochpancreatography may be performed.

Treatment

Treatment is very unsatisfactory. Pancreatic enzymes and a high calorie, high protein diet may help.

Surgical procedures undertaken for pain or persistent jaundice include division of the sphincter of Oddi. Total or subtotal pancreatectomy may be undertaken and continued alcoholism is the most important factor in predicting failure to improve.

CARCINOMA OF THE PANCREAS

(i) In the head; usually presenting with progressive obstructive jaundice.
(ii) In the body and tail — persistent pain is the prominent symptom.

The diagnosis is made only following isotope scanning, duct canalisation, duct aspiration, cytology and coeliac axis arteriography or even lapartomy.

Treatment

If jaundiced the patient will require vitamin K and mannitol preoperatively (p. 384). Anastomosis of the gall-bladder to the duodenum relieves the jaundice (cholecystoduodenostomy). Should the growth be operable, it may be excised 3 weeks later. This is a long, difficult operation and carries a high mortality rate.

Islet cell tumour

A tumour of the islet cell results in an excessive secretion of insulin. The patient suffers from recurrent hypoglycaemic attacks. Cure is effected by excision of the tumour.

Gastrin-secreting tumour

This tumour causes intractable duodenal and jejunal ulceration. The treatment is removal of the tumour if it can be located or total gastrectomy to cut off the acid response to gastrin.

BIBLIOGRAPHY

Williams K G, Dawson J L 1979 British Medical Journal 2: 766

37
Diseases of the small intestine

Inflammation of the small intestine is common but with the notable exception of Crohn's disease the response to medical treatment is usual. Carcinoma, so prevalent in the gastro-intestinal tract is a rare finding in the small bowel. The dominant surgical lesion is intestinal obstruction which has been considered in Chapter 33. Its causes and the special features of one or two particular conditions are reviewed here.

Injury

Abdominal injury may result in a tear of the small intestine. The symptoms and signs are a combination of those of internal haemorrhage and peritoneal irritation. After resuscitation laparotomy is undertaken.

INFLAMMATORY CONDITIONS OF THE SMALL INTESTINE

Meckel's diverticulum

In the last 60 cm of the ileum a diverticulum of the bowel (Fig. 35.3) not unlike the appendix, may be present. It varies in length from 5 cm to 50 cm and, like the appendix, it may become inflamed. The symptoms, signs, and treatment are similar to those of appendicitis. On other occasions it may be the cause of intestinal obstruction by ensnaring a loop of the intestine, and the clinical features are those of intestinal obstruction. An important feature of the histology of Meckel's diverticulum is the frequent presence of ectopic epithelium such as gastric and pancreatic tissue. Ectopic gastric epithelium is very apt to cause the adjacent epithelium to ulcerate and bleed. A bleeding Meckel's diverticulum is one of the commonest causes of rectal bleeding in children.

Crohn's disease or regional enteritis

This is an inflammatory condition originally described in the terminal ileum. It is now accepted that it is a generalised disease involving any part of the gastrointestinal tract, the commonest sites being the terminal ileum and the large intestine including the rectum. The cause is unknown. It may give rise to symptoms similar to appendicitis due to inflammation, or it may give rise to obstructive symptoms. Ninety per cent of all cases come to surgery eventually. Corticosteroids and immuno-suppressive drugs such as azathioprine may be prescribed but are of doubtful value. Obstruction, perforation or fistula formation are complications which occur.

The diagnosis is more often made after investigation by radiology, rectal biopsy and endoscopic examination of the colon and biopsy to distinguish it from proctocolitis.

Acute obstruction usually subsides on treatment with nasogastric suction and intravenous fluids so that if operation is necessary it can be performed as an elective procedure. Resection is the usual procedure but the recurrence rate is 40 per cent per year throughout the lifetime of the patient. Yet most sufferers from the disease remain cheerful and hopeful that things will not get much worse from a condition which is virtually a life sentence.

Intestinal obstruction

The main clinical features and treatment of acute intestinal obstruction we have already considered in Chapter 33. Chronic intestinal obstruction is a condition in which the obstruction is incomplete, and usually terminates in acute obstruction.

Causes

The bowel may be obstructed because:
1. Its lumen is blocked by a foreign body or a gall-stone.
2. Its wall is altered by disease such as Crohn's disease, a stricture due to an old tuberculous ulcer, or drugs such as potassium chloride in certain preparations, or to an intussusception.
3. The wall is constricted by something outside it; by a loop twisting around itself — adhesions or connective tissue bands. The neck of a hernial sac is the commonest cause of all.

1. Blockage by a foreign body. One cause is a gall-stone. The fundus of the gall-bladder becomes adherent to the duodenum, and slowly a fistula between the two organs is formed (Fig. 33.4). A large gall-stone may pass through the fistula and become impacted in the narrowest portion of the small intestine, the ileum. If the stone is small it may pass without difficulty. An impacted stone is removed after incision of the bowel and then the wall is re-sutured.

In some conditions of intestinal hurry, digestion has not time to occur and inadequately chewed food may block the lower ileum. This may result after gastrectomy or gastrojejunostomy. Swallowed foreign bodies such as marbles are occasionally the cause of blockage in the case of children.

2. The wall is altered by disease. Crohn's disease, which has already been discussed, is one cause. An important cause, particularly in infants under 12 months, is intussusception.

Intussusception. This is due to a small portion of the bowel becoming invaginated into the portion distal to it. As a result of peristalsis, the process is carried further until, as it were, the bowel, instead of being a single tube, now has three layers. The bowel is, in fact, telescoped into itself (Fig. 37.1).

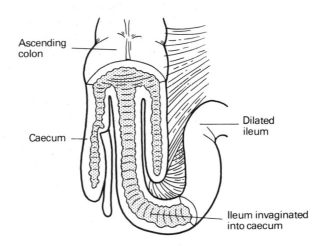

Ascending colon

Caecum

Dilated ileum

Ileum invaginated into caecum

Fig. 37.1 An intussusception.

Symptoms and signs. The child is usually a healthy male infant about 9 months old. His good health is probably the cause of excessive peristalsis driving one loop of bowel into the one below. The change of diet at the time may be a causal factor, and in the infant the Peyer's patches are enlarged so that they form a small tumour-like mass, disturbing the normal peristaltic wave. An alternative theory is that it is due to enlargement of Peyer's patches from an adenovirus which could account for its seasonal occurrence. The child screams with pain, which is typical of intestinal colic. The face becomes very pale when the colic is at its height and brightens in the intervals between the spasms. Vomiting is invariably present, and the passage of a small amount of bright red jelly-like blood clot per rectum is almost diagnostic. Careful examination of the abdomen reveals a sausage-like mass. Treatment consists of reduction of the bowel usually by operation, but retrograde pressure by barium enema may effect reduction. It should be given only under X-ray screening control. The nurse must watch especially for recurrence of symptoms on the first night after operation.

In the adult, intussusception occasionally occurs due to an adenoma, a Meckel's diverticulum, or a growth.

3. Lesions outside the bowel.

Causes
  Strangulated hernias
  Bands
  Adhesions.

Bands and adhesions may form as a result of previous operations or from tuberculous peritonitis. As in all acute obstructions, urgent operation is essential.

Mesenteric thrombosis

This condition presents with acute abdominal pain, circulatory collapse, the passage of blood from the rectum and abdominal tenderness. It is increasingly common as a manifestation of atherosclerosis. The main vessel or branch of it may be involved with gangrene of the segment of intestine supplied. The outlook is very poor however it is treated. Treatment includes resection, removal of the thrombus and anticoagulant therapy.

OPERATIONS ON THE SMALL INTESTINE

Enterostomy

1. *For feeding purposes.* This is performed:

(a) Sometimes for inoperable cancer of the stomach.
(b) Very occasionally for intractable gastric ulcer where the condition of the patient is too poor for radical operation, yet relief from medical treatment is very slight.
2. For ulcerative proctocolitis. The ileum is brought to the surface—an ileostomy (Ch. 33).

Resection

A loop of bowel is removed. The continuity of the intestine is then restored by suture.

This is usually performed for a gangrenous small intestine or for injury. Postoperatively the important points are the relief of flatus by the passage of a flatus tube and aspiration of the stomach to relieve any distension above the anastomosis as well as parenteral fluid replacement.

Enteroanastomosis

This is the short-circuiting or bypassing of one portion of the bowel into another beyond a pathological lesion without removing the cause.

This is frequently performed for an obstruction which is not causing gangrene of the intestine, such as tuberculosis of the small intestine, severe adhesions, or Crohn's disease.

Ileojejunal bypass

This has been performed for obesity. The immediate mortality is 5 per cent and the complications are many—wound dehisence, chest infection, pulmonary embolism, polyarthritis, electrolyte depletion and bypass enteritis. Weight loss is due not to malabsorption but to loss of appetite from a dilated bowel. The long-term results are poor.

Reversed loop in short gut syndrome

The short gut syndrome follows massive bowel resection in such conditions as mesenteric occlusion and internal strangulation. A loss greater than 75 per cent results in rapid intestinal transit, diarrhoea and malabsorption. If medical measures fail reversal of a $7\cdot5-14\cdot0$ cm segment of the more distal small intestine is undertaken.

BIBLIOGRAPHY

Alexander-Williams J, Fielding J F, Cooke W T 1972 Gut 13: 973
Gazzard B G, Price H L, Libby G W, Dawson A M 1978 British Medical Journal 2: 1117

38

Stoma care

Stoma care commences when the decision to form a stoma has been taken. The successful management of a stoma (literally a mouth or opening) on the abdominal wall demands surgical and nursing skills, the cooperation of the patient as well as assistance from the pharmacist, the social worker, the housing authorities and maybe those responsible for refuse disposal. The support of the patient's family and the skill of the community nurse are essential. The indications, the choice of stoma and the perioperative management are discussed in Chapters 39, 40 and 42.

Surgically attempts have been made to make stomas continent. The continent reservoir ileostomy has been designed but the complications associated with it have been too serious to commend it for general use. The magnetic ring implant (p. 404) in colostomies also has special complications.

TYPES OF STOMAS

1. Ileostomy. The terminal ileum is fashioned to project as a spout 5 centimeters long onto the skin of the abdominal wall (Figs. 38.1 and 38.2). The effluent is semi-fluid and corrosive.

2. Colostomy. The faecal discharge from an iliac colostomy is semi-solid but may be more fluid from a transverse colostomy.

3. Ileal conduit. A loop of ileum is isolated from the bowel, the upper part of the loop is closed and the ureters transplanted into the lumen. The lower end is brought out as a stoma. The small intestine is restored in continuity. (Fig. 38.3).

4. Cutaneous ureterostomy. The ends of one or both ureters are attached to the skin surface.

The problem facing the patient with a stoma of whatever type is that he is to have an opening which has no sphincter and an effluent for collection and disposal. This requires a mechanism in which leakage is prevented, damage to the stoma and surrounding skin is avoided and is also odour-proof.

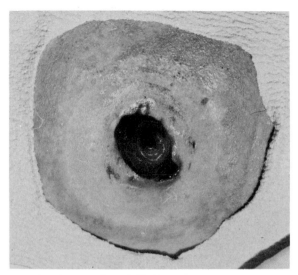

Fig. 38.1 Ileostomy showing coaption of skin to mucosa.

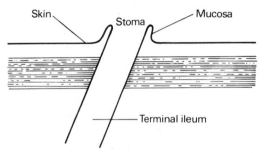

Fig. 38.2 Diagram showing the terminal ileum brought through the abdominal wall. The mucosa of the ileum is everted and sutured to the skin.

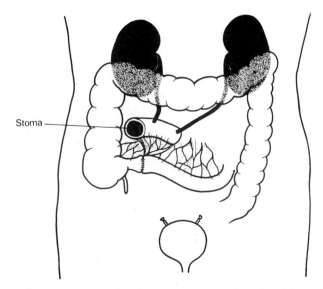

Fig. 38.3 Urinary conduit. The ureters are implanted into the isolated loop of the ileum. As shown the ileum is restored in continuity.

There are three essential preoperative steps:

1. Acceptance by the patient. The patient is often very ill, which is precisely the reason that major surgery terminating with an ileostomy is advised.

To the desperately ill patient with severe proctocolitis or severe intestinal obstruction any relief is welcome. The patient suffering from a lesion such as carcinoma of the rectum who feels comparatively well finds a stoma difficult to accept.

The surgeon should preferably see the patient alone and satisfy himself that not only is consent obtained but that the patient understands to what he is consenting. His approach will depend on the personality of the patient and vary according to his age, intelligence, work and other relevant factors. He will be told that the stoma is a projecting moist and red spout of normal bowel. He must be reassured that he will be taught how to look after it and will not be discharged home until he is proficient in its care, and that afterwards he will have the support and care of the unit. He can be reassured that he need not worry about odours and other people will be unaware that he is wearing a bag. Potency is worth mentioning at this stage. All potency is abolished in the male following total cystectomy and it may follow abdominoperineal resection of the rectum or a total proctocolectomy. Nonetheless, the thought of a stoma is very distressing to most patients but their fears about eating, ability to work and partake in normal activities can be allayed.

The next person to discuss the problem with the patient is the stoma care nurse (stomatherapist). Her specialised knowledge and support in the hospital and in the future will inspire confidence. She may arrange a meeting with an ileostomy patient of the same sex who can encourage and help. The patient's relatives should also be involved at this stage.

2. Siting the stoma. This is marked on the abdominal wall a day or two before the operation by the surgeon and stoma care nurse together. An ileostomy flange is fixed to the skin, avoiding scars, creases of fat and boney prominences with the patient lying in bed and standing. The bag is then fitted. The site chosen is usually midway between the umbilicus and the anterior superior spine but avoiding the patient's belt line. It is then indelibly marked on the skin of the abdominal wall. This disc of skin is removed as the first step at operation before the abdominal wall is distorted by major incision. The siting for a temporary colostomy is not usually as important because it is done as an emergency and hopefully it would be closed before too long. The ongoing problems should not arise.

3. Allergy testing. The patient should be tested for allergy to the materials used in the appliance to avoid allergic reactions at a stage when they can be most inconvenient.

THE APPLIANCES

There is a wide choice of appliances available for all types of stomas and continuous research is in progress to improve them. The final choice will be made by the patient, assisted by the stomatherapist. This can be decided only when the oedema and swelling of the stoma subside and the patient finds a technique of management at which he is efficient. He is in no way committed to use what has been applied in the immediate postoperative period. It is explained to the patient that the bag with which he comes back from the theatre is for the convenience of nursing observations like drainage and not for the patient's convenience. That will come later when he is going home.

The shape of the stoma may change as time progresses and it should be noted that while most are rounded some stomas are almost square.

The *two main types* of appliance are 'closed' and 'drainable' which can be in either a single piece or in two pieces (Fig. 38.4). The one piece consists of a bag and an attached adhesive square which sticks to the skin around the stoma. The two piece consists of a flange which adheres to the skin and a bag which can be removed from the face of the flange without disturbing the skin.

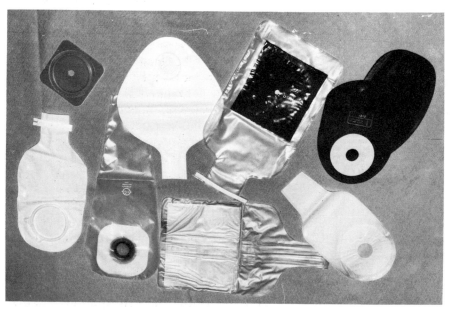

Fig. 38.4 Types of drainable stoma bags showing type of outlet and closures. Suitable post operatively or for an ileostomy.

The closed bag would be used for a patient with a reasonably well formed stool and the drainable for one that requires frequent draining of the effluent such as an ileostomy, a caecostomy or transverse colostomy. The urobags have a different kind of seal at the bottom to reduce the risk of leakage.

All stoma bags fitted at operation should be drainable and transparent so that the stoma can be inspected and the effluent drained without disturbance. Later, opaque bags may be used to conceal sight of the effluent and a cover of cotton-polyester conveniently absorbs sweat from the skin. The bags are odourproof and disposable bags are usually preferred. A belt may be worn with the appliance while the abdominal muscles are still weak but with experience the patient may decide it is unnecessary. For those who engage in heavy work or sporting activities stronger non-disposable materials may be used and a belt is essential.

ILEOSTOMY

At the end of the operation the wound and the skin around the stoma may be protected by stomadhesive and an appliance is fitted. As soon as possible the patient is taught to look after the stoma. The stoma is insensitive but delicate and easily traumatised. The surrounding skin has to be kept in good condition and will become sore if leakage occurs. The basic problem is to maintain a perfect seal between the skin and the appliance which may be changed as often as the patient feels it is necessary but, in any case, not longer than every 7 days.

Normally the rule for aseptic technique is — 'from clean area into dirty area' but in the case of a stoma patient any soiling — due to a leaking bag etc., should be cleaned up and a fresh bag applied prior to any aseptic technique being carried out.

This method allows the stoma bag to be undisturbed for several days should the surgical dressing encroach on the adhesive area of the bag.

If stomadhesive is put on top of a surgical dressing, leakage will inevitably follow because an inadequate seal has been achieved.

Postoperative care of the stoma

1. The abdominal dressing will have to be changed if it is soiled. The stoma bag should be changed before the midline dressing because the bag can stay on for several days whereas the dressing may need changing more frequently. If the bag is put on after the dressing overlapping will occur and this would lead to leakage.

2. The stitches. Some surgeons prefer to remove the stitches after 5–6 days even if they are of catgut to avoid 'bumpy' healing around the stoma which predisposes to leakage. This is especially so in urinary stomas.

3. Baths. While still in hospital the patient can get into the bath with an appliance on if the wound is unhealed. Once it has healed a bath may be taken without the appliance and the skin would benefit from washing.

4. Skin soreness and leakage are discussed below.

Surgical complications at the stoma

1. Skin soreness is discussed below but, in addition to the causes mentioned, poor siting of the stoma may require revision.

2. Prolapse, recession or fistula formation, as well as obstruction may necessitate surgical refashioning of the stoma.

3. Bleeding is usually due to damage by the flange and will clear up as soon as the cause is recognised and corrected.

4. Recurrent disease does not occur in proctocolitis but may be the cause if the stoma was fashioned for Crohn's disease and further investigation is indicated.

5. Hernia formation adds to the difficulties of secure healing. It may be controlled with a suitable belt.

Changing the appliance

The final choice of the type of appliance will be made by the patient with the advice of the stoma nurse and amongst the factors to be considered will be the general condition of the patient. A bag which at first sight may seem to be unsuitable because it is too large and without stomadhesive may be advised. An elderly person with arthritic hands and poor eyesight may find it difficult to manage stomadhesive and positioning the bag correctly over the stoma. Someone with a poor prognosis would be given a bag they can stick straight on. Their condition and their ability to manage are going to deteriorate.

In a two piece appliance the bag is detached, the stoma wiped free of mucus or faecal material with a soft paper tissue and the bag attached to the flange. When the whole appliance is changed, whether it is a one or

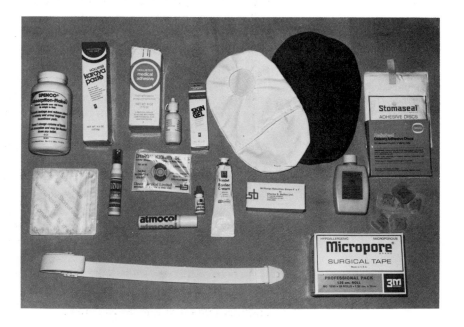

Fig. 38.5 Ileostomy accessories:
Skin protection Adhesives
Deodorants Karaya Paste
Bag covers Flatus filter
Spenco flakes (render very fluid output more solid and lessen risk of leakage.

two piece, the following equipment is necessary:-
1. A new appliance.
2. Warm water.
3. White tissues.
4. Double sided plaster, stomahesive, Karaya washers or paste.
5. A pair of scissors.
6. A bowl lined with newspaper for discarded tissues and the appliance.
The new appliance is prepared and the old appliance removed by gently peeling it off. The stoma and the surrounding skin is wiped with soft tissue to remove old Karaya or faecal material. Adhesive material still adherent to the skin is best removed by the patient taking a bath rather than by using solvents. Otherwise the area is washed with warm water using no soap. The skin is thoroughly dried with tissues and adhesive is applied only when the skin is absolutely dry. The new appliance is fitted and the old appliance and soiled tissues wrapped in newspaper for disposal.

Leakage and skin soreness

This may occur because, —
1. The skin was not completely dry.
2. The plaster was wrinkled.
3. The flange was not fitted correctly over the stoma or the hole in the appliance was not the correct size. This may also cause bleeding from injury to the spout of ileum. The stoma contracts for several weeks following the operation and it is essential to measure the size. Discs are provided by the manufacturers for this purpose.
4. The patient has increased in weight so the appliance is ill-fitting.
5. Air from the bag has not been expelled.
6. The bag has been allowed to overfill or a bag which is too large has been used so that the flange is soaked in effluent.
7. The site of the stoma is poor.
8. *Allergic reaction* even on occasions to the Karaya gum, the adhesive as well as other materials.
9. *Monilial infection of the mouth* can extend to the skin around the stoma. Many patients have been on antibiotics which, as well as diarrhoea, may induce a monilial infection.
As soon as skin soreness appears every effort is made to discover and correct the cause. Assuming the preoperative allergy tests (p. 396) negative skin soreness is treated by application of stomadhesive with Karaya gum to the excoriated skin so that it acts as a second skin on which the appliance can be placed. In severe reactions hydrocortisone cream may be prescribed but stomadhesive can be used on top to act as a surface on which to put the appliance. The cream content may prevent the bag sticking but there are barrier creams which will allow the adhesive to stick. Soreness sufficiently severe to require hydrocortisone while the patient is in hospital should have been investigated and corrected before it became so severe. It should be borne in mind that hydrocortisone is absorbed by the stoma.
If leakage is due to old scars, skin folds or creases, Karaya paste is used to mould the equipment over them to secure a tight fit.

Other requirements of the patient

1. Access to the advice of a stomatherapist.
2. A bathroom in his home.
3. Ready access to a supply of new equipment.
4. A settled method of disposal of used appliances and wipes. The bag's contents can be emptied into the lavatory but the bag is wrapped in newspaper, placed in a plastic bag which is tied and disposed of in the dust bin. If this is not possible other arrangements are made with the authorities. They should not be burnt in an open fire as plastic gives off nasty acid fumes.

ILEAL URINARY CONDUIT

The ureters are implanted into a free isolated loop of ileum (Fig. 38.3). The stoma, which looks identical with an ileostomy stoma, discharges urine and a little mucus but no faecal material (Fig. 38.6). The management of the appliance and the care of the stoma is identical to that of an ileostomy. Immediately after the operation a Foley catheter is inserted into the loop, the balloon inflated and the catheter brought out through the flange of the appliance into the collecting bag. Ureteric catheters may have been inserted and drain in the same way. Seven days later, if they have not been extricated previously they are removed. A bag with a non-return valve should be used and at night a drainage bag with tubing can be attached if necessary (Fig. 38.7). Complications are similar to those of an ileostomy stoma but, in addition, the following may develop:—

1. Obstruction of the stoma. It will be noticed that the urinary volume has diminished and the flow is slow. A gloved finger passed into the stoma

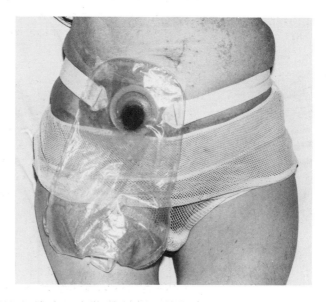

Fig. 38.6 Urinary ileal conduit with bag attached.

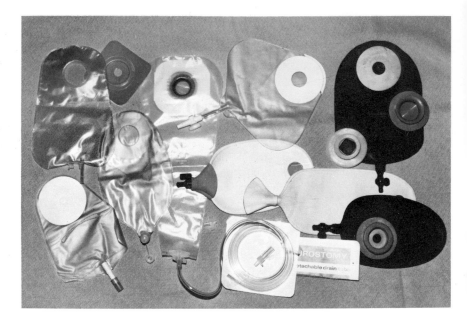

Fig. 38.7 Equipment for urostomy. Note the outlet on the bags, one of which shows night drainage tube attached.

is all that is usually necessary. A catheter may be inserted to drain the loop.

3. **Urinary infection** is a constant hazard. A specimen of urine is taken from the stoma with a sterile catheter for bacteriological examination — one from the bag is of no value. Mucus found in the urine from an ileal conduit is quite normal and not indicative of a urinary infection.

3. **Phosphatic deposits and encrustation** from infected urine may occur on the stoma. The urine is acidified with ascorbic or mandelic acid and the appropriate antibiotic administered. The patient is confined to bed and a wet dressing of half strength vinegar dissolves the deposits and reduces the oedema in a few days. The bag needs to be a neat fit otherwise leakage will occur.

Cutaneous ureterostomy

The ureters are stitched to the skin and urine collected by means of stick-on bags. The problems are much greater than those of an ileal conduit as leakage is more likely.

COLOSTOMY AND CAECOSTOMY

The formation of an artificial anus entails bringing a portion of the large intestine to the surface of the abdominal wall so that its contents are diverted to the exterior.

This may take the form of either a colostomy or a caecostomy. Of the two, the colostomy is undoubtedly preferable because the faeces become more solid as they approach the rectum.

The faecal discharge from a caecostomy is thin and extremely irritant, so that, as a permanent arrangement, it is unsatisfactory. It is occasionally performed as an emergency measure in a patient who is so ill from obstruction of the distal bowel that exploration of the abdomen is impossible. After a low anastomosis in the distal bowel it may be performed as a temporary 'safety valve'.

A colostomy is performed either as a temporary or permanent measure for growths of the pelvic colon or rectum. It is almost invariably performed in cases of wounds of the rectum, so that the faecal flow is deviated from the wound. Congenital absence of the rectum or paraplegia in young adults is occasionally an indication.

CAECOSTOMY

A caecostomy is performed by the insertion of a tube into the caecum. The opening is usually valvular in type and frequently closes spontaneously after the tube has been removed.

The tube is connected to a Bardic bag by the bedside so that the drainage is dependent and the discharge does not irritate the skin. After 24 hours when the caecostomy site is sealed off by inflammatory adhesions twice daily irrigation of 50 ml normal saline is commenced. As much as possible of the colonic contents as well as the irrigating fluid is withdrawn and drainage continues.

After 10 days, however, the tube drops out, and every effort must be made to prevent the skin from becoming inflamed and excoriated. Moist and petroleum jelly dressings tend to make the skin soggy. Stomadhesive with a good seal will protect the skin.

A permanent caecostomy is almost unmanageable from the patient's point of view and if at all possible it is avoided by anastomosis of the ileum to the transverse colon.

COLOSTOMY

The varieties of colostomy are illustrated in Figure 38.8.

1. Loop colostomy. A loop of colon is brought to the surface of the abdominal wall and held in position by a thin rod passed through the

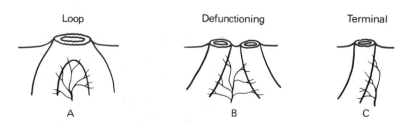

Fig. 38.8   Types of colostomy.

mesocolon. The wound is then sutured. The colostomy is opened immediately.

2. Defunctioning colostomy. The loop is exteriorised and then divided so that there is no communication between the two orifices which are now separated by a bridge of skin. This provides complete rest to the distal colon.

3. End or terminal colostomy. The colonic mucous membrane is sutured to the skin. Since this is usually performed only when all the distal bowel has been removed there is only one orifice. It is performed in conditions such as abdomino-perineal resection of the rectum and there is no possibility of subsequent closure. The patient should not be given any false hope that the colostomy can be removed.

A colostomy may be performed in the ascending, transverse or pelvic colon. The more distally it can be placed the better as the contents become more solid. A loop colostomy has a rod which is very slender and is brought out subcutaneously so that when the colon is opened and the mucosa sutured to the skin a colostomy appliance can be fitted immediately. The rod is removed about the tenth day.

As all colostomies are now opened at once a colostomy bag is fitted at the end of the operation. Suitable ones are transparent disposable bags with a Karaya gum seal which can be emptied from the bottom without disturbing the seal. In the immediate postoperative period the effluent is usually very fluid and large in amount. Inspection of the colostomy is possible without disturbing the appliance. The stools become more solid after 4 or 5 days. The patient is now instructed in the use of a colostomy appliance. The choice is between a stick-on bag which is more liable to cause skin irritation and a disposable bag with a flange which has to be changed once or twice a week.

A magnet continent colostomy device. A magnetic ring may be implanted subcutaneously and the colon is drawn through it at the operation to make the colostomy. The stoma is treated on conventional lines for 3 to 6 weeks, when the magnetic cap is fitted. It is still under trial but is not without complications.

The orifices of a colostomy

A loop colostomy has two orifices (Fig. 38.9):

1. The 'active' orifice through which faecal material is discharged and which leads proximally away from the growth.

2. The 'non-active' orifice, which leads distally towards the growth. Usually only mucus is discharged from this opening.

The nurse should be able to recognise the 'active' orifice, because it is through this opening that washouts are normally given. The 'active' orifice in an iliac colostomy is usually the upper opening, the 'non-active' one the lower. In a transverse colostomy the opening towards the right side of the abdomen is the active orifice and towards the left the non-active. A terminal colostomy has only an active orifice as the bowel below it (usually the rectum) has been removed. If the nurse is in any doubt, or the colostomy performed is not one with which she is familiar, she should have no hesita-

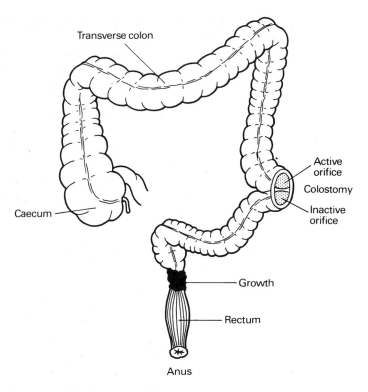

Fig. 38.9 Diagram of the orifices of a loop colostomy.

tion in asking the surgeon which is the active orifice.

A washout should be given through the non-active orifice:

1. Before a second stage operation for excision of the rectum or colon. (In this case the active orifice must, of course, also be washed out).

2. If the patient with a colostomy is troubled by excessive mucus or pus from a fungating growth.

Postoperative management and complications

1. The rod is removed about the tenth postoperative day.

2. The sutures are removed about the fifth or sixth day if the wound has healed.

3. Regulation of the bowel. Normally the bowel will act without any special measures. If the bowel is obstinate a Dulcolax suppository may be inserted into the opening of the colostomy and this usually produces a good result. Exceptionally, a washout through the colostomy may be given in the same way as rectal washouts are performed.

Once the bowel has been regulated, washouts and enemas are unnecessary. Some authorities find that about half their patients prefer washouts for control of the stoma. The appropriate apparatus has now made this procedure safe.

Diarrhoea may occur as a reaction to one or more components of the diet which must be traced and eliminated. Natural wheat bran is helpful.

Diarrhoea may be checked by the administration of kaolin opiates, codeine or amphetamine sulphate. If it is persistent, however, it should be investigated. If this shows no obvious cause and severe 'looseness' persists, spironolactone may be given.

4. Dressing. Provided full control has been obtained gauze or lint smeared with petroleum jelly is all that is necessary. A disposable plastic bag is worn attached with adhesive. The skin around the stump should be washed with warm soapy water.

Complications of a colostomy

1. *Sepsis* in the wound.

2. *Prolapse of the bowel*. In this condition a loop of bowel above the colostomy is blown out through the wound. It is usually due to a technical error in selecting the wrong portion of the bowel at operation. The doctor will usually be able to reduce it in the ward.

3. *Retraction*. The loop may slip back into the abdomen, particularly if the mesentery is very short. Another cause for this complication is too early removal of the rod.

4. *Intestinal obstruction*. A loop of small bowel may become ensnared at the side of the colostomy. The symptoms are those of small bowel obstruction, and urgent laparotomy is indicated.

5. *Contracture of the colostomy orifice*. This is usually prevented by excision of an area of skin when performing the colostomy opening. Occasionally it may be necessary to dilate the opening by inserting a gloved finger.

6. *Bleeding* may occur from injury to the junction of the colonic mucous membrane and the skin. The usual cause is a flange that is too small and this should be corrected. Sometimes small granulomatous patches develop and can be cauterised with a silver nitrate stick. If there is no obvious local pathology to account for the bleeding reinvestigation of the colon is undertaken by the usual methods — radiography and endoscopy.

7. *Sore skin* is usually due to leakage, an ill fitting appliance or reaction to an ingredient in one of the appliance's components. In order to heal the skin the cause must be established — then steps taken to remove or reduce it.

The size of the appliance may need altering — erosion can occur if the appliance rubs against the stoma whilst excoriation can occur if skin is exposed to the bag's contents. Faulty application e.g. stoma not central in gasket can result in both these conditions occurring together.

Appliances that have a precut gasket only offer a circular opening thus an elipse of skin will be exposed in the case of a double barrel colostomy. This area can be protected by the use of barrier cream or stomahesive which has been carefully cut to the correct shape. Leakage can be prevented by careful application of the bag using agents such as Karaya paste and Karaya powder to fill in gullies or flatten ridges as necessary.

Where reactions to substances has occured then contact with that substance must cease. A different appliance may be the answer, or the patient may prefer to keep their now familiar appliance but to introduce stomahesive and/or barrier cream. Castellani's paint has been found to be very effective in helping to heal a sore skin but, as it is spirit based, it will cause some considerable discomfort if the skin is broken — this effect can be resolved by diluting the solution with ordinary water.

Early detection and treatment saves much time, effort and pain.

Instructions to the patient

There are 100 000 patients with colostomy in Great Britain. Certain basic amenities are essential for the management of colostomy, and these include an indoor lavatory, a bath and hot water. A patient with a colostomy should have top priority for housing. They also require more home help and modern cleaning and laundry methods. Some form of incineration is necessary for dressings. The laundry service for the incontinent should be used but, in most areas, it does not function at the weekend. The community services can be a tremendous help to the patient with a colostomy.

The patient should be taught how to attend to the colostomy. A colostomy is compatible with a useful and happy life but the initial training is most important. Routine washouts are unnecessary and harmful. There is a danger of colitis or perforation. With training the colostomy will function once or twice a day. Fruit and pips usually irritate the colostomy but what the patient can eat is largely a matter of intelligent investigation by himself. An agent which retains water and renders the stool soft but formed may be advisable. Agar or methyl cellulose in granules taken with water in the morning may be helpful.

GENERAL ADVICE TO THE STOMA PATIENT

1. Diet. The patient can eat what he fancies and discovers what is unsuitable by trial and error. Digestion and absorption are largely unimpaired. Natural wheat bran helps to regulate the bowel. Many patients find onions, beans and peas keep the bowel very loose. The patient should drink as much fluid as before, alcohol is not forbidden but beer may need to be restricted because the large volume increases the quantity of the effluent.

2. Work and exercise. The majority of patients return to their previous occupation and resume sporting activities. When swimming a plastic disc cup may be fitted over the flange or stoma.

3. Drugs. Many drugs affect stoma function. Oral antibiotics may cause diarrhoea while the tricyclic antidepressants by their anticholinergic action cause constipation as will analgesics.

4. Washing the bag. The bag can be washed out instead of removal daily. A 50 ml syringe or a jug may be used to fill the bag with warm water. The bag is shaken and drained so that the patient is left with a clean bag.

5. Unsuitable lotions which produce skin irritation include Savlon and Tinc Benz, nor should Dettol be used to wash out a bag.

6. Rectal bowel action. Where the rectum has not been excised and is still in continuity with the bowel the patient will have an occasional bowel action. The patient who has had a total colectomy and ileostomy performed but in which the rectum has been closed from above should be warned that he may occasionally pass a little mucus.

7. Sexual advice. When all the wounds have healed normal sexual activities may be resumed and many ileostomists become parents.

8. Societies are self help groups formed by the patients themselves and groups include the Ileostomy, Colostomy and Urinary Conduit Associations. They will make domiciliary and hospital visits pre and post operatively and help mostly with day to day living whereas the medical staff are better able to give advice on appliances. By attending the meetings that are held the patient can obtain samples of new appliances without bothering their general practitioner.

The closure of a colostomy

When it is anticipated that a colostomy will ultimately be closed it is advisable to train the patient to perform sphincter exercises each day, so that there is no atrophy of the anal sphincter when it comes into action again.

The closure of a colostomy may be a dangerous operation unless the bowel is carefully prepared. It is essential to be certain that the bowel between the colostomy opening and the anus is not obstructed. A barium enema is administered through the anus and the barium is allowed to run out of the colostomy opening. Radiographs will confirm the patency or otherwise of the segment of bowel.

Preoperative preparation

The colostomy wound must be firmly and completely healed before the operation can be attempted. The lower bowel must be completely free of hard faecal material. Rectal washouts are given after the instillation of olive oil to soften the material. A further X-ray is taken to ensure no barium remains in the colon or rectum.

Postoperative treatment

A flatus tube should be passed every 4 hours, but enemas must *not* be given for fear of perforating the sutured bowel.

A careful watch must be kept for the symptoms of peritonitis.

BIBLIOGRAPHY

Care of Stoma Patient Conference 1975. Abbott Laboratories Royal College of Nursing Stoma Care Forum 1979. Abbott Laboratories Stoma Care 1973.

39

Diseases of the caecum and the colon

The main diseases of the large intestine are inflammatory conditions and new growths. New growths of the colon are one of the more favourable sites for treatment.

INFLAMMATORY CONDITIONS OF THE COLON

Ulcerative proctocolitis

Non-specific ulceration of the colonic and rectal mucous membrane is a condition which is usually treated medically. The aid of the surgeon is sought when it is considered that the bowel is so diseased that excision is advisable. The usual operation consists of making an artificial opening in the terminal ileum known as an ileostomy (Fig. 38.1) after total colectomy or total proctocolectomy. An alternative procedure is anastomosis of the ileum to the rectum.

The patient may present with:

1. Acute fulminating disease which is a desperate emergency. Medical measures have failed, the patient is loaded with cortisone and is dying from a combination of severe haemorrhage and gross toxic absorption. Total removal of the colon has to be undertaken as a life-saving measure.

2. Relapsing proctocolitis although requiring the same extensive surgical ablation presents the opportunity to correct anaemia, fluid and electrolyte imbalance as well as vitamin deficiency. The problems arising from the formation of an ileostomy can be discussed with the patient.

At the end of the operation the main wound is sealed off and protected from the ileostomy. Postoperatively, resuscitation may be exacting, particularly following an operation for fulminating disease, and should be treated in an intensive care unit. The care of the stoma is an important procedure and has been discussed in detail in Chapter 38.

Antibiotic colitis

Diarrhoea is a fairly common sequel to antibiotic therapy. Occasionally it may herald the onset of:-

1. *Staphylococceal enterocolitis*. See Chapter 35.

2. *Pseudomembranous colitis* which may develop after antibiotic therapy and after surgical operation. Diarrhoea which is profuse but usually not bloodstained may occur during, or even a week or two after the antibiotic treatment is discontinued. The patient may be toxic, disorientated and collapsed. Sigmoidoscopy reveals the characteristic pseudomembrane. The disease is caused by *Cl. difficile* which secretes a powerful necrotising toxin. The administration of vancomycin is usually curative.

Ischaemic colitis

This condition is due to arterial insufficiency in the colon and is usually diagnosed after investigation by a barium enema. The splenic flexure area is the portion most usually involved, and when the disease is localised to a short segment resection and end to end anastomosis may be performed.

Crohn's disease (See chapter 37).

DIVERTICULAR DISEASE OF THE COLON

This is a condition of disorder of muscle function of the bowel. There is an increase in the tone of the longitudinal muscle and contraction of the circular muscle. The result is muscular hypertrophy. Diverticulum formation is a complication of this muscle abnormality and infection is a complication which may occur in a diverticulum. The corrugations of the bowel are very striking in a dissected specimen (Fig. 39.1). A diverticulum may perforate causing peritonitis or several diverticula may form a conglomerate inflamed mass, sometimes with abscess formation. The inflammatory mass may form a stricture and obstruct the bowel, and can be easily mistaken for a new growth. The inflammatory process may involve the bladder, and a fistula between the colon and the bladder is most commonly due to this condition (Fig. 33.4C).

Clinical features

The patient is usually past middle life, and, according to the course of the disease, the clinical features vary.

1. *Peritoneal symptoms* may be most prominent:
   (a) Pain, particularly in the left iliac fossa.
   (b) Constipation and some urgency of micturition.
   (c) Vomiting is usually present.
   (d) The temperature and pulse rate are elevated.
   On examination a localised mass may be felt in the left iliac fossa.

2. *Obstructive symptoms*. A fibrous stricture may form, and the symptoms are those of large bowel obstruction (p. 351).

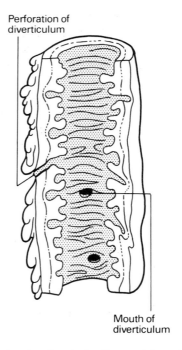

Fig. 39.1 Segment of colon showing diverticular disease of the colon complicated by perforation.

Treatment

The majority of acute episodes subside with rest in bed and a low residue diet during the acute phase. As a long term measure a low residue diet is undesirable because it causes constipation and obesity and, therefore, a normal or high residue diet is advised.

If a palpable mass is present the Ochsner-Sherren regime (Ch. 34) is instituted. A front perforation of the colon causes faecal peritonitis and after resuscitation resection of the affected segment and a colostomy is performed. The peritoneal cavity is drained and peritoneal lavage (Ch. 34) instituted. The bowel continuity is restored by a subsequent operation.

An elective resection of the colon with end to end anastomosis is indicated for fistula formation, recurrent abscess, haemorrhage and intractable disease.

Hirschsprung's disease

This is a congenital lesion, probably genetic in origin, due to the absence of ganglion cells of the myenteric nerve plexuses (of Auerbach and Meissner) in the rectum and colon (Fig. 39.2). The bowel is paralysed, peristalsis does not occur and the contents of the gut cannot move. The normal bowel proximal to the paralysed section becomes very distended with gas and faeces. The baby's abdomen is distended, he passes little or no meconium and soon vomits. If a little finger is passed into the rectum the baby may deflate and be well for a few days before the symptoms recur.

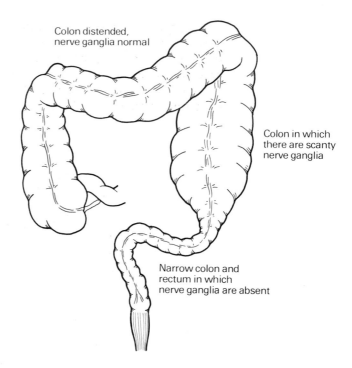

Colon distended,
nerve ganglia normal

Colon in which
there are scanty
nerve ganglia

Narrow colon and
rectum in which
nerve ganglia are absent

Fig. 39.2 Hirschsprung's disease.

Treatment

Treatment depends on the severity of the obstruction. Babies with only a short length of abnormal colon may be treated by the frequent passage of a soft rectal tube or small saline washouts. Diagnosis can then be confirmed by a radio-opaque enema and rectal biopsy. Babies with a long segment require an emergency laparotomy and a colostomy is performed in the normal colon. Once the wound has healed and feeding established, the child can go home. There is no urgency to proceed to the next stage of treatment, which should be deferred until the baby weighs about 11·4 kg. He is then readmitted for the operation of rectosigmoidectomy.

NEW GROWTHS OF THE COLON AND CAECUM

Carcinoma of the large bowel causes 14 000 deaths each year in the United Kingdom. It is commoner in north-west Europe and North America. The areas of large incidence of disease have a high standard of living. Several studies indicate a possible relationship of large bowel cancer to diet, either excess of fat or protein. The theory is that intestinal bacteria produce carcinogens from the dietary fat and from the bile steroids.

Familial polyposis of the colon is a condition in which carcinomatous change is inevitable and only a total proctocolectomy will save the patient. It should be undertaken before malignant changes occur and all members of the family must be examined regularly.

Malignant growths, usually carcinomas, are extremely common. They may occur in any portion of the large bowel, but the most common sites in order are the rectum, the pelvic colon, and the caecum. Although some growths, particularly in the caecum, are soft and proliferative, the vast majority grow around the bowel and eventually cause obstruction by forming a ring stricture (Fig. 39.3).

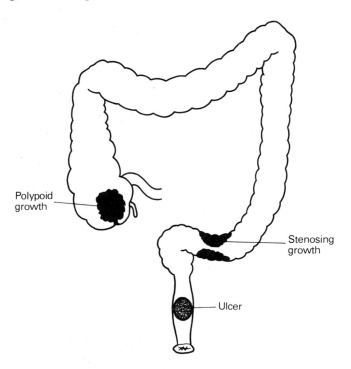

Fig. 39.3   The commonest sites and types of malignant growths in the large intestine.

Symptoms and signs

Increasing constipation is the most important symptom. At first, aperients give relief. Later the dose has to be increased, with a diminished effect, and finally the bowel action ceases. Many patients present themselves suffering from acute obstruction.

Pain is not prominent, and is usually described by the patient as being due to 'wind'. This is quite an accurate description, since his difficulty arises in his inability to pass flatus. The passage of small quantities of blood is an occasional complaint, but severe haemorrhage is uncommon.

Anaemia particularly hypochromic in type may be the presenting and only symptom of carcinoma of the caecum.

A lump in the right iliac fossa felt by the patient is unfortunately not an uncommon symptom in carcinoma of the right colon and caecum.

Other symptoms may occur. The increasing size of the abdomen is a frequent complaint, and is due to distension of the bowel. In later cases the distension is further increased by secondary deposits which cause ascites (free fluid in the peritoneal cavity).

Diarrhoea with mucus, particularly alternating with constipation, is not uncommon and is due to ulceration of the bowel above the growth by retained faeces. Loss of weight appears slowly.

Examination of the abdomen may reveal a palpable mass or a distended large bowel. In early cases nothing abnormal can be made out on abdominal or rectal examination.

Investigations

Radiographic examination of the colon after the administration of a barium enema or barium meal may be performed. Exfoliative cytology (p. 197) may be undertaken.

Preparation of the patient for a barium enema. Preparation may be for 48 hours, or shorter preparation (an enema given the previous night, and a colonic washout next morning at least 2 hours before examination) may be satisfactory. Occasionally in the ambulant patients preparation by Dulcolax suppositories is satisfactory.

Sigmoidoscopy is of value for growths in the lower bowel 30 cms from the anus.

Fibreoptic colonoscopy (Fig. 39.4) enables the whole of the large intestine to be visualised. The examination is performed under sedation and is aided by image intensification X-ray control to check the position of the

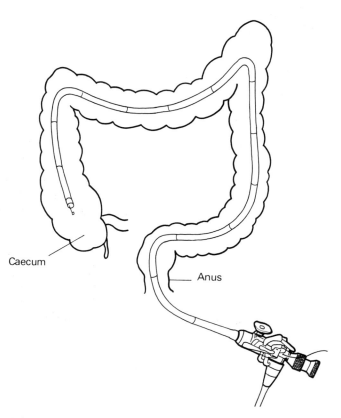

Caecum

Anus

Fig. 39.4 Colonoscopy.

instrument. The examination may take up to an hour and should always follow a barium enema study. In addition to diagnosis polyps can be removed with the diathermy snare without the patient having to undergo open surgery. A colonic anastomosis can be inspected to detect recurrence following resection for carcinoma. The colon should be clean and empty for a satisfactory examination.

Treatment

Treatment consists of a partial colectomy depending on the site of the growth (Fig. 39.5.) A growth which cannot be removed is short circuited (Fig. 39.6) to prevent the onset of intestinal obstruction.

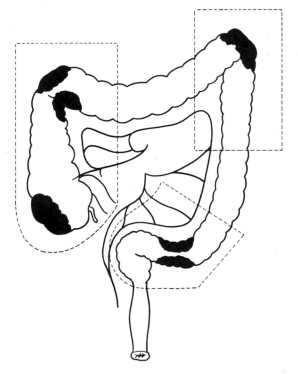

Fig. 39.5 Colectomy: extent of resection of bowel and lymphatic field for carcinoma in various parts of the colon.

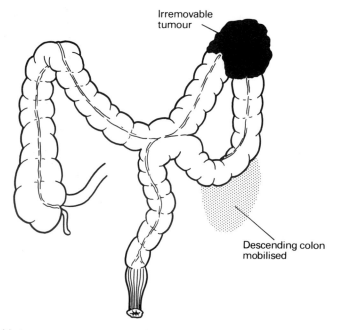

Irremovable tumour

Descending colon mobilised

Fig. 39.6 Colocolic anastomosis short-circuiting an irremovable tumour.

THE CARE OF THE PATIENT FOR COLONIC OPERATIONS

The principal procedures for colonic diseases are:

1. Colostomy which has been reviewed in detail in Chapter 38. If at all possible and if colectomy is not feasible a short circuiting procedure is preferable.

2. Colectomy. The preoperative care has in addition to the usual preparations for a major abdominal procedure two special aims:

(a) *The relief of mild obstructive symptoms* if present so that a one stage procedure with restoration of continuity of the bowel can be undertaken. A light non-residue diet and repeated enemas and washouts over several days may be required to clear the bowel.

(b) *To prevent infection* at the anastomosis and in the abdominal wound. Colectomy involves cutting across and suturing the large intestine the lumen of which is normally teeming with bacteria. The single most effective procedure is to ensure that the bowel is empty of faecal material at operation. The diet is reduced and for the 2 days before operation only fluids are allowed by mouth. The bowel is washed out the day before operation and again on the morning of the operation until the effluent is clear. An hour immediately preoperatively a rectal tube is passed to recover any residual fluid.

Antibacterial substances are taken by mouth to reduce infection and suppress E.Coli but at the expense of propagating dangerous non-clostridial anaerobes which infect the anastomosis causing leakage and breakdown of the abdominal incision. These are more effectively controlled by the administration of metronidazole (500 mg) given intravenously in 100 ml of saline in the anaesthetic room over a period of 20 minutes and repeated in similar dosage 8 and 16 hours later (Eykyn et al).

In addition systemic antibiotics may be prescribed. The nasty foul smelling pus in infected wounds following colectomy is caused by the non-clostridial anaerobes and not by E. Coli which produces *odourless* pus.

The after care

Enemas which may rupture the anastomosis should not be given but the passage of a flatus tube helps to relieve distension. Some surgeons perform a three finger dilatation of the anus for a similar purpose.

The general postoperative care described in Chapter 4 is necessary.

A low residue diet is consumed until the bowel has healed. Drains are removed when ordered and any signs suggestive of the development of a fistula, for example gas bubbles or a faecal discharge, reported at once.

Late complications include:

1. Bowel frequency is sometimes distressing after right hemicolectomy due to reduced water absorption. Isogel 5 ml t.d.s. or codeine phosphate 30–60 mg t.d.s. may help. In some cases lactose intolerance is the problem and a week's trial of excluding milk from the diet may be prescribed. When a considerable portion of the ileum has been removed as part of the operation bile salts may not be absorbed and watery diarrhoea may be produced. Cholestyramine 1–4 g may be advised.

2. Vitamin B$_{12}$ deficiency. As vitamin B$_{12}$ is absorbed from the lower ileum a careful watch should be kept for the onset of macrocytic anaemia, and intramuscular vitamin B$_{12}$ may be required indefinitely.

BIBLIOGRAPHY

Barlett J G, Te Wen Chang, Onderdonk A B 1978 Lancet 1: 338

40

Diseases of the rectum and the anus

The management of diseases of the rectum and anal canal demands considerable nursing skill. Unlike most operative wounds healing is by secondary intention because primary suture is usually impossible.

Rectal examination

This procedure is usually carried out by a doctor. A small tray is prepared, (Fig. 40.1) containing:

 Disposable glove (e.g. Dispos-A-Glove)
 Lubricating jelly (e.g. KY)
 Kleenex wipes
 Paper bag (disposal)
 Proctoscope—with light, leads and battery, if available
 Torch or portable light.

 The patient is informed, privacy is ensured and the patient assisted to lie, if possible, in the left lateral position, with the knees well flexed and the buttocks near to the edge of the bed. The bedclothes are turned back to

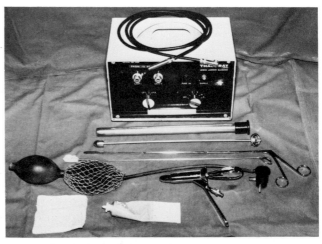

Fig. 40.1 Equipment for rectal examination.

expose the buttocks and anal region and personal clothing is rearranged.

The person carrying out the examination puts on a Dispos-A-Glove, lubricates the tip of the index finger and anus and gently carries out the examination. If proctoscopy is to follow, the nurse assists in this procedure.

On completion of the examination, the anus is wiped with tissues and these, together with the used glove, are discarded into the paper bag. The patient is repositioned and made comfortable.

Used equipment is removed, the tray is cleaned. If the proctoscope is of the electrical variety, the leads are disconnected. The proctoscope is washed and soaked in Savlon 1 per cent for at least 30 minutes.

Perianal abscess

Infection in the rectal or anal wall from an inflamed haemorrhoid or abscess may spread into the perianal fossa or ischiorectal tissues (Fig. 40.2) or the infection may be blood borne.

Pain may be severe because the pus is under considerable tension. Pain on defaecation is usually present. The affected area is swollen, red, and indurated.

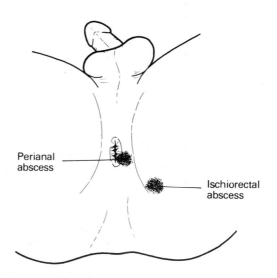

Fig. 40.2 Abscess formation around the anus.

Treatment

Very free drainage is necessary, and, as in all wounds around the anus, healing must occur from the depth of the abscess cavity. This is achieved by frequent baths and keeping the wound well open with a corner of a square of gauze soaked in Eusol. If this is not carried out meticulously the skin heals over and one or more septic tracks are left in the depth, with resultant fistula formation.

Fistula-in-ano

A fistula is a track lined with septic granulation tissue connecting two epithelial lined surfaces. The surfaces which the track connects in this region are the skin of the buttock and mucous membrane of the anal canal. The commonest cause is an ill-treated or neglected perianal abscess. Rarely multiple fistulae are present when the condition is tuberculous. Fistula-in-ano may be a complication of Crohn's disease, ulcerative colitis or diverticular disease of the colon.

A radiograph of the chest should be taken in all cases of fistula to exclude pulmonary tuberculosis.

Symptoms and signs

A mucous or purulent discharge occurs around the anus. There is usually no pain until the opening becomes blocked and an abscess forms in the track behind.

Treatment

The two openings are found with a fine probe, and the track is excised. A wide raw area is left to granulate, and the same care is essential as in the case of an abscess to see that healing takes place slowly from the floor of the cavity. The specimen which has been excised is sent for pathological examination to exclude tuberculosis and new growth formation. The detailed preparation and aftercare are discussed later in this chapter.

Fissure-in-ano

This is the most painful of all rectal conditions. As a result of pressure from hard dry faecal material, a small crack (or fissure) appears in the posterior portion of the anal wall. There is severe pain on defaecation, and this persists for several hours afterwards. The patient dreads another bowel action; the faeces as a result become still harder and drier. When the bowel has to act the pain is more severe than ever. A small pile, known as a 'sentinel pile', is usually present.

Treatment

In acute cases three-finger dilatation of the anus under an anaesthetic is sufficient to effect a cure. Dilatation greater than three fingers may result in a tear of the anus. This requires admission for only half a day. If the fissure is thickened, excision of the crack and partial division of the internal sphincter is necessary.

Pilonidal sinus

This is a very common cause of recurrent abscess formation in the area between the tip of the coccyx and the anal margin (Fig. 40.3). Fine tracks lead from the skin into the tissues down to the coccyx.

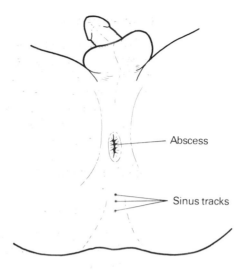

Fig. 40.3 Pilonidal sinus.

Treatment

1. *Acute stage*. An abscess may form, and incision is necessary. Any area seen to contain hair is laid open.

2. *Radical treatment* consists of wide excision of the area. A few millilitres of methylene blue are injected into the track by means of a syringe and cannula—*not a needle*. The wound is closed by uniting the skin and the cavity obliterated by means of several deep nylon sutures tied over a roll of gauze. The wound is left undisturbed for 14 days. After this time it has healed. The patient is nursed lying on the side or the prone position.

More usually, however, surgical treatment is limited to opening up and laying open all visible tracks. The hairy skin of the buttock is shaved and kept shaved postoperatively. Special care is taken to remove any visible hair which may be seen in the granulating wound. A tiny nylon bottle brush is used for extracting hairs and debris present. The patient is advised to bath at least once daily, particularly following defaecation. He is also instructed to wipe the anus in a direction away from the sinus and not towards it. He should continue permanently with careful personal hygiene.

Pruritus ani

Severe irritation and itching (pruritus) around the anus may occur from many causes. The commonest cause is threadworms. Other causes are a vaginal discharge, gross uncleanliness, haemorrhoids and diabetes. It may occur without any obvious cause. This is known as idiopathic pruritus ani.

Symptoms and signs

Severe irritation causes great distress, particularly at night in bed. The buttock area is covered with multiple scratch marks and the loss of sleep results in extreme weariness.

Treatment

The urine is tested for sugar because the condition may be caused by mild infection of the skin in diabetic subjects. Any obvious focus of irritation is treated. Warm baths of sodium bicarbonate and painting with 1 per cent gentian violet solution give considerable relief. An antipruritic cream such as Teevex is of value. The injection of local anaesthetic into the affected area may be advised.

Haemorrhoids

Internal haemorrhoids contain an artery in the pedicle. The exact nature of a haemorrhoid is still a matter of doubt. They have been stated to be dilated veins, arteriovenous fistulas or merely, according to Thomson, displaced or prolapsed cushions of mucous membrane extruding from disruption of the supporting tissue. Great confusion has arisen from a lack of understanding of the terms 'internal' and 'external' haemorrhoids.

External haemorrhoids are small dilated veins covered by redundant folds of skin, and are situated on the anal margin. The only complication is a small haemorrhage into the skin folds. This causes severe pain which can be relieved by simple incision through which the haematoma is evacuated. No special preparation is necessary, and evacuation of the haematoma gives immediate relief. A simple gauze dressing is all that is necessary and it can be removed the next day. The patient has a bath and no further dressings are required.

Internal haemorrhoids. Internal, or true, haemorrhoids always originate inside the bowel (Fig. 40.4). There are three stages (degrees) of increasing severity.

1. Early in their development they are soft and bleed readily.
2. Later they become thickened and descend outside the sphincter on defaecation, but return spontaneously afterwards.
3. Still later they remain outside (prolapsed haemorrhoids).

Constipation and excessive straining at stool are important causes of haemorrhoids in a substantial proportion of patients. Burkitt has noted the rarity of haemorrhoids in rural Africans who consume a high residue diet which produces bulky stools. A patient with a history of passing hard stools or difficulty in defaecation should be advised to increase his intake of fluids and the bulk of fruit and vegetables.

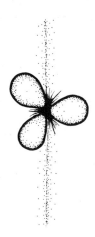

Fig. 40.4 The sites of the three primary haemorrhoids. With the patient in the lithotomy position these are 3, 7 and 11 o'clock.

Symptoms and signs

Bleeding is the earliest symptom, and severe anaemia may result if it is profuse. The blood is bright red and occurs on defaecation. As they progress, irritation and distress during prolapse are prominent complaints. Prolapse may occur suddenly or gradually. Sudden prolapse is extremely painful, and if the piles cannot be returned the patient is unable to walk. The anus and lower rectum may be examined visually by means of a proctoscope.

Treatment of prolapsed haemorrhoids

Treatment is directed to the relief of pain and the reduction of the inflammation locally. Rest in bed, preferably with the lower end of the bed raised and the patient lying on his side, is essential. Compresses of lead and opium or cold sodium sulphate are soothing as well as warm baths. Morphia (15 mg) eight-hourly should be prescribed, and the diet should be confined to fluids. Anal dilatation may be advised and in many is effective even in painful prolapsed haemorrhoids.

Treatment by injections

Injections can be given only when the haemorrhoids are inside the anal canal. This is most effective for early bleeding haemorrhoids. Five per cent phenol in almond oil is injected by means of a haemorrhoid syringe. The patient is placed in the left lateral position or in the knee elbow position and a proctoscope is passed. Apart from a tiny amount of bleeding complications are unusual.

Anal dilatation

Lord believes that the primary defect is narrowing of the outlet of the anal canal. The anal sphincter is unable to dilate to whatever size is necessary to allow the stool to pass and faecal material has to be expressed. The rise in intraluminal pressure obstructs the venous return from the haemorrhoidal area. The haemorrhoidal plexus dilated with blood further obstructs the outlet. The aim of dilatation is to break this vicious circle.

1. Procedure. Dilatation of the anal sphincter up to eight fingers is undertaken under a general anaesthetic in an operating theatre. When dilatation has ironed out the constriction a sponge is placed in the anal canal to reduce the risk of haematoma formation. It is removed 1 hour later and the patient can go home.

2. Postoperative dilatation by the patient at home. The patient is instructed to pass a specially designed dilator 1½ inches long each day for 2 weeks after a hot bath before retiring, and on alternate days for the following month. It should be left in position for 1 minute. After this time the patient should pass the dilator only if there is any tightness.

Complications:

(a) Haematoma.

(b) Splitting. There is a danger of infection so the patient must be kept in hospital and antibiotics prescribed.

(c) Prolapse occurs occasionally and should be reduced.

(d) Incontinence. If it occurs it usually clears up in 2 weeks, but more recently some more persistent cases of sphincter dysfunction have been noticed and it would appear that for patients with a patulous anus dilatation is an unsuitable method of treatment.

Operative treatment

This is a very satisfactory operation and consists of ligation of the three primary haemorrhoids. The preparation and after-treatment are considered on p. 425. Ligation with rubber bands is an alternative to formal operative ligation. It requires no anaesthetic and the patient is back at work next day. Discomfort is mild apart from transient mucus leakage. Complications are rare. In the presence of Crohn's disease the incidence of complications is high and if at all possible operative interference is best avoided.

Cryosurgery

The need for operation for haemorrhoids has diminished considerably since the introduction of Lord's dilatation. An alternative to surgical ligation is cryosurgery which necessitates hospitalisation for only 2 days.

Prolapse of the rectum

Conditions which predispose to rectal prolapse are chronic cough, constipation, phimosis, whooping cough, torn perineum from childbirth, and occasionally threadworms. The essential aim of treatment in these conditions is to treat the cause.

Rectal prolapse may be:

1. *Incomplete.* In this form only the mucous membrane prolapses. This condition is usually seen in infants. In the adult it may be associated with haemorrhoids and is cured at the same operation. In infants, regulation of the bowels is usually all that is necessary. If the condition persists the buttocks are strapped together after the prolapse has been reduced, and the child is kept in bed.

2. *Complete prolapse* is a distressing condition associated with ageing, weight loss and decreasing muscle tone.

Treatment

If possible, the prolapse is replaced and the patient confined to bed. The foot of the bed should be elevated. If the patient's condition is satisfactory cure by operation may be undertaken. This consists of anchoring the rectum by an abdominal approach. In more feeble patients a suture of silver wire or nylon may be inserted around the anus to leave an aperture the size of the base of the operator's index finger. This is sufficient to allow a motion to pass but small enough to prevent the mucosa prolapsing.

Simple stricture of the rectum

Simple stricture of the rectum may occur as a result of a gonococcal proctitis, ulcerative proctocolitis or as a complication of an operation for haemorrhoids or radiotherapy. Administration of an enema which is too hot may give rise to rectal stricture and it cannot be stressed too often that the temperature of all fluids used must be taken with a thermometer. Dilatation with special rectal bougies may be advised.

Proctitis

Inflammation of the rectum or anal canal unassociated with haemorrhoids or a new growth may be:

1. Non-specific. This is part of the condition of ulcerative proctocolitis (p. 409) in which the rectum is involved in about 70 per cent of cases.

2. Specific. Causes include bacillary and amoebic dysentery, gonococcal and tuberculous infection. The treatment is that of the cause.

Rectal biopsy

Biopsy of a rectal lesion is of great value in the diagnosis of rectal tumours, whether simple or malignant in nature, and in the differentiation of Crohn's disease from ulcerative proctocolitis. It is also of value in the confirmation of the presence of amyloid disease.

RECTUM AND ANUS (excluding removal of the rectum)

The rectum, the anus, and the surrounding skin are teeming with vast numbers of pathogenic organisms. By any method of preparation it is impossible to have a sterile operating field. It is none the less important to render the area as free of organisms as possible, and operation in this area must be carried out under strict conditions of asepsis so that fresh forms of infection are not introduced. Because absolute asepsis is impossible, all wounds in this area require free drainage, and healing always occurs by secondary intention.

General preoperative treatment

1. The bowel. The bowel should be emptied before the operation. A mild aperient is given 2 nights before the operation, followed by an enema in the evening and a washout on the morning of the operation day. A rectal washout is given not later than 6 hours before the patient goes to the theatre.

Rectal washout. An enema saponis is given to ensure that the bowel is empty of faeces.

Equipment required (on a trolley):

Rectal tube or catheter

Connection tubing 0·6 m (2 ft) in length

Funnel

Small jug — 1 litre

Large jug containing 4 l fluid (tap water) at 37·8°C (100°F)
Bucket
Incopad
Large polythene sheet
Disposable gloves
Lubricating jelly
Medical wipes/tissues.

The procedure is explained to the patient, and he is told that it may take 15 to 20 minutes. He is allowed to pass urine. He is placed in the left lateral position, with an Incopad under the buttocks. The polythene sheet is spread on the floor, and the bucket placed on it.

The small jug is filled with fluid. The funnel, connection tubing and catheter are assembled. The tip of the catheter is lubricated. Some fluid is run through to expel air, and then stopped. The patient is asked to take a deep breath, and the catheter is inserted about 6 cm (2½ in) into the rectum. The funnel is raised above the level of the buttocks; 300 ml (half pint) of fluid is run into the rectum. Before the funnel is empty it is inserted over the bucket and the fluid siphoned back. The process is repeated until the fluid returns clear, or the 4 litres of prepared fluid have been used.

Afterwards, the tube is withdrawn. The anal region is cleansed. If the patient desires, he is allowed to use a bedpan or commode. He is left comfortable in bed.

Used equipment is discarded. The fluid siphoned back and also that passed into the bedpan are measured and added together—the total amount thus returned is usually equal to the amount given.

After washing and drying her hands, the nurse reports on the amount of fluid given and returned, whether the final washout was returned clear, and any untoward effects.

2. The perianal region. The skin around the anus, groin, and supra-pubic area should be shaved and washed with soap. In painful conditions such as perianal abscess this is carried out after the patient has been anaesthetised.

3. The diet. During the 2 days before the operation the diet should be light, nutritious, and of the non-residue type.

A sigmoidscopy is performed to exclude carcinoma before a haemor-rhoids operation is commenced. The usual position for operation is the lithotomy (Fig. 40.5).

Postoperative treatment

Pain. This is usually severe, and repeated morphia injections are neces-sary. Hot baths are valuable for the relief of pain following an operation for haemorrhoids, and many patients like to spend several hours a day lying in a hot bath.

Haemorrhage may occur, and will be severe if the ligature of a haemor-rhoid base has slipped. It must be reported at once and arrangements made for return to the theatre to secure the bleeding point. A rare but occasional complication is a secondary haemorrhage about the tenth day—this requires the administration of antibiotics, securing the bleeding point in the

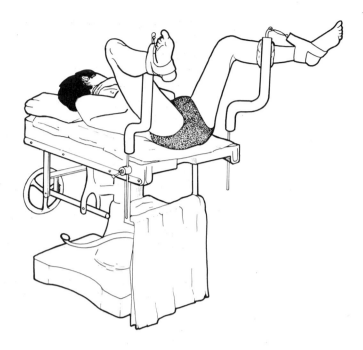

Fig. 40.5 Lithotomy position.

theatre and, if necessary, blood transfusion.

A tube covered with petroleum jelly is frequently left in the anal canal at the end of the operation for haemorrhoids, partly for the passage of flatus and partly lest haemorrhage should occur and not be revealed owing to the sphincter ani being in spasm.

The packs. The original packs in cases of fistula are usually removed at the end of 24 hours and replaced, after irrigation of the wound, by a light pack. In most cases flat packs are used, but one corner can be tucked into the wound to ensure that the skin edges are not allowed to fall inwards. Firm, deep packing with ribbon gauze is avoided.

A normal diet with an adequate fluid intake is allowed as soon as the patient desires it. The bulk of the stool is increased by giving bran or a hydrophilic laxative such as Isogel 10–20 ml/daily or Normacol 10–20 ml/daily. In addition, to keep the faecal material lubricated and ease bowel movement, a lubricant laxative such as Mil-Par (15 ml at night) is prescribed. If the bowel has not moved by the third or fourth day two glycerine suppositories may be given or an olive oil enema, followed by a soap and water enema. A bath is taken after every bowel action.

Digital dilatation of the anus. This is a particularly important after-treatment following a haemorrhoid operation. It is commenced on the sixth day and performed daily for 2 days. Its purpose is to separate the 'sticky' surfaces so that stricture formation does not occur.

Acute retention of urine. This is particularly liable to occur after a haemorrhoid operation, and, if the simpler methods fail, catheterisation must be undertaken (Ch. 43).

NEW GROWTHS

Simple new growths include polyps and adenomas. The main symptoms are similar to those of haemorrhoids, and the treatment is excision.

Carcinoma of the rectum

Malignant new growths are very common.

Symptoms and signs

1. *Constipation.* Increasing constipation alternating with diarrhoea is not uncommon.

2. *Bleeding.* The blood is bright red in colour and is so important a symptom that it must not be attributed to haemorrhoids until carcinoma has been excluded. Pain in the rectum is a late symptom in most cases, but appears earlier in growths situated in the anal canal.

3. *Tenesmus.* With a polypoid growth of the rectum, the patient has a constant sensation of fullness associated with the desire to defaecate, which is not relieved by bowel action.

4. *Sciatic pain* is sometimes the presenting symptom, and is due to infiltration of the sacral plexus by the growth.

5. *Intestinal obstruction* may develop acutely if the lumen of the bowel has been narrowed by the growth.

6. *Mucus and pus.* The discharge of mucus and pus may occur in a large fungating growth filling the rectum.

7. *Digital examination* of the rectum will reveal a palpable growth.

8. *Sigmoidoscopic examination.* The higher reaches of the rectum and the lower colon may be examined by means of a sigmoidoscope and a portion of the growth taken for biopsy. The bowel should be emptied by a gentle aperient, followed by a Dulcolax suppository, 6 hours before examination. Some surgeons prefer no preparation at the first attempt.

Treatment

The standard procedure for most patients suffering from carcinoma is abdominoperineal resection of the rectum and the results are excellent. A more conservative procedure may be possible where the growth is situated in the upper third. The sphincter is preserved, end to end anastomosis performed and a colostomy avoided. Local excision only may be all that is necessary if the tumour is small and pathological examination shows removal to have been complete and the grade of tumour not poorly differentiated. For abdominoperineal resection two surgical teams combine, one operating in the abdomen and the other in the perineum at the same time. Resection of the rectum is always a severe operation.

Blood transfusion is commenced before the operation. The bowel should be emptied by aperients and enemas. After the patient has been anaesthetised a Gibbon or small Foley catheter is inserted into the bladder. This is left in place for 4 to 10 days as temporary disturbance of bladder function

results from removal of the rectum. A washout of the rectum with antican-
cerous agents may be undertaken *in the theatre*. It minimises the risk of
implantation as well as diminishing the risk of recurrence at the suture line
if a sphincter preserving operation is possible.

Postoperative care

The abdominal wound is closed and covered with Elastoplast. To the colostomy is attached a disposable bag.

Immediate postoperative treatment

The patient is laid on his side and the head is kept low (on one pillow)
until he recovers consciousness. Blood transfusion is continued until the
general condition is satisfactory.

Systemic antibiotic therapy is commenced after the operation.

Strain by coughing or attempting to pass urine must be limited to the
minimum.

There is a great loss of blood serum into the large wound of the
perineum, and the patient must have a very high protein diet to compensate for this. Eggs, meat, milk, and cheese are necessary. A transfusion of
blood plasma for this specific purpose may be necessary about the seventh
or eighth day.

The bladder. A catheter is left in the bladder and connected to a closed
drainage. About the fourth to fifth day the catheter can be removed. A
good sign that the bladder will function is to see the patient passing urine
around the catheter before it is removed.

Fluids should be taken as soon as possible by mouth and the diet
increased as soon as the bowel sounds are heard. The colostomy frequently does not work for a day or two after operation and, if necessary, a
gentle washout through the colostomy opening affords considerable relief.
He must be instructed in the care of his colostomy (Ch. 38.).

The perineal wound

In women with malignant disease the posterior vaginal wall is excised
because the recto vaginal septum is the commonest site of recurrent disease. A year later it is impossible to tell whether the vaginal wall has been
removed or not. As it is not sewn up the vagina remains normal in size and
epithelialises. The perineal wound is sewn up and a corrugated drain is
brought out through the vagina. For inflammatory disease the vaginal wall
is not excised and the wound which remains can be closed completely as
it is in the male for carcinoma or inflammatory disease. Sometimes it is
impossible to close the wound completely and the wound is left open
around a drainage tube. In closed wounds a Shirley drain with immediate
suction drainage is inserted for 5 days.

Closed wound. The amount of the discharge is recorded over a 24 hour
period. The stitches are removed about the tenth day and at all times the
wound is kept dry.

Open wound. The drainage tube is removed in 48 hours and the wound irrigated with Eusol or hydrogen peroxide until the granulation appears. The centre of the wound must be kept open, inserting a finger if necessary but the suture line should be kept dry using dry pads.

Pressure on the wound is avoided by the patient lying on his side. With help the patient can stand or sit out of bed.

Conservative resection

A sphincter preserving operation is possible for growth of the upper third of the rectum. The postoperative care is similar to a colectomy but special care must be taken to see that the flatus tube is passed no further than 2 cm beyond the anal sphincter.

Adjuvant chemotherapy such as 5-fluorouracil may be used in the presence of metastases, or immunotheraphy in the form of BCG. The results, however, are poor.

BIBLIOGRAPHY

Bartlet J G et al 1977 Gastroenterology 73: 772
Burkitt D P 1973 Recent advances in surgery no 8. Churchill Livingstone, Edinburgh p. 257
Thomson W H F 1975 British Journal of Surgery 62: 542

41

Hernia

A hernia is a pouch of lining membrane protruding itself through a weak point in the covering structures. The most common site of a hernia is the abdominal wall. The term, however, includes a weakness at any point, for example, a defect of the skull results in what is known as a hernia cerebri.

The weak points in the musculature of the abdomen are the canals and the scars through which certain structures normally run. The hernias which occur at these sites (Fig. 41.1) are named accordingly:

1. Inguinal.
2. Femoral.
3. Umbilical, in the adult usually paraumbilical.

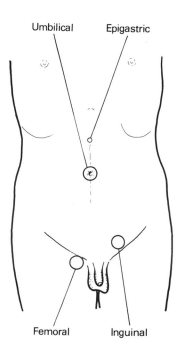

Fig. 41.1 The sites of hernias on the abdominal wall.

4. Epigastric.
5. Incisional, known as ventral, if arising on the anterior abdominal wall.
6. Obturator.
7. Hiatus hernia (Chapter 32).
8. A rarer type of hernia is the diaphragmatic. The abdominal contents herniate into the chest.

The constituents of an abdominal hernia are:

(a) The sac. This is the protruding pouch of peritoneum.

(b) The contents. The most frequent are loops of the small intestine and the great omentum. They slip in and out, provided the hernia is not strangulated or obstructed. Long-standing friction results in adhesion of the contents to the sac. Almost any abdominal organ except the pancreas may be found in a hernial sac.

(c) The coverings include all the tissues superficial to the hernia· and consist of the stretched muscles and aponeurosis, the fascia, and the skin.

The cause of hernia

A hernia may be congenital or acquired.

The commonest hernia in an infant is an umbilical hernia, from the failure of the umbilicus to seal off satisfactorily. The majority of small congenital umbilical hernias in infants cure themselves and reassurance of the parents is the only treatment necessary. In the larger ones a simple operation is necessary if they do not close spontaneously. In gross cases the whole of the intestines are outside the abdomen, a condition known as exomphalos. This condition requires urgent operation. Combined with an undescended testicle, congenital inguinal hernia is not uncommon in male children.

Hernias are frequently acquired as a result of tearing of the muscles due to strenuous work or play.

SYMPTOMS AND SIGNS OF UNCOMPLICATED HERNIA

Small hernias are noticed by the patient only after coughing or standing up. A swelling, with a slight dragging ache, is the commonest complaint. The skin over a large hernia may be in folds which tend to become eczematous as a result of friction.

On examination there is an expansile impulse on coughing.

Complications of a hernia

1. Irreducibility of the contents occurs in long-standing hernias.

2. Strangulation. The blood supply to the loop of bowel is cut off, and, in addition to the local pain, the symptoms and signs of intestinal obstruction are present (p. 351). There is no impulse on coughing, and the hernia is irreducible and tender. Unrelieved, the strangulated loop of bowel becomes gangrenous.

3. Progression. Increase in size is usual.

4. Intertrigo of the skin, i.e. abrasion due to two folds of skin rubbing together.

Treatment

Operative repair is the treatment of choice and many uncomplicated hernias are suitable for 'day' surgery and patients can get up next day at home. The sac is excised after the contents have been reduced into the abdomen and the weakness repaired by suture of the muscles or by the introduction of special suture material if the muscles are weak. The patient is kept in bed for only one day, but in large recurrent hernias 3 to 4 days in bed are advisable. He is advised against very heavy lifting for 3 months. There are special cases, however, when this ideal course of treatment is not possible:

1. In the presence of special aggravating factors recurrence of the hernia is inevitable so these must be treated before operation on the hernia is contemplated. They are:
    (a) Enlargement of the prostate.
    (b) A urethral stricture.
    (c) Constipation.
    (d) A persistent cough.

2. The patient is temporarily unfit for operation
    (a) In an infant the operation for hernia is undertaken at 3 months or even earlier.
    (b) During pregnancy, provided the hernia is reducible, operation is best deferred until after parturition.
    (c) After a severe illness such as pneumonia.
    (d) Chronic bronchitis with an acute exacerbation.

3. The patient is unfit for operation
    (a) Extensive pulmonary tuberculosis.
    (b) Extreme age.

In all these conditions a truss may be advised, provided the hernia can be reduced and is not a femoral hernia. No truss so far designed will control a femoral hernia.

In babies an umbilical hernia is reduced by supporting with strapping. This is the only type of hernia support which may 'cure' the hernia, because obliteration of the umbilicus is a physiological process and adequate support may enable it to proceed to completion.

Special advice to a patient wearing a truss

Careful washing and powdering of the skin are necessary. The pad must be maintained in good repair, and if a spring is used in the truss it must be renewed before it becomes too weak.

The patient must be instructed to apply his truss while he is lying down in bed after the hernia has been reduced.

The care of the patient for a hernia operation

Careful shaving of the suprapubic area and cleansing of the skin are essential. Slight cuts from shaving are very likely to give rise to infection, which will ruin the operation.

Abdominal exercises are commenced on the day following the operation. Retention of the urine may occur and must be relieved. Abdominal distension must be prevented by passing a flatus tube.

If the patient is very fat and the hernia is large it is usually wise to prescribe measures to reduce his weight before the operation.

Some patients have two very large hernias, and it is frequently decided to operate on them one at a time as the sudden reduction of the contents of two large hernias into the abdomen may give rise to cardiorespiratory embarrassment.

Certain terms connected with hernia operations give rise to some difficulty:

1. *Herniotomy* means opening of the sac.

2. *Herniorrhaphy* refers to the repair of the defect in the musculature.

3. *Hernioplasty* is a heniorrhaphy in which extra material, such as monofilament nylon or implants of teflon are introduced for wide deficiencies.

Recurrence which is in the order of 10 per cent is due to faulty technique (failure to remove the sac), infection, straining, coughing and heavy lifting.

42

Diseases of the kidney and ureter

The kidneys are situated on the posterior abdominal wall behind the peritoneal cavity. The right kidney lies below the liver and behind the second part of the duodenum, while the left kidney, which is higher placed than the right is situated behind and below the spleen. There are two major calices in each kidney which empty into the renal pelvis which has a capacity of 5 to 8 ml. The ureter, which joins the renal pelvis to the bladder, is about 25 cm long and its muscular coat provides the vermicular (peristaltic) movement. The ureter enters through the bladder muscle on an oblique course and terminates at the base of the trigone. In the female the ureter is only 0·5 cm from the cervix of the uterus.

The surgical significance of these facts is:

1. The surgery on the kidney and ureter is performed behind the peritoneal cavity whenever possible to avoid contaminating it with urine. If the peritoneum has been opened inadvertently at operation or if the approach has been transperitoneal a careful watch has to be kept for signs of peritonitis (Ch. 34).

2. The oblique entry of the ureter through a tunnel in the bladder musculature prevents the reflux of urine from the bladder. It does not prevent the ascent of bacteria from the bladder into the ureter and thence to the kidney.

3. The proximity of the ureters to the cervix of the uterus enables a cervical growth to spread and obstruct the ureters.

The kidneys have a rich blood supply from the aorta through the renal arteries and the level is a critical one in resection of an abdominal aneurysm (Ch. 23). The renal veins drain directly into the inferior vena cava so that a renal tumour may spread rapidly to the lung.

The main functions of the kidney are the control of water and electrolyte balance, the excretion of nitrogenous waste products and the elimination of drugs.

The kidney may be damaged and ultimately destroyed by failure of its blood supply, prolonged hypotension, toxins, bacterial infection, a mismatched blood transfusion, a new growth or any lesion obstructing the flow of urine down the ureter or the lower urinary tract.

INVESTIGATIONS

The repeated collection of specimens of blood and urine, intravenous urography involving abdominal compression in a darkened X-ray room, catheterisation and cystoscopic examination before a definitive operation is undertaken are a demanding ordeal for any patient. Unfortunately the only certain method of assessing progress or cure afterwards is a repetition of some or all of these procedures. These patients evoke special sympathy. The purpose as well as the details should be explained to the patient and, as far as possible, discomfort eliminated.

The objects of investigation

1. To determine the precise anatomy. One kidney may be absent, the ureter may be reduplicated or other anomaly may be present.
2. To assess renal function, bladder evacuation or exclude reflux into the ureter.
3. To localise the site and extent of disease.

RENAL INVESTIGATIONS

1. Collection of specimens

Urine for routine examination is collected in a clean urinal or bedpan. Observations of colour, smell, deposits, specific gravity and pH are made. Tests for abnormalities (glucose, ketones, albumin, bile and blood) are carried out in the ward.

If bacteriological examination is required, a midstream specimen of urine is collected from a male patient. Prior to this the genital area is cleansed with soap and water. The male patient is instructed to retract the foreskin and to pass a little urine into the urinal, to interrupt the stream and pass a little urine into a sterile container, and then to complete micturition into the urinal. Female patients, who usually require assistance, are asked to pass urine directly into the sterile container or a sterile receiver. The container is then sealed, labelled and sent to the laboratory.

If the patient has an indwelling catheter a fresh specimen is obtained by spigotting the catheter for 20–30 minutes and then releasing the spigot and collecting the urine in the sterile container. The specimens may be collected in two portions for routine examination and specimens kept for inspection in two separate glasses.

2. Residual urine

The presence of residual urine is a most valuable sign of prostatic enlargement. The correct method of estimating residual urine is as follows:

(a) The patient is requested to empty his bladder completely by his own efforts. The normal bladder is empty at the end of micturition, and if a catheter is passed no urine will be obtained.

(b) If, after the patient has emptied his bladder to the best of his ability, a catheter is passed and urine is obtained, this is known as 'residual urine'.

The volume should be measured and charted.

If for any reason it is undesirable to pass a catheter this can be estimated by an intravenous pyelogram which on the 'postmicturition' film will show an outline of the residual urine.

3. Examination of the urine

This will include a search for the presence of red blood corpuscles, pus, cancer cells, and organisms, as well as abnormal chemical constituents such as albumin and sugar.

4. Blood urea

The normal is 2·50–6·67 mmol per litre (15 to 40 mg per cent). A more accurate test, because it is uninfluenced by diet or the state of hydration, is the serum creatinine, normal value 53–106 μmol per litre (0:6–1:2 mg per 100 ml).

5. X-ray examination

Straight, or direct, X-ray examination will in 90 per cent of cases reveal the presence of stones.

An intravenous pyelogram (a urogram) will reveal most abnormalities of the kidneys and, in addition, is a valuable test of renal function. A damaged kidney will not secrete the dye in sufficient strength to give a radiographic shadow.

In preparation for X-ray examination of the renal tract, the bowels should be emptied by the administration of vegetable aperient on each of the two previous nights. The passage of a flatus tube will reduce gas shadows, which so frequently interfere with a good film of the kidneys. The bladder is emptied.

On the morning of the examination no fluid or food is given. Films are taken at 5, 10, and 30 minutes or longer after the injection of 20 ml of 50 per cent solution of a medium containing an iodine compound. A small amount of leakage outside the vein in the arm is very painful, and if it should occur a hot fomentation is applied. The risk of idiosyncrasy to iodine should be anticipated by always having at hand 1 ml of hydrocortisone and a solution of dextrose for immediate intravenous injection.

Many patients complain of pain from the abdominal compression used in the examination to demonstrate the ureters more adequately.

6. Cystograpy

The bladder may be visualised when the dye injected for a pyelogram reaches the bladder, or alternatively a more adequate picture of the bladder may be obtained by passing a catheter and filling the bladder with dye. An X-ray taken when the patient is micturating—micturating cystourethrogram—will reveal whether there is reflux of urine into the ureters from the bladder.

7. Cystoscopy

This is visual examination of the interior of the bladder.

Preparation of a patient for cystoscopy.

(a) The suprapubic area need not be shaved in the male unless the examination is likely to be followed by open operation.

(b) The patient should be encouraged to drink freely so that the secretion of urine can be observed from each ureteric orifice. There is no objection to the patient consuming plenty of fluid up to 3 hours before the anaesthetic unless the anaesthetist gives further instructions.

(c) The patient should attend for the examination with the bladder fairly full, so that the surgeon is able to examine the gross appearance of the urine as it flows from the bladder. In the male, phimosis is sometimes present, and a dorsal slit may be necessary before the cystoscope is passed.

(d) Radiographs and notes must be available in the theatre.

(e) For every cystoscopic examination urethral dilators should be sterilised and at hand in case the condition should turn out to be complicated by a urethral stricture.

8. Ureteric catheterisation and retrograde pyelography

A ureteric catheter may be passed up the ureter of either kidney to collect a specimen of urine secreted by that kidney. To ensure that the label on the specimen is correct it should be written out at once and care must be taken of the specimen, since damage or loss necessitates a repetition of the whole procedure.

If a retrograde pyelogram is to be performed the catheter is left in position and the patient is taken to the X-ray department, unless a special cystoscopy room equipped with X-ray apparatus is available. The radio-opaque medium is injected into the ureteric catheter with a syringe and the kidney and ureter X-rayed.

Instructions may be given for the catheter to be left in position until it falls out spontaneously. This procedure is frequently of value in aiding the patient to pass a small stone from the kidney or ureter. Two millilitres of sterile liquid paraffin may be injected into the catheter two-hourly for 12 hours to aid the passage of a stone. All specimens of urine which are voided must be retained for straining and examination in case a stone has been passed.

9. Ultrasonography

Ultrasonography is a noninvasive investigation easy to perform and repeat. Valuable information concerning the size and consistency of the kidney can be obtained.

10. Aortography

The renal arteries are visualised by injecting the radio-opaque medium directly into the aorta. This helps to distinguish a cyst from a neoplasm and would help to identify an aberrant renal artery.

11. Renal biopsy

This may be occasionally performed.

12. Radioisotope studies

Radioisotope studies of the kidney may be undertaken to determine further information about renal blood flow, function or the presence of a lesion obstructing a portion of the kidney.

RENAL FAILURE

Failure of the kidneys to clear the blood of waste products may be due to inadequate blood flow, damage to the kidneys or obstruction to the outflow of urine from the renal pelvis, from the ureters or from the lower urinary tract. It may occur suddenly or it may be the result of long-standing and progressive destructive disease. Uncontrolled, the patient will die.

Renal failure, whatever the cause, is aggravated by:
1. Incorrect fluid balance which causes waterlogging of the tissues.
2. Infection which causes tissue breakdown.
3. Ingestion of protein.
4. Excessive breakdown of protein such as occurs in starvation.
5. Potassium imbalance.

ACUTE RENAL FAILURE

Causes

1. Prerenal hypotension which will recover as shock is treated.
2. Renal tubular obstruction by:
   (a) Mismatched blood transfusion. The tubules are obstructed by agglutinated (clumped) red blood cells.
   (b) Myohaemoglobin produced in muscles which have been severely crushed (the crush syndrome).
   (c) Precipitation of drugs such as crystals of sulphonamides.
   (d) Bile pigments, particularly when associated with a fall in blood pressure such as following operations on patients with obstructive jaundice (the hepatorenal syndrome).
3. Tubular necrosis.
   (a) Following operation and concealed accidental haemorrhage.
   (b) Certain metallic poisons.
   (c) From acute pyelonephritis.
   (d) Bacteraemic shock.

4. Post-renal or obstructive, for example a stone or other lesion blocking the ureter of the only functioning kidney which the patient possesses.

Clinical picture

The patient may remain well for several days. The striking feature is oliguria (300 ml or less), leading to complete anuria. The blood urea and the serum potassium rise each day. After about 6 to 10 days vomiting, breathlessness and increasing acidosis are evident. Before death, twitching and convulsions may occur.

Management

For low blood pressure the appropriate treatment to overcome these conditions is instituted. An obstructive lesion is relieved.

If the patient is anuric the most important nursing features are:

1. To stop all fluids until a satisfactory regime is instituted.
2. To stop all antibiotics and drugs because many of them are not now being excreted and cumulative effects are liable to arise.
3. All foods should be forbidden.

The patient may be kept alive for a very long time and the longer the time he is kept alive the greater is the chance that the kidneys may recover or regenerate provided the correct treatment is undertaken. Basically this consists of the fluid intake being limited to the amount lost by sweating and respiration. This amounts to 1 litre a day, but the body produces 500 ml of water which accumulates. Therefore the total amount of fluid which can be given to the anuric patient is 500 ml. To prevent the breakdown of body protein a high carbohydrate diet is essential and must contain about 2000 calories and should be mineral-free. The fluid and carbohydrates are best combined in a solution in 500 ml of Hycal (a flavoured liquid dextrose concentrate) which provides 2100 calories. This can be administered by drinking or by a nasogastric tube into the stomach. If the patient is unable to tolerate either method 500 ml of 50 per cent dextrose is administered every 24 hours by a polythene catheter into the inferior vena cava.

Because the patient's diet is lacking in vitamins they can be administered as a supplement.

When a diuresis occurs a volume of fluid equal to the amount of urine secreted plus 500 ml is given as potassium-rich fruit juice. The precise amount of fluid and its nature should be determined over 24 hours following blood and urine electrolyte estimations at least once daily.

In all cases of oliguria or anuria of sudden onset, mannitol 50 g in 500 ml of 5 per cent dextrose, is given in 30 minutes. If there is a response by diuresis, intravenous fluid and mannitol up to 100 g daily are given. A careful watch on the serum sodium is kept as mannitol tends to depress it. If.there is no response to mannitol, structural damage has occurred and a modified Bull's regime is instituted. If this fails, peritoneal dialysis may be undertaken.

CHRONIC RENAL FAILURE

Causes

1. Chronic nephritis.
2. Polycystic disease of the kidneys.
3. Kidneys destroyed by calculi.
4. Hypertensive kidney disease.
5. Bilateral hydronephrosis.

The onset of disease is gradual, the patient is anaemic, the skin dry and retinitis is usually present. Vomiting, nausea and terminal intermittent respiration occur. The treatment is a low protein diet and dialysis. A renal transplant may be undertaken.

Dialysis

1. Peritoneal dialysis. Dialysis means the transfer of solutes across a semipermeable membrane. Substances in solution pass from areas of high concentration to areas of low concentration by diffusion.

During peritoneal dialysis, fluid of a known concentration is introduced into the peritoneal cavity. Blood vessels and the fluid in the cavity are separated by peritoneum which acts as a semipermeable membrane. The concentration of certain solutes in the dialysing fluid is lower than that in the blood and, therefore, salts for excretion diffuse into the peritoneal cavity.

Dialysing fluids contain a mixture of the normal plasma electrolytes in a 1·36 per cent solution of dextrose. A hypertonic solution (6·36 per cent dextrose) may be used to withdraw fluid. Heparin and antibiotics may be added as prescribed by the doctor.

The danger of infection makes sterility during any part of the process essential, and a bacterial filter is fitted to the inflow tube. Prior to the procedure the bladder must be emptied as there is a possibility of perforation of a distended bladder. The abdomen is shaved and cleaned with an antiseptic. A local anaesthetic is given. A catheter is then inserted into the peritoneal cavity and connected by tubing to two bags of dialysing fluid. The fluid is allowed to flow rapidly into the peritoneal cavity (1–2 litres in 10–15 minutes), it remains there for 20–30 minutes and is then allowed to drain.

It is essential that accurate fluid balance records are maintained as the amount of fluid introduced and that drained should correspond approximately. Patients should be weighed daily and observations of temperature, pulse and blood pressure maintained. Blood for urea and electrolyte estimations and dialysis fluid for culture and sensitivity are sent daily to the laboratory.

2. Haemodialysis. The artificial or mechanical kidney is basically a semipermeable membrane of Cellophane.

    (a) On one side of the membrane is a bath of fluid. The composition of the fluid is such that the substances which it is desired to attract into the bath are absent or of lower concentration than in the blood.

(b) One the other side is the patient's blood.

The process is one of dialysis. The essential ions are kept in the blood by maintaining an identical concentration in the bath. The substances which it is particularly desirable to attract from the blood, in cases in which this is used, are urea and potassium (K^+).

The patient is connected to the machine by canalising an artery and vein. The blood passes along one side of the Cellophane and is returned to the previously filled reservoir of venous blood before being returned to the body by a vein.

The machine requires the undivided attention of a team — including a biochemist.

Renal transplantation

Renal transplantation has been discussed in Chapter 26.

Anabolic hormones

Breakdown of protein tissue (catabolism) increases the amount of nitrogenous and potassium products in the blood. Synthesis or building up of lean tissue is know as anabolism. Occasionally these anabolic hormones (Deca-Durabolin is one) are of value, particularly in:

1. Some cases of acute renal failure, by depressing the formation of nitrogenous and potassium end products.

2. To counter the protein breakdown (catabolic) phase following acute illness, trauma, or major surgical interference.

SYMPTOMS AND SIGNS OF URINARY DISEASE

Pain

1. Renal pain. This may be of two varieties:

(a) A fixed dull aching in the loin. Lesions which distend the kidney frequently give rise to pain of this type. If the outer surface of the kidney is inflamed, as is commonly the case in pyonephrosis, adherence of the organ to the muscles in the loin may give rise to very severe pain.

(b) Renal colic or, more strictly, ureteric colic. The pain commences in the loin and radiates to the testicle in the male or the vulva in the female. It is severe and violent (Fig. 42.1). The expression of a small stone or clot frequently results in this type of pain.

2. Bladder pain. Bladder pain may be felt as a suprapubic discomfort, but more commonly is felt as a burning pain in the urethra at the end of micturition.

Haematuria

The passage of blood in the urine is known as haematuria. Haemorrhage arising in the bladder usually results in the passage of bright red blood, more marked at the end of micturition. Bleeding originating in the kidney

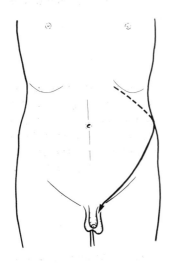

Fig. 42.1 Ureteric colic radiates from the loin to the groin.

is more intimately mixed with the urine, and the urine passed is usually described as 'smokey'. In addition to gross bleeding, the presence of small quantities of blood may be discovered only by microscopic examination of the urine.

Causes

1. **Renal:**
   (a) Injury to the kidney.
   (b) Haemorrhage into a cyst of a congenital cystic kidney.
   (c) Acute nephritis.
   (d) A stone.
   (e) Tuberculosis.
   (f) A neoplasm, e.g. innocent — angioma; malignant — hypernephroma, or nephroblastoma.
2. **Extrarenal:**
   (a) Hypertension.
   (b) Anticoagulants in excess.
   (c) The sulphonamide drugs.
   (d) Certain blood diseases.
3. **The Bladder:**
   (a) Foreign body.
   (b) Severe cystitis.
   (c) A stone.
   (d) Neoplasms.
   (e) An enlarged prostate.
4. **Urethra**
   (a) Trauma.
   (b) A stone.
   (c) Urethritis.

Following operation on any portion of the urinary tract haematuria is common and aggravated if clot formation occurs.

Increased frequency of micturition

Under nervous strain increased frequency of micturition is not an uncommon symptom. Irritation of the mucous membrane of the trigone of the bladder by infection, a stone or a growth are the usual urological causes. In tuberculosis of the urinary tract the mucous membrane is not only damaged but contraction of the bladder may result in unbearable frequency. Increased frequency is a prominent symptom of overflow retention (p. 445).

Difficulty in micturition (dysuria)

Difficulty with micturition is usually due to an enlarged prostate or to urethral stricture in the male. In the female it may be due to a painful urethral caruncle, a retroverted gravid uterus, or an impacted pelvic tumour.

Strangury

Strangury is the desire to pass urine when only a few drops are present in the bladder and is unrelieved by micturition. This symptom is fairly commonly associated with ureteric colic.

Scalding

Scalding, or pain on micturition, is usually due to infection.

Retention

Retention is the inability to pass urine.

Oliguria

Oliguria means that the urinary output is diminished — usually less than 300 ml in 24 hours.

Anuria

This is a condition in which no urine is formed by the kidneys or if glomerular filtrate is formed it is totally reabsorbed so the patient passes no urine, and on catheterisation none is recovered from the bladder. It is frequently due to a stone or other lesion blocking the ureter of the only kidney which the patient possesses.

Other causes are:

Acute tubular necrosis.

Shock. The urinary output is diminished, but as the patient responds to treatment kidney function is resumed.

Nephrotoxic durgs such as gentamicin.

The sulphonamide drugs. The crystallisation of the sulphonamide drugs in the renal tubules is liable to occur if the patient does not drink sufficient fluid when taking the drugs.

INCONTINENCE

Incontinence is the patient's inability to control emptying of the bladder. It may be:

1. True incontinence

The sphincter is damaged, or the nerves eliminated so that coordinated micturation is impossible.

Incontinence is a cause of much suffering. The patient is always wet and damage to the skin occurs very rapidly. Many silently accept their misery from a sense of shame. Until recent times incontinence has been regarded as a disease to be treated instead of looking at continence as the result to be achieved whenever possible. Acute illness, injury or immobility may result in incontinence and will pass as soon as the patient recovers strength. Impacted faeces in the rectum may cause acute retention with overflow incontinence. These forms may be treated by catheterisation and the catheter is removed as soon as the underlying precipitating factor is cured or corrected.

Following cerebrovascular accidents the nervous control to inhibit micturition is diminished but not entirely destroyed. This results in urge incontinence and is aggravated by emotional stress. The most important need is to be able to empty the bladder without delay so that a bedside commode is essential by night as is physical proximity (a few yards on a level surface) to a lavatory by day. In addition habit training to establish a regular frequency pattern of bladder emptying is necessary. An alarm with a flashing light to remind the patient and staff unobtrusively for the need for a further visit to the lavatory is described by Rowe.

When habit training fails there is a variety of equipment available which includes disposable incopads and napkins. Marsupial pants invented by Dr F.L. Williams hold an absorbent pad in a waterproof pouch on the outside of the garment. They are made of one way water repellent fabric which remains dry while allowing urine to pass through into the disposable pad. Because the pad is on the outside there is no need to remove the pants when the pad is changed.

Catheterisation with emptying in a bag or other device is a last resort.

2. False or paradoxical incontinence

The patient suffering from prostatic obstruction may develop acute retention (Fig. 42.2) with the result that a litre or more of urine may accumulate

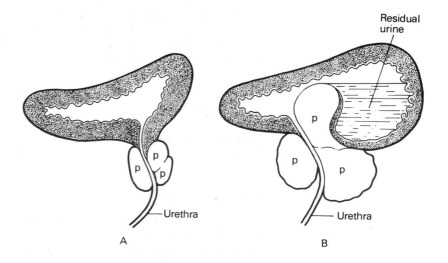

Fig. 42.2 A. Normal bladder after micturition.
B. Bladder obstructed by an enlarged prostate. (p. on the diagram).

in the bladder. After a certain point 60 or 90 ml may overflow. The condition is really one of retention, and the incontinence is only a complication of this condition. Retention with overflow is a common description of this condition. This condition may also occur in women with an incarcerated gravid uterus.

3. Stress incontinence

Stress incontinence is a condition, usually seen in women, in which coughing, sneezing, laughing, or any condition which increases intra-abdominal pressure results in some escape of urine from the bladder. It occurs because the supports of the sphincter have been damaged, usually due to injuries sustained during childbirth, and some element of cystocele is present.

DISEASES OF THE KIDNEYS AND URETERS

CONGENITAL ABNORMALITIES

Congenital abnormalities of the urinary tract are legion. The commonest are:

Polycystic disease of the kidneys
Horse-shoe kidney
Absence of one kidney
Ectopic kidney.

1. Polycystic kidney (congenital cystic kidney). This condition is probably due to failure of complete fusion of the cortex of the kidney with the medulla. Clinically, the disease is usually seen about the age of 40. Both kidneys are enlarged and irregular. The patient's symptoms are those of incipient renal failure from which, at a later date, he will die unless a renal transplant is successful.

2. Horseshoe kidney. The kidneys are joined together across the midline, usually at their lower poles. The importance of the condition lies in the necessity for recognising it prior to operation. A horseshoe kidney is liable to all the diseases which may occur in an anatomically normal organ.

3. Absence of one kidney. This may occur as a result of failure to develop. Such knowledge is vital in cases of disease of the only kidney which is present.

4. Ectopic kidney. The kidney may be situated in the pelvis instead of in its usual position in the loin.

INJURIES TO THE KIDNEYS

Injuries to the kidney may occur as a result of a fall or kick, usually taking the form of rupture of the organ. If the peritoneum in front of the organ is torn, peritonitis may occur. In some cases the condition is one of bruising.

Clinical features

Following a severe rupture of the kidney there is obvious haematuria, swelling, and pain in the loin combined with the general signs and symptoms of internal haemorrhage. An IVP should always be performed.

Treatment

In severe cases exploration of the kidney is carried out. When the condition is one of bruising, healing usually occurs if the patient rests in bed. All urine voided is kept and the time of evacuation marked on the label so that the amount of blood in each specimen can be compared.

SURGICAL DISEASES OF THE KIDNEYS

The various surgical lesions of the kidneys are a source of great confusion to the nurse. Their names are complicated and sometimes bewildering. Very simply:

Hydronephrosis (pyelectasis) is a condition in which the renal pelvis is distended due to partial obstruction, usually at the expense of the parenchyma of the kidney which, in extreme cases, is no more than a thin sac and the number of functioning renal units may be very small indeed.

Pyelonephritis is an infection of the renal pelvis and of the solid or parenchymatous portion of the kidney, often with small abscesses which destroy its substance.

Pyonephrosis is a condition in which a hydronephrotic kidney has become infected, and the kidney may be no more than a bag of pus.

Hydronephrosis

Hydronephrosis is a condition of dilatation of the renal pelvis. In an extreme case the kidney is simply a sac of clear fluid. The condition develops as a result of intermittent obstruction to the outflow of urine. Complete obstruction results in atrophy of the kidney.

The obstruction is sometimes caused by failure of nervous coordination in the ureter, but most cases are secondary to some other condition. If the primary cause is unilateral, one kidney is affected. If the cause is bilateral, both kidneys may be affected. The term pyelectasis is gradually replacing hydronephrosis in common usage and the affection of the ureter inaccurately described as dilatation is known as ureterectasis.

Conditions causing unilateral hydronephrosis

1. A stone in the ureter.
2. The pressure of tumours on the ureter.
3. Kinking of the ureter from bands or aberrant blood vessels (extra vessels to the kidney in addition to the normal renal ones).

4. Nervous inco-ordination at the junction of the renal pelvis with the ureter. This may become bilateral.

Conditions causing bilateral hydronephrosis

1. Prostatic obstruction.
2. Urethral stricture and congenital urethral valves.
3. Phimosis.
4. Carcinoma of the cervix uteri.
5. Bilateral renal or ureteric calculi.
6. Retroperitoneal fibrosis.

Complications

1. Renal failure (particularly in bilateral cases).
2. Infection (pyonephrosis).

Treatment

Treatment of most cases will be that of the primary cause.

In severe unilateral cases a plastic operation or nephrectomy may be necessary.

INFECTIONS OF THE KIDNEY

Pyelonephritis

Acute pyelonephritis is a pyogenic infection of the renal pelvis and the kidney surrounding it. Unless treated seriously and with great care chronic pyelonephritis will occur. The causal organisms are *Escherichia coli* or any of the common pyogenic organisms.

Pyelonephritis may occur in pregnancy and is predisposed to by progestin causing interference with the muscular contraction of the ureter rather than the effect of pressure of the uterus.

Clinical features

1. Pain in the loin and in the lower abdomen. The pain may resemble that of acute appendicitis. In addition there is usually frequency of micturition with scalding pain.
2. Pyrexia of the order of 39° C (103° F) is usually present. A rigor may be the presenting symptom.
3. Vomiting and the signs of a general febrile condition may be marked. On examination there is tenderness on the affected side in the region of the kidney. The urine contains pus and organisms.

Treatment

The causal organism is isolated and its sensitivity determined. While this is in progress the reaction of the urine to litmus must be determined. If it is acid an alkaline mixture is given, e.g. mist. potassium citrate. Antibacterial therapy is commenced and when the laboratory sensitivities are to hand any change of preparation which is indicated is made. Three litres of fluid must be taken daily. The dosage of antibacterial substances is based on an intake of 3 l of water.

When the acute stage has subsided full investigation of the urinary tract is carried out to determine any causal condition for the inflammation. The urine should be repeatedly examined for organisms when there has been apparent cure, otherwise chronic pyelonephritis will occur.

Chronic pyelonephritis is often slow to respond to treatment. Many cases in adults have had their origin in repeated urinary infection in infancy and childhood. Children who have had more than one attack of urinary infection should be investigated. Many will be found to have congenital anomalies of the renal tract. Some have neurological disturbances of the bladder leading to urinary retention and infection, while others will have anomalies of the junction of the ureter and bladder which allow reflux to occur up the ureters when the bladder contracts. This reflux can be minimised by instructing the patient in the art of double micturition — the child micturates, waits for a few minutes until the ureters drain into the bladder and then empties the bladder again. Reflux can be cured by a plastic operation in which the new valvular mechanism is constructed at the junction of the ureter and bladder.

Perinephric abscess

A perinephric abscess is an infection beneath the fatty capsule surrounding the kidney. The infection may arise as a result of the rupture of a small abscess in the kidney, but more usually it is blood-borne from a boil, carbuncle, or septic finger.

Symptoms and signs

The patient who has recently recovered from a staphylococcal infection runs a temperature for which no obvious cause can be found. There may be a dull ache in the loin. Later, the pain increases in severity and the loin becomes swollen and bulging.

Treatment

Incision of the abscess and drainage is usually required. The drainage tube will be left in position for at least a week, and in most cases a little longer. Antibiotics are usually unnecessary. Disease of the kidney may have to be dealt with subsequently.

Tuberculosis of the kidney

The kidney may be infected with tubercle bacilli from the blood stream or from a tuberculous lesion in some other portion of the genito-urinary tract. Unchecked, the disease is disseminated into the ureters, the bladder, and the opposite kidney.

Symptoms and signs

1. Frequency of micturition is the outstanding symptom.
2. Pain may be present in the loin, or true ureteric colic and haematuria may occur, due to small portions of granulation tissue passing down the ureter.
3. Painless haematuria.
4. The symptoms and signs of tuberculosis may be present elsewhere.

Investigation

Intravenous pyelogram may reveal distortion of the renal pelvis, and the typical cystoscopic appearance is a 'golf' hole appearance of the ureteric orifice.

Urine. The urine is acid in reaction, contains pus and is sterile on routine culture. Tubercle bacilli may be found on examination of the urine, early morning specimens being sent on three successive days or only after culture on special media.

Treatment

Antituberculosis chemotherapy (Ch. 9) is commenced. If resolution is not complete on chemotherapy, partial or total nephrectomy may be undertaken provided the disease is now limited to one kidney.

Pyonephrosis

Pyonephrosis is a condition of inflammation of the kidney and renal pelvis in which the renal substance has been almost completely replaced by a bag of pus. The patient complains of severe pain in the loin, which is swollen and tender. Rigors may be present and the temperature is often elevated to 39° C (103° F).

Treatment

Drainage of the abscess by nephrostomy or removal of the kidney will be necessary. Nursing treatment is similar to that of acute pyelonephritis.

URINARY STONES

Kidney stones

Most stones are secondary to infection (recurrent pyelonephritis), but parathyroid overactivity may be shown to play an increasingly important part in their formation. Due to the concentration of the urine, the condition is said to be commoner in tropical climates. Patients who excrete abundant calcium in the urine, for example patients suffering from tuberculous arthritis of the spine with marked decalcification, are more likely to form a stone. Excessive intake of calcium and vitamin D also increases the likelihood of stone formation. Its formation can, to a large extent, be prevented by regular change in the position of the frame to which the patient is secured. The consumption of abundant fluid is a further preventive measure which may be undertaken in these patients but in other patients a large fluid intake seems to be largely ineffectual. Hypercalcaemia is often idiopapathic (i.e. cause unknown).

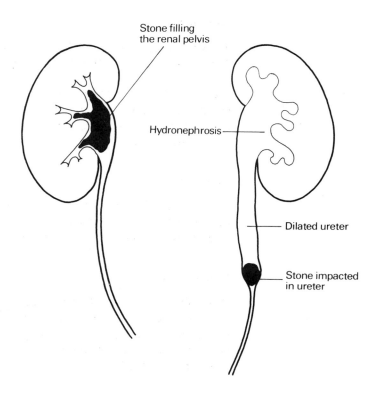

Fig. 42.3 Stones in the upper urinary tract.

Types of stone

Renal stones may be:
    1. Solitary.
    2. Multiple.
They may be composed of:
    (a) Oxalates (of calcium).
    (b) Phosphates (of calcium).
    (c) Uric acid.
    (d) Urates.
    (e) Fibrin.
    (f) Cystine.
    (g) Xanthine.

Symptoms and signs

Small stones give rise to prominent symptoms. A large stone may form quietly, but cause greater damage to the kidney.

1. Pain. Typical ureteric colic is extremely painful. The pain in the loin is sharp and biting and radiates with greater severity to the testicle in the male or to the labia in the female. The patient writhes about in pain and may vomit.

2. Strangury. There is a great urge to pass urine every few minutes, but only a drop or two is voided.

3. Haematuria. The urine may be tinted with blood or there may be frank haemorrhage.

A small stone may be passed by the patient as a termination of the violent pain with considerable relief. When large fixed stones are present the pain is a more constant dull ache in the loin. Occasional bouts of pyrexia occur as a result of infection.

Investigations should be full and complete and may include a calcium balance, which may reveal the presence of hyperparathyroidism (Ch. 28).

Treatment

1. Treatment of the acute attack. This consists of rest in bed and the relief of pain by the injection of pethidine.

2. In the quiescent stage. Antispasmodics are prescribed and the patient is advised to walk about. The passage of a ureteric catheter may aid the passage of the stone, or at the ureteric orifice it may be removed endoscopically with a device such as Dormier's basket. If the stone fails to pass, its removal from the kidney (nephrolithotomy) or ureter (ureterolithotomy) will be undertaken, and if the damage to the kidney has been severe, removal of the organ may be necessary.

3. Dissolution is possible by using an irrigating procedure but while cystine, phosphate and uric acid stones can be dissolved the commonest type of stone composed of calcium oxalate is refractory. Percutaneous nephrostomy using a catheter large enough for irrigation avoids the need for open surgery. It is a method to complement rather than compete with surgical removal and may be appropriate for patients unfit for surgery or a patient who has undergone several previous operations for renal stones.

NEW GROWTHS OF THE KIDNEY

Simple tumours, although they do occur, are not very common. Malignant new growths are the nephroblastoma (Wilms' tumour) which is seen in infants and the hypernephroma (carcinoma of the kidney) of the adult. Both tumours are extremely malignant, and blood-borne metastases to other organs are early and extensive.

Carcinoma of the renal pelvis may occur in association with carcinoma of the ureter or bladder.

Symptoms and signs

Painless haematuria is the commonest symptom. In addition, there may be pain in the region of the affected kidney. Intravenous pyelogram is essential in localising the disease. More refined techniques include angiography, isotope scans and ultrasonic detection.

Treatment

Removal of the kidney is the treatment of choice, but the end results are poor, since spread by the blood stream, particularly to the bones, occurs at an early stage in the disease. Radiotherapy may be given postoperatively and chemotherapy using actinomycin is also used.

THE CARE OF PATIENTS FOR OPERATION ON THE KIDNEY

Operations on the kidney consist of:

1. Nephrolithotomy, that is, removal of a stone.
2. Nephrostomy. (Insertion of a tube into the kidney to drain pus or urine.)
3. Nephrectomy. (Partial or total removal of the kidney.)
4. Pyeloplasty to correct hydronephrosis.

Preoperative care

Infection in the kidney should be reduced as far as possible by the administration of antibacterial drugs according to the results of the sensitivity tests. The urinary function must be at the highest possible level, and the blood urea reading is a fairly satisfactory rough guide. In most cases a figure of under 6·5 mmol per litre is desirable.

Preparation of the skin

The loin, back, abdomen, and chest are shaved in the usual way. A large cross may be made on the leg with a skin pencil by the doctor to indicate the side of the operation. Preoperative drugs are given as prescribed and the bladder is emptied. The bowel is emptied with suppositories the night previous to surgery.

Radiographs and notes must be brought to the theatre and arrangements are made for an X-ray to be taken on the theatre table during the operation if this proves to be necessary. In cases of stone the patient is X-rayed immediately before going to theatre as the stones are sometimes passed 'silently' or change their position in the urinary tract while awaiting operation. Most cases will be operated on lying on the opposite side with the lower leg flexed, the upper leg straight, and the trunk secured to the table by a strap and maintained by sandbags or rubber cushions (Fig. 42.4).

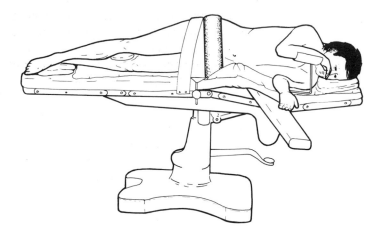

Fig. 42.4 Usual position for operations on the kidney.

Postoperative care

On return to bed the patient should be laid on the affected side. Later, he should be propped up to encourage drainage from the kidney down the ureter to the bladder. A careful watch must be kept for haemorrhage from the wound and in the urine. Some blood staining of the urine is inevitable for a day or two postoperatively except of course when the kidney has been totally removed.

The signs and symptoms of renal failure must be carefully watched for, and, in addition, the supervention of chest complications. Urinary antiseptics must be continued.

Pain must be relieved by analgesics.

The amount of urine, the presence of blood, or the onset of retention must be carefully noted. A fluid balance chart is essential.

Some degree of sepsis is almost inevitable if the wound has been drained. The sutures are removed when the wound has healed, usually the 8th to 10th day. Paralytic ileus sometimes occurs following surgery in the retroperitoneal space. This should be treated as previously described (p. 346).

The tube left in the perinephric space is usually removed on the 3rd day, but if a tube has been inserted into the renal pelvis it is left until it loosens itself—about the 10th day. It should be connected to a Bardic bag outside the bed. A primary leak may occur from the drain site. This usually stops spontaneously.

The period in bed varies from 2 to 3 days in most cases.

THE URETER

The only condition which requires special consideration is the presence of a stone in the ureter. If the stone fails to pass spontaneously, or after the passage of a ureteric catheter, the stone may have to be removed by operation. The preparation and aftertreatment are similar to that of an operation on the kidney. The only special points of importance are:

1. *Skin preparation*. The whole abdomen should be prepared on both sides, as well as the usual kidney area, since a ureteric stone may be removed through a lower midline incision.

2. *X-ray* immediately before the operation is essential and the patient must not be allowed to stand up or walk about after it has been taken. A stone which was in one portion of the ureter may have changed its position since the previous X-ray.

3. *The tube*. The wound usually seeps urine for several days, and special care is necessary to control infection in the urine and in the wound.

URINARY DIVERSION

Transplantation of the ureters

This operation may be performed for carcinoma of the bladder, after severe crush injuries, or for a severely contracted tuberculous bladder. An occasional indication is an ectopic bladder, a condition in which the pubic bones fail to fuse and the bladder mucous membrane lies on the abdominal wall, dribbling urine continuously from the exposed ureteric orifices. The ureters may be transplanted into:

1. The pelvic colon and the patient passes urine by the rectum. This operation carries the risk of ascending urinary infection and also of excessive reabsorption of chloride ions from the rectal mucosa. Before operation the rectal sphincter should be examined for continence.

2. An isolated loop of ileum. This avoids both complications of colonic transplants.

A common indication in children for transplantation of the ureters into an ileal loop is a paralysed bladder with a myelomeningocele. The operation may be necessary to gain continence or to prevent renal deterioration in the chronically infected neurogenic bladder. Transplantation into an ileal loop rather than the colon has the advantage of less electrolyte disturbance but is also necessary because the anal sphincters are paralysed. The main disadvantage is the need of a urinal bag.

Preparation and aftercare

The mental preparation of the patient who is to undergo ureteric transplant either to the pelvic colon or into an isolated loop of ileum is extremely important. The change in habit following surgery must be fully explained to the patient.

Electrolyte balance and kidney function are corrected as far as possible. The bowel is further prepared by enemas and colonic washouts.

Postoperative care

The care is that of any patient returning to the ward following major surgery.

Points applicable to ureteric transplant to the pelvic colon:

1. Rectal tube in situ. Continuous drainage into a Bardic or Aldon bag should be set up. This tube is inserted while the patient is in theatre and should be watched very carefully postoperatively to ensure that drainage is constant. Should drainage be negligible this should be immediately reported to the medical staff.

2. A nasogastric tube is aspirated hourly as required.

3. Intravenous fluids should be given and correct fluid balance is very important.

4. Sedation.

5. There may be a urethral catheter in situ but this is only acting as a drain. There may also be a wound drain.

6. Aperients and enemas postoperatively are withheld as for any other type of intestinal surgery.

7. Dietary modifications may be necessary depending on electrolyte and blood urea levels both in the postoperative and convalescent stages. Table salt is avoided and sodium bicarbonate 1 g and potassium bicarbonate 1 g daily are given to counteract acidosis and hyperchloraemia.

Patients who have had an ileal loop transplant have less rigid dietary restrictions.

The care of and problems arising from an ileal conduit have seen discussed in Chapter 38.

Retroperitoneal fibrosis

Retroperitoneal fibrosis is a rare condition, sometimes caused by drugs like methysergide or some analgesics taken in excessive amounts. It may cause obstruction to the ureters or the inferior vena cava. Steroids may be used in treatment. Surgical relief of the obstruction is often necessary.

43

Diseases of the bladder, and the male genital organs

The normal bladder has a capacity of about 360 ml.

ACUTE RETENTION OF URINE

The patient is unable to pass urine and he complains of severe pain. The cause may be:

1. Reflex. Postoperative retention is very common. Following operations on the rectum and anus great difficulty with micturition, if not actual retention, is usual.

2. Organic nervous diseases. These are often slow in onset with no pain. Lesions of the central nervous system may affect the bladder centre in the spinal cord.
   (a) Fractures of the spine with damage to the spinal cord.
   (b) Multiple sclerosis, and other diseases of the central nervous system.
   (c) Children with myelomeningocele.

3. Mechanical causes.
   (a) Rupture of the urethra.
   (b) Prostatic obstruction.
   (c) Urethral stricture and urethritis.
   (d) A stone, a foreign body, or a growth obstructing the neck of the bladder or urethra.
   (e) A retroverted gravid uterus.
   (f) Phimosis.

Clinical presentation

1. Sudden acute retention may occur in men with no previous history of urological disorder. The causes include drunkenness and hysteria.

2. Retention as a culmination of previous dysuria, increasing frequency and voiding a decreasing volume of urine. The attack is precipitated by cold or being unable to empty the bladder at a convenient moment.

In both types the patient is in severe pain and a firm, distended bladder is easily palpable.

3. Acute-on-chronic retention. This is the most dangerous form. The patient has had long-standing urinary symptoms and his general health has deteriorated because of renal failure. There is usually no complaint of pain and a complete unawareness of the severity of his condition. The large atonic bladder is painless.

Treatment and nursing care

The patient must never be catheterised and sent home forthwith. He should always be admitted to hospital, and the following measures instituted:

1. Analgesics and rest. The patient is in pain and anxious. Morphia (15 mg) is prescribed.

2. Attempted micturition. This is attempted when the pain has been relieved. A dose of mist. potassium citrate. (15 ml), a hot pack to the abdomen, or a hot bath into which the patient can pass urine, should all be tried. If these fail the retention must be relieved.

3. Mechanical relief. Mechanical relief is given by:

(a) Urethral catheterisation is the usual method which is employed. It is a common and important surgical procedure and will be considered in detail.

(b) Suprapubic catheterisation, by open method or by puncture with a trocar and cannula, will be performed only when it is impossible to pass a catheter by the urethra.

(c) Suprapubic needle puncture of the bladder. This is generally undesirable, but it may be the only method if catheterisation has failed and surgical aid is not available.

4. The maintenance of the excretion of urine by the kidneys is provided for by the administration of liberal quantities of fluids.

5. Investigation of the cause includes clinical examination of the urine, the blood, and an intravenous pyelogram is undertaken as soon as possible.

CATHETERISATION

Catheterisation can be mechanically simple, but on occasions it is extremely difficult or impossible. The management of the catheterised patient and the prevention of infection are always difficult and require great care and patience. The problems which arise from catheterisation may be summarised according to the part of the urinary tract which is affected.

1. The urethra.

(a) Trauma. The catheter may tear the delicate lining of the urethra and this is more likely to occur the more frequently the catheter has to be passed. A water-soluble lubricant is used. The more rigid the catheter the greater the trauma.

(b) The wider the catheter the greater is the pressure against the cells of the lining wall.

A large catheter is more traumatic, but a small catheter once passed is more readily blocked by blood clot or debris.

Urethritis is more likely to develop from catheterisation and infect the bladder causing cystitis, and the kidney causing pyelonephritis.

2. The penis.

(a) Meatal stricture is liable to develop from the combined effects of a large catheter made of irritating material and from infection.

(b) Balanitis and meatal ulceration. If the prepuce cannot be retracted a dorsal slit will have to be performed to avoid balanitis. Strapping the catheter to the glans penis may cause irritation. It is preferable to use a self-retaining catheter (Fig. 43.1).

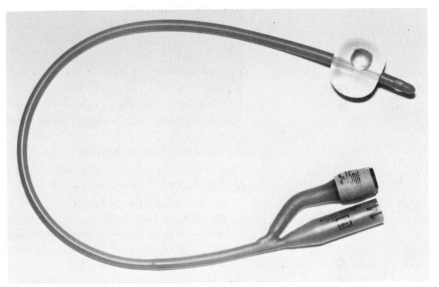

Fig. 43.1 Foley's catheter showing balloon inflated.

3. The bladder. The bladder may be infected by:

(a) Careless catheterisation including neglect of asepsis.

(b) Infection creeping up the lumen of the catheter and, in this connection, air bubbles are particularly important as a source of infection. Closed drainage using an Aldon bag prevents airborne infection.

4. The kidneys. The kidneys are particularly easily infected in cases of long-standing chronic retention of urine in which hydronephrosis has developed and the ureteric orifice mechanism in the bladder is no longer adequate to prevent regurgitation back into the ureters.

The choice of catheter will be determined by consideration of all the factors which have been mentioned above together with consideration of the cause of retention.

The size of catheter is determined by what one expects to recover from the bladder. In increasing size:

Clear urine—	the smallest
Pus—	intermediate
Blood—	the largest

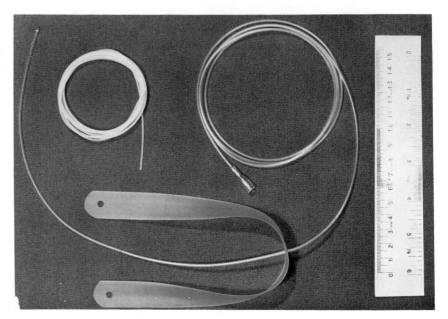

Fig. 43.2 Gibbon catheter.

The 'Portex' Gibbon catheter (Fig. 43.2) constituted a major advance because:

(a) It is easy and safe to pass.

(b) It eliminates urethritis by its small size and non-irritant nature.

(c) It requires the minimum of attention since changing and washouts are usually unnecessary; its main disadvantage is that it does not accommodate a bladder washout if one is required.

The catheter is supplied presterilised by gamma rays.

In a case of suspected rupture of the urethra or bladder a catheter must never be passed in the ward.

Catheterisation can be an extremely dangerous operation. Force must not be used and unless full asepsis is maintained the patient may lose his life.

Many of these patients are agitated, in pain and dirty, so that the initial treatment consists of morphine or pethidine intramuscularly and giving the patient a hot bath. He may pass urine into the bath, obviating the need for a catheter. The majority do not, so catheterisation has to be undertaken.

A good light, an assistant and all the equipment necessary, including at least a second catheter (in case one is dropped) should be available.

1. The genitalia are washed.
2. After masking, a full scrub-up is undertaken and sterile gloves are put on.
3. The genitalia are cleansed with 0:25 per cent chlorhexidine.
4. The patient is draped with sterile towels.
5. A whole tube of gel containing lignocaine 1 per cent and chlorhexidine 0·25 per cent is injected into the urethra, the tube being previously immersed in an alcoholic solution of chlorhexidine for 10 minutes.

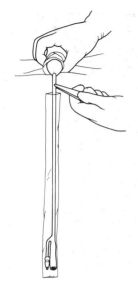

Fig. 43.3 Method of passing catheter.

6. A penile clamp is attached to keep the gel in the urethra. About 3 minutes is necessary to produce adequate analgesia.
7. A catheter is passed using a no-touch technique (Fig. 43.3).
8. The catheter is connected at once to bag (Fig. 43.7).

If the catheter is to be left indwelling it should be connected at once to to a drainage bag with a non-return valve and a tap at the base for emptying. A specimen of urine is taken as soon as the bladder is entered. Further specimens are taken by inserting a needle low down in the connecting tube before it enters the bag so that the seal is not broken. At a similar point the connecting tube is clamped off when the bag is changed. This prevents the ascent of air bubbles carrying possible infection into the bladder. The connecting tube is attached to the inner side of the thigh. The need for care to prevent infection is as great when changing the bag as in any other part of the procedure.

On the very rare occasion when it is impossible to withdraw fluid from the balloon of a Foley's catheter, chloroform should be injected through the side tube.

Catheter care

The external urinary meatus and the catheter as it enters the urethra should ideally be cleansed with 0·25 per cent chlorhexidine 4 hourly. This is sometimes impractical but it should be done at least twice a day. Chlorhexidine cream should be applied around the meatus. A small sterile dressing or a small ring of sponge over the catheter should be placed around the meatus. All this is to remove urethral discharge which accumulates around the meatus and to prevent infection entering alongside the catheter.

Suprapubic cystotomy

This procedure consists of opening the bladder by an incision in the lower abdomen. It may be performed for acute retention of urine if it is impossible to pass a urethral catheter or if there is gross infection of the urine.

A self-retaining catheter may be inserted through a bladder perforator in certain cases of retention.

DISEASES OF THE BLADDER

RUPTURE OF THE BLADDER

A blow on the lower abdomen, especially if the bladder is full, is the commonest cause of rupture. Through the tear, urine seeps into the peritoneum (intraperitoneal rupture). As a complication of a fracture of the pelvis the bladder may also be ruptured, but the tear is extraperitoneal and in this variety there is no danger of peritonitis.

Both injuries are severe. Untreated, the patient with an intraperitoneal rupture develops peritonitis, while the patient with an extraperitoneal rupture develops extensive fulminating cellulitis as a result of extravasation of urine over the tissues of the abdominal wall and the perineum.

Clinical features

1. The patient is usually in a state of shock.
2. The lower abdomen is tender and rigid.
3. No urine has been, or can be, passed. The patient should be discouraged from attempting to pass urine because it flows through the rupture.
4. Catheterisation (which should be performed in an operating theatre) recovers only a small quantity of bloodstained urine.

Treatment

Shock is treated and a laparotomy performed. The bladder is sutured and the peritoneal cavity may be drained if the rupture has been intraperitoneal.

A urethral catheter or occasionally a suprapubic catheter is inserted to keep the bladder empty during healing as well as a tube in the retropubic space.

CYSTITIS

Cystitis is a condition in which the bladder mucosa is inflamed. Many patients, particularly women, attribute any symptom, such as dysuria or scalding pain on micturition, to 'cystitis'. In many instances pyelography and examination of mid-stream specimens of urine reveal no abnormality. Only an initial specimen of urine or a urethral swab will contain pus and organisms.

Acute cystitis may be part of a general urinary infection. Chronic cystitis is usually associated with obstruction to the outflow of urine. The presence of a foreign body, such as a stone passed from the kidney, or an abnormality of the bladder, e.g. a diverticulum or cystocele, predisposes to infection.

Infection may pass down the ureter from a diseased kidney and give rise to a similar type of infection in the bladder. The organisms may be pyogenic or tuberculous. Ascending infection from the urethra is a common cause of cystitis.

Most infections arise by ascent of bowel organisms from the perineum — haematogenous infections are rare except in the neonatal period. Since the incidence of urinary infection is greater in females, it seems reasonable to suggest that the shortness of the female urethra facilitates the entry of organisms.

Urethral stricture and prostatic obstruction as well as spinal injuries, all of which interfere with the effective drainage of the bladder, predispose to infection.

Symptoms and signs

The principal symptoms are suprapubic pain, scalding pain on passing urine and frequency of micturition. Haematuria may be present if the inflammation is severe.

In some cases an underlying neoplasm gives rise to the symptoms of cystitis. Examination of the urine reveals the presence of pus, organisms, and possibly red blood corpuscles.

Treatment

The most important single factor in treatment is to encourage the patient to empty the bladder completely. In acute cases the patient has to be in bed, and consume 3 litres of fluid daily. The reaction of the urine if acid is changed by giving mist. potassium citrate. Antibiotics are prescribed only after bacteriological examination and sensitivity tests. Personal hygiene and care of the general health are important in overcoming the condition. When the symptoms subside a full investigation, particularly to discover any cause of defective bladder emptying which can be remedied, is under-taken. If bladder neck obstruction is present in the female endoscopic resection will be necessary.

Bladder washouts (lavage) are not usually performed unless specially ordered. Fluid must not be forced into the bladder under pressure, and bladder washouts should be of the correct temperature: 37°C (100°F). Normally 180 to 210 ml of fluid are instilled, but if the patient complains of pain before this volume has been used no attempt should be made to force a further quantity into the bladder. The common solutions used are:

Silver nitrate 1/15 000 to 1/5000.

Acetic acid 0·5 per cent.

Hibitane 1/5000, in pure aqueous solution — not the form in which it is sent for ward stock.

Noxyflex 1 per cent for continuous irrigation, 2·5 per cent for instillation.

Bladder lavage: irrigation

Bladder washout (irrigation) may be ordered for:

Chronic cystitis.

Haematuria with clot formation as the presenting sign of disease.

Haematuria following operation on the bladder or prostate. ⌐

The fluid usually used is saline 0·9 per cent, sterile, and at room temperature.

1. Continuous lavage — or closed system. The irrigating fluid is suspended from a drip stand, passes down a giving set, and enters the bladder through one arm of a three-way catheter. Together with the urine it drains out of the bladder via the other arm of the catheter into a drainage bag (Fig. 43.7). The rate of the flow of the irigating fluid is prescribed by the doctor, e.g. immediately after operation it may free-flowing, or 1·5 litre in 1 hour.

Before putting up a fresh container of irrigating fluid the drainage bag is allowed to empty into a jug, then respigotted or reconnected and the contents are measured. The nurse washes and dries her hands. The litre of fluid is checked and put up, and the flow regulated as prescribed. The amount of irrigating fluid and of drainage is recorded/charted. Whilst the irrigation is in progress, the nurse observes:

N.B. (a) that urine is being secreted.
    (b) that the fluid is flowing into the bladder at the prescribed rate
    (c) that it is draining out of the bladder into the drainage bag
    (d) whether any bleeding is increasing or decreasing
    (e) the presence of any clots
    (f) any distension of or discomfort in the bladder or abdomen
    (g) the amount flowing in as compared with the amount draining out
    (h) the condition of the suprapubic wound and its dressing.

The irrigation continues until the urine is clear — usually, for not less than 48 hours and often for 3 to 4 days. The drainage system is changed as necessary. When the continuous irrigation is to cease, the patient is informed and made ready by being given privacy and by having personal and bedclothing rearranged.

The flow of the irrigating fluid is stopped, the giving set disconnected and the catheter arm spigotted — sterility being maintained — leaving continuous drainage of urine via the catheter and drainage tubing and bag. A note is made on the fluid chart to this effect, i.e. irrigation ceased. The patient is repositioned, encouraged to drink fluids in abundance, and all intake and output carefully measured and recorded. Used equipment is disposed of in the soiled dressing bag.

If requested, 24 hours after discontinuation, a catheter specimen of urine is collected and sent to the laboratory.

2. Hand irrigation. A basic dressing trolley is prepared, with the addition of a 50 ml catheter-tip syringe, irrigating fluid, bowl, receiver, spigot.

The patient is informed of what is going to happen and his cooperation obtained. The trolley is taken to the bedside, privacy is ensured, and the patient is placed in a comfortable position with his legs apart.

Using the aseptic technique, the dressing packet is opened and prepared. Outer packs are opened, the contents are placed on the sterifield. Some irrigating fluid is poured into the bowl. A towel is placed under the catheter, the receiver is placed between the legs. The spigot is removed and discarded, or the drainage bag is disconnected and its end covered with a sterile swab.

Using gentle pressure on a syringe 30 ml of fluid is instilled and then sucked back, noting the amount, colour, presence of clots, etc. It is repeated as necessary until no clots return.

A clean spigot is put in, or the drainage bag is reconnected. The receiver is removed.

N.B. If after instillation of the first 30 ml no fluid is drawn back, the medical officer is notified at once, no attempt being made to introduce more fluid at this stage.

The meatus and nearby catheter are swabbed. The patient is dried and made comfortable. The trolley and its contents are removed. A report/record is made of the result.

STONES IN THE BLADDER

Bladder stones develop as a result of infection.

The stone may form in the bladder or may enlarge in the bladder after being passed from the kidney. The main symptoms are pain, frequency of micturition by day, haematuria and strangury.

X-ray reveals the presence of the stone, which is removed by the introduction of a crushing instrument *per urethram*, or, if too large and very hard, by the suprapubic route. Very occasionally a stone is not opaque and can be diagnosed only on cystoscopic examination.

NEW GROWTHS OF THE BLADDER

A new growth in the bladder (Fig. 43.4) may be malignant from the beginning. If it is simple (papilloma) there is a strong tendency to recur in spite of treatment, and eventually to become malignant. Because of this the condition is now usually called papillomatous disease of the urinary tract. The disease is multicentric in origin so that even a small lesion confined to the mucous membrane is to be regarded as the first manifestation of the disease. Because lesions may erupt and may invade the bladder wall a patient suffering from the disease must be cystoscoped at regular intervals for the remainder of his life.

Workers in certain industries of which rubber manufacture is an example should be screened for disease by cytological examination of the urine at regular intervals.

Symptoms and signs

1. Painless haematuria is the most constant symptom. At the end of micturition almost pure blood may be passed.

2. Increased frequency and scalding on micturition develop if secondary infection occurs.

3. Pain may be intolerable in the late stages of carcinoma, and frequently takes the form of severe sciatica from infiltration by the growth, of the sacral plexus.

4. Bimanual examination of the bladder, with the finger in the rectum and the hand on the abdominal wall, may reveal a swelling.

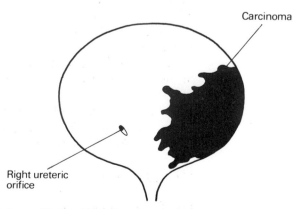

Fig. 43.4 Carcinoma bladder. The left ureteric orifice has been invaded and the left kidney will be non-functioning.

Treatment

In addition to a full urinary investigation, cystoscopy is performed to confirm the diagnosis and a biopsy may be taken. The growth is removed by endoscopic resection or if small by cystodiathermy. More extensive lesions are treated by:

1. Megavoltage radiotherapy.
2. Partial cystectomy (not often).
3. Total cystectomy with urinary diversion (Ch. 42).

DIVERTICULUM OF THE BLADDER

A diverticulum (Fig. 43.5) may occur in the bladder secondary to obstruction in the urethra or as a result of inherent weakness of the musculature of the bladder. The condition is frequently complicated by sepsis, stone formation, and the occurrence of a new growth.

The treatment is that of the causal condition combined, if necessary, with excision of the diverticulum.

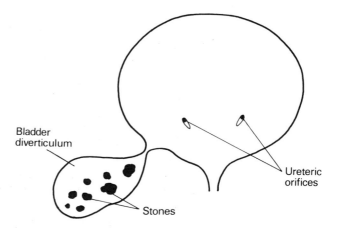

Fig. 43.5   A diverticulum of the bladder complicated by stone formation.

DISEASES OF THE PROSTATE

The prostate is a gland about the size of a walnut, situated in the proximal portion of the male urethra.

The commonest lesion is prostatic obstruction. This results in increasing urinary disturbance and damage to the kidneys. The bladder is never completely emptied, so that back pressure causes hydronephrosis (Fig. 43.6). The patients are usually advanced in years, 60 or over being the usual age. Disturbance of the patient's general health may be very great.

Causes

1. *Simple (benign) enlargement.*   This is the commonest type.

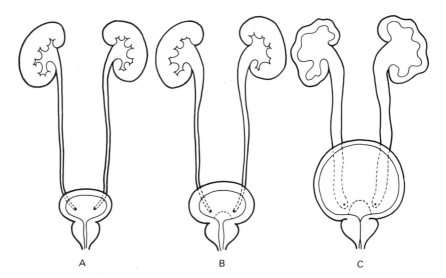

Fig. 43.6 The effects of prostatism. A. Normal. B. Moderate enlargement, hydronephrosis and hypertrophy of the bladder. C. Gross enlargement, extensive hydronephrosis and an atonic distended bladder.

2. Prostatic fibrosis in which the internal meatus is almost closed by narrowing.

3. Carcinoma of the prostate.

Symptoms and signs

1. Increased frequency and difficulty of micturition are prominent complaints. The patient's sleep is disturbed. The general health and well-being deteriorate from lack of sleep.

2. Haematuria may occur in some cases as a result of congestion.

3. Pain and scalding on micturition develop from infection of the residual urine.

4. Acute retention of urine may develop. About 1 in 10 patients present with acute retention. In a neglected case renal failure will set in, and the patient may be admitted to hospital in coma or in a semicomatosed state.

5. Enlargement of the gland may be felt on rectal examination.

Treatment

If at all possible prostatectomy in some form, or even in stages, is carried out. If the patient's condition is too poor then an indwelling catheter may be all that is possible and a Foley catheter, preferably made of inert silastic material, would seem to be the one of choice. Occasionally a permanent suprapubic catheter has to be left in place. The precise method of treatment will depend on:

1. *The nature of the obstruction*
2. *The effect it produces.* Most important are those on:
   (a) The kidneys.
   (b) The bladder.

Stone formation, infection or diverticulum formation may be extensive.

3. *General health of the patient.* Many patients have associated disease like myocardial insufficiency or chronic bronchitis. In such patients spinal or epidural anaesthesia can be used satisfactorily.

Choice of operations

Transurethral resection of prostate. Gland resected *per uretheram* by resectoscope. No abdominal wound.

Retropubic (Millin). The prostate is removed by operation in the space between the back of the pubis and the bladder (which is not opened).

Suprapubic-transvesical (Freyer, Harris, Wilson-Hey). The bladder is opened and the prostate enucleated. Freyer's original type — Wilson-Hey — improved haemostasis.

Perineal approach rarely used in the U.K.

The most satisfactory operation for prostatic obstruction is endoscopic resection. In expert hands 95 per cent of all enlargements can be dealt with by this method. There are no tubes beyond a urethral catheter which has to be observed to ensure that the effluent is draining and kept clear. There is no wound in the abdominal wall, in the bladder or the prostatic capsule and the patient can usually be discharged on the fifth day passing urine satisfactorily.

Preparation for operation

The preparation and aftercare of all types of operations for the relief of prostatic obstruction are basically similar. It is the details which confuse the nurse. Consideration of the two basic problems serves to show the lines along which treatment should be directed. They are:

1. *The maintenance of adequate renal function.* The best general test of renal function is the level of the blood urea — normal 2·50–6·67 μmol per litre (15 to 40 mg per cent). Whatever the level it will be raised by:
- (a) Blood loss which is sufficient to lower the blood pressure because the kidneys fail to excrete in conditions of hypotension.
- (b) Infection which prevents the kidneys from functioning satisfactorily.

It will be lowered by:
- (a) Control of infection.
- (b) Free drainage of the bladder which also means that the kidneys can work without back pressure.
- (c) A large intake of fluids resulting in a correspondingly large output of urine.

2. *Postoperative bleeding.* It is impossible by any method of prostatectomy to stop all the bleeding in the theatre and, for this reason, the nurse has a very special responsibility in the postoperative care of these patients. There are two dangers:
- (a) Haemorrhage may increase on return to the ward and
- (b) The blood lost may form clots in the bladder, causing bladder dis-

tension. This in turn prevents retraction of the blood vessels and increases further the amount of bleeding. The clots may block the drainage tube or catheters and the patient is in severe pain. To aggravate matters already bad the consequent hypotension causes diminution or cessation of renal excretion and increases the likelihood of renal failure. For all these reasons the following lessons emerge:

1. Renal function should be as good as possible as measured by the blood urea or blood creatinine. Preferably it should be normal and the higher it is above normal the greater the risk of operation.

2. The patient should be in the best possible general condition and have a haemoglobin reading of at least 12 g per dl.

3. Postoperatively all measures should be taken to prevent clot formation.

General care

1. Renal function is improved if necessary by catheter drainage and by urinary antiseptics, and bladder washouts are given if the urine is grossly infected.

2. Large fluid intake is encouraged. Tea, coffee, lemonade, cocoa, or other drinks to which glucose has been added may be given. A jug of fluid should be available on the top of the patient's bedside locker and the nurse must encourage the patient to drink with unrelenting persistence. Sufficient fluid must be taken to keep the patient's tongue moist and a careful fluid balance chart must be kept.

3. A specimen of urine is sent to the laboratory for examination and the blood urea and blood creatinine are estimated.

4. The scrotum is supported on a broad piece of Elastoplast strapped across the thighs. This simple procedure diminishes the risk of epididymo-orchitis, which is a an occasional complication in these cases.

5. Breathing exercises improve the patient's general condition and diminish the risk of postoperative pulmonary complications.

6. The pressure areas require meticulous care. Faulty junctions of the drainage apparatus result in a wet bed, and every effort must be made to keep the patient dry.

7. The blood pressure is estimated.

The patient is fit for operation when the blood urea is about 6·67 μmol per litre (40 mg per cent) or below, and the urine is almost free of pus.

The general condition of the patient must, of course, be considered in assessing fitness for an operation.

Postoperative care

The principal complications are:
1. Haemorrhage.
2. Infection.
3. Renal failure.
Other complications which are liable to occur are:
1. Pulmonary complications.

2. Epididymo-orchitis.

3. Obstruction of the bladder neck.

Careful preliminary treatment considerably reduces the risk of postoperative complications. However, prostatectomy is a severe undertaking, the majority of patients being men of advanced years.

On return from the theatre the patient is positioned recumbent in bed. The foot of the bed should be elevated and a slow transfusion of blood is continued if necessary. Fluids of a diuretic nature such as mannitol may be given intravenously.

There must be a careful check on the respiratory movement and oxygen is administered if necessary. If the patient is collapsed the blood transfusion is usually speeded up by the house surgeon until the blood pressure is satisfactory. Bacteraemia as a cause of hypotension should be excluded if the patient's condition does not improve. Hydrocortisone may be prescribed and a blood culture taken.

The patient is usually nursed on a siliconised mattress. He is moved frequently in bed to prevent the onset of chest complications, and is allowed to sit out of bed as soon as possible if his general condition is satisfactory.

Care of the drainage tubes

The number and arrangement of the drainage tubes will usually vary with the type of operation.

1. Endoscopic resection. As there is no wound the only drainage is through a three way Foley or similar self-retaining catheter.

2. Millin or Wilson-Hey (Fig. 43.7). There is an abdominal wound. A small piece of corrugated rubber is left in the retropubic space to drain the sutured incision in the prostatic capsule or bladder. This can be removed in 48 hours. A catheter similar to that used in endoscopic resection is used to drain the bladder.

Removal of the catheter. The catheter is removed at a varying period between 2 and 10 days. After removal of the catheter the patient should pass urine every hour so that the bladder does not become distended and stretch the healing wound. On the first night after removal he should be woken every 2 hours to pass urine.

In all forms of prostatectomy:

The scrotum must be carefully supported if the risk of epididymo-orchitis is to be diminished.

The fluid intake must be abundant and the consumption of fluids must be encouraged by the nurse. The blood urea often rises after the operation, since prostatectomy 'upsets' the kidney functions temporarily, and if fluid is not supplied these patients become uraemic, have no pain, are sleepy, and lie quite still as they die gradually from renal failure. Urinary antiseptics, including antibiotics, are of the greatest value in controlling infection and thereby diminishing the risk of renal failure.

The sutures. The superficial sutures are removed about the eight to tenth day.

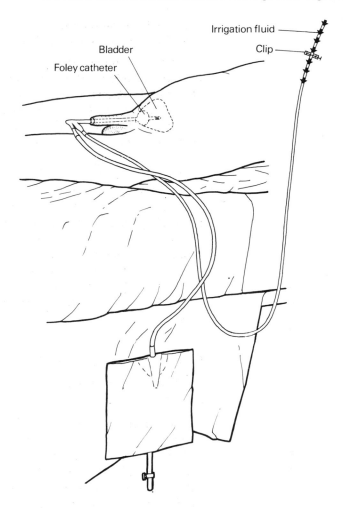

Bladder

Foley catheter

Irrigation fluid

Clip

Fig. 43.7 Closed drainage of the bladder by a urethral catheter into an Aldon bag. The irrigating solution can be run through the other channel in the catheter.

Most patients after open protatectomy are fit for discharge about 10–14 days after the operation, provided no complication has arisen.

Complications

1. *Clot retention*. If clot retention occurs the bladder should be irrigated gently with 3·8 per cent sodium citrate by means of a large bladder syringe. e-Aminocaproic acid (p. 103) may be used to diminish bleeding. If the patient develops a clot retention which it is impossible to clear by mechanical means the bladder may have to be reopened.

2. *The patient pulls out the catheter*. This will have to be reinserted, sometimes under a further anaesthetic.

3. *Circulatory collapse* is prevented by adequate blood transfusion and keeping the drainage tubes free so that clot retention does not occur.

4. *Infection and septicaemia.*

5. *Suprapubic leakage* may occur after the catheter has been removed. It usually clears up after three or four days further catheter drainage. Intermittent drainage should be instituted before removal of the catheter.

6. *Epididymo-orchitis*: The scrotum should always be well supported.

7. *Secondary haemorrhage* is an occasional complication about 8 days postoperatively and requires bladder washouts, free drainage and antibiotics.

8. *Stricture formation* may cause a diminishing stream of urine and bougies may have to be passed.

9. *Incontinence.* Some incontinence is very likely to be present in the early days after removal of the catheter. It is prevented and diminished by urethral exercises. The patient is instructed to commence passing urine and then to stop and start again three or four times during the day. This promotes tone in the sphincter muscle. The patient who is temporarily incontinent will be greatly helped by a condom urinal.

10. *Persistent pyuria* is common after the operation and is not significantly diminished by operating under an antibiotic umbrella. Antibacterial substances are only given if there is evidence of gross infection.

CARCINOMA OF THE PROSTATE GLAND

Carcinoma of the prostate is not uncommon. An established carcinoma of the prostate is usually too fixed to be removed. Occasionally a focus of malignancy is discovered on pathological examination of an enlarged prostate which has been removed for what was believed to be simple enlargement.

The signs and symptoms are similar to those of simple enlargement, but pain is more prominent. Spread of the growth to the bones occurs early in the disease and the serum acid phosphatase is elevated.

Investigations include estimation of the serum acid phosphatase, skeletal X-ray, lymphangiography and needle biopsy as well as the usual tests to assess renal function.

Treatment

It may be decided to take no further steps in treatment beyond observation when a localised focus of malignancy had been discovered in a gland believed to be clinically simple. In other patients the preparations most commonly used are stilboestrol or dienoestrol by mouth which are given indefinitely. A dosage of 1 mg t.d.s. is as effective in it's response as a larger dosage and diminishes the risk of thrombosis. Thrombosis is a calculated risk of oestrogen therapy but is worth taking in view of the gravity of the condition. Stilboestrol diphosphate (Honvan) or Tace may be prescribed if stilboestrol is ineffective. Occasionally bilateral orchidectomy may be performed.

Endoscopic resection is frequently performed for temporary relief in this condition. A channel is cut by means of a resectoscope, using diathermy coagulation.

After the operation a catheter is left in the urethra for 3 days. Radiotherapy may be undertaken in some cases but radical surgical removal is rarely advised.

If the patient's growth is resistant to hormones the outlook is gloomy.

Prostatic calculi

Prostatic calculi may occur as a result of infection or small abscess formation and usually require no treatment.

THE PENIS AND URETHRA

CIRCUMCISION

This operation is usually performed for phimosis (Fig. 43.8). If balanitis (infection under the prepuce) is present the prepuce is slit on its dorsal surface, since circumcision in the presence of infection is likely to be followed by extensive skin sloughing. In the infant circumcision is a very minor procedure, but in the adult it is a more severe undertaking.

Many infants are referred to clinics for advice on circumcision but only in a few is it necessary. The baby's prepuce is naturally tight and it may not retract easily until he is 3 or 4 years old. A common cause of reference is the ulcerated foreskin associated with ammoniacal dermatitis (napkin rash). For this condition, circumcision is strongly contra-indicated and will remove nature's protection for the glans and external urinary meatus and so allow ammonia to burn the glans. This will produce stenosis which is a complication of a meatal ulcer. Ammoniacal dermatitis is caused by bacteria from faeces fermenting the urea in wet napkins, with the production of ammonia. The treatment is to allow the child to be without a napkin as much as possible.

In many cases, when the foreskin is too tight, a dorsal slit, and not circumcision, is all that is required.

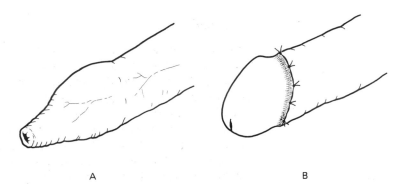

A   B

Fig. 43.8 A. Phimosis.
B. Circumcision.

Complications of circumcision

1. Haemorrhage.
2. Infection.
3. Urethritis, particularly damage to the external urinary meatus.
4. Meatal ulcer.

Balanitis

This requires repeated saline baths, antiseptic dressings such as eusol, and the provision of free drainage by dorsal slit if necessary.

Carcinoma

Carcinoma of the penis occurs occasionally, and treatment necessitates removal of the organ and the lymphatic glands in the groin.

The wounds

After the extensive dissection which is necessary to remove the glands in both groins it is usually difficult to secure healing of the wounds. The skin flaps are thin and lymph accumulates beneath. Firm pressure dressings are most important. Lymph which accumulates may be aspirated, with every care taken to avoid infection. Less effective is continuous suction.

Pin-hole meatus

This condition causes urinary obstruction. The treatment is enlargement of the meatus.

RUPTURE OF THE URETHRA

Rupture of the urethra is a serious injury usually caused by a fall astride a spike or the sharp edge of a kerbstone. Frequently it is associated with a fracture of the pelvis.

Clinical features

1. Pain is present in the perineum, which is swollen and tender.
2. Bleeding occurs from the urethral orifice.
3. There is retention of urine.

Treatment

The patient is advised not to pass urine, because it would only flow into the tissues and add to the dangers. Morphia (15 mg) is prescribed to relieve the pain of retention until he can be taken to the theatre.

The urethra is explored by an incision in the perineum with the patient in the lithotomy position. The divided urethra is sutured and the wound is left open so that irrigation can be carried out and infection prevented. The bladder is drained suprapubically to divert the flow of urine until the urethra has healed.

In the immediate postoperative period the sulphonamide drugs, urinary antiseptics, and fluids are given. As soon as healing occurs dilatation is performed, and the patient is advised to return one to two months later for further dilatation and examination. A grave complication is urethral stricture.

URETHRAL STRICTURE

The vast majority of urethral strictures used to be due to gonorrhoea but, with the easy cure of this disease by the antibiotics, instrumentation and injury are now probably the commonest causes. The urinary stream gradually diminishes until the patient is almost unable to pass urine. Back pressure results in hydronephrosis of the kidneys and hypertrophy of the bladder. Periurethral abscess is an occasional complication.

The treatment consists of repeated dilatation with bougies. In refractory cases the stricture may have to be divided by operation. Following urethral dilatation rigors are liable to develop, due to bacteraemic shock. For this reason urethral dilatation is one of the few procedures which should be performed under the cover of a broad-spectrum antibiotic.

DISEASES OF THE TESTICLE, THE SPERMATIC CORD AND ITS COVERINGS

Undescended testis

The testes develop near the kidneys *in utero*, and at birth both testicles are in the scrotum. The maldescent is frequently associated with a hernia and gives rise to symptoms only if recurrent nipping of the testicle occurs at the external abdominal ring.

Treatment

The testicle should be brought down by operation before the age of 7. Hormones may be prescribed to encourage normal descent and development but their value is questionable.

If a hernia is present operation will be necessary for this condition at about the age of 4 years, and should conservative measures fail to bring about the descent of the testis operative replacement of the organ in the scrotum will usually be performed.

The nurse must take care of any special stitch or retentive apparatus which may be fitted to secure the testicle in position. The operating surgeon will give precise instructions about the postoperative care of the stitches and their date of removal.

Acute epididymo-orchitis

Inflammation of the testis and epididymis is known as epididymo-orchitis.

Aetiology

In adolescents the commonest cause is its occurence as a complication of mumps. In the adult the commonest organism is the *E. coli*. The gonoccocus is the second commonest cause of infection.

Symptoms

The testicle is tender and swollen and the scrotal skin may be oedematous. In many cases the condition is combined with a urinary infection, and increased frequency and scalding of micturition may be present.

Treatment

The patient should be confined to bed and the scrotum supported on a sling of broad strapping attached to the thighs. Urinary antiseptics, together with a course of sulphonamide therapy, are prescribed. The urine should be examined for bacteria, antibiotic sensitivity, or other abnormal constituents.

Resolution is usual and drainage is rarely necessary. The acute stage subsides rapidly, but complete resolution takes two or three months, and recurrent attacks are not uncommon.

Ligation of the vas deferens may be advisable for recurrent attacks.

Chronic epididymo-orchitis

Causes

1. Tuberculosis.
2. Syphilis.

Tuberculous epididymitis may be part of a tuberculous infection of the urinary tract, or it may occur as a solitary lesion in the genito-urinary tract.

Treatment. Antituberculous chemotherapy (p.70) is commenced. In refractory cases the epididymis may be excised.

Syphilis. A gumma gives rise to a large painless swelling of the testicle. At puberty a congenital syphilitic may develop epididymo-orchitis. The treatment is that of syphilis.

Torsion of the testis

Torsion of the testis gives rise to severe pain and acute swelling. Immediate operation is desirable and, because the same condition may occur on the other side, the opposite testicle should also be fixed in the scrotum.

Hydrocele

A hydrocele is a collection of serous fluid in the tunica vaginalis or sac

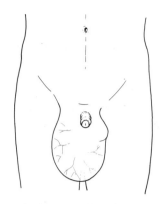

Fig. 43.9 Right hydrocele. The left side of the scrotum is normal.

surrounding the testicle (Fig. 43.9). The condition may be secondary to disease of the testicle, but usually develops without any obvious cause.

Treatment

Aspiration by means of a needle and syringe inserted into the hydrocele under local anaesthesia.

The only preparation necessary is the cleansing of the skin with Savlon. A torch is essential to transilluminate the swelling so that the surgeon can select an area of skin between the large veins and thereby obviate the formation of a haematoma. The puncture hole in the skin is covered by collodion gauze dressings.

Tapping is only a palliative measure and the sac refills, so that the procedure will have to be repeated fairly frequently.

Radical cure. This is effected by excision of the sac or by turning the sac inside out. Diathermy is frequently used during the operation, so the nurse must remember to adjust the bandages and clothing so that a bare area of skin is easily available on the patient's thigh for the diathermy electrode.

A drain will be inserted in the scrotum for 48 hours, and the scrotum must be supported on strapping across the thighs for ten days after the operation. This is most important if a massive haematocele is to be avoided.

Haematocele

A haematocele is a collection of blood around the testicle. The condition is sometimes due to trauma and sometimes to a new growth. Aspiration or open drainage may be necessary.

New growths of the testicle

New growths are not common but are intensely malignant. The primary lesion rapidly results in ulceration and fungation. Secondary deposits occur high in the abdomen.

Treatment

The testicle is removed and megavoltage therapy is prescribed for the abdominal glands.

THE SPERMATIC CORD

Funiculitis or inflammation of the spermatic cord may occur as a complication of epididymo-orchitis. The treatment is similar to that of infection of the testicle.

Varicocele (Fig. 43.10)

Varicocele is a condition of varicosity of the veins in the spermatic cord,

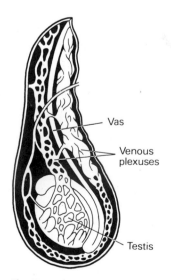

Vas

Venous plexuses

Testis

Fig. 43.10 Varicocele.

and occurs almost invariably on the left side. A slight dragging pain or, more usually, routine medical examination calls attention to the condition.

Treatment

The vast majority of cases require no treatment at all. A suspensory bandage is advised if the patient complains of pain. Operation may be undertaken and consists of excising the dilated veins.

Vasectomy (Fig. 43.11)

Vasectomy is division of the vas deferens. It may be undertaken for:
1. Recurrent epididymo-orchitis.
2. As a method of family planning.

The surgeon must satisfy himself that the patient understands the nature of the operation, the difficulties of reversal and have the consent of the patient's wife. Before all these criteria are satisfied there is much to be said for a doctor specially interested in marriage counselling interviewing the couple before a decision is taken.

The operation is usually performed under local anaesthetic without the necessity for hospital admission.

The vas is divided through a small incision at the upper end of the scrotum on each side. Minor sepsis in the wound and a haematoma (which may require aspiration) are occasional complications. Semen examinations are essential until they show no living spermatozoa and until three negative tests are obtained vasectomy is not a safe method of contraception.

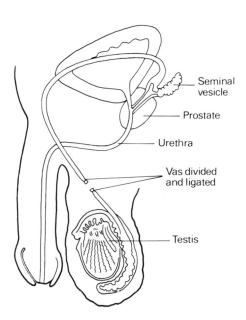

Fig. 43.11 Vasectomy.

THE SCROTUM

A sebaceous cyst is probably the commonest lesion of the scrotal skin and is excised in the usual way.

Carcinoma of the scrotal skin is now extremely rare.

BIBLIOGRAPHY

British Medical Journal Editorial 1978 1: 61
Dretler S P, Pfister R C, Newhouse J H 1979 New England Journal of Medicine 300: 341
Roe P F 1977 Age and Ageing 6: 238–239

44

Injuries and diseases of the central nervous system

The central nervous system consists of the **brain** and the **spinal cord**.

STRUCTURE

THE BRAIN

The brain lies within the bony skull which provides it with some protection against injury. The largest part of the brain is made up of the two **cerebral hemispheres**, each with a surface folded into small crests (**gyri**) and grooves (**sulci**). Each hemisphere is divided into four lobes: The **frontal lobe**, lying anteriorly, is separated by the central **sulcus** from the **parietal lobe**, with the **occipital lobe** behind. The **temperal lobe** beneath the frontal and parietal lobes is separated by a deep groove, **the Sylvian fissure**.

The cerebral hemispheres

The surface of the cerebral hemispheres, the **cerebral cortex**, contains millions of nerve cells which give it a greyish pink colour (grey matter). Just beneath the cortex lies the white matter which consists of nerve fibres supported by a framework of connective tissue (neuroglia). Deep within each hemisphere, embedded in white matter are clusters of grey matter known as the **basal ganglia**, the **thalamus**, and the **hypothalamus**.

The brainstem

The brainstem, a single midline structure mostly made up of nerve fibres, extends from beneath the cerebral hemispheres to the spinal cord (Fig. 44.1). It is subdivided into:

1. The midbrain
2. The pons
3. The medulla oblongata.

The **cerebellum**, comprising two laterally placed hemispheres and a midline vermis lies on the back of the brainstem. The **cranial nerves**, excepting the first pair, enter or emerge from the front of the brainstem.

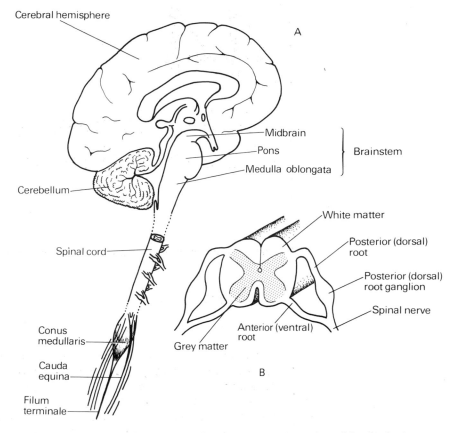

Fig. 44.1 A. Median section of the brain, showing the relationship of the cerebral hemispheres and cerebellum to the brainstem. The spinal cord is continuous with the medulla and ends in a bulbous swelling, the conus medullaris.
B. The spinal cord in cross-section.

The blood supply

The brain derives its blood supply from the two **internal carotid** and two **vertebral arteries** in the neck. On the undersurface of the brain, branches join each other to form a ring, the **circle of Willis** (Fig. 44.2). From here major blood vessels (the anterior, middle, and posterior cerebral arteries) leave to supply well-defined parts of the cerebral hemispheres.

The meninges

The brain and the spinal cord are completely surrounded by three membranes — the meninges.

The dura mater, the outer membrane, is tough and fibrous. It is plastered to the inside of the skull, but also extends into the cranial cavity as folds separating the components of the brain. A midline fold, the **falx cerebri**, extending from the front of the head to the back separates the two cerebral hemispheres, while a horizontal sheet (the **tentorium cerebelli**) slips between the cerebral hemispheres above and the cerebellum below. The brainstem descends through a gap in the tentorium, the **tentorial hiatus**.

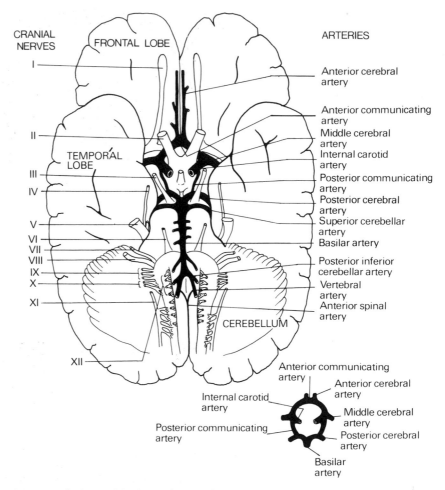

CRANIAL NERVES

FRONTAL LOBE

ARTERIES

I

II

TEMPORAL LOBE

III

IV

V

VI
VII
VIII
IX
X

XI

XII

CEREBELLUM

Anterior cerebral artery

Anterior communicating artery
Middle cerebral artery
Internal carotid artery
Posterior communicating artery
Posterior cerebral artery
Superior cerebellar artery
Basilar artery

Posterior inferior cerebellar artery
Vertebral artery
Anterior spinal artery

Anterior communicating artery
Internal carotid artery
Posterior communicating artery

Anterior cerebral artery
Middle cerebral artery
Posterior cerebral artery
Basilar artery

Fig. 44.2 The base of the brain, showing the cranial nerves and major arteries. *Inset*: the circle of Willis.

The arachnoid mater lies beneath the dura and is a much thinner membrane.

The pia mater is very fine and closely applied to the brain itself. The arachnoid and the pia are separated by the **subarachnoid space**.

The ventricles

The brain is hollow, each cerebral hemisphere containing a large cavity, the **lateral ventricle**, filled with colourless watery **cerebrospinal fluid** produced by fronds of vascular tissue, the **choroid plexuses**.

The lateral ventricles join a third ventricle in the midline, and from here cerebrospinal fluid passes down the midbrain in a narrow **aqueduct of Sylvius** to reach the fourth ventricle (Fig. 44.3). Through three small openings in the roof of this ventricle, the fluid escapes to the subarachnoid space, bathing the outside of the brain. It circulates to the top of the head where it is finally absorbed into the **superior sagittal sinus**, a venous channel lying within the falx and draining into the internal jugular veins.

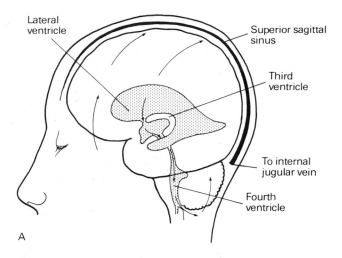

A

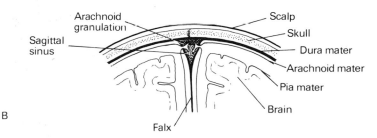

B

Fig. 44.3 A. The circulation of the cerebrospinal fluid.
B. Cross-section through the superior sagittal sinus. Cerebrospinal fluid drains from the subarachnoid space into the sagittal sinus through the arachnoid granulations.

THE SPINAL CORD

The spinal cord is continuous with the medulla oblongata and extends down the spinal canal to the level of the lower border of the first lumbar vertebra. It consists of a central core of grey matter surrounded by a shell of white matter. At regular intervals along its length, the spinal cord gives off paired **anterior** and **posterior nerve roots** which join to form **spinal nerves**. These leave the spinal canal segmentally between adjacent vertebrae, and at the lower end are quite long resembling a horse's tail (the **cauda equina**). A gentle expansion, the **conus medullaris**, marks the end of the spinal cord which is attached to the coccyx by a fine fibrous strand, the **filum terminale**. The subarachnoid space extends down to the sacrum.

FUNCTION

The left cerebral hemisphere controls the right side of the body and vice versa. Furthermore in each hemisphere there are relatively discrete areas

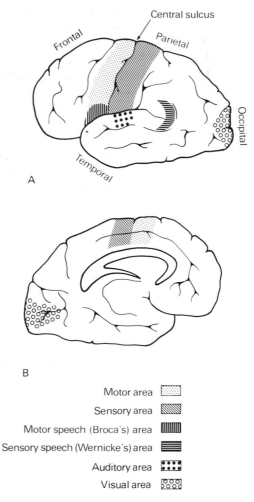

Motor area   ▦

Sensory area   ▨

Motor speech (Broca's) area   ▥

Sensory speech (Wernicke's) area   ▤

Auditory area   ⊡

Visual area   ⊙

Fig. 44.4 Localisation of function in the left cerebral hemisphere
A. lateral aspect.
B. medial aspect.

which appear to have specific functions (Fig. 44.4). Thus the gyrus just in front of the central sulcus (the **motor cortex**) has a predominance of cells which, when stimulated, induce movement on the opposite side. The gyrus behind the central sulcus (the **sensory cortex**) subserves general bodily sensation. The **visual cortex** lies in the occipital lobe.

Other aspects of brain function are represented in one hemisphere only. In right-handed people, speech (which involves both comprehension and expression) is organised in the left cerebral hemisphere, as is the ability to read, write, and do arithmetic.

The basal ganglia appear to be involved in the organisation of involuntary movements associated with change in posture and with emotional reactions. The thalamus, on the other hand, is principally a relay station through which nerve impulses are transmitted to and from the hemisphere. The hypothalamus takes part in the control and regulation of the visceral and metabolic activities of the body. The cerebellum has a controlling influence on posture and coordinates muscle tone to allow smooth voluntary movements.

At the cellular level, when a nerve cell (**neurone**) is stimulated, it gives off a small electrical discharge which travels along its length. It seems that the influence of one nerve cell over another is dependent on chemical transmitter substances. These are released when a neurone is excited, and may have a stimulating or inhibiting effect on adjacent nerve cells. There therefore exists a mechanism whereby electrical activity can be passed up and down the central nervous system through relays of nerve cells. In this way the brain receives information from the outside world (as well as from within the body), is able to make sense of it, and coordinates any action that may be appropriate.

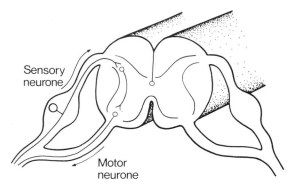

Sensory neurone

Motor neurone

Fig. 44.5 The reflex arc.

The reflex arc (Fig. 44.5) is the simplest example of this mechanism. Taking a pinprick as an example, this stimulus excites a sensory nerve which reaches the spinal cord through a posterior nerve root. From here, further neurones are excited and a chain reaction follows up to the brain where the pain is appreciated. Meanwhile, within the spinal cord, other neurones directly stimulate a motor nerve leaving the cord through an anterior nerve root. Stimulation of this nerve causes muscle contraction, and the limb is smartly removed from the source of pain. All this, of course, happens in a fraction of a second, indeed before one becomes consciously aware of the pain.

THE NURSE, THE PATIENT, AND THE RELATIVE

ARRIVAL

Admission to a neurosurgical ward is a worrying time for the patient and his relatives. Much of the anxiety is generated from ignorance. The belief that neurosurgery comprises operations on patients helpless and hopeless is still widespread, and the fear of having one's faculties disturbed by surgery is understandable. The truth of the matter is that the neurosurgeon today is concerned with the management of a large number of eminently treatable conditions, and he aims to restore affected patients to a full and active life. Naturally he is also involved in serious and life-threatening conditions such as major head injuries and inoperable tumours, and he has his share of disappointment, frustration, and sadness.

First impressions are important, and a friendly welcome shown to a new arrival and his relatives does much to reassure a patient. He may be tired and hungry after a long journey. He may be worried by seeing other patients on the ward who are confused, restless, or perhaps have some difficulty with speech. People with bandaged heads provide an unfamiliar and sometimes distressing sight.

While the nurse is completing the various admission forms and settling the patient in bed, it is courteous to tell him the names of the ward sister and medical staff. Relatives require reassurance as much as patients, particularly when the patient is unconscious or has been admitted without their knowledge after an accident. They are frequently able to provide much of the patient's history and can amplify a referral letter from another hospital.

EXAMINATION

The houseman will wish to speak with the patient and his relatives as soon as possible after their arrival. He will build up a history of the patient's complaint which will help to establish the diagnosis. If the patient has been admitted unconscious from an accident and there are no eye-witnesses, the ambulancemen may have useful information.

After taking the history, a doctor will wish to examine the patient. Most of the examination will be conducted with the patient on his bed, but abnormalities of posture and gait will require room to stand and walk. The doctor will need the following equipment in the examination tray:

1. Scents for testing the sense of smell, e.g. oil of cloves, camphor, coffee, asafoetida.
2. Ophthalmoscope.
3. Torch.
4. Charts for testing visual acuity.
5. Solutions for testing the sense of taste, e.g. sweet—sugar, sour—citric acid, bitter—quinine, salty—salt.
6. Auroscope.
7. Tape measure, to assess muscle wasting or head circumference.
8. Patellar hammer.
9. Test tubes containing hot and cold water to assess temperature sensation.
10. Pins and cotton wool to assess pinprick and light touch sensation.
11. Tuning fork.
12. A pair of geometrical dividers to estimate two-point discrimination.
13. Some small familiar objects, e.g. keys, a spoon, a pen, to assess any speech disturbance (nominal dysphasia) and stereognosis.

By the time the examination is complete, the doctor should have a good idea of the diagnosis, but he will usually want to support his bedside assessment with appropriate investigations.

INVESTIGATION

Urinalysis

Chemical analysis, a cell count, and culture for organisms are performed on the urine of all patients. Further tests, such as specific gravity, urinary osmolarity and electrolytes, are performed should the need arise.

Blood tests

Every patient has blood taken for a full blood picture, ESR, electrolytes and urea, and grouping. Liver function tests, plasma proteins, calcium and phosphorus, and serological tests for syphilis may be indicated.

Lumbar puncture

Indications

1. **Diagnostic**. To establish the presence of blood and pus in the cerebrospinal fluid.
2. **Therapeutic**. To inject appropriate antibiotics in the treatment of meningitis.
3. **Anaesthetic**. For spinal anaesthesia.

Technique

A lumbar puncture may be performed with the patient sitting upright or lying on a bed in the left lateral position. Reassurance of the patient by the attending nurse is very important to the speedy successful performance of the puncture.

The skin over the back from the rib margin to the buttocks is first cleaned with antiseptic. Local anaesthetic is injected along the proposed course of the lumbar puncture needle, usually between the spinous processes of the 3/4 or 4/5 lumbar vertebrae. With the patient's spine well flexed to open the space between the vertebrae, the needle is inserted into the spinal subarachnoid space. The pressure of the cerebrospinal fluid is measured with a manometer. If the nurse now compresses the jugular veins in the neck, she will increase the intracranial pressure which registers as a rise on the manometer (Queckenstedt's test). Release produces a fall. Failure of the fluid to rise and fall freely in this test implies obstruction to its flow, perhaps by a spinal tumour. The cerebrospinal fluid is collected in three specimen bottles, and sent to the laboratory for cell count, culture, and protein, glucose and chloride estimation.

The cerebrospinal fluid is normally clear and colourless. If the puncture has been traumatic, the fluid will be bloodstained, but clears rapidly in successive specimen bottles. Fluid that is uniformly bloodstained in all three bottles confirms a subarachnoid haemorrhage. In meningitis, the fluid has a cloudy, even milky appearance.

At the end of the procedure, the needle is withdrawn and the puncture site is sealed and covered with a dressing. Drainage of cerebrospinal fluid lowers the intracranial pressure and post-lumbar puncture headache is occasionally a problem avoided by nursing the patient flat in the prone position for 6 hours. If headache is severe, the foot of the bed should be raised.

It is important to avoid lumbar puncture when there is suspicion of raised intracranial pressure. Removal of fluid in this situation may induce 'coning' (see Head Injuries) with fatal results.

Fields of vision

This involves the formal charting of blind spots in the centre or at the edge of the visual field. Disturbance of normal function at different points along the visual pathway from the eyeballs to the occipital cortex produces certain well-defined visual field defects.

Radiographic examination

Plain X-rays

A chest X-ray is performed on all patients, and may reveal a primary lung cancer or secondary deposits from a tumour elsewhere. Skull X-rays may show evidence of raised intracranial pressure, thickening or erosion of bone, a calcified tumour, or displacement of a calcified pineal gland. The majority of skull fractures can be seen on X-ray. Cervical spine X-rays should be performed on patients with all but the most trivial head injuries.

Contrast studies

1. Air-encephalogram. Air injected into the subarachnoid space by lumbar puncture rises into the head and provides silhouette pictures of the ventricles and the surface of the brain. Headache, sometimes severe, usually follows this investigation.

2. Ventriculogram. This involves the injection of air or carbon dioxide directly into the lateral ventricle through a burrhole (or anterior fontanelle in an infant). Again a silhouette picture of the ventricular system is obtained. Injection of Myodil or water-soluble metrizamide provides positive contrast studies.

3. Cerebral angiogram. The injection of iodine-containing contrast into the bloodstream outlines the cerebral blood vessels. The injection is made directly into the carotid and vertebral arteries, or a catheter is passed from the femoral artery in the groin up the aorta to the great vessels in the neck. The procedure is usually performed under general anaesthesia.

4. Myelogram. Myodil or a water-soluble contrast medium is injected into the spinal subarachnoid space by lumbar puncture or occasionally a puncture in the neck. The contrast outlines the spinal cord, the roots of the cauda equina, and the spinal theca.

The information provided by these contrast studies is gleaned mainly from the displacement and distortion of normal structures and the demonstration of filling defects.

Electroencephalography (EEG)

This investigation records the electrical activity of the brain. It may prove helpful in localising irritative lesions.

Isotope brain scan

Many intracranial lesions cause a breakdown of the blood brain barrier allowing leakage of substances from the bloodstream into the brain substance. Because of this, they may be revealed by scanning the head after the intravenous injection of a radioactive isotope, technetium$_{99}$.

Computerised tomography (CT)

This non-invasive technique has become available in many neurosurgical centres. It is quite painless, and merely demands that the patient should keep still during the investigation which is completed in a few minutes. The head is scanned as a series of horizontal or vertical cross-sectional slices of pre-selected thickness by a narrow beam of X-rays. Detectors mounted opposite the X-ray tube measure the rays after the beam has passed through the head. The machine gradually works its way around the head, and the information obtained is displayed on a television monitor. Intracranial structures are identified according to whether they are of high or low density compared with normal brain tissue. Appearances may be enhanced by the intravenous injection of iodine-containing contrast.

Intracranial pressure monitoring

In recent years, interest has grown in the direct monitoring of intracranial pressure. The pressure is conveyed from inside the head along a column of fluid to a transducer which allows the information to be presented on a chart or as a digital display. Pressure may be measured in the ventricles, the subarachnoid space, or outside the dura. Rising pressure can be detected before there is any change in a patient's physical signs.

OBSERVATION

Careful observation of patients with neurological conditions is of central importance to patient welfare. Clinical deterioration may develop rapidly; if not appreciated early and dealt with promptly, the outcome may prove fatal. The nurse's responsibility in this respect is therefore considerable, and if she has any particular concern about a patient, she should share this immediately with the sister or nurse in charge.

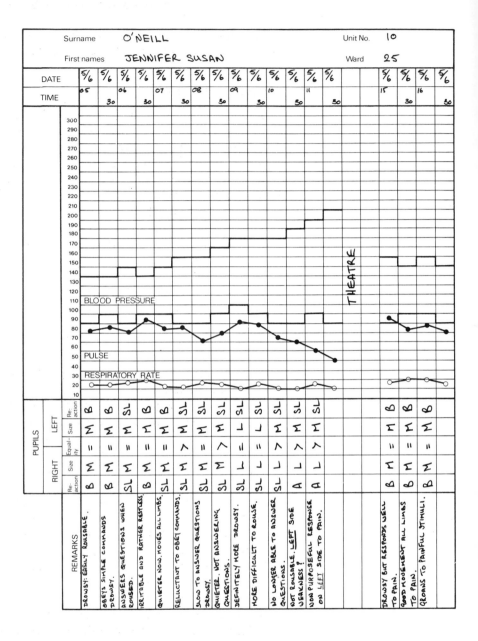

44.6 A CNS observation chart, showing the features of cerebral compression in a patient whose head injury was complicated by an extradural haematoma.

The letters on the pupil chart are:–

Reaction	B	—	brisk
	SL	—	sluggish
	A	—	absent
Size	M	—	medium
	L	—	large
Equality	=	—	equal
	>	—	right larger than left

The observations required of a nurse comprise a simple neurological assessment and a note of the vital signs (Fig. 44.6).

Neurological assessment

1. Level of consciousness. This is really the level of responsiveness. It is the single most important observation a nurse can make, and a little care in its recording is well worthwhile. Words like 'coma' and 'stupor' are best avoided, for they have different meanings for different people. Far better is to use simple words which everyone can understand. Thus, is the patient fully alert and cooperative? Is he confused and disorientated? Is he drowsy but rousable? Is his response to your remarks inappropriate because he is dysphasic and cannot understand you?

A patient with a more depressed level of responsiveness will not respond to verbal commands. His reaction to painful stimuli should then be noted. Does he respond purposefully to pain, localising the site of pain and pushing away the noxious stimulus? Does he react by flexing or extending his upper limbs (decorticate and decerebrate responses)? Does he respond at all?

The level of consciousness should be recorded at the time of admission so that a baseline is drawn to appreciate subsequent changes. Increasing intracranial pressure from any cause produces progressive deterioration in a patient's conscious level.

2. Pupillary changes. The size, equality, and reaction of the pupils to light must be recorded. In the early stages of cerebral compression, distortion of the brainstem may irritate the third (oculomotor) nerve and produce pupillary constriction, although this observation may easily be missed. With increasing compression, the third nerve fails to function, and the pupil dilates and becomes less responsive to light. If the cerebral compression is the result of a unilateral space-occupying lesion, then the pupil on this side is the first to become paralysed. The opposite pupil soon follows a similar pattern until ultimately both pupils are fully dilated and unresponsive to light (Fig. 44.7).

Pupil inequality by itself, as an isolated finding, is quite meaningless. The important point is the *progression* of pupillary signs combined with the overall assessment of the patient.

3. Limb movement. A unilateral weakness of the arm and leg (**hemiparesis**) or weakness of both legs (**paraparesis**) is easily demonstrated

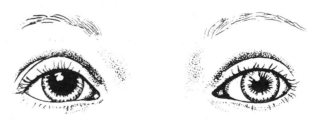

Fig. 44.7 Unequal pupils in cerebral compression. The right pupil is dilated and does not react to light.

in a conscious and cooperative person. But if a patient cannot obey commands, a note should be made of any asymmetry of spontaneous movements of the limbs implying an underlying weakness. Likewise the response to painful stimuli may be different on the two sides of the body. Was this present on admission or is it a new finding?

Vital signs

1. Pulse rate. Cerebral compression characteristically produces a slow bounding pulse.

2. Blood pressure. Raised intracranial pressure would normally drive blood out of the brain, so to ensure its adequate perfusion and nutrition, there is a compensatory rise in the blood pressure.

3. Respiratory rate. Usually the respiratory rate slows and breathing becomes deeper in the presence of cerebral compression.

4. Temperature. Blood in the subarachnoid space produces a moderate pyrexia. Temperatures in excess of 40°C may occur where there is damage to the hypothalamus or midbrain.

The frequency of these observations is decided by the doctor in charge. It should be emphasised that we seek to record the patient's *progress* with carefully documented observations; isolated findings are of little value.

As the nurse becomes familiar with the technique of recording a patient's signs, she will acquire further useful information which may never appear on a chart. Thus she will be able to tell a doctor about inappropriate behaviour, any speech problem, any tendency to ignore one side of the body, difficulty with coughing or swallowing, incontinence, fits, and many other observations which may prove helpful in the patient's management.

PREOPERATIVE NURSING CARE

All patients have some fear of surgery, and a neurosurgical operation is particularly worrying for those aware of their surroundings. There is anxiety about possibly not waking from the anaesthetic, or sustaining irreparable brain damage.

A patient is frequently reluctant to share these fears. He may also be worried about threatened unemployment, the care of his family, financial responsibilities, and religious beliefs. He may have understood very little of what he had been told by his doctors. All these problems snowball in many patients' minds, and a kind reassuring nurse who has time to talk can do more than anyone to help a patient approach his operation with calmness and greater understanding. The conduct of the nursing and medical staff does much to inspire (or undermine) a patient's confidence.

It is important that relatives should be kept abreast of a patient's progress. They at least must be told the diagnosis and prognosis as far as they are known. Relatives of patients recently rendered unconscious for one reason or another are often bewildered and frightened, and may place blind trust in nursing and medical staff in a desperate attempt to reverse events. They need comfort and reassurance, with the facts explained as simply as possible.

Unless an operation is an emergency, it is worthwhile spending a little time beforehand trying to improve the patient's physical condition. Smoking should be discouraged and any chest infection treated vigorously with physiotherapy and antibiotics. Debilitated patients may require rehydration and perhaps feeding by a nasogastric tube or intravenous line. Attention to pressure areas is of the greatest importance and repeated incontinence may make catheterisation desirable.

Consent for an operation is obtained by a doctor, who should at the same time explain the proposed operation in simple terms and outline any possible risks. The nurse may later be able to go over any points which are still unclear. She will introduce the anaesthetist the day before surgery, and explain the need for preoperative fasting. Reassurance of rapid regrowth of hair does much to make the shaving more tolerable for women, and the loss may be disguised with a scarf or wig. The patient should be told that he will come round from his anaesthetic with his head bandaged and an intravenous line in his arm.

POSTOPERATIVE NURSING CARE

Of supreme importance in the postoperative period is an open airway. The anaesthetist will only remove an endotracheal tube when he is satisfied that the patient can look after his own airway. He may wish to check the patient's blood gases, and is likely to give oxygen by face mask.

The patient recovering from an anaesthetic is at great risk of airway obstruction from secretions, vomit, and his tongue falling backwards. For this reason, he should be nursed semiprone (Fig. 44.8) or on his side, but never

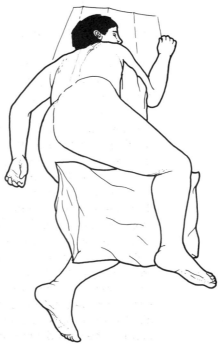

Fig. 44.8 The semiprone position.

on his back. Regular suction of the mouth and throat removes secretions and stimulates the cough reflex which helps to keep the airway clear.

As soon as a patient enters the recovery ward after his operation, his condition must be recorded on the observation chart. Failure to regain consciousness and any new abnormal signs must be noted and reported at once.

A note is made of the operative findings, and details concerning drains, catheters, intravenous fluids, and drugs are recorded, together with any special remarks from the surgeon or anaesthetist. When the patient's conscious level has improved sufficiently to allow safe transfer, he is returned to his ward.

Thereafter his neurological condition continues to be observed carefully. Occasionally patients are confused and restless, particularly at night time. They may require the protection of cot sides and their hands may need to be bandaged to prevent injury. Restlessness may indicate a full bladder requiring catheterisation.

Analgesia rarely needs to be strong after operations on the head, but should be given in adequate doses after spinal surgery. Intravenous lines are taken down once the patient is drinking normally and not feeling nauseated. Drains are usually removed 24 to 48 hours after the operation. At the same time, the patient may be encouraged to sit out of bed for a short period. The physiotherapist has a very important contribution to make throughout the patient's admission, but never more so than in the postoperative period. She will help with the care of the chest, and with the gradual remobilisation of the patient. Removal of sutures, from the head on the fifth and from the back on the tenth postoperative day, is always an important milestone for the patient.

Relatives should be kept informed of a patient's postoperative progress. They will discuss the final diagnosis with the doctor and the ongoing management. Foreseeable problems should be explained and solutions implemented where possible.

THE CARE OF THE UNCONSCIOUS PATIENT

There is a similarity between the unconscious patient and a newborn child. Neither can indicate his needs or desires, and the nurse does well to realise her patient is totally dependant on her.

The airway. The importance of a clear airway cannot be overstressed. If it is compromised, the resulting rise in the blood carbon dioxide and fall in the blood oxygen encourage swelling of the brain and a rise in intracranial pressure which may prove fatal. The patient should be nursed in the semi-prone position so that secretions and vomit will drain out of the mouth and the tongue cannot fall back. Regular removal of secretions by suction backed up with physiotherapy provides reasonable insurance against disaster. An oropharyngeal airway is useful to allow access to the mouth even when the jaws are clenched.

If there is any doubt at all about the airway, the safest procedure is to insert a cuffed endotracheal tube. This is mandatory, of course, if the patient is to be electively ventilated. If it seems as though a patient is going to require an endotracheal tube for more than a few days, he should undergo a tracheostomy since prolonged intubation encourages erosion or stenosis of the trachea.

The position. A pillow under the chest prevents a patient in the semi-prone position from rolling onto his face. Another pillow between the knees with the upper leg drawn up keeps the patient stable. There is no need for a pillow under the head (Fig. 44.8).

Nursing observations. The importance of careful observation has already been underlined (p. 491). The chart must record:

1. The level of consciousness.
2. The size, equality and reaction of the pupils to light.
3. Limb movements.
4. The pulse, blood pressure, respiratory rate, and axillary or rectal temperature.
5. The frequency and nature of any fits.

Skin care. The patient should be turned every 2 hours to relieve pressure areas and prevent the development of sores.

Limb care. Two hourly passive movement of all the limbs helps to improve the circulation and may prevent contractures.

Nutrition. The unconscious patient may be fed very satisfactorily through a nasogastric tube. An adult usually requires 2·5 litres of fluid in 24 hours, but a pyrexia or hot environment may increase this figure. There are numerous proprietary feeds currently available which provide a balanced diet of proteins, fats, and carbohydrates with vitamin supplements. Occasionally a patient may require intravenous feeding.

Mouth care. Regular toilet is very important in preventing infection of the mouth and salivary glands. Swabs of glycerine of thymol and ordinary toothpaste on a toothbrush suffice. Cracked lips need a lip-salve.

Bladder and bowel care. Urinary incontinence is best managed by catheterisation although in the male patient, Paul's tubing may be strapped to the penis. The alternative is the frequent changing of sheets. Wet sheets encourage the rapid appearance of pressure sores.

Retention of faeces will require the assistance of suppositories and enemas. Diarrhoea is sometimes a problem with patients on synthetic feeds.

Eye care. The unconscious patient may not blink and the eyes should be kept moist with methyl cellulose drops. Dried secretions and lashes should be removed by irrigation with saline. The cornea should be protected by keeping the eyes closed with gauze pads soaked in saline. Infection usually responds to chloramphenicol ointment.

Other points. The hair should be kept clean and groomed. The nails should be clean and clipped. Pyjamas and nightdresses need to be changed. Most important of all, the patient needs to be spoken to with words of comfort and encouragement.

DEPARTURE

When a patient is considered fit for transfer, he will either be discharged home or returned to his referring hospital to continue convalescence. At times he may be a little reluctant to venture out of the unit he has come to trust over the previous few days. He should be reassured that his surgeons will continue to keep in touch with him on an outpatient basis, and if there are any specific problems, his family doctor can refer him back at any time. Instructions on any medication must be clearly understood, and an adequate amount supplied.

HEAD INJURIES

Head injuries are exceedingly common, and the majority are so trivial as never to be seen in hospital. Nevertheless there are over 150 000 hospital admissions for head injury each year, and most of these are treated in general surgical wards. Only a small minority require transfer to neurosurgical centres for specialised care and treatment of complications.

Injuries to the scalp

The scalp has a rich blood supply, and a wound will bleed profusely. Pressure on the wound with a firm bandage or the fingertips will usually control the haemorrhage, but a patient may be severely shocked from blood loss before he can reach medical help.

Injuries to the skull

Fractures of the skull may be simple (closed) or compound (open), single or multiple. They may affect the vault, or the base, or both:

(a) **Fractures of the vault** may be fissured (a simple crack) or depressed (where a fragment of bone is driven into the head).

(b) **Fractures of the base** may damage the cranial nerves with resulting impairment of function. Thus there may be weakness (paresis) or complete paralysis of muscles supplied by the cranial nerves (e.g. ocular muscles, facial muscles), and impairment or loss of sensation (e.g. smell, sight, hearing).

Anterior cranial fossa fractures may cause haemorrhage from the nose (**epistaxis**), leakage of cerebrospinal fluid down the nose (**CSF rhinorrhoea**), and a **subconjunctival haemorrhage** in the eye. This bright red haemorrhage characteristically has no posterior border for it results from blood tracking forwards from behind.

A *middle cranial fossa* fracture is suggested by bleeding and escape of cerebrospinal fluid from the external auditory meatus (**otorrhoea**), and the appearance of a dark bruise behind the ear (**Battle's sign**) a day or two after the injury.

Injuries to the brain

The brain is a soft organ with the consistency of porridge, enclosed in a rigid skull. Damage to the brain in a head injury may be local at the site of impact, and/or distant on the opposite side. If the moving head strikes an unyielding object, such as a road, movement of the skull ceases abruptly but the brain undergoes a slower deceleration and so becomes compressed at the site of impact. There follows a recoil movement of the brain which then strikes the opposite side of the skull thereby sustaining a second injury (**contrecoup** phenomenon).

Damage to the brain may be obvious to the naked eye (contusion and laceration), or only microscopic (diffuse neuronal damage). The severity of the lesion does not necessarily correlate with the patient's clinical condition; patients may be fully conscious and orientated with contused or lacerated brain, yet there may be prolonged unconsciousness with no macroscopic injury.

Further damage may be inflicted on the brain as a result of the initial injury. Swelling from **oedema** is a normal sequel to damage to any part of the body, and is part of the inflammatory response. Such swelling leads to raised intracranial pressure because of the unyielding nature of the skull. Pressure may be further raised by **intracranial haemorrhage** from vessels torn at the time of injury. Both oedema and haemorrhage can lead to serious cerebral compression. Because of this high pressure state, the brain tends to be thrust down (i.e. herniate) through the opening at the base of the skull (the foramen magnum) compressing vital centres of the brain controlling the heart and respiration. This herniation is known as **coning** and may occur rapidly, demanding prompt treatment if the patient is to survive. If the signs of cerebral compression are to be picked up at the earliest possible moment, patients with head injuries require careful and continual observation by the nurse.

ASSESSMENT OF HEAD INJURIES

This relies on recording the sequence of events following a head injury. The time and details of the injury are important. Was the patient unconscious from the outset? When did the patient reach hospital? What was his condition on arrival? Are there any other injuries?

Nursing observations, described on p. 491, are begun immediately, and continued throughout the patient's stay in hospital. All patients who have lost consciousness from their injury are admitted to ensure that any complications that might arise are quickly discovered and promptly treated. The vast majority of patients admitted to hospital are conscious on arrival and make an uneventful recovery, returning home after 24 hours. Very frequently patients cannot remember events immediately preceding the accident (**retrograde amnesia**) or following the accident (**post-traumatic amnesia**). An estimate of these periods of amnesia should be made; the severity of the head injury appears to correlate with the duration of post traumatic amnesia.

TREATMENT OF HEAD INJURIES

We have seen that the majority of patients admitted to hospital with a minor concussion make a rapid and complete recovery and are discharged after 24 hours. Patients who have sustained a major head injury provide a much greater challenge.

Resuscitation

The first necessity in the treatment of a major head injury is to ensure that the airway is preserved. Blood, secretions and vomit should be removed from the mouth and throat and the patient placed in the semiprone position. It may be necessary, after a rapid clinical examination, to paralyse the patient with muscle relaxants, and insert an endotracheal tube. Simultaneously an intravenous line is set up to replace lost fluids. Blood is taken for a full blood picture, blood gases, and grouping and cross-matching. The patient's head injury and neurological deficit are assessed, and a search made for any other injuries. Profuse haemorrhage from the scalp may be controlled with local pressure or an artery forceps. The nurse detailed to the patient records her observations.

X-rays

Once the patient's condition is stable, it is safe to move him to the X-ray department. Skull X-rays may reveal a fracture, intracranial air, and perhaps a shift of the pineal gland away from the midline. The paranasal and mastoid air sinuses may be opacified with blood. X-rays of the cervical spine may show an associated fracture or subluxation. A chest X-ray should be always be done for it may reveal rib fractures, a pneumothorax or haemothorax, or pneumonitis from aspiration of vomit. It will also show the position of the endotracheal tube if this has been inserted.

Further management

Further management depends largely on the condition of the patient:

If he has now regained consciousness

   1. Closed head injury. It is legitimate to admit him to the ward for continued observation.
   2. Open head injury:
      (a) *Leakage of cerebrospinal fluid from the nose or ear* usually indicates a compound skull fracture. The fluid should be allowed to drain freely, and the patient should be instructed not to sniff or blow his nose if there is a rhinorrhoea. Prophylactic antibiotics are prescribed against the development of meningitis or a brain abscess. CSF rhinorrhoea and otorrhoea usually cease spontaneously, but if persistent, repair of the dural tear with a fascial graft may be necessary.
      (b) If there is a *scalp wound*, the scalp must be shaved to provide a good exposure. After infiltration of local anaesthetic and preliminary toilet, the wound is carefully examined with a finger to see if it communicates with a deeper injury. If the edges are ragged, they are excised. The wound is then sutured. The patient's immunity to tetanus should be

checked and brought up-to-date if necessary. Scalp defects may require rotation of large skin flaps and split-skin grafting.

(c) *A compound depressed skull fracture* requires elevation and usually removal of the indriven fragments. If the dura is torn, this should be repaired, if necessary with a fascial graft. A large postoperative skull defect can later be corrected by the insertion of a metal plate (**cranioplasty**).

If he remains unconscious or his condition deteriorates

The great concern here is whether or not the patient is suffering cerebral compression from a surgically treatable cause (viz. an extradural or subdural haemorrhage, Fig. 44.9). The simplest means of establishing this is by burrhole exploration of both sides of the head. The side of the fracture, or if there is pupillary inequality, the side of the larger pupil, is examined first. If a surface collection is found, then a **craniectomy** (removal of bone) or a **craniotomy** (cutting a bone flap) may be performed to remove the clot and stop the bleeding. If there is easy access to a CT scanner, then a

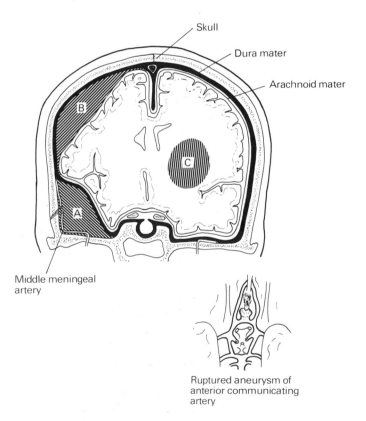

Fig. 44.9   Intracranial haemorrhage
   A. Extradural haematoma
   B. Subdural haematoma
   C. Intracerebral haematoma
Extradural, subdural and intracerebral haematomas are all space-occupying, unlike a subarachnoid haemorrhage.
Inset: A ruptured aneurysm of the anterior communicating artery.

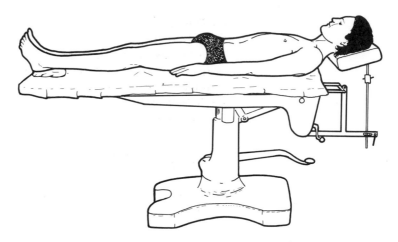

Fig. 44.10 Position for craniotomy.

haematoma can usually be excluded without recourse to surgery.

In the majority of patients there is no surface clot but the brain is swollen. Measures to counteract this include:

(a) Intravenous mannitol (10 or 20 per cent)
(b) Intravenous frusemide
(c) Intravenous hypertonic urea (90 G in 200 ml of invert sugar)
(d) Elective hyperventilation.

Intravenous dexamethasone is very frequently given, sometimes in high dosage, but there is little evidence that it has a useful part to play in the treatment of head injuries.

The facility exists in some centres to monitor the intracranial pressure. This records the patient's response to treatment and may help in forming a prognosis.

The important role of the nurse in the ongoing management has already been described (see The care of the unconscious patient, p. 494).

Assuming consciousness is regained, the patient now embarks on a carefully planned programme of rehabilitation. The physiotherapist, occupational therapist, speech therapist, and medical social worker all have very important parts to play if the patient is to make full use of his abilities and return to a useful life.

COMPLICATIONS OF HEAD INJURIES

1. Complications of the unconscious state

(a) Early. Airway obstruction by vomit, blood or secretions; shock from other injuries.

(b) Late. Infection of the lungs and urinary tract; pressure sores; weight loss.

2. Intracranial haemorrhage (see Fig. 44.9)

(a) Extradural
(b) Subdural
    (i) Acute — first 48 hours
    (ii) Subacute — 2nd to 14th day
    (iii) Chronic — after 14th day
(c) Subarachnoid
(d) Intracerebral

3. Infection

(a) Meningitis
(b) Abscess

4. CSF leak

From:
(a) Nose (rhinorrhoea)
(b) Ear (otorrhoea)

5. Epilepsy

(a) Early onset — during the first week after head injury
(b) Late onset — after the first week

RESIDUAL DISABILITY

1. Physical disability

This occurs from damage to:
(a) Cerebral hemispheres
    (i) Dysphasia
    (ii) Hemiparesis
(b) Cranial nerves
    (i) Anosmia
    (ii) Visual field defects
    (iii) Squints
    (iv) Facial weakness
    (v) Deafness and vertigo

2. Mental disability

There may be alteration of personality, and impairment of intellect and memory. Headache, dizziness, fatigue, irritability, and pain at the site of injury are common features of the normal recovery process following a head injury. When properly managed, they are short-lived, but they may persist for weeks or months (**post-concussional syndrome**).

DISEASES OF THE BRAIN

The neurosurgeon is commonly concerned with the management of patients with intracranial tumours, aneurysms and vascular malformations, hydrocephalus, and abscesses. Much of his work deals with spinal pathology—tumours, degenerative disease of the spine including prolapsed intervertebral discs, and vascular anomalies. He may also be asked for help in the management of intractable pain, epilepsy, and unwanted movements, e.g. in Parkinson's disease.

Intracranial tumours

The minority of these tumours are benign, e.g. meningioma. Those that are malignant may be primary (gliomas), or secondary (the result of metastatic spread from elsewhere).

Such tumours usually present with symptoms and signs of raised intracranial pressure:

1. Headache, often severe and frequently occurring in the early morning.
2. Vomiting, unrelated to food.
3. Increasing drowsiness.
4. Papilloedema (swelling of the optic disc in the eye).

In addition there may be localising signs, e.g. dysphasia, hemiparesis, visual field defects, according to the site of the tumour. Sometimes the patient presents with fits.

Many benign tumours can be completely removed and the patient cured. Surgical treatment for malignant tumours is less rewarding. Depending on its site and the patient's neurological deficit, a primary malignant tumour may be removed as far as the naked eye can see (macroscopic removal) or a palliative decompression may be all that can be offered. There may be a case for just obtaining histological confirmation of the tumour by burrhole biopsy. Whichever approach is adopted, it is usual for surgery to be followed by a course of radiotherapy.

Cerebral metastases, when multiple, are not amenable to surgical treatment, but occasionally a solitary secondary deposit can be removed with considerable relief of a patient's symptoms.

Aneurysms and vascular malformations

Subarachnoid haemorrhage, characterised by sudden onset of very severe headache frequently accompanied by vomiting and loss of consciousness, is most commonly caused by rupture of an intracranial aneurysm (Fig. 44.9 inset). The condition carries a high mortality rate (30 to 35 per cent in the first 3 days). The minority of patients who recover well from their haemorrhage are candidates for angiography to localise the source of their bleeding. Subsequent surgery is aimed at reducing the likelihood of further, perhaps fatal, haemorrhage. The approach may be:

1. *Direct*, by protecting the aneurysm with a clip or by wrapping it with muslin or muscle, or

2. Indirect, by clipping or tying the parent vessel to reduce the pulse pressure of the blood to which the aneurysm is exposed.

Subarachnoid haemorrhage may also result from an arteriovenous malformation, but the haemorrhage is usually less severe and carries a lower mortality. Generalised or focal epilepsy is a more common presenting symptom while migrainous headache occurs less frequently. There may be an audible bruit, and diagnosis is confirmed by angiography. Where feasible, treatment is by surgical excision.

Hydrocephalus

Hydrocephalus describes enlargement of the head resulting from the impaired circulation and accumulation of cerebrospinal fluid. It is more commonly congenital than acquired, and there may be other associated malformations. As the head enlarges, the fontanelles and scalp veins become prominent, the face appears relatively small, the eyes appear downcast ('sunset eyes'), and percussion of the head yields a crackpot note. X-rays of the skull confirm widening of the suture lines.

Treatment

Treatment is directed towards bypassing the obstruction to the circulation of cerebrospinal fluid. Most commonly, the fluid is diverted into the bloodstream (ventriculo-atrial shunt) or peritoneal cavity (ventriculo-peritoneal shunt), where it is rapidly reabsorbed. A catheter is inserted through a burrhole into a lateral ventricle of the brain and passed subcutaneously behind the ear to the neck. If the fluid is to be diverted into the bloodstream, the lower end of this catheter is passed down the internal jugular vein and superior vena cava to the right atrium (Fig. 44.11). Otherwise the catheter is threaded subcutaneously to the epigastric region where the abdomen is opened to gain access to the peritoneal cavity. Retrograde flow of blood or cerebrospinal fluid up the shunt is prevented by a valve system, e.g. the Pudenz valve (Fig. 44.12), which also provides a means of testing the patency of the shunt; an incompressible valve implies a distal obstruction, while a proximal obstruction is suggested by a valve that fails to refill after emptying.

Occasionally hydrocephalus may be treated by:
1. A direct attack on the site of the block.
2. Removal of a choroid plexus papilloma producing excessive CSF.
3. Short-circuiting a block by passing a catheter from the lateral ventricle to the cisterna magna (Torkildsen's ventriculocisternostomy).
4. A thecoperitoneal shunt (from lumbar theca to peritoneal cavity).

Cerebral abscess

A cerebral abscess is usually caused by staphylococci or streptococci. It may result from direct extension of infection from the middle ear or paranasal air sinuses, from infected head injuries, or occasionally it may arise from blood-borne infection from distant sources, e.g. bronchiectasis and pneumonia.

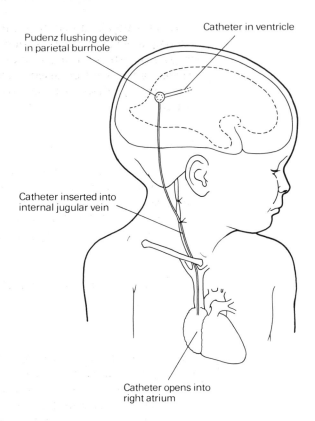

Fig. 44.11 Pudenz-Heyer ventriculo-atrial shunt.

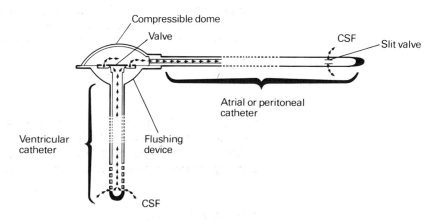

Fig. 44.12 The Pudenz-Heyer shunt system.

There is usually a history of preceding infection. A mild pyrexia may be accompanied by signs of meningeal irritation — neck stiffness and resistance to passive extension of the knee with the hip joint flexed (Kernig's sign). There may be signs of raised intracranial pressure with focal disturbance of function, e.g. dysphasia, hemiparesis, visual field defects. Fits may be a feature.

Treatment

Treatment consists of repeated drainage of the abscess by aspiration through a brain needle, and injection of appropriate antibiotics. At the same time, a radio-opaque medium is injected to follow the progress being made with serial skull X-rays. Antibiotics should also be given systemically. At a later date it may be appropriate to excise the abscess remnant.

INJURIES OF THE SPINE AND SPINAL CORD

THE SPINE

Cervical

The cervical spine may be injured by excessive flexion, extension, lateral flexion, or rotation. Flexion injuries tend to produce wedge compression fractures which are stable and unlikely to injure the spinal cord. Rarely there may be posterior prolapse of an intervertebral disc. Flexion-rotation injuries may cause subluxation (unstable), dislocation, or fracture dislocation (very unstable with likelihood of spinal cord injury). Hyperextension may produce a subluxation unstable in extension, with possible cord injury.

Thoracic and lumbar

Most fractures result from excessive flexion of the spine, producing stable wedge compression of the vertebral bodies without threat to the cord. Less commonly, flexion combined with a rotation force produces a dislocation or fracture-dislocation that is very unstable and usually injures the cord or cauda equina.

Treatment

Reduction is unnecessary in stable fractures. A collar for the neck and gradual remobilisation for the back are all that is needed. Subluxations and dislocations first require controlled reduction by traction, if necessary by open operation, followed by immobilisation in a plaster collar or jacket.

THE SPINAL CORD

The cord or cauda equina are damaged in only a small proportion of spinal injuries. Injury in the thoracic and thoraco-lumbar region is most common.

Complete transection of the cord is usual in thoracic injuries and may occur in the neck. There is a complete flaccid paralysis, sensory loss, and suppression of sphincter control below the site of injury. This state of **spinal shock** fades over days or weeks as the paralysis becomes spastic and visceral reflexes return uncontrolled by higher centres.

The neurological deficit may be patchy in incomplete transection of the cord. Severe injury to the cauda equina causes a permanently flaccid paraplegia and sensory loss, with no return of the visceral reflexes, unless the nerve fibres recover their function.

Treatment

The fracture. Bony displacement in the cervical spine should be reduced. If there is evidence of a disc prolapse on emergency myelography, this demands removal. Paraplegia from thoracic injuries is deemed to be the result of complete transection of the cord, and nothing is gained from attempts at reduction. In the thoraco-lumbar and lumbar regions, where the neurological injury is likely to be incomplete, immediate reduction and internal fixation should be considered.

Nursing Care

The patient is nursed on his back and on his side, being turned every 2 hours. The skin requires special attention and a sheepskin under the patient reduces the risk of pressure sores. The limbs require full passive exercise and massage to encourage the circulation and prevent contractures. Breathing exercises reduce the risk of developing hypostatic pneumonia. An indwelling catheter drains the bladder. Within about 3 months of complete transection, the bladder begins to empty as a reflex as soon as it has reached capacity—the **automatic bladder**. Injury to the sacral segments of the cord or the cauda equina interrupts this reflex arc, and emptying of the bladder is dependant upon a local reflex in the bladder wall itself. This **autonomous bladder** can be encouraged to empty by abdominal compression or straining.

The patients are fully aware of their neurological deficit, and encouragement and confidence in their ability are the corner-stones of their rehabilitation. Patients with complete cord transections learn to lead a useful life from a wheel chair, while many of those with injuries to the cauda equina are able to get about with elbow crutches or walking sticks. The contribution of the physiotherapist during this difficult time cannot be overstressed.

DISEASES OF THE SPINE AND SPINAL CORD

CONGENITAL DISEASES

Spina bifida

1. Spina bifida occulta
2. Meningocoele
3. Myelomeningocoele

These conditions are due to incomplete closure of the vertebral canal, particularly in the lower portion of the spine.

1. Spina bifida occulta is a condition in which the bony arch of the spinal canal is deficient. In mild cases there are no symptoms or signs, and the condition is diagnosed as an accidental finding on X-rays. Sometimes there is a sacral pit, and the overlying skin may be covered with a soft tuft of hair. There may be partial paralysis of the feet due to tethering of the nerves of the cauda equina. Club foot deformities may occur.

An operation may have to be undertaken to release tethered nerves, and deformity of the feet may require correction.

2. Meningocoele (Fig. 44.13). Here the meninges bulge on to the skin, so that there is a large bluish cyst which becomes more tense as the baby coughs or cries. The spinal cord itself is not involved. The condition is evident at birth.

Unless the greatest care is taken, the meninges may rupture, with the escape of cerebrospinal fluid. There is then a risk of infection, and meningitis may prove fatal.

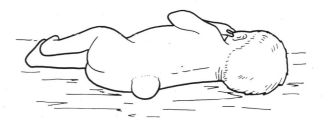

Fig. 44.13 Lumbar meningocoele.

Treatment. If the skin overlying the meningocoele is healthy, there is no urgency to operate. It is essential that the skin be very carefully protected — maceration from wet napkins must be avoided. Wool or lint may be used to pad the swelling which should be washed, dried and powdered at each napkin change. If the covering is very thin, or has ruptured, a decision must be made whether or not to close the defect. The operation involves excision of the membranes and repair of the back by mobilising fascia and skin.

Most of these children will grow up to be normal adults after closure of the defect, although some will have minor neurological defects in the legs or difficulty with the anal or bladder sphincters.

3. Myelomeningocoele. This is a condition in which nervous tissue bulges through the bony defect and the spinal cord is exposed on the surface as a flat ribbon. It is usually associated with some paralysis below the level of the lesion. Paralysis may be minor or in the most severe cases complete paraplegia may exist. In addition, there may be deformities of the lower limbs, deformities of the vertebral column, dribbling incontinence, and hydrocephalus.

Treatment. The decision on whether or not to repair a myelomeningocoele is often difficult but should be made as early as possible. The baby should be handled gently to avoid rupture of the delicate sac. A moist saline pad should be placed over the lesion and lightly bandaged in position.

If it is agreed to close the defect, a specimen of the mother's blood as well as details of the pregnancy and labour should be sent with the baby on transfer to another hospital for operation. Surgery aims at mobilising and burying the exposed cord which is then covered with fascia and skin. Postoperatively the baby is nursed on his side in an incubator, being changed from side to side every two hours, or alternatively partly suspended face downwards in elastic slings passed under the abdomen. Babies are nursed with the head low for the first few days to minimise leakage of cerebrospinal fluid from the wound. The baby should be handled as little as possible and should be fed in the incubator. There is a high risk that he will go on to develop hydrocephalus which willl require the insertion of a shunt.

As these children grow, they impose an increasing strain on the family. Help from various social service organisations and the educational authority is usually invaluable.

ACQUIRED DISEASES

Tumours

(a) **Tumours of the vertibral column**.

Primary tumours, e.g. myeloma are unusual.

Secondary tumours are very much more common, and have usually spread from the lung, breast, thyroid or prostate. Vertebral erosion and collapse lead to cord compression.

(b) **Tumours of the spinal cord and meninges**.

Primary tumours of the spinal cord, e.g. ependymoma, are not common

Secondary tumours are exceedingly rare.

Tumours arising from the root sheaths (**neurofibromas**) and the meninges (**meningiomas**) are relatively common and benign. Malignant tumours are rare.

Clinical features

Tumours of the spine and spinal cord present with symptoms and signs of cord compression:

1. At the level of compression: a lower motor neurone lesion with flaccid weakness and wasting, depressed tendon reflexes, and local sensory root irritation producing pain and hyperalgesia.

2. Below the level of compression: an upper motor neurone lesion with spastic weakness, increased tendon reflexes, and sensory impairment.

3. Loss of bladder and bowel control, and sexual function in men.

Treatment

For tumours of the vertebral column, decompressive laminectomy (Fig. 44.14) may be indicated in an effort to prevent increasing paraparesis

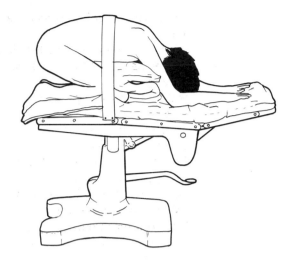

Fig. 44.14   The Moslem praying position for laminectomy.

and preserve sensation and bladder function. Surgery may be followed by radiotherapy. Tumours of the spinal cord are usually irremovable; histological confirmation is obtained by biopsy, and treatment is by subsequent radiotherapy. Neurofibromas and meningiomas can frequently be removed intact and the patient cured.

Laminectomy is performed with the patient in the Moslem praying position or prone on a Wilson frame. This reduces bleeding from venous congestion due to pressure on the abdomen.

Nursing care is similar to that described for injuries of the spine.

Degenerative disease of the spine

Degenerative changes in an intervertebral disc may encourage herniation (prolapsed intervertebral disc) or stimulate new bone formation and hypertrophy of ligaments (spondylosis).

Cervical spondylosis is the commonest cause of pain in the neck and upper limbs in middle and later life. New bone formation (osteophytes) may encroach on an intervertebral foramen, compressing a spinal nerve and producing lower motor neurone symptoms and signs, and perhaps some sensory impairment. Narrowing of the spinal canal may lead to cord compression with spastic weakness, increased tendon reflexes, and possibly sensory impairment. If symptoms are rapidly progressive, a cervical fusion or decompressive laminectomy may be indicated.

Degenerative disc disease of the **thoracic spine** is comparatively rare, but early recognition and treatment is important if permanent paraplegia and loss of sphincter control are to be avoided. The disc is reached by a posterolateral approach.

In the **lumbar region**, roots of the cauda equina may be compressed by stenosis of the spinal canal, but more commonly by a prolapsed intervertebral disc. The patient complains of lumbar backache with pain radiating through the buttock, down the back of the thigh and outer side of the calf to the outer border of the foot (sciatica). There is often a history of injury to the back. Pain is characteristically worsened by movement and straining, and eased by rest. A central disc prolapse may produce pain in both legs precipitated by exercise and relieved by rest (intermittent claudication of the cauda equina). Examination reveals a rigid lumbar spine, resistance to passive straight-leg raising, wasting and weakness of the leg, impaired sensation, and depressed tendon reflexes. Treatment is initially conservative with bed rest on a firm mattress and analgesics. Traction to both legs may prove beneficial, and frequently a corset or plaster jacket is helpful. If pain persists despite an adequate trial of conservative treatment, operative removal of the prolapsed disc may be indicated. After subsidence of the acute attack, the patient should be advised to:

1. Avoid heavy lifting.
2. Sleep on a firm bed.
3. Avoid sitting in too low a chair and rising too suddenly.
4. Perform spinal exercises daily and swim if at all possible.

A change of occupation may be necessary.

Infections

Extradural abscess. This is usually the result of spread of infection, often trivial, from elsewhere in the body. The patient has a fever and complains of severe back pain. Neurological signs rapidly develop. Surgical drainage is urgent if permanent damage to the spinal cord is to be avoided.

Tuberculous osteitis (Pott's disease). This condition is now rare in the U.K. A blood-borne infection, it most commonly affects the thoraco-lumbar spine. The spine is rigid, and local back pain may be referred to the abdomen or chest, mimicking appendicitis or pleuritic pain. There may be vertebral collapse classically producing a kyphosis. Neurological signs may appear as the disease progresses and are due to cord compression; there may be a complete paraplegia. A local abscess may form, and rarely pus may track down beneath the psoas fascia to point in the groin (psoas abscess). Antituberculous therapy (rifampicin, ethambutol, INAH, pyridoxine, perhaps streptomycin and PAS) and a good diet should be combined with complete rest of the spine, if necessary in a plaster bed. Abscesses require drainage through an anterolateral approach, and subsequent spinal fusion may be indicated. Paralysed limbs require the care outlined under Injuries of the Spinal Cord.

FURTHER READING

Potter J M 1974 The practical management of head injuries, 3rd edn. Lloyd-Luke (Medical Books) London
Jennett B 1977 An introduction to neurosurgery,   edn. Heinemann Medical Books, London

45

The peripheral nerves

The peripheral nervous system comprises the **cranial nerves** related to the brain stem, and the **peripheral nerves** related to the spinal cord.

INJURIES TO THE PERIPHERAL NERVES

There are three types of injury:

1. **Division**, which may be complete or partial.
2. **Contusion**, in which the nerve fibres are bruised but eventual recovery can be expected.
3. **Compression** from adjacent bone or soft tissue.

An injury to a nerve results in loss of function in the area supplied. If a division is complete, the loss of function is complete, producing:

1. *Motor changes*, i.e. immediate loss of power and later wasting of the muscles supplied by the nerve.
2. *Sensory changes*. Pain, touch and temperature sensation are lost in the area of skin supplied by the nerve.
3. *Trophic changes*. By this is meant the curious undernourished appearance which the skin develops. At first white, dry and scaly, the skin later becomes shiny and bluish, and painless ulceration may occur.

Partial division produces an incomplete disability.

Prevention

The nurse must take every precaution to avoid injury to the nerves. This just requires a little thought in the general nursing care. Important examples are:

(a) The arms of an unconscious patient must never be allowed to hang over the edge of the bed or operating table as this may compress the radial nerve causing a wrist drop.

(b) Intramuscular injections in the buttock should be given in the upper outer quadrant, well away from the sciatic nerve.

(c) Skin traction on a Thomas's splint or abduction frame must avoid the neck of the fibula. Compression of the adjacent lateral popliteal nerve may produce a foot drop.

Treatment

The vast majority of nerve injuries are not operated upon until the surgeon is certain that division has occurred. In many instances he will advise waiting to see if spontaneous recovery takes place.

In all cases he will require that the paralysed and/or anaesthetic area be kept in good condition to make full use of any recovery that may take place. The following general principles are fundamental:

Paralysed muscles must not be overstretched. For example, a drop wrist should be held in a cock-up splint, and a drop foot should be splinted at a right angle. Massage is valuable in encouraging the local circulation. Passive exercises help to avoid contractures. Electrical (galvanic) stimulation is useful in maintaining circulation and movement.

Insensitive skin requires special care. Insensitive fingers are easily burnt quite painlessly by cigarettes. The patient must be warned of the danger, and it may be wise to cover the fingers or hand with a kid glove to increase the margin of safety. Hot-water bottles, bed cradles, radiant heat lamps, and other ward furniture may all constitute similar hazards.

TUMOURS

Tumours may arise in the nerve cells themselves or in the nerve sheaths. Multiple tumours of the nerve sheath are characteristic of neurofibromatosis (Von Recklinghausen's disease — Fig. 45.1).

Tumours present as a tender lump that can be felt beneath the skin, or there may be intermittent pain radiating to the periphery of the nerve associated with impaired motor or sensory function.

Treatment is excision where possible.

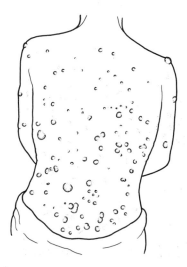

Fig. 45.1   Neurofibromatosis.

NEURALGIA

This describes paroxysmal pain along the course of a nerve. Examples are trigeminal and glossopharyngeal neuralgia, postherpetic neuralgia, and phantom limb pain.

Surgical treatment aims at intercepting the sensory pathway. Numerous procedures are described but relief is by no means guaranteed.

LESIONS OF INDIVIDUAL NERVES

THE CRANIAL NERVES

Number	Name	Function	Lesion
I	Olfactory	Mediates the sense of smell	Commonest cranial nerve to be damaged in head injuries. Avulsion causes loss of the sense of smell (anosmia).
II	Optic	Mediates sight	Injury or compression produces partial or complete blindness.
III	Oculomotor	Controls constriction of the pupil, movement of the lens, and inward, upward and downward movement of the eyeball	Injury or compression produces a dilated pupil and a divergent squint.
IV	Trochlear	Controls downward and outward movement of the eyeball	Injury or compression produces an inability to look downwards and outwards. Rarely occurs as an isolated finding.
VI	Abducens	Controls outward movement of the eyeball	Injury or compression produces a convergent squint.
V	Trigeminal	Mediates facial sensation. Controls muscles of mastication	Impaired function may result from injury or compression. The cause of trigeminal neuralgia is unknown.
VII	Facial	Controls muscles of facial expression	Injury or compression produces a lower motor neurone facial weakness (Fig. 45.2). The cause of Bell's palsy is unknown.
VIII	Vestibulo-cochlear	Mediates balance and hearing	Injury or compression produces deafness and imbalance.
IX	Glosso-pharyngeal	Mediates sensation from the back of the tongue and throat	Rarely injured. Compression may produce difficulty in swallowing.
X	Vagus	Controls palate and vocal cord movement, heart rate, and movement and secretions in the gastrointestinal tract	Compression may produce difficulty in speaking, swallowing and coughing. Vagotomy reduces gastric acid secretion (Chapter 35).
XI	Accessory	Innervates sterno-mastoid and trapezius muscles	Damage interferes with head, neck and shoulder girdle movements.
XII	Hypoglossal	Innervates the tongue	Damage produces wasting and weakness.

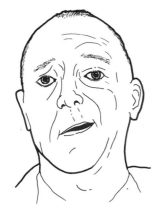

Fig. 45.2 A lower motor neurone facial weakness affecting the right side of the face.

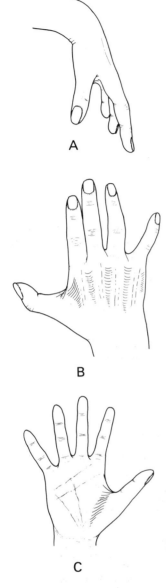

Fig. 45.3 Peripheral nerve palsies
A. Radial nerve palsy — wrist
   drop.
B. Ulnar nerve palsy — claw
   hand, note the wasting of small
   muscles between extensor
   tendons to digits.
C. Median nerve palsy note the
   wasting of the small muscles of
   the thumb (thenar eminence).

THE PERIPHERAL NERVES

1. Axillary nerve. May be injured in trauma around the shoulder joint, resulting in wasting of the deltoid muscle and weakness of shoulder abduction.

2. Radial nerve. May be injured in fractures of the humerus, causing a wrist drop from paralysis of the extensor muscles. (Fig. 45.3A).

3. Ulnar nerve. Injury or compression at the elbow leads to wasting and weakness of some of the forearm muscles and small muscles of the hand. In addition, sensation may be impaired over the inner one-and-a-half fingers and medial border of the hand (Fig. 45.3B).

4. Median nerve. Injury causes wasting and weakness of the small muscles of the thumb, and sensory loss over the lateral aspect of the hand and outer three-and-a-half digits. (Fig. 45.3C).

5. Sciatic nerve. This may be injured by trauma or by the nurse with misplaced injections into the buttock. Infiltration of the nerve roots by primary or secondary tumours in the pelvis may cause sciatica. There is weakness of the foot and impaired sensation over the foot and lower leg.

6. Lateral popliteal nerve. Compression at the head of the fibula produces a foot drop and impaired sensation between the big and second toes.

7. Femoral nerve. Weakness of the quadriceps femoris and pain and parasthesiae over the front of the thigh may occur as femoral neuritis complicating diabetes mellitus. Occasionally the cause is a retroperitoneal tumour. A similar clinical picture may result from prolapse of the L3/4 intervertebral disc, when surgery may be indicated.

46

Diseases of bone

Diseases of bones and joints cannot be properly understood without a sound knowledge of the anatomy, and a study of Figure 46.1 would be well worth while before reading further.

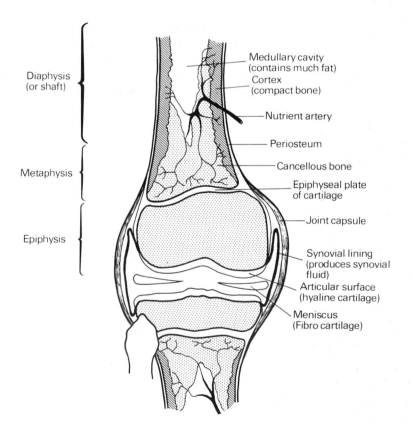

Fig. 46.1   Knee joint to show anatomy of typical bone and synovial joint.

Diseases of bones can best be classified as follows:
1. Congenital
2. Traumatic
3. Infective
4. Metabolic
5. Neoplastic

CONGENITAL DISEASES OF BONE

Babies may be born with mild or severe failure of development of the bones and in some cases bones which are normally present may be completely absent. This is best seen in the tragic results of thalidomide therapy where the complete absence of one or more limbs was not unusual. Lesser degrees of deformity such as a congenitally short femur or a congenitally short radius (producing a radial club hand known as Madelung's deformity) are also occasionally seen. A rare condition which leads to severe disability is that known as congenital pseudarthrosis of the tibia where the junction between the upper two thirds and lower third of the tibia fails to develop properly and gives rise to a false joint in the middle of the bone. These children may need years of treatment before they are able to walk on the tibia without splintage. Another type of congenital abnormality is the group in which hamartomata form. These are areas in the bone which do not develop in the normal way and may give rise to bone cysts or areas of fibrous dysplasia in the bone. These most commonly occur in the metaphysis or the epiphysis of the bone.

TRAUMATIC LESIONS OF BONE

These have been covered in Chapter 20 under the heading of fractures.

INFECTIVE DISEASES OF BONE

Bone may be infected by the ordinary pus forming bacteria giving rise to the condition known as osteomyelitis, which may be acute or chronic. Other infecting agents are the tuberculosis bacillus and the organisms which affect the bowel such as brucella, typhoid and dysentery. The usual mode in which the bacteria gain access to the bone is through the blood stream and this is known as haematogenous spread. Bones can however be infected directly from compound wounds into the bone.

Acute osteomyelitis

This is a common condition in young children and must be suspected whenever an ill child with a high temperature presents and diagnosis is not immediately obvious.

It is worthwhile considering symptoms and signs of this condition in

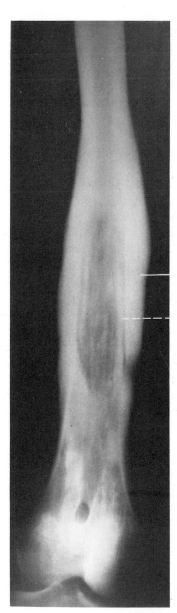

Fig. 46.2 X-ray of femur affected by chronic osteomyelitis, Involucrum shown by continuous line. Sequestrum shown by dotted line.

parallel with the pathology of the disease. The initial infection gains access to the bone via the blood stream, having entered the circulation from some other septic focus in the body, such as a boil or a sore throat. The bacteria settle in the bone in the metaphysis where the blood vessels are branching into finer and finer arterioles and capillaries. If the body's defences do not contain the bacterial infection then the bacteria begin to multiply and a small abscess develops in the bone close to the cortex. As is usual with abscesses oedema soon develops around the abscess and the pressure in the bone is increased. At this stage the child is feverish with no particular localising signs. There are certainly no changes on X-ray at this stage. As the bone abscess spreads so the infected oedema passes through the tiny channels in the cortex of the bone and starts to elevate the periosteal lining from the outer aspect of the cortex. At this stage the child might begin to complain of some localised pain in the affected area and as the disease progresses so there might develop clinical tenderness on palpation of the site of bony infection. If this remains untreated the bone from which the periosteum has been elevated will die because its blood supply has been damaged. The abscess may then enlarge through the soft tissues and eventually discharge through the skin giving rise to a discharging sinus. At this stage the acute disease has become a chronic infection. A small or large area of bone may be deprived of its blood supply and die. Dead bone eventually becomes separated from live bone and it is then known as a sequestrum. The infective process and the presence of dead bone excites the living bone to produce new bone to repair the damage and it is not unusual for the new bone formed completely to surround the various dead pieces of bone rather like an envelope surrounds a letter. It is for this reason that the new bone formed is known as an involucrum (Fig. 46.2).

Treatment of osteomyelitis

The treatment of acute osteomyelitis is aimed at preventing the spread of the abscess and bone death. One of the ways of combating infection is the use of antibiotics. In these modern days many bacteria are resistant to commonly used antibiotics and it is always helpful to find out which particular organism is causing the infection. Blood cultures are therefore essential in any child with a high temperature and an undiagnosed condition, as these will often tell the surgeon which organism is causing the infection. If the organism is not known it is quite common to use a combination of antibiotics such as Fucidin and Erythromycin to cover as wide a spectrum of bacteria as possible. The limb should also be rested in a splint.

If the signs of infection begin to settle with the child's affected limb splinted then surgery may not be necessary. However, if the infection remains clinically active and the child's temperature high, and if the site of infection can be accurately localised then some surgeons will operate on the bone to relieve the tension in it by drilling the bone and allowing the pus to escape.

The initial treatment therefore is rest and antibiotics and the second treatment which may be necessary is surgical drainage, just as in any other surgical infection elsewhere in the body.

Once the disease has reached the chronic stage with the formation of sinuses and sequestrae it is necessary to remove the dead sequestrae by surgical operation before the chronic osteomyelitis will heal up.

Tuberculous osteitis

This once very common disease is now much less common. Tuberculosis is still however seen occasionally and one of its favourite sites is the spine. Tuberculous infection does not progress as quickly as does pyogenic infection and the physical signs are not so dramatic. Generalised constitutional debility is often present together with localised pain or discomfort. The abscess which is formed does not excite the body's defence mechanism to such an extent so that there is little local hyperaemia and therefore little localised warmth. This is why a tuberculous abscess is often known as a cold abscess (Ch. 9). However the damage it can do is considerable and if the abscess bursts from the vertebral body through into the spinal canal it can cause paraplegia, — the so called Pott's paraplegia.

The treatment of tuberculous osteitis whether in the spine or elsewhere is complete rest of the affected part and the exhibition of antituberculous drugs such as Pasinah and Rifampicin. Streptomycin is little used these days because of its dangerous side-effects upon the ear and its tendency to produce a severe fibrotic reaction.

In earlier days patients with tuberculous osteitis were often kept in hospital for many years until the infection became quiescent but nowadays most surgeons would treat the lesion initially with rest and chemotherapy but would be much more ready to perform a surgical excision of the affected area if the disease failed to settle fairly quickly.

Other infections of bones

Infections of bone by other organisms are treated by means of suitable antibiotics or chemotherapy which kill the bacteria or prevent them from multiplying. In the case of those organisms which normally infect gut it is often difficult to isolate the bacteria themselves but fortunately there are various blood tests which can be done which will give the surgeon considerable help in making the diagnosis. These tests estimate the amount of the natural body defence protein which is mobilised to agglutinate the infecting organisms so that antibrucella, antityphoid or antidysenteric titres are often helpful in reaching a diagnosis. Once the diagnosis has been made then the appropriate treatment can be ordered.

METABOLIC DISEASES OF BONE

Bone, like any other tissue, is living and therefore the normal biochemical processes of living tissues go on within the bone. Thus bone is constantly being remodelled, the blood stream brings new chemicals to the cells and takes away used ones. These chemicals may be organic (proteins and carbohydrates) or inorganic (calcium and phosphorus). It is estimated that the calcium content of the human body is completely changed every seven years. It is not surprising therefore that occasionally things go wrong with the living processes (metabolism) in bone.

Parathyroid diseases

One of the ductless glands that controls the calcium and phosphorus metabolism of the body is the group of glands known as the parathyroids. These small glands are situated on the posterior surface of the thyroid gland and produce parathormone. If an excess of parathormone is produced, e.g. should an adenoma of the parathyroid gland develop, then the calcium in the bones is rapidly mobilised and is lost to the body through the kidneys. This may give rise to an acutely painful illness where the bone becomes extremely thin and weak and there is a danger of formation of kidney stone. The treatment is to remove the offending parathyroid tumour. A more chronic parathyroid disease may give rise to the formation of multiple cysts in the bone, a condition known as osteitis fibrosa cystica.

Rickets and osteomalacia

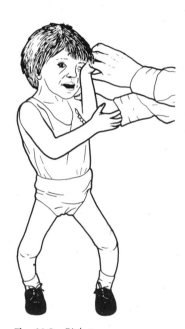

Another of the chemical agents responsible for the control of the calcium metabolism is vitamin D and an absence of vitamin D in a growing child will give rise to a condition known as rickets. Rickets can also be caused by a failure to take in an adequate amount of calcium through the gut or by an excessive amount of calcium being excreted through the kidneys. Rickets can therefore be caused by inadequate calcium in the diet, by an insufficient vitamin D intake or by an excessive excretion of calcium by the kidneys (renal rickets). Whatever the cause the bones do not develop properly, they become soft, there is swelling of the epiphyses and widening of the epiphysial plates of cartilage and the shafts of the bones will bend (Fig. 46.3).

The treatment of rickets requires correction of the basic metabolic defect and if bone deformity has occurred this will need correction either by manipulations and plaster or by osteotomies to straighten the bones. Once the epiphyses have fused and bone becomes adult then deficiency of vitamin D or calcium gives rise to softening of the bone which in adults is known as osteomalacia. The treatment is the same as for rickets. These two diseases are becoming more common in temperate climates as more dark skinned people emigrate from their own sunny warm countries. This is because sunlight is essential to the formation of vitamin D within the body when the diet is deficient in this vitamin.

Fig. 46.3 Rickets.

Paget's disease

Paget's disease of the bone is an affliction of the elderly and is very common indeed. The causation of the disease is unknown but it is well known that a great increase in the blood supply of the bone occurs and a great increase in the rate of calcium changeover within the bone also occurs. This gives rise to considerable new bone formation so that the bones

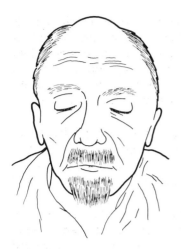

Fig. 46.4 The skull of a patient with Paget's Diseases.

become thicker, but because of the lack of calcium they also became softer. Sufferers slowly develop the bowed legs and the enlarging skull which are typical of the disease (Fig. 46.4). Pathological fractures in this condition are common. Because of the increased blood channels within the bone the action of the heart is put under strain and congestive cardiac failure may occur. Sarcomatous change is much more common in Pagety bone than in normal bone.

Gout

Gout is an abnormality of metabolism which causes the deposition of sodium urate crystals within the ends of the bone and within the joint linings. These crystals may become so large that they burst through the skin overlying the bone giving rise to what is known as a tophus. An acute attack of gout can be one of the most painful experiences in life but fortunately it can be treated easily and effectively by means of anti-inflammatory agents and can be prevented by means of special drugs to increase the excretion of uric acid.

NEOPLASTIC DISEASES OF BONE

Tumours of bone may be benign or malignant. If malignant they may be:
1. primary
2. secondary

As will be seen from the diagram at the beginning of this chapter, bone is composed of a number of tissues including bone itself, cartilage, blood vessels, nerves and fibrous tissues, e.g. the periosteum. Primary tumours may develop in any or in a combination of these tissues, whereas secondary tumours deposited in bone via the blood stream from primary cancer in other organs, will have the same characteristics as the primary growth from which they were derived.

Benign tumours of bone

These are quite common and usually require no treatment unless they are interfering with joint movements or causing pressure symptoms on neighbouring organs. Such tumours may be osteomas (pure tumours of bone tissue), chondromas (pure tumours of cartilage tissue), or fibromas (pure tumours of fibrous tissue) or they may be mixed, e.g. osteochondroma which has some bone tissue and some cartilage tissue within the growth.

Malignant tumours of bone

The primary malignant tumours of bone are largely diseases of younger people and the most malignant of all unfortunately affect children before growth has ceased. Because the bone is not a glandular tissue malignant disease of the bone is not known as carcinoma but as a sarcoma. Again the malignant tissue may arise in any of the components of bone.

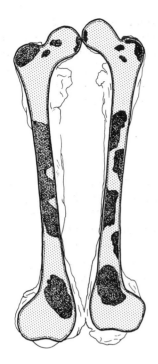

The most common primary malignant tumour of bone in children is osteogenic sarcoma which arises from the cells which are actively producing bone. Such tumours give rise to new bone formation which is often laid down in a radial manner giving the so-called 'sunray appearance', on X-ray. These tumours are highly malignant and give rise to pain and swelling. They metastasise rapidly via the blood stream to the lungs and are usually fatal within a very short period (Fig. 46.5).

Modern methods of treatment are however giving rise to hope that better results may be obtained in the future. If the tumour is accessible it is excised, often by means of amputation, and the surgical treatment is followed up by serial treatments with a mixture of cytotoxic drugs to try and control the secondary spread of the tumour.

Another rare tumour which is distressing in its rapidly fatal course is the so called Ewing's tumour which is thought to arise from the endothelial cells of the blood vessels in the bone. This tumour is more usually treated by local excision followed again by serial cytoxic therapy and radiotherapy. Other primary malignant tumours such as chondrosarcoma and fibrosarcoma in bone usually arise in a later age group and are not so rapidly fatal, and in fact there are many instances of 20 years survival after such lesions have been treated.

Fig. 46.5 Drawing of a femur cut longitudinally to show the spread of osteogenic sarcoma within the bone.

Secondary tumours of bone

Secondary deposits may be laid down in bone from cancers elsewhere in the body. By far the most common primary tumour to give rise to secondary bone deposits is cancer of the breast and secondary deposits of breast cancer in bone are the commonest bone tumour that is seen. However secondary deposits may also present in bone from carcinoma of the bronchus, the prostate, the kidney, the thyroid and the uterus. They are often only diagnosed when a pathological fracture occurs through them but are sometimes diagnosed by X-ray after the patient complains of persistent pain.

Cancer of the breast and the prostate are sometimes 'hormone dependent' and secondary deposits from such cancers are often treated by exhibiting hormones to the patient. Thus a secondary cancer from the prostate may be treated by performing an orchidectomy and treating the patient with Stilboestrol. In most circumstances secondary bone tumours are treated by means of radiotherapy and occasionally by cytotoxic drugs.

47

Diseases of joints, muscle and tendons

Joints may be freely mobile, in which case there is a cavity between the bone ends which is lined by a synovial membrane producing fluid to lubricate the movement of the joints (see Figure 46.1). Such joints may be of several mechanical types such as the ball and socket joints seen in the very mobile joints such as the hip and the shoulder; hinged joints moving freely in one plane only such as the elbow and the knee; pivoting joints such as that between the head of the radius and the lower end of the humerus, which allow rotation of one bone on the other; or gliding joints such as the joints between the small bones of the wrist (the carpus) or the foot (tarsus.) The less mobile joints are those in which the bone ends are joined by fibrous tissue or cartilage and this situation is seen in the discs between the vertebral bodies, or the fibrocartilage between the two pubic bones at the front of the pelvis. The ribs have synovial joints between their posterior ends and the vertebral column but have flexible areas between the front ends of the ribs and the costal cartilages joining the ribs to the sternum anteriorly.

Diseases of joints may be classified into the following four groups:
1. Congenital
2. Inflammatory
3. Traumatic
4. Degenerative

CONGENITAL JOINT LESIONS

The most important condition to consider under this heading is congenital dislocation of the hips. The causation of this condition is not fully understood but a very important factor in its production is the position of the baby's legs whilst in the womb. Extended breech deliveries, where the legs are acutely flexed with the knees lying straight up the front of the trunk, give rise to congenital dislocation of the hips much more commonly than do the normal vertex deliveries. The neonatal paediatrician will test new born babies hips for stability within the first few hours of birth and if there is any suggestion that the hips may be unstable the babies are usually nursed in double nappies to keep the legs abducted so that the head of the femur is positioned securely within the acetabulum. If the hip instability persists then special splints may be used to keep the legs in the abducted position at the hip joints. By the use of this treatment a large percentage of dislocated hips are stable by the time the baby starts standing and walking. However if the hips remain dislocated by the time the child is of standing age then treatment must be instituted to reduce the hip and keep it reduced until the acetabulum is fully developed. This may require nursing on special abduction frames with traction on the legs followed by a period in a plaster of Paris spica. Should this treatment fail to keep the hips well in position then surgical treatment may be necessary in the first years of life in order to stabilise the head of the femur within the acetabulum (Figs. 47.1 and 47.2).

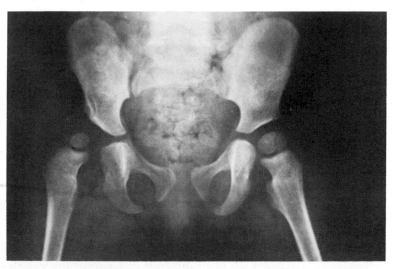

Fig. 47.1 An X-ray showing congenital dislocation of the right hip.

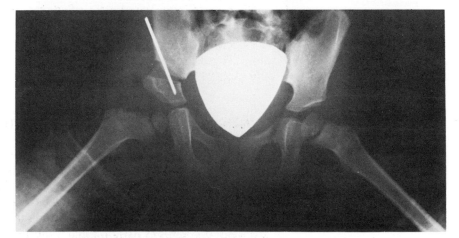

Fig. 47.2 The same patient as Fig. 47.1 after operative reduction and stabilisation by osteotomy of the pelvis immediately above the acetabular roof. The osteotomy is held open by a wedge of bone fixed by a Kirschner wire. A gonad shield is in place to protect the ovaries from irradiation during the X-ray.

An open reduction of the dislocated hip may be necessary and this is sometimes combined with osteotomies of the pelvis on that side to tilt the acetabular roof well over the head of the femur. This position is then maintained until the bone and soft tissues have healed after a period in a plaster spica.

INFLAMMATORY LESIONS OF JOINTS

Inflammatory lesions may be caused by infecting organisms such as bacteria or they may be caused by non-infective conditions such as rheumatoid arthritis.

INFECTIVE JOINT DISEASE

Infection gives rise to a hot, swollen and acutely painful joint which the patient will protect by muscle spasm, and will avoid moving at all costs because of the pain. As in acute osteomyelitis the temperature will be raised and in fact infective arthritis is often caused by osteomyelitis close to the joint.

An important cause of acute infective arthritis in new born babies is infection reaching the joint through an infected umbilical cord. In older patients the infection reaches the joint through the blood stream or by direct infection from a compound wound of the joint. The treatment is to rest the joint completely, to isolate the causative organism and to treat the infection with the appropriate antibiotic. In some cases operative drainage of the joint becomes necessary just as in osteomyelitis or in any other severely infected surgical lesion.

As in the case of fractures the muscles which control the affected joint must be kept as strong as possible by regular static exercises (i.e. exercises without moving the joint).

Tuberculous infection of joints is less common than it used to be but it still occurs. The treatment of such joints follows exactly the same principles, i.e. rest, muscle exercises, appropriate chemotherapy and occasionally surgical drainage.

NON-INFECTIVE INFLAMMATORY CONDITIONS OF JOINTS

Rheumatoid arthritis

This disease is one of the most widespread and crippling in the world. It consists of inflammatory synovitis in which the inflamed synovium spreads over the joint surface and eats its way into the articular cartilage thus causing great pain and deformity. It may affect the patients at any age although it is more common in early middle age.

Its cause is unknown but, for some reason, the body defence mechanisms fail to recognise protein molecules produced by the body, and attack these proteins with antibodies at certain sites. This causes the release of toxic products which damage the affected tissues. The synovium is one of the major targets of such a reaction but rheumatoid arthritis also affects the walls of blood vessels, the lungs and the eyes, so that a patient with a severe form of rheumatoid arthritis may become extremely ill.

Treatment of rheumatoid arthritis

Many different types of anti-inflammatory drugs have been produced in order to treat this painful condition and it is wise to start treatment with the simpler drugs such as salicylates and to progress to the more complicated drugs with their larger proportion of side-effects only if the condition fails to respond to simple treatment, including splintage where necessary and physiotherapy.

A course of gold injections is sometimes given as it has been found that the injection of heavy metals is sometimes helpful. Systemic steroid treatment is also sometimes prescribed in the event that no other drug seems to be having any effect. However the serious side effects of long term steroid therapy must always be borne in mind. More recently drugs such as penicillamine and immuno-suppressive drugs have been tried with good effect in some patients. The surgical treatment of rheumatoid arthritis consists of one of several methods:

(a) Injections of radioactive substances such as radioactive gold or Yttrium into the larger joints has recently been shown to be very effective.

(b) Excision of the affected synovium. This operation (synovectomy) is practiced quite frequently when an accessible joint is persistently painful and swollen.

(c) Excision of the whole joint and replacement with an artificial joint is practiced more and more when the disease has destroyed the affected joint.

Other conditions resembling rheumatoid arthritis

'Rheumatism' is a lay term for a very large number of diseases which may cause inflammatory synovitis of joints. Such conditions as psoriasis, gout, pseudogout (inflammation of joints caused by crystals other than uric acid) and joint inflammations associated with various bowel diseases are some examples. A particular condition which may present in a similar way to rheumatoid arthritis is ankylosing spondylitis. This is a condition which affects the spine mainly but can also affect other joints in the body. It is characterised by pain and increasing stiffness so that eventually the spine may become completely rigid — the so-called poker back.

TRAUMATIC LESIONS OF JOINTS

Acute dislocations and compound joint injuries have been dealt with in Chapter 20. Internal derangements of joints may be caused by trauma such as the very common torn meniscus in knee joints.

This is almost always caused by acute rotation strains usually during

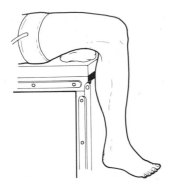

Fig. 47.3 Position of table for menisectomy or exploration of the knee joint.

  (i) The tourniquet position, high up on the fleshy part of the thigh to diminish pressure on the large nerves to the lower leg.
 (ii) The calf is several inches away from the bottom leaf of the operating table.
(iii) The knee joint is lifted by a sand-bag under the lower thigh and the surgeon can flex and extend the joint during surgery if necessary.

sporting activities and the two classical symptoms of this condition are locking of the joint and giving way of the joint. If these symptoms occur frequently then the meniscus requires removal. The operative position is shown in Figure 47.3.

The patient who has a torn meniscus removed must be encouraged to perform quadriceps exercises from the moment he recovers from the anaesthetic. A splint or plaster cylinder is usually applied to the knee for the first 10 days or so after operation and the patient encouraged to walk as soon as possible.

RECURRENT DISLOCATIONS

A damaged joint may become so unstable that it dislocates on frequent occasions during normal movement. This happens particularly to the freely mobile shoulder joint and also to the patella.

A shoulder joint which dislocates recurrently requires surgical stabilisation and several operations have been devised to prevent further recurrence.

In the same way a patella which dislocates frequently is a considerable disability and again requires surgical stabilisation. This is usually done by transferring the attachment of the patellar tendon from its central point on the upper tibia to a position more medially placed on the upper shaft of the tibia.

SLIPPED UPPER FEMORAL EPIPHYSIS (Fig. 47.4).

Before the epiphysial plate of cartilage between the head of the femur and the neck of the femur has become ossified there is considerable mechanical strain upon it because of the amount of weight it bears and because of

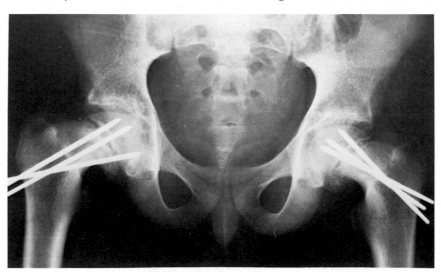

Fig. 47.4 X-rays showing fixation of bilateral slipped upper femoral epiphyses.

its rather vertically placed position. The head of the femur sometimes slips upon the epiphysial plate and a deformity occurs in the hip joint. This condition is more likely to happen in fat children with poorly developed sexual characteristics. Should a slip occur then the treatment is to reduce the slip by slow gentle traction and then fix the head to the neck of the femur by means of pins passed up the femoral neck.

PERTHE'S DISEASE

This is a condition occurring in children between the ages of six to ten which results in softening of the epiphysis of the head of the femur. It gives rise to a painful limp and the treatment is to rest the child in bed on traction until the pain diminishes. The pathological process in the head of the femur takes 2 to 3 years to complete its cycle, and it is important that the head of the femur should be well contained within the acetabulum during this period.

Treatment is only necessary if the head of the femur is partly outside the acetabulum. In this case treatment consists either of an operation to position the head of the femur in the acetabulum or else the child is kept in a special type of splint which achieves the same object.

The pathological process in Perthe's Disease is known as osteochondritis and this process occurs in many other parts of the body during the growing period. One of the more common places is at the upper end of the tibia where the tendon is attached. The condition is then known as Osgood Schlatter's disease.

PROLAPSED INTERVERTEBRAL DISC

An intervertebral disc is a form of joint between the bodies of the vertebrae and consists of an outer tough elastic annulus fibrosus and an inner semi-fluid nucleus pulposus. When the annulus fibrosus is ruptured by trauma the central nucleus can bulge out through the weakened spot. This can often be shown by a myelogram. If this traumatic bulge presses upon one of the lumbar nerve roots it gives rise to sciatica. The treatment of this condition is dealt with in Chapter 44. An alternative operative position to that shown in Chapter 44 is illustrated in Figure 47.5. This is also used for operations on the spine.

DEGENERATIVE DISEASES OF JOINTS

Like any mechanical joint the joints of the body wear away with increased use and increased age. Therefore heavy people who lead active lives are more liable to develop arthritic changes than are slightly built persons who take a less active part in life. Again, like any mechanical joint, a human joint which has been damaged by disease or injury when the patient is young will wear away more quickly than a normal joint so that degenerative

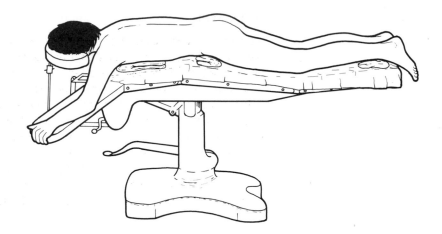

Fig. 47.5 Position on table for spinal operations.
 (i) The body is in a comfortable, relaxed position as spinal surgery may take several hours.
 (ii) The pelvis is supported by sand-bags and the chest by a pillow so that there is no pressure on the abdomen. This means that there is no pressure on the vena cava so that the spinal veins do not become engorged with blood.
 (iii) One (or two) arms are easily accessible for I.V. drips, B.P. measurement or for injections by the anaesthetist.
 (iv) This position can be used for operations on the cervical spine, the thoracic and lumbar spine or the sacrum.
 (v) Note the special head-rest attachment on the table.

changes also occur in patients who have had fractures into joints, patients who have had diseased joints, e.g. rheumatoid arthritis or septic arthritis, and in patients who have had cartilages removed, Perthe's disease or slipped epiphysis. Degenerative changes in joints give rise to friction instead of the usual smooth movement and this causes pain, synovial inflammation and swelling together with a tendency for the bone to become irregular in shape and to give rise to irregular outgrowths from the side of the joint known as osteophytes. These changes occur not only in synovial joints but also in the less flexible joints such as the intervertebral discs and the sacroiliac joints. They may give rise to quite severe deformities of the joints such as those seen in hallux valgus.

TREATMENT OF DEGENERATIVE JOINT DISEASE

Nonoperative treatment consists of resting the joint, reducing the weight of the patient — and this is a most important aspect as a reduction in weight obviously will reduce the stress upon the joint — various forms of physiotherapy and occasionally appropriate splinting. However as a rule surgical treatment usually becomes necessary and such treatment usually is one of three types of operation:
 (a) arthrodesis,
 (b) arthroplasty,
 (c) osteotomy.

Arthrodesis

Arthrodesis consists of the excision of the joint surfaces and the apposition of the raw bony ends so that the bones join together and the joint no longer exists. This has the effect of relieving the pain permanently and providing a stable mechanical structure. It has however the great disadvantage of permanently restricting mobility of that part of the body. This may not be very important in such areas as the spine but it becomes increasingly important in the mobile limbs. Arthrodesis is therefore used mainly in the spinal column to treat degenerative arthritis, in the toes to treat deformities and occasionally in the hip and the knee in the younger patient. When the joint is arthrodesed it requires to be immobilised in the same way as a fracture until the bone is soundly fused.

Arthroplasty

Arthroplasty means repair of a joint. A joint may be rendered mobile and painless merely by excising the joint and allowing the space between the bones to fill with blood clot which becomes organised into fibrous tissue. This is the principle behind such common procedures as Kellers' operation, where the proximal two thirds of the proximal phalanx of the big toes is removed, or the less common practice, Girdlestone's operation, where the head and neck of the femur are excised leaving the hip joint as a rather elastic flail joint. Such arthroplasties are known as excision arthroplasties and the postoperative care consists of a period of immobilisation until the blood clot is organised followed by mobilisation exercises and encouragement of normal activities as far as possible.

In more recent years surgeons have concentrated not only on excising the affected joints but on replacing them with prosthetic materials. These materials, be they metal, plastic or silicone rubber, are either impacted into the bone or are secured to the bone by means of an acrylic resin cement. Practically all joints in the body can be replaced except those in the spinal column, but the indications for such operations are mostly to be found in the ball and socket hip joint. The hip joint can be replaced by a metal socket and a metal ball, the former being screwed into the ileum and the latter impacted into the femur (Ring). The metal components may be secured to the bone by cement (McKee) but the more commonly used hip arthroplasty now is that where a metal femoral prosthesis articulates with a polyethylene acetabular component both of them being secured to the bone by cement (Charnley and other types, Figures 47.6 and 47.7).

Whichever method is used great care is placed upon preoperative skin preparation, the eradication of any septic focus within the body and antibiotic cover for the operation. Many surgeons prefer to perform such major joint replacement surgery in a hyper-sterile theatre so that orthopaedic surgeons often appear like spacemen operating in plastic tents. All these precautions are designed to reduce the risk of infection to a minimum as infection deeply placed within the body in relation to foreign material will give rise to persistent sepsis and loosening of the prosthesis which will then have to be removed.

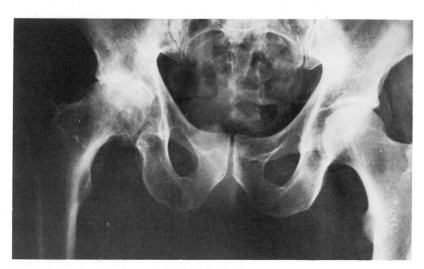

Fig. 47.6 X-ray showing osteoarthritis of right hip joint.

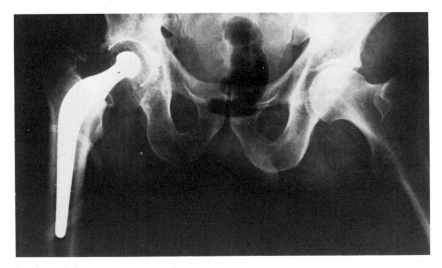

Fig. 47.7 The same patient as in Fig. 47.6 showing that the hip has been replaced with a Charnley total hip prosthesis.

Postoperatively the antibiotic cover is continued for several days, the patients are prevented from sitting or walking for several days and precautions are taken to reduce the other great danger in operation, i.e. pulmonary embolus from thrombosis of the deep veins in the leg or the pelvis. Many regimes are adopted to prevent this complication such as the use of plasma expanders, e.g. Dextran 40, mechanical massage for the calves, small doses of anticoagulants and active foot and ankle exercises by the physiotherapist. The patient is usually able to be discharged from hospital walking between sticks about a fortnight after the operation. Other joints which are commonly replaced are the metacarpo-phalangeal joints of the fingers and for this operation very flexible silicon rubber prostheses are used. A large variety of artificial knee joints has been produced but to date none has become more popularly used than another because the merchanical action of a human knee joint is very difficult to reproduce. Shoulder joints, elbow joints and ankle joints are also occasionally replaced where necessary.

Osteotomy

Division of a bone close to a joint either above it or below it produces relief of pain. The reason for this is poorly understood but part of the answer must lie in the relief of mechanical strains upon the joint and part of the answer in the division of nerves running from the joint.

An osteotomy of the upper tibia is an extremely useful operation to halt the progress of degenerative disease in a knee which has developed either valgus or a varus deformity. The limb requires immobilisation in plaster for a few weeks until the bone is joined after which rehabilitation is begun. Osteotomy of the upper femur between the lesser and greater trochanters (the so-called intertrochanteric osteotomy) has been used for many years to relieve the pain of osteoarthritis of the hips and it is still used by many surgeons in the treatment of the younger patient with an osteoarthritic hip (Fig. 47.8). If the operation of osteotomy fails to produce the desired effect then arthroplasty can still be carried out whereas if arthroplasty had been the first choice, followed by complications, then there is no other operation to fall back upon. Osteotomy is also quite frequently used in younger patients for deformity and early degenerative changes in the big toe joint. It should not be forgotten that the big toe joint is an extremely important joint in the body as it is one of the major weight bearing joints.

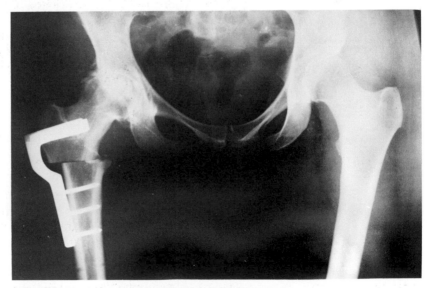

Fig. 47.8 X-ray showing treatment of an osteoarthritic right hip in a younger patient by inter-trochanteric osteotomy.

MISCELLANEOUS

There are many conditions which are not strictly joint lesions but which occur in the peri-articular tissues.

Bursitis and tenosynovitis

Bursae are sacs of fluid placed in the tissues to lubricate movements of tendon or skin over bone and these bursae quite often become inflamed; a typical example is housemaids knee (Fig. 47.9). The tendons themselves are closely surrounded by filmy sheaths which are similar in structure to the synovial linings of joints. Inflammation of these sheaths is known as tenosynovitis and such an inflammation may cause thickening of the tough outer sheath enclosing the synovial sheath causing constriction of the tendon. Such a condition requires release of the tendon by incision of the thickened sheath.

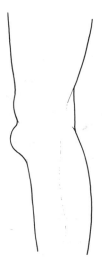

Fig. 47.9 Pre-patellar bursitis (housemaid's knee).

INJURIES OF MUSCLES AND TENDONS

These injuries are discussed in this chapter because muscles and tendons are closely associated with bones and joints.

Muscles are frequently partially torn, in which case they bleed and large haematomas may develop in their sheathes, or they may be severely bruised by direct violence with a similar end result. The treatment is rest followed by restoration of function when the pain and swelling subside.

Tendons may rupture either through injury (e.g. Achilles tendon rupture in athletes) or because of disease (e.g. the extensor tendons of the fingers in rheumatoid arthritis). The usual treatment of these injuries is surgical repair of the ruptured tendons.

When the flexor tendons of the hand are accidentally severed, primary suture is usually only undertaken by expert surgeons in special hand surgery centres. Most accident surgeons find they get better results by suturing only the skin as a first measure and then inserting a tendon graft to replace the severed tendon some weeks later. All patients who have had hand surgery require nursing with the hand elevated for the first few days to avoid postoperative swelling. This complication is the main cause of poor results.

There is a circular cuff of muscle tendons which surrounds the shoulder joint from the front to the back passing across the top of the joint. This is known as the rotator cuff and tears and inflammatory lesions of this are extremely common occurrences. They are best treated by local injection of hydrocortisone into the tender area and by various forms of physiotherapy. A similar condition occurs at the elbow, either on the medial or the lateral side but more usually laterally. This is an inflammatory lesion of the muscle origin from the bone and has acquired the colloquial name of tennis elbow.

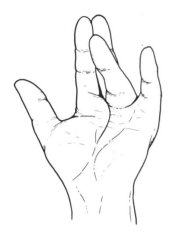

Fig. 47.10 Dupuytren's contracture of the palm and left ring finger.

Dupuytren's contracture

This condition causes curling up of the fingers because of contracture of the tough tissue underlying the skin of the palm. It is an inherited condition and is progressive. The skin of the palm becomes infiltrated by the thickened palmar fascia and it becomes nodular and ridged (Fig. 47.10). The treatment of this condition is excision of the thickened tissue deep to the palmar skin.

Ganglion

A ganglion is a tense, painful cyst arising from the synovial lining of a joint or tendon sheath. It is full of jelly-like material and can sometimes be burst and dispersed by direct pressure or a sharp blow. If not, excision is the usual treatment.

Ingrowing toenail

This painful condition should more properly be described as an overgrowth of the skin fold at one or the other, or both, sides of the great toenail. At all events a deep groove, or sulcus, develops between the nail and the skin which inevitably collects dirt and skin secretions, subsequently causing inflammation and often purulent infection (Fig. 47.11).

This chronic, painful condition can be prevented by wearing well-fitting shoes and by careful attention to foot hygiene. It can sometimes be cured by skilled foot care, but often avulsion of the nail is necessary to drain the infection, and sometimes radical excision of the nail bed, preventing further growth of the nail, may be needed.

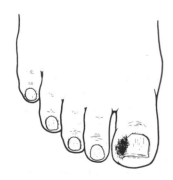

47.11 An ingrowing toe-nail.

POLIOMYELITIS

Mention must be made of this condition although it is becoming increasingly uncommon in those countries where an active immunisation programme is under way. The disease is caused by a small virus which attacks the anterior horn cells in the spinal cord; hence its name. This causes inflammation, swelling and eventual destruction of the nerve cells affected so that the muscles supplied by these nerves become paralysed. The disease is characterised by a high fever, indistinguisable at first from fever caused by any other disease, but the diagnosis becomes clear once the paralysis develops after forty-eight hours or so. The disease may affect practically every muscle in the body or may be highly selective affecting a few muscles here and a few there. In the more severe forms of the disease the patient will often require assisted respiration and indeed this may become necessary as a permanent measure. However more commonly the patient survives with his respiratory mechanism intact and is left with varying degrees of paralysis.

Surgical treatment of poliomyelitis

Surgical treatment is confined to stabilising unstable joints by various methods, by strengthening the action of various weak groups of muscles, by transferring the tendons of strong muscles to reinforce the action of the weaker ones and to correct deformities which may have been allowed to develop during the acute illness.

If a lower limb is paralysed whilst the patient is young then it does not grow so quickly as the unaffected opposite limb and because of this a difference in leg lengths may be one of the more disabling affects of an attack of poliomyelitis. Surgical treatment can help to lengthen the affected joint by means of slow and continuous traction on a divided bone over a period of 2 to 3 weeks or surgery may be directed towards preventing growth of the longer limb. This can be done by preventing growth at the epiphysial plates of cartilage. The operation is known as epiphysiodesis if bone is placed across the epiphysial plate or as epiphysial arrest if metal staples are placed across the epiphysial plate.

48

Diseases of the ear, the nose, and the throat

Diseases of the ear, the nose, and the throat are considered together because these structures are linked anatomically and are affected by the same pathological processes. Until recently, surgery in this area was aimed at eradicating the common infections but the emphasis has now moved towards reconstruction. Hearing can often be restored and function can be re-established even after major resections for malignancy.

SYMPTOMS OF EAR DISEASE

1. Deafness means that the patient has a hearing loss which may be mild or severe. If the cause of the deafness lies in the outer ear or the middle ear, it is said to be a conductive deafness. If the cause lies in the inner ear or the auditory nerve, it is a sensori-neural deafness. The most common cause of deafness in childhood is serous otitis media whereas in adults, presbycusis is most common. Presbycusis means the deafness of the elderly and it is a sensori-neural hearing loss caused by the degeneration of nervous tissue.

2. Pain. Earache or otalgia is a very common complaint. In children, the commonest cause is acute otitis media whereas in adults it is otitis externa. The pain may arise from the ear itself or from an adjacent site with a shared nerve supply. The commonest site for referred pain is the throat, where infections or, more rarely, malignant tumours are responsible.

3. Discharge. A discharge from the ear may be mucoid, purulent or bloody. It must be distinguished from the escape of wax which is a normal process. Commonly, the cause of a discharge is otitis externa or otitis media and in the latter event, a perforation will be present in the tympanic membrane.

4. Vertigo is a form of dizziness where the patient experiences a spinning sensation. It is a common symptom when the balance, or vestibular system of the inner ear is diseased. It is accompanied by nausea and vomiting and it is difficult to treat.

5. Tinnitus, or noise in the ear, is a very common complaint. Its quality varies from a high-pitched whistle to the clanging of bells or recognisable snatches of music. It is a distressing symptom and although it can some-times be alleviated, it can seldom be cured.

DISEASES OF THE OUTER EAR

Bat ear

The pinna protrudes from the side of the head because the ridge of the antihelix has not formed. The child may be the object of derision and the antihelix can be reconstructed fairly easily through an incision on the back of the pinna.

Wax

Wax or cerumen is a normal substance produced in the external ear canal. It is made up of epithelial scales mixed with the secretions from special glands in the skin of the outer ear. In most people, the wax escapes as it is formed but in some, it remains in the ear canal, obstructing it and causing deafness. Olive oil or liquid paraffin ear drops will soften the impacted wax which is then removed by syringing.

It is important that the water in the syringe should be at body tempera-ture so as not to stimulate the inner ear and cause dizziness. The jet of water is directed at the wall of the ear canal and the wax is washed out. A receiver is held beneath the ear and the patient's clothing is protected by a mackintosh sheet. The ear must be dried gently after the syringing and it should be examined by a doctor to exclude any damage to the tympanic membrane.

Foreign bodies

These are commonly found in the ears of children and the variety is immense. Sometimes they can be removed by a probe or syringing but the child is often frightened and uncooperative and a general anaesthetic will be necessary. The ear must always be checked to exclude any underlying damage.

An insect in the ear is treated similarly.

Otitis externa

This is an inflammation of the outer ear which is lined by skin. The condi-tion is usually bilateral and the symptoms start with itching. The patient scratches the ear which becomes infected, painful, and sometimes blocked by a thin muco-purulent discharge. Allergy, stress, and the presence of infected water may all play a part but the treatment is the same. Any pre-cipitating cause is removed and a swab is taken for culture and sensitivity. The ear canal is cleaned gently, thoroughly, and frequently using a wisp of cotton wool on the tip of a suitable probe. Drops are then instilled directly or used to impregnate a small wick of ribbon gauze which is left in the ear for one or two days. The drops may be simple disinfectants or may be combinations of topical antibiotics (to kill the bacteria) and steroids (to reduce the inflammation). The condition tends to recur.

Boils

A boil, or furuncle, is found in the outer hair-bearing skin of the ear canal. It is very painful because the skin at this site is firmly tethered to the underlying cartilage. Like boils elsewhere, it is caused by the staphylococcus and the relevant antibiotic is only necessary when the symptoms are severe. Analgesics are necessary and the possibility of underlying diabetes must be excluded.

Tumours

Malignant tumours of the ear are commonest in the outer ear where both basal cell carcinoma and squamous carcinoma are found. The small lesion is treated with radiotherapy but the larger will need surgical excision.

MIDDLE EAR DISEASE

In order that sound may pass efficiently through the ossicles, the Eustachian tube must allow air to enter the middle ear from the nasopharynx. In children particularly, the tube becomes blocked and this obstruction is responsible for many conditions in the middle ear.

Serous (secretory) otitis media

When the Eustachian tube becomes blocked, the air trapped in the middle ear is absorbed into the surrounding tissues and is replaced by thin fluid. In time, small glands appear in the lining of the middle ear and the mucus which they secrete, explains the popular name of 'glue ears' which is given to this condition. It is seen most in those children where an immature musculature and repeated upper respiratory tract infections, predispose to tubal obstruction.

The child develops a hearing loss which may pass unnoticed. However, the parents may have noted that the child's school work has deteriorated or that he turns up the television. There may also be associated episodes of earache. An examination of the ear will reveal the presence of fluid behind the tympanic membrane and a simple whisper test or an audiogram will confirm the presence of a hearing loss.

If the condition is temporary or intermittent, nothing need be done since most children outgrow the condition. If it is more severe, an alternative means of allowing air into the middle ear, must be found. A hole is made in the tympanic membrane (a myringotomy) and the hole is prevented from healing by inserting a small plastic tube (grommet, dottle or stopple) (Fig. 48.1). At the same time, any underlying cause (sinusitis or enlarged adenoids) is treated.

As long as the grommet remains in place and remains unblocked the

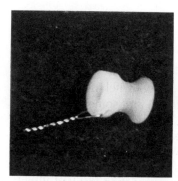

Fig. 48.1 A grommet for insertion in secretory otitis media. Ten times the normal size.

hearing is normal. However, the grommet drops out after an average period of 6 months. It is hoped that the patient will have outgrown the problem by then, but a grommet may need to be reinserted if fluid reaccumulates.

Acute otitis media

The middle ear is in continuity with the nasopharynx and is therefore very prone to infection from it. This is especially so in the presence of serous otitis media when a convenient culture medium is available for the invading bacteria. The middle ear mucosa becomes inflamed and the cavity fills with pus which escapes by bursting out through the tympanic membrane into the external ear.

The patient, who is usually a child with a cold, develops an earache of increasing severity which ceases when the membrane bursts. The perforation usually heals after 2 to 3 days but this should be checked after one month and the presence of an underlying serous otitis media excluded.

The patient should be confined to bed and given analgesics. A covered hot-water bottle applied to the ear is helpful and warm olive oil drops will soothe the inflamed membrane. If a patient is seen before the perforation occurs, penicillin should be given and should be continued for at least 5 days and until the inflammation has settled. A swab should be taken from the discharging ear and sent for culture and sensitivity. Complications may arise but these are now rare. The commonest was acute mastoiditis, a condition in which an abscess develops in the mastoid bone and bursts out behind the ear. It is now only seen in children whose natural defence mechanisms are not functioning normally.

Chronic otitis media

When a middle ear infection becomes persistent it is called chronic otitis media. Permanent damage is done to the tympanic membrane and to the ossicles and the patient may be very deaf with a large central perforation and a persistent discharge. The discharge is particularly likely to occur when the patient has a cold because infected secretions pass up the Eustachian tube.

An attempt is made to remove any source of infection in the nose or nasopharynx and the local discharge can be controlled by regular toilet and the instillation of ear drops. When the ear has been dry for several months it is suitable for a surgical repair of the perforation. A piece of fascia is taken from the surface of the temporalis muscle and the thin tissue is grafted over the perforation. The graft may be laid on the inner or the outer surface of the tympanic membrane and the operation is known as a myringoplasty (myrinx is Greek for the tympanic membrane). Similarly, any loss of ossicular continuity can be corrected by repositioning a damaged ossicle or by replacing it with a piece of bone or a prosthesis. This operation is called a tympanoplasty. More recently it has become possible to remove the tympanic membrane and its attached ossicles, in one block from a cadaver. These homograft tissues can then be implanted into a suitable patient but the operation is technically very difficult.

Cholesteatoma

This is a cyst lined by squamous epithelium and filled with layers of epithelial scales. The cyst forms from an in-pouching of the upper segment of the tympanic membrane, into the middle ear cavity. Initially the epithelial scales escape into the external canal, but as the mouth of the pouch narrows, they are retained and accumulate. The cholesteatoma is unique in that it has the property of eroding most of the tissues which it encounters. The contents of the cyst become infected and the condition may be regarded as a form of chronic otitis media.

The extent of the damage is determined by the direction in which the cholesteatoma enlarges. Usually the ossicles are damaged, but an upward extension will produce a brain abscess or meningitis. Similarly, a medial extension may produce a facial paralysis or damage the inner ear.

The patient complains of deafness and an offensive scanty discharge. There may be evidence of a complication and an examination of the ear will reveal a marginal perforation with white epithelial scales protruding. The treatment of a cholesteatoma is surgical and some form of radical mastoidectomy is necessary for its removal.

There are two forms of mastoidectomy operation. In a simple or cortical mastoidectomy, a hole is drilled from the surface of the mastoid bone into the mastoid antrum and the localised disease is removed. The operation does not interfere with the middle ear and postoperatively, the external canal and tympanic membrane may appear normal. For a cholesteatoma, this operation alone would be unsuitable because the middle ear itself is involved. A simple mastoidectomy is done first and then the bony wall between the simple cavity and the external canal is removed. The remnants of the tympanic membrane and the ossicles are also removed and we are left with a large cavity which can be seen on postoperative examination. This is the radical mastoidectomy and the ear will be safe although the patient will still be deaf and may still have a discharge. There will also be good access for toilet.

Otosclerosis

In otosclerosis, abnormal bone grows across the margins of the oval window and on to the footplate of the stapes which can no longer vibrate. The condition is commoner in women; it begins in early adulthood and the deafness progressively worsens. The treatment is a choice between a hearing aid and surgery and the operation is known as a stapedectomy. The mobile part of the stapes is removed and a hole is made in the fixed footplate. A piston (or a similar prosthesis) is placed in the hole and hooked around the incus to re-establish sound transmission. The inner ear is at risk during the operation and this must be clearly explained to the patient. Some dizziness almost always occurs temporarily and this is countered by a drug such as Stemetil.

DISEASES OF THE INNER EAR

Any disease affecting the inner ear causes damage to the delicate nerve endings responding for hearing and balance and the patient may complain of vertigo, deafness, or tinnitus. Surgery is rarely of any assistance but a hearing aid will help the deafness which is very common in old age.

Trauma, loud noises and some drugs may damage the inner ear and they should be avoided if possible. In Meniere's disease, there is an accumulation of endolymph in the inner ear and the patient suffers from episodes of severe vertigo. If the hearing is good, certain specialised operations can be attempted but the results are not often convincing. If the hearing is bad, the inner ear can be destroyed in an operation known as a total labyrinthectomy and the result is often very beneficial.

A tumour known as an acoustic neuroma may occur in the internal auditory canal and its symptoms will mimic those of inner ear disease. The ear, nose and throat surgeon carries out many investigations to distinguish between these in an attempt to diagnose a neuroma at an early stage.

DEAFNESS

Deafness is a disability which separates the sufferer from society. Communication becomes difficult and there is a tendency for the non-aggressive personality to become a recluse. Although hearing aids may help, they never provide normal hearing and they may aggravate the disability. When speaking to deaf people, especially the elderly, the speaker should face his companion and speak clearly and distinctly. It must be remembered that deafness varies for sounds of different pitch and the patient may hear some sounds normally. Shouting usually distorts speech even more and it often causes distress and acute discomfort.

Points of interest in ear surgery

Incisions for ear operations may lie behind, or in front of, the pinna. Since the hair often encroaches on the operation site, it is usually necessary to shave a narrow band in order to allow the application of an adhesive sterile towel.

The examination of the ear is carried out with a head mirror, a head light or an electric auriscope. Since the middle ear structures are so small, a binocular operating microscope is employed for middle ear operations (Fig. 48.2). The instruments used in middle ear surgery are angled so that the manipulating hand does not obscure vision down the narrow external canal (Fig. 48.3).

DISEASES OF THE NOSE

Symptoms of nasal disease

1. Bleeding. The medical term for a nose bleed is epistaxis. The blood

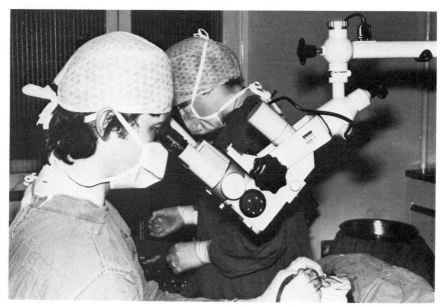

Fig. 48.2   An ear operation using the operating microscope.

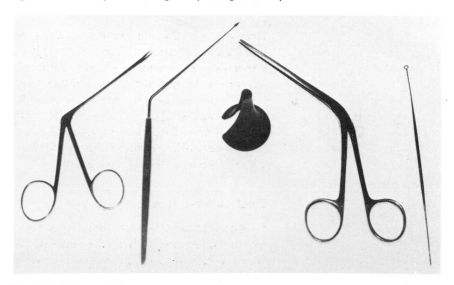

Fig. 48.3   Instruments in ear surgery
Left to right — Crocodile forceps Myringotomy knife Aural speculum Tilley's aural dressing
forceps Jobson Horne probe

may escape through the nostrils or it may run backwards into the
nasopharynx and throat.

2. Obstruction.   This may be fluctuant or permanent and it is caused by
mucosal congestion, a deviated septum or nasal polyps. The congestion
may be infective or allergic. The patient with nasal obstruction, snores and
mouth-breathes.

3. Discharge.   This is usually watery in allergic conditions and purulent
in infective conditions. A unilateral persistent discharge is caused by a for-

eign body (in children) or a tumour (in adults). A discharge which passes backwards into the throat is known as a postnasal drip.

4. Loss of the sense of smell. This is an under-rated disability and is little understood.

NASAL LESIONS

Fractured nasal bones

The nasal bones are flattened or deviated to one side following trauma. If the patient is seen within 3 weeks, the deformity may be corrected under general anaesthesia. If treatment is sought much later, a rhinoplasty becomes necessary. In this operation, the skin of the nose is separated from the underlying nasal skeleton and the shape is corrected as desired.

Septal Abscess

Trauma causes bleeding between the septal cartilage and the overlying muco-periosteum. This haematoma will cause nasal obstruction and unless it is drained it will form an abscess with subsequent destruction of the cartilage.

Deviated nasal septum

A significant deviation of the septum causes nasal obstruction and interferes with the drainage of the sinuses. It is corrected by one of the two following operations.

1. Sub-Mucous Resection (S.M.R.) of the nasal septum. The muco-periosteum is raised and the deviated portion of cartilage is removed.

2. Septoplasty. The offending cartilage is straightened and repositioned in the mid-line.

Epistaxis

A nose bleed presents in two ways. In the young patient, bleeding occurs from a superficial septal blood vessel lying just inside the nostril on a spot known as Little's area. Bleeding is initiated by the slightest trauma or infection and it is usually trivial. The first aid treatment is to grip the tip of the nose between thumb and forefinger and to exert firm pressure over the bleeding point for 3 minutes. If the epistaxes occur regularly, the offending vessel is cauterised under local or general anaesthesia and any underlying nasal infection is treated.

In the elderly patient, bleeding is often heavy and arises from larger vessels at the back of the nose. There is a history of hypertension and access to the responsible vessels is poor. The nose is packed with ribbon gauze impregnated in paraffin or a suitable disinfectant and this is left in place for one or two days. Pressure can also be exerted on the bleeding area by inflating a special balloon. A blood transfusion may be obligatory and the surgical ligation of the arteries supplying the nose, sometimes becomes necessary.

It must be emphasised that an epistaxis is often a sign of some underlying systemic disease.

Infection

The common cold or coryza is the commonest nasal infection. It is an acute viral rhinitis which presents with sneezing, mucosal congestion and a mucoid discharge. After 2 days, a secondary infection by various bacteria results in a purulent discharge and the condition settles within 1 week without any treatment.

Allergic rhinitis

An inflammatory congestion of the nasal mucosa can be caused by an allergy as well as by an infection. The symptoms, although similar, present in varying patterns. In hay fever, the nasal mucosa is allergic to grass pollen and the symptoms of sneezing, obstruction and a watery discharge are only present during the early summer months. With perennial rhinitis, the symptoms are present throughout the year and numerous allergens, such as feathers and house dust, may be responsible.

If possible, the allergen should be identified and avoided, and in some cases a course of desensitisation injections is helpful. Anti-histamine drugs suppress the symptoms but produce unwanted drowsiness as a side-effect. Many patients respond well to steroid nasal sprays such as Beconase, but these should be prescribed with care.

Nasal polyps

Allergic rhinitis is sometimes associated with the appearance of polyps in the upper part of the nose. Localised areas of mucosa become swollen and droop downwards into the nasal cavity to give the appearance of skinned grapes. They cause nasal obstruction and there is no treatment apart from surgical removal which is carried out under local or general anaesthesia. Nasal polyps are harmless but they tend to recur because the underlying problem has not been treated.

Vasomotor rhinitis

When the nasal mucosa becomes swollen and congested without any evidence of infection or allergy, the condition is known as vasomotor rhinitis. It is caused by an alteration in the behaviour of blood vessels supplying the mucosa and it is sometimes believed to have a psychological basis. The main symptom is nasal obstruction and it is difficult to treat.

Decongestant nasal sprays or drops are not advocated since they aggravate the condition when used persistently. When the mucosa overlying the inferior turbinate bone is particularly swollen, it may be reduced in volume by the application of surface cautery or sub-mucosal diathermy. A polluted

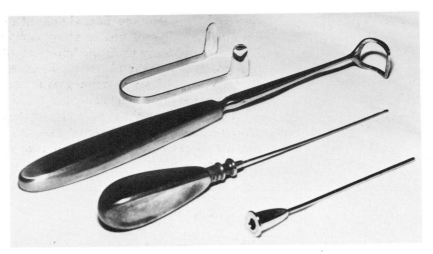

Fig. 48.4 Instruments for nasal surgery
Nasal speculum
An adenoid curette
Trocar and cannula for sinus wash outs.

or centrally-heated environment makes the condition worse and the patient should be encouraged to take a healthy diet, plenty of fresh air and exercise.

THE ADENOID

This is the name given to the pad of lymphoid tissue which lies on the roof of the nasopharynx behind the nose. In the past, it has been held responsible for a variety of symptoms in children but its role as a scapegoat has recently become much diminished. The adenoid is normally enlarged between the ages of four and seven and on rare occasions it may be so large as to obstruct the nasal passages and affect the opening of the Eustachian tube. The adenoid gradually atrophies after the age of eight.

The removal of the adenoid is still carried out for nasal obstruction and in the treatment of serous otitis media although its role in these conditions has not been proven. The operation of adenoidectomy is done with the mouth held open by a special gag and with the patient in the supine position. The adenoid curette (fig. 48.4) is guided behind the soft palate and the pad of lymphoid tissue is scraped out. Care must be taken not to damage any other structures during this blind procedure. Since the main complication is haemorrhage, it is imperative that the patient is carefully observed during the postoperative period.

Points of special interest

The nose is examined by raising the tip and shining a light inside. The view may be improved by retracting the margins of the nostril with a nasal speculum. The back of the nose is examined by placing a small mirror through the mouth and behind the soft palate. When a light is directed at the mirror, the reflection of the nasopharynx and posterior nose is seen. Nasal operations occur at the upper end of the respiratory tract and special emphasis is therefore placed on the protection of the lower airway. As in the ear, the instruments are angled to permit better vision and a headlight is employed to concentrate light at the site of operation.

Postoperatively, the nose is almost always blocked by oedema, and the obstruction is eased by nasal douches using warm sterile saline. The patient inevitably mouth-breathes and regular mouth-washes prevent the resulting dryness.

THE SINUSES

There are four sets of air sinuses on each side of the skull; the maxillary sinus (or antrum), the frontal sinuses, the ethmoid sinuses and the sphenoid sinuses. They are placed around the nose and are therefore called paranasal sinuses. Each sinus is an air-filled space in the skull and each drains into the nose by a small opening, the ostium. The largest sinus is the maxillary antrum which lies in the cheek bone and it is this which is most often infected. If all the sinuses are infected, the condition is known as pansinusitis. Sphenoid sinusitis is very rare.

Maxillary sinusitis

When the nose is infected by the common cold, the lining of the maxillary antrum is involved in the same way. As long as the ciliated epithelium which lines the antrum, remains healthy and as long as the ostium stays open, there is no problem. Once the ostium blocks, mucus and pus accumulate in the antrum and the patient is said to have acute maxillary sinusitis.

The patient is pyrexial and ill and there is a throbbing pain over the affected cheek which is also very tender to pressure. The nose is often blocked and examination will show the presence of pus which is swabbed and sent for culture. The patient is kept in bed and given suitable analgesics and the symptoms usually settle on antibiotics, penicillin being the treatment of choice.

In some patients, the infection becomes chronic and the lining mucosa becomes thickened, polypoid and partially destroyed. The patient has a blocked nose and a postnasal drip. The antrum is no longer able to drain via the ostium and surgical treatment is necessary.

The first step is to carry out an antral washout. A trocar and cannula (fig. 48.4) is introduced into the antrum via the nostril and the thin layer of bone below the inferior turbinate. The trocar is removed and a syringe is applied to the cannula which is flushed out with saline. The accumulated pus is removed and the ostium is unblocked. This procedure may need to be repeated but if it is inadequate, it will be necessary to construct a permanent drainage opening below the inferior turbinate. This is known as an intranasal antrostomy and it gives the antral mucosa the opportunity to return to normal. If the situation is irreversible, the infected mucosa is removed through an opening constructed in the front of the antrum beneath the upper lip. This is known as a Caldwell-Luc operation and it allows good access to the antrum.

Ethmoiditis

There are several small ethmoid sinuses which lie between the orbit and the upper nose. They are often involved by chronic infection in conjunction with the antrum. Acute ethmoiditis is unusual and it is only seen in children. Oedema of the soft tissues around the eye, is seen and it is treated with penicillin.

Frontal sinusitis

An acute infection of the frontal sinus is dangerous because it is so near to the brain. The patient should therefore be admitted to hospital and given systemic penicillin. A nasal swab is taken for culture and if the condition does not settle, the sinus is drained through the roof of the orbit. Chronic frontal sinusitis is difficult to eradicate and it tends to recur in spite of surgical treatment.

Tumours

Malignant tumours can reach a considerable size in the maxillary antrum before they produce symptoms. The symptoms, when they appear, depend upon the direction of spread. Problems may arise with the eye, the teeth or the nose and there may be a swelling of the cheek. It must be emphasised however, that the commonest cause of a swollen cheek is an infected tooth of the upper jaw. The treatment is by radiotherapy, surgery or a combination of the two. Surgery may involve the removal of an eye and considerable cosmetic deformity results. The prognosis for malignant tumours in this area is poor.

THE THROAT

The trachea and the oesophagus meet at the hypopharynx which continues upwards into the oropharynx. At its junction with the pharynx, the structure of the trachea has become modified to form the larynx. These three structures, the larynx, the hypopharynx and the oropharynx, constitute the throat (see Fig. 48.5).

Symptoms and signs of throat disease

Dysphagia or difficulty in swallowing is a serious symptom if it persists for longer than a few days. Together with pain, it is commonly found in tonsillitis but a more serious cause is a malignant tumour or an impacted

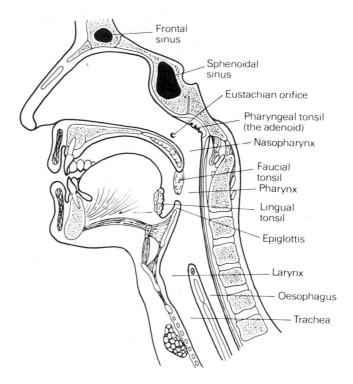

Fig. 48.5 The pharynx, the larynx and trachea.

foreign body.

Pain usually presents on swallowing and it often radiates to the ear.

Hoarseness. This means that there is a roughness of the voice, caused by some factor which prevents the smooth approximation of the vocal cords. Infections are the commonest cause but an early tumour of the vocal cords should always be suspected.

Cough. This is an explosive release of air through the vocal cords and it suggests the presence of an irritation in the larynx or trachea.

Stridor or noisy breathing. It may be present during inspiration, expiration or both. It implies that there is a narrowing of the respiratory tract.

Examination of the throat

The throat is examined by indirect or direct laryngoscopy. An indirect laryngoscopy is done by pressing a warmed mirror against the soft palate and observing the reflection of the larynx and hypopharynx. It can be difficult to do this when the patient has a sensitive throat and a direct laryngoscopy becomes necessary. This involves the insertion of an illuminated metal tube into the pharynx under general anaesthesia. The larynx is then examined directly through the tube. A narrower and longer tube is employed for an oesophagoscopy.

DISEASES OF THE THROAT

Infections are very common especially in childhood, where they may be serious. However, surgery is only important in the treatment of tumours in the larynx and pharynx.

Tonsillitis

When the surface of the tonsil and the oropharynx becomes inflamed, the patient has pharyngitis. He has a sore throat but he is not ill. When the deep tissues of the tonsil are acutely infected, the patient has acute tonsillitis. He has a sore throat but he is also ill and runs a high temperature. The infecting organism is commonly a virus but secondary bacterial infection occurs especially with the streptococcus. Whatever the infecting organism, the clinical features are the same and the examination findings vary with the stage of the illness. The tonsils are usually large, red and covered with patches of purulent debris which have been extruded from the tonsillar crypts. The upper cervical and sub-mandibular lymph glands are often enlarged and tender. In the very small child there may be no sign apart from a refusal to take food.

The condition is commonest in childhood between the ages of five and eight but it does occur in young adults who have not gained immunity. The patient is ill for 2 or 3 days and gradually improves over the next 5 days.

Treatment consists of rest in bed and isolation of the patient. He is encouraged to drink, and swallowing is made easier by the administration of an analgesic such as aspirin. Antibiotics are not usually necessary because most episodes are viral in origin and the natural course of the condition is short. In the more severe attack or where a complication is feared, an antibiotic is advisable and penicillin is probably best.

If the acute attacks recur five or six times a year and there is a significant interference with schooling or work a tonsillectomy should be considered. If the child is around the age of seven or eight when first seen, it is worthwhile postponing surgery for 1 year because most gain immunity around this age. A simple enlargement of the tonsils is not an indication for their removal. It must be appreciated that tonsillitis and other upper respiratory tract infections are so common around the age of five that they must be considered as part of the normal process of growing up.

The operation is carried out under general anaesthesia and the tonsil is dissected from the underlying pharyngeal tissue. The adenoids are no longer removed routinely at the same time and the operation is never done while the tonsil is inflamed.

Postoperatively the patient should be nursed on the side with the head down so as not to inhale blood or a tonsil fragment (Fig. 48.6). The main complication is haemorrhage and its early recognition is essential. Observations are made on the respiration, colour, pulse and blood pressure and any excessive swallowing should be reported to the surgeon who will examine the patient. If bleeding occurs, the patient is returned to the theatre for ligation of the bleeding point.

The following day the patient is encouraged to eat and drink and an

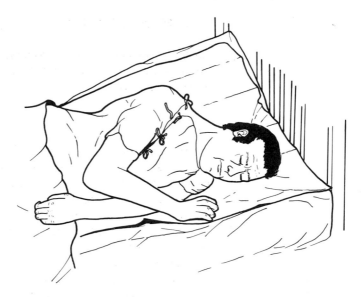

Fig. 48.6 Position after tonsillectomy. Pillows are placed behind the mattress on one side.

analgesic such as soluble aspirin is given before each meal. The throat is very sore and the pain may radiate to the ear. Children are normally kept in for about 3 days and adults for a day or so longer. Secondary bleeding may occur about 1 week after the operation but this is due to infection and it responds well to penicillin.

Peritonsillar abscess (quinsy)

Rarely in adults, the tonsillitis does not settle and the infection spreads on one side, into the adjacent pharyngeal wall and soft palate. A unilateral abscess forms and the swelling pushes the tonsil up to, or even across, the mid-line. The patient cannot open his jaws and the saliva which he cannot swallow, dribbles from the mouth.

The treatment of this peritonsillar abscess is to incise it and the patient is given a course of penicillin. The tonsils are removed 6 weeks later to prevent a recurrence.

Most patients sent up to hospital with a suspected quinsy are usually found to have a persistent bilateral tonsillitis as part of the picture of glandular fever.

THE LARYNX

Acute laryngitis

The larynx may be involved in any acute upper respiratory tract infection. In adults, this causes hoarseness and the best treatment is to rest the voice. In children, however, the larynx is smaller and any additional narrowing by inflammatory oedema interferes with the airway. Initially the child has stridor (croup) but severe respiratory obstruction can result. Admission to hospital, humidity in an oxygen tent, naso-tracheal intubation or a tracheostomy may all become necessary if the symptoms are severe.

Chronic laryngitis

The patient is persistently hoarse in this condition and a tumour may be suspected. The vocal cords are red and thickened and the patient often follows an occupation which demands an over-use of the voice in a smoky environment. Treatment is notoriously difficult because the patient may need to lose his job in order to achieve the essential voice-rest.

Vocal nodules are small swellings which occur on the vocal cords and are thought by some to be a form of chronic laryngitis. They cause hoarseness and if large, they can be removed by direct laryngoscopy.

Tumours of the larynx

Benign. Laryngeal papillomata are small viral warts which grow in the larynx of the small child. They produce hoarseness, stridor and respiratory obstruction and they are removed by suction diathermy, cryosurgery or more recently by the laser. A tracheostomy is done if the symptoms are severe but the papillomata eventually disappear when immunity is gained by the host.

Malignant. A patient suffering from a laryngeal tumour presents with hoarseness. In the early stages he may be treated by radiotherapy with preservation of the voice and a good prognosis. In the later stages and for those tumours which recur after radiotherapy, a laryngectomy is carried out.

The larynx produces speech and prevents the entry of food into the trachea. Both these functions are lost after a laryngectomy. After the removal of the larynx one is left with the cut end of the trachea and a defect in the pharynx. The latter is sutured up while the trachea is brought out through the middle of the neck and sutured to the skin.

Postoperative care of the laryngectomy

1. The care of a tracheostomy has been discussed in Chapter 17.
2. A laryngectomy is a major procedure because the patient loses his main organ of communication. He can no longer ask for attention and initially he requires the constant presence of a nurse. Many patients are not accustomed to writing and they become intensely anxious, frustrated and depressed. Great demands are therefore made upon the patience and sympathy of the attendant nurse. The patient is provided with a pencil and pad and a bell is placed within easy reach. A selection of word-cards is also useful (Fig. 17.2). In time many patients learn a new form of speech whereby air is swallowed and regurgitated to produce a vibration in some suitable piece of tissue. This is a similar mechanism to that of the 'belch'. The degree of clarity achieved by this technique, varies with the motivation of the patient.

3. Feeding is initially achieved through a naso-gastric tube while the pharyngeal defect is healing. An adequate liquidised diet is given and a close eye is kept on the patient's weight and upon his fluid output.

Basic nursing care is at a high premium because the patient is often elderly and in poor physical condition. However, the rewards are great because the patient is sometimes totally rehabilitated.

Tumours of the pharynx

These tumours present with dysphagia or with a gland in the neck. Radiotherapy is often the first treatment of choice but many come to need surgery. Pharyngeal tumours often involve the adjacent larynx and so an adequate excision includes the larynx as well as the pharynx. It is no longer possible to suture the defect in the pharynx as after a laryngectomy and a method has to be found to bridge the gap. This continuity is provided by the transference of a section of gut or by employing grafted tubes of skin. The patient commonly develops fistulae and stenosis at the site of the operation and the postoperative period is a protracted one. A block-dissection of the lymph glands in the neck is commonly done with a pharyngo-laryngectomy.

The postoperative care is the same as that after a laryngectomy although the problems are worse because of the bleeding difficulties. Much effort is needed in preventing the patient from becoming depressed.

49

Diseases of the eye

REFRACTIVE ERRORS

In the normal eye at rest, parallel rays of light are brought to a focus on the retina, and such an eye is called emmetropic. Other eyes are abnormal in that they cannot bring parallel rays of light to a clear focus on the retina when at rest, because these eyes have an error of refraction and are therefore ametropic. Correcting spectacles will allow such an eye to achieve a clear focus when at rest. This refractive variation between eyes depends upon the length of the eye, the curvature of the cornea and, to a lesser extent, the position and refractivity of the lens in the eye. Defective or uncomfortable vision may be due solely to an error of refraction. This can be corrected by spectacles and is not regarded as a disease. The important part of the examination is to exclude defects in the eye or its associated areas of the brain which are due to disease.

Common refractive errors are:

1. **Astigmatism** in which the image focused on the retina is indistinct due to unequal refraction of the eye in different refractive planes. For example, the horizontal lines of an object may be seen clearly whereas the vertical outlines are blurred.

2. **Myopia** is a condition of short-sightedness. Near objects can be seen clearly whereas distant ones are indistinct. Myopic eyes are often large eyes, although not necessarily so.

3. **Hypermetropia** commonly called long-sight. The distant vision is more easily achieved whereas near vision is much more difficult. The lens in the eye can to some extent be used to overcome this disability by exercising accommodation which is carried out by using the ciliary muscle of the eye to alter the curvature of the lens. The extra effort put into accommodation in this condition also leads to excessive convergence effort and may play an important part in the development of convergent squint of the accommodative type.

4. **Presbyopia** is a progressive failure of accommodative power from the age of about 14 years, when it is very large, to the age of 70 to 80 when there is virtually no accommodative power remaining. For most people at the age of 45 the loss of accommodation is such that reading spectacles are

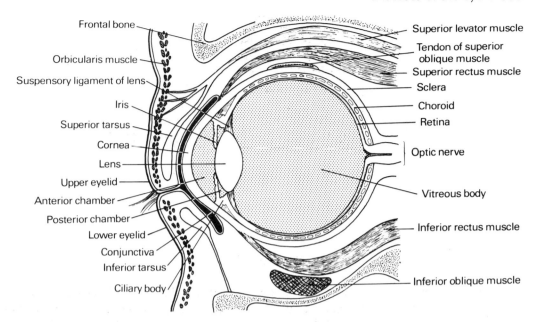

Frontal bone

Orbicularis muscle

Suspensory ligament of lens

Iris

Superior tarsus

Cornea

Lens

Upper eyelid

Anterior chamber

Posterior chamber

Lower eyelid

Conjunctiva

Inferior tarsus

Ciliary body

Superior levator muscle

Tendon of superior oblique muscle

Superior rectus muscle

Sclera

Choroid

Retina

Optic nerve

Vitreous body

Inferior rectus muscle

Inferior oblique muscle

Fig. 49.1 Section of the orbit showing internal structure of the eye.

required. The hypermetropic patient who is already using his accommodation for distance purposes will be affected by the need for reading glasses at an earlier stage, whereas a myope may be able to defer the use of reading glasses until well after his 45th birthday.

Contact lenses are lenses worn on the eye and have some advantages over the normal types of spectacles in certain cases as they can reduce the irregularity of the cornea after disease of this structure. They do not cause the large differences in the size of retinal images seen by each eye as happens with normal spectacle lenses where there is a large difference of refraction in the two eyes (anisometropia).

THE EXAMINATION OF THE EYE

A good light is essential and a strong lens is of assistance in focusing the light. Various procedures may be adopted. A brief outline is given of what may occur, although different diseases of the eye may require different procedures for their elucidation.

General examination

1. Examination of the eyelids and face may reveal diseases such as acne rosacea or herpes zoster ophthalmicus which may be associated with disease in the eye.
2. Estimation of the tension or pressure of the eye by gentle palpation with the fingers. The normal pressure is 10 to 20 mmHg.
3. The movements of the eye to elucidate different forms of squint.
4. Examination of the surface of the conjunctiva and pressure on the

lacrimal sac to note any regurgitation from the sac which may indicate the tear duct being blocked.

5. The examination of the surface and transparency of the cornea. A localised abrasion may be noticed by watching for any distortion of the image reflected from a light or window on the surface of the cornea when the eye is moved in different directions. This can be shown much more readily by the use of fluorescein, which stains corneal defects green. This is best applied with sterile paper strips impregnated with sterile fluorescein, obtained in single dose dispensers and moistened with sterile saline and touched on the conjunctiva of the lower lid or the patient's own tears may be used to release the fluorescein from the strip.

6. The depth of the anterior chamber, that is the distance between the cornea in front and the iris behind, should be noted. A deep anterior chamber may indicate the absence or dislocation of the lens. A shallow anterior chamber may indicate a leak from the anterior chamber, for instance through a small wound or leaking ulcer, or that the eye is predisposed to angle closure glaucoma.

7. The movements of the pupil and the appearance of the iris must be noted. The pupil reactions are tested first by shining a light into each eye in turn. The direct reaction is the contraction of the pupil in the eye illuminated and the indirect reaction to light is the contraction of the pupil in the other eye when one is illuminated. The reaction to convergence is the contraction of the pupils when the person looks at an object which is held close to the face.

8. Examination of the lens either by oblique illumination or by the use of the ophthalmoscope with a $^{+}12$ dioptre lens in the viewing aperture when the lens may be seen against the underlying red fundus reflex. Opacities indicate cataract.

9. A rapid and useful estimation of the visual field (confrontation) can be carried out by comparing the visual field of each eye of the patient in turn with the visual field of the examiner's opposite eye.

Instrumental examination

1. Examination of the interior of the eye with an ophthalmoscope. This may be made easier by dilating the pupil with a mydriatic drop. Atropine should not be used in routine examination except in children. When the pupil is dilated, a full examination of the interior of the eye is made consisting of the lens, vitreous body, and retina in turn.

2. Optical examination for the estimation of refractive errors.

3. Examination of the fields of vision with a perimeter, and for a more detailed examination of the central part of the field of vision a Bjerrum screen is used.

4. Detailed examination of the eye with a slit lamp. In this procedure, a thin beam of light is thrown into the eye and the various structures are examined with a low power binocular microscope. The retina, the intraocular tension (applanation tonometry) and the angle of the anterior chamber (gonioscopy) may be examined by the use of extra attachments.

5. Swabbing of the conjunctival sac in infective states to ascertain the

types of organism present and their sensitivity to various antibiotics.

6. Estimation of colour vision by use of the Ishihara plates or colour lanterns.

7. Tonometry. Estimation of the intraocular pressure by the use of a calibrated instrument that indents the cornea (Schiotz tonometer) or by the applanation tonometer attached to a slit lamp.

BASIC NURSING OF EYE CONDITIONS

The following general principles are of special importance in the nursing of patients suffering from disease of the eye.

1. Attention to minute detail is essential.

2. An aseptic or no-touch technique should be maintained when carrying out treatment.

3. The droppers should never touch the eye or lids, otherwise they will become contaminated, which can lead to infection within the drop bottles. Because of this, single dose dispensers are advised or, where a bottle is to be used more than once, then each patient should have his own bottle of drops and preferably the drops should be transferred from the bottle to the patient's eye with a disposable sterile dropper which is never returned to the bottle a second time.

4. The drops should be double-checked as the instillation of the wrong drops may lead to a disaster. Particularly, drops which dilate the pupil may, in certain patients, produce acute glaucoma with serious risk of damage to the vision. Single dose containers pose a special risk because they all look alike and the printing is very small. It is therefore most important that the name be carefully read.

5. In general, where there is a purulent discharge, the eye is not covered in order to allow the discharge to escape.

6. Where there has been an abrasion or wound of the eye either accidental or planned, as in surgery, then the eyelid may be kept closed by the fixing of a pad over the eye. If there is a large wound, then further protection may be given by using a strong shield (cartella) which fits over the pad and by abutting on the bone above and below can protect the underlying eye against an accidental knock, for instance by the patient's hand when he is sleeping.

7. The majority of patients require covering of the affected eye only. In certain circumstances, however, both eyes may be bandaged when it is essential that the eyes be kept still in order to prevent complications.

8. If the patient is totally blindfolded, then it is important not to surprise him and he should be spoken to gently as you approach and before touching him.

DISEASES OF THE EYELIDS

Stye (hordeolum)

A stye is a staphylococcal infection of an eyelash follicle. The pus under pressure produces pain and the lax eyelid tissues allow great surrounding swelling (oedema).

Treatment

Local heat. Local antibiotic treatment.

Blepharitis

An inflammation of the lid margins, prone to recur after cessation of treatment.

Treatment

The crusts are removed with moist swabs of saline or weak sodium bicarbonate lotion. Antibiotic ointment is rubbed into the lid margin for several weeks and reinfection excluded by rigorous personal hygiene, the use of antiseptic soap, naseptin ointment in the nose and clearing the scalp of dandruff.

Meibomian cyst (Chalazion)

This is not a true cyst but is a swelling in the lid varying from lentil to large pea size, caused by accumulation of scavenger cells (macrophages) packed with oily material from a Meibomian gland. Normally the oil is secreted on the lid edge and thus on to the surface of the tear film covering the conjunctiva and cornea.

Treatment

Treatment consists of incision of the lesion and curettage under local or general anaesthesia.

Entropion

Entropion is a turning in of an eyelid. This causes the eyelashes to rub on the cornea, giving discomfort but more seriously, corneal ulceration may be produced. Irritation in the eye or tight bandaging may produce spastic entropion. This is relieved by curing the primary condition or removing the bandage as appropriate. Common causes of entropion are changes in the lid due to age (senile), scarring or mechanical factors.

Treatment

Treatment is by surgery.

Ectropion

In this condition the eyelid turns outwards. The tears cannot reach the lacrimal punctum and the patient will be troubled by watering (epiphora). The exposed conjunctiva becomes inflamed and thickened, giving the more severely affected an unsightly appearance. Weakness of the lid muscle due to age or paralysis (facial palsy) may be the cause. Contracture due to skin disease or injury can readily produce this eversion.

Treatment

Treatment is by surgery.

WOUNDS OF THE EYELIDS

Careful repair is required to avoid complication by ectropion or entropion. The lid edge is particularly important to avoid notching and consequent watering or exposure of the cornea. Poor repair may cause trichiasis (eyelash rubbing on the eyeball) and in the inner sixth the canaliculus is liable to damage and requires skilful repair.

Ptosis

Ptosis of the upper eyelid is a dropping of the lid and may be due to increased weight of the lid or weakness of the muscle that elevates the upper lid. The muscle weakness may be a failure in development, may be due to acquired disease or injury affecting the muscle, the nerve-muscle junction (myasthenia gravis), or the nerve supply which is partly from the third cranial nerve and partly from the sympathetic nervous system.

TUMOURS OF THE EYELIDS

The common malignant lesion is basal cell carcinoma (rodent ulcer) which is usually suitable for local excision but radiotherapy is effective provided the cornea, eyeball and canaliculi are shielded from damage.

DISEASES OF THE CONJUNCTIVA

Inflammation of the conjunctiva is called conjunctivitis and this may be due to infection or allergy, or physical or chemical irritants. Infective conjunctivitis may be due to: Koch-Weeks bacillus, Pneumococcus, Streptococcus, Staphylococcus, Gonococcus, Diphtheria bacillus and also various viruses.

Clinically there is an increased redness of the conjunctiva and the eyes are uncomfortable, and, depending on the type and severity of the organism causing the condition, different types of discharge may occur from the eyes — mucoid, mucopurulent, purulent, or sanious (blood-stained). In some cases a membrane forms on the conjunctiva and then diphtheria may be considered as a possible cause, though in recent years diphtheria has been very rare. Ophthalmia neonatorum is a conjunctivitis occurring in the newborn and is due to the infection of the eyes at birth. In a number of

cases the infecting organism is the Gonococcus and the condition produced is that of severe purulent conjunctivitis which, by implication of the
cornea and secondary corneal ulceration and possible infection of the
interior of the eye, may lead to blindness. In parts of the world where
Gonococcus is common, then prophylactic treatment such as sulphacetamide or penicillin may be given to the eyes at birth, but where this
organism is rare, for instance here in Britain, then the eyes are swabbed
clean with sterile moist swabs and only if there is any evidence of infection
is a swab taken to send to the laboratory and treatment commenced with
local and systemic antibiotics.

In Britain the majority of ophthalmia neonatorum is not caused by
Gonococcus. *Staphylococcus aureus* is a frequent cause and, where the
onset is delayed for a few days, inclusion conjuncitivitis may be found.
Inclusion conjunctivitis belongs to the same group of viruses as trachoma.

The treatment is similar to that of gonococcal conjunctivitis.

Phlyctenular conjunctivitis

This is a disease of young people, characterised by the appearance of small
grey nodules in the conjunctiva, which may easily spread on to the cornea
and cause marked deterioration in vision by subsequent vascularisation
and scarring of the cornea.

The conjunctivitis is often complicated by secondary infection which
requires treatment in the usual way.

This disease is now thought to be a form of allergy of which tuberculous
infection is one possible cause.

Trachoma

Trachoma is a disease caused by a virus so large in size that it shares some
characteristics with bacteria in so far as it can be seen with the ordinary
microscope after staining and it can be affected by antibiotics. The disease
is endemic in many parts of the world, particularly the Middle East, Far
East and South America, where a large part of the population has the infection at some time. The effects can be mild or severe. The disease may also
occur in epidemic form. It can be carried to temperate countries where it
may be passed on, thus occasional cases are found in Britain. The acute
stage is a very red eye with discharge and large follicles in the conjunctiva
lining the eyelids to give an appearance almost like sago grains. The upper
part of the cornea may also be affected and later the lining of the lids
(palpebral conjunctiva) becomes scarred, leading to an entropion, and
further damage is caused by the eyelashes rubbing. Secondary infection
may be a further cause of serious corneal damage so that in a worldwide
context, this is the cause of blindness for thousands of people.

New growths

At birth, small dermoids may be found at the junction of the conjunctiva
and cornea, and dermolipomas may be found in the posterior parts of the

conjunctiva. Other benign growths are small pigmented naevi. Malignancy is rare, though there is a type of malignant melanoma is situ and there may be a spread of basal cell carcinoma from the lids. An epithelioma may occur at the junction with the cornea.

DISEASES OF THE CORNEA

Corneal ulcers

Corneal ulcer is a loss of the covering epithelium. Such loss may be caused by injury, where it is called an abrasion. An abrasion usually heals rapidly and the eye is normal again within 24 to 48 hours. However, infection delays the healing and may cause advancing invasion of the substance of the cornea and then it is called a corneal ulcer.

An ulcer of this type can be due to infection with the ordinary pus-forming organisms, such as Staphylococcus and Pneumococcus, but some varieties of the Gram-negative organisms may also enter the substance of the cornea if the covering epithelium is damaged. The bacteria will rarely penetrate the intact cornea, though occasionally do so in a severe purulent conjunctivitis. Viral infections will, however, penetrate the cornea even when it is intact. Fungi are always secondary invaders after preliminary damage has been done by viruses, bacteria or injury. Drying of the cornea due to inability to close the lids because of prominence of the eye or failure of the eyelid closure (facial palsy) will lead to ulceration. Loss of the nerve supply also carries great risk of ulceration (neurotrophic keratitis).

Symptoms and signs

The eye is red and painful with watering and photophobia. The vision is impaired. The ulcerated area may show as a grey patch on the cornea, but in milder cases it is more easily shown by staining with fluorescein. Treatment is by antibiotics locally either by surface application or by subconjunctival injection, and sometimes systemic treatment also is required if there is a danger of the infection spreading into the interior of the eye. Severe corneal ulceration may lead to iritis and this also requires its own treatment. Virals infections may require treatment with chemical cauterisation, though now some antiviral agents are available. Treatment is also aimed at preventing secondary infection by other invaders. Fungus may be a secondary invader, and then, if it will not respond to antifungal agents, local excision or even corneal grafting may be indicated. Corneal ulcer may heal by scarring which, if it is in the central part of the cornea, can seriously affect the vision. Failure to heal may lead to perforation of the cornea and loss of contents of the eye. On other occasions, infection spreads to the interior of the eye with serious damage and even loss of the eye.

Interstitial keratitis

This is deep inflammation in the cornea with an intact epithelium, i.e. there is no ulceration. There is more than one cause for this, but the term is most commonly used to describe the inflammation of the cornea occurring in congenital syphilis. Treatment consists of general antisyphilitic remedies plus local atropine and corticosteroids.

Deep inflammation also occurs as a complication of viral infections of the epithelium.

Keratoplasty

Keratoplasty means corneal grafting. In this operation part of the diseased cornea is replaced by healthy corneal tissue either from the eye of a dead person or from an eye that has been removed for some pathological condi-toin yet has an intact cornea. The grafting may take the form of the replacement of a small area of the cornea in its entire thickness (a penetrat-ing graft) or the replacement of a circumscribed area of the cornea in part of its thickness only (lamellar graft). By this means, an opaque cornea inter-fering with vision is replaced by clear tissue.

DISEASES OF THE IRIS

Iritis

The uveal tract comprises the iris, ciliary body and the choroid. Inflamma-tion of the various parts is called iritis, cyclitis and choroiditis respectively, and in the usual course of events one tissue is involved with the others so that an iritis has some degree of cyclitis with it and a choroiditis is likely to be accompanied by some degree of cyclitis as well. Uveitis may be due to many causes. The cause may be transmitted from outside, for instance as an indirect infection carried in by a perforating injury (exogenous). The disease may develop because of organisms or allergy spread via the blood steam (endogenous uveitis). Iritis may also develop as a reaction to other local eye disease, for instance corneal ulcer or scleritis (secondary). Infec-tive organisms in the form of bacteria or viruses, fungi and protozoa may be involved. However, sometimes the iritis is a state of reaction in an allergic manner.

In iritis the blood vessels of the conjunctiva around the cornea are inflamed. The iris is swollen and inflamed and the pupil is small leading to adhesions between the posterior surface of the iris and the lens behind. Inflammatory cells appear in the anterior chamber, and if these are profuse an exudate may be seen with the naked eye. Iritis is accompanied by a varying amount of pain and impairment of vision. Severe pain usually indi-cates some complication, for instance secondary glaucoma. In choroiditis, inflammatory cells enter the vitreous humour producing cloudy vision.

Treatment

Ideally, this is directed at the systemic cause in the first instance, but it is also important to give local treatment to the eye in the form of atropine drops to dilate the pupil and keep it dilated, plus local corticosteroids in most instances. Systemic corticosteroids may be necessary.

Melanoma

This is a malignant tumour that arises in the uveal tract, usually the choroid. Dissemination occurs widely throughout the body, but the commonest site of secondary deposits is the liver.

DISEASES OF THE RETINA

Detachment of the retina

The retina becomes separated in part from the choroid. The condition may arise as a result of trauma but usually there is a predisposing weakness in the retina, which leads to holes in the retina and spontaneous detachment. It may be secondary to other disease in the eye when it is displaced by tumour or exudate. Sometimes there are general systemic causes. Partial loss of the field of vision or distorted vision are prominent symptoms and complete blindness of the affected eye may ensue. Myopic eyes are more liable to retinal detachment than normal eyes.

Treatment

If the detachment is secondary then the ideal is to treat the cause, for instance uveitis or scleritis. If the detachment is secondary to tumour of the retina then the tumour is treated. Where this is untreatable the eye may need to be removed. Detachment of the retina due to tears or holes is called a simple retinal detachment and this is treated surgically. Scarring is caused by diathermy, by cyrothermy or by light coagulation. In most cases a shortening or infolding operation may be necessary on the outer scleral part of the eye—scleral resection or plication. Plastic materials are now being used to cause indentation. Both eyes are usually bandaged for a period afterwards so as to prevent movements of the eyes and strict bed rest is essential. Afterwards the patient is warned to avoid bending and stooping, or any severe exertion that might cause a recurrence of the detachment.

Retinoblastoma

Retinoblastoma is a malignant growth of the retina that occurs in young children, usually in the first few years of life. The condition may necessitate the excision of the eye, but irradiation from cobalt plaques and chemotherapy, plus sometimes light coagulation, may enable the eye to be preserved with safety. The condition may be bilateral, particularly with the dominant inherited variety. Spontaneous retinoblastoma due to a somatic mutation usually affects one eye only.

Retrolental fibroplasia

Retrolental fibroplasia is a condition that sometimes occurs in premature babies treated with oxygen at a concentration exceeding 30 per cent. It affects both eyes and is characterised by the formation of fibrous tissue behind the lens and detachment of the retina is often present.

Retinopathy

A number of conditions previously described as retinitis are not inflammations and are now classed as 'retinopathy'.

Hypertensive. The most severe changes appear in malignant hypertension. Using the ophthalmoscope, oedema of the optic disc (optic nerve head) appears as a swollen disc with blurred margins, loss of the normal central pit (physiological cup) and the vessels may be obscured on the disc by exudates. The retina near the disc shows flame-shaped haemorrhages and exudates of cotton wool appearance. The oedema affects the retina also and in severe forms the central retina is affected causing a drop in visual acuity and later hard exudates in a star distribution may appear at the macula (centre of the retina).

Arteriosclerotic. The vessels show thicker walls than normal and alter the veins where the retinal artery crosses a vein. Lesser degrees of hypertensive changes may be shown and the veins may be obstructed leading to multiple retinal haemorrhages and oedema in the area of the retina served by the vein. Arterial obstruction which may be due to an embolus or to failure of the blood supply to the ophthalmic artery may occur.

Diabetic. The individual features visible with the ophthalmoscope can be found in other conditions, but the overall pattern is typical enough to suspect the diagnosis. Tiny round (dot), or slightly larger (blot) haemorrhages can be seen in the retina. Some of these are microaneurysms of the capillaries not haemorrhages. Hard-edged white or yellow exudates appear, particularly in the macular area. In general, the younger patients show a tendency to the formation of new blood vessels on the retina and optic disc producing vitreous haemorrhage and retinal detachment. Diabetic retinopathy is the largest cause of blindness in young adults in Europe and North America. Proliferative diabetic retinopathy may now be treated by extensive ablation of the retina using photocoagulation or laser applications.

AFFECTIONS OF THE LACRIMAL APPARATUS

The lacrimal gland secretes tear fluid which is shed as a fine film over the conjunctiva and cornea. The fluid drains by way of the lacrimal punctae into the canaliculi to the lacrimal sac and duct into the inferior meatus of the nose. If there is blockage in any of these structures, then the tears are unable to drain away and pour on to the face, resulting in epiphora. The stagnation of tears may become secondarily infected causing a lacrimal abscess, or a mucocele may result, and the infection may cause a unilateral conjunctivitis. Treatment consists of treating the secondary infection. If this is unsuccessful, then a new drainage channel may be made into the nose (dacryocysto-rhinostomy), or in some cases removal of the infected duct altogether (dacryocystectomy). In small children, probing the tear duct may be sufficient.

Glaucoma

Glaucoma is a term that indicates an increase of pressure within the eye above the normal limits. Where the rise of tension is associated with some known pathological event, such as a dislocated lens or an intraocular tumour, then the condition is known as secondary glaucoma, but when no cause can be found, the condition is called primary glaucoma.

Primary glaucoma. (a) Acute closed angle glaucoma or (b) an insidious quiet type chronic glaucoma called open angle glaucoma. The increased pressure in the eye can, if unrelieved, lead to blindness.

Acute glaucoma. Occurring most often in elderly subjects, the onset is sudden, accompanied by severe pain and redness of the eye. Rainbow haloes around white lights may be an early warning symptom. The cornea is 'steamy' due to alteration within the cornea and the pupil may be fixed and dilated. The intraocular pressure is markedly raised. Miotic drops should be used. Usually pilocarpine is given intensively. The intraocular secretion of fluid should be reduced by the systemic use of drugs such as acetozolamide. If the tension still remains high then some form of drainage operation has to be done urgently on the eye, as the vision can fail rapidly and permanently. If the pressure comes down with medical treatment then an iridectomy is performed which prevents recurrence of the acute attacks.

Chronic glaucoma. The onset of this condition is gradual with the result that the extent of permanent damage to vision may be very great before the condition is noticed. The eye may appear superficially normal, but curtailment of the field of vision may be very marked and blindness may result.

Treatment consists of the use of miotic drops, Beta-blocking drugs in drop form, 1% neutral adrenalin drops singly or in combination. The patient must be kept under observation. If the raised pressure in the eye is not controlled, then surgery is advised.

OTHER AFFECTIONS OF THE EYE

Strabismus

Strabismus or squint is due to many causes. It may be paralytic, due to damage to the nerves supplying the extrinsic muscles of the eyeball, or it may be due to maldevelopment of one group of muscles or their faulty insertion. It may follow an uncorrected refractive error or be a manifestation of some cause of defective vision in an eye such as a corneal scar or congenital cataract. A concomitant squint is one in which the degree of convergence or divergence of the eyes is the same in all positions of gaze. In a paralytic or incomitant squint, the degree of deviation varies with the direction of gaze. Squints are common in children and if uncorrected may lead to grave deterioration of vision in the squinting eye (amblyopia).

Treatment

Paralytic squint requires treatment of cause where possible, but where not possible amelioration.

In the acute phase one eye may be covered to prevent double vision and subsequently the eyes may have surgery to return them to single vision. Some correction may also be made by prisms in the spectacles.

A non-paralytic squint is treated by the provision of glasses to correct the refractive error, orthoptic treatment to reverse any amblyopia which may develop and surgery on the extraocular muscles if there is any remaining squint.

Nystagmus

Nystagmus is the name given to oscillatory movements of the eyes. These movements may be in any direction, but most often occur laterally. The condition may be due to many causes. It may be congenital, be a manifestation of some defect of vision such as congenital cataract or defect in the retina, part of a nervous disease such as disseminated sclerosis or cerebellar tumour, or follow some disease of the inner ear when the semicircular canals are implicated. It can also arise as an occupational condition in miners.

Cataract

The normal lens is a soft, clear structure. With age it becomes harder but remains clear. The development of opacity is the condition known as cataract.

A cataract may occur as a congenital condition, and infection of the mother with rubella in the early stages of pregnancy is one such cause. It may be secondary to some underlying disease of the eye such as iridocyclitis, glaucoma, retinal detachment or injury, and may occur as a manifestation of some general disease such as diabetes. Most commonly, cataract arises as a senile condition.

As the cataract extends, light is unable to penetrate into the eye and vision becomes worse.

Treatment

Removal of the lens is usually necessary in advanced cases. This results in inability to focus so that strong lenses must be supplied in spectacles after operation.

Care of the patient for cataract surgery

The general condition is improved as much as possible, paying attention particularly to diabetes mellitus. Conjunctival swabs are no longer carried out routinely but the eyes must be carefully examined to exclude possible infection and some surgeons give broad spectrum antibiotic drops for at least 48 hours preoperatively. The operation is carried out under local or general anaesthetic.

Postoperative care of the patient

This has been simplified by the increased suturing of the cataract wound so that it is now possible to mobilise the patient more or less immediately and only the operated eye is covered. It is useful to have the eye covered with a pad, a shield, and with a bandage at night in order to reduce the risk that the patient may knock his eye during sleep. The eye is dressed daily and a local antibiotic drop instilled. Other treatments are given according to the decision of the surgeon.

Complications

1. Postoperative mania is not uncommon in elderly patients. It may subside with sedatives, but may require the uncovering of the eye.

2. Prolapse of the iris may occur, and the importance of avoiding straining is very great in the prophylaxis. Further operation is necessary if it occurs, and consists of the excision of the prolapsed portion and resuturing.

3. Intraocular infection is damaging and can lead to the loss of the eye.

4. Chest complications may arise as in any operation performed on a patient of advancing years who, of necessity, has been confined to bed.

5. Haemorrhage into the eye may result from sudden movement, clumsy application of eye drops, or squeezing of the eye after instillation.

Orbital cellulitis

The whole orbit may be involved in a severe infection which may require drainage and systemic treatment.

INJURIES AND FOREIGN BODIES

Injuries occur commonly as a result of lodgment of small foreign bodies like dust particles on the cornea.

Treatment

Early removal of the foreign body is very important since corneal ulceration may develop. All cases are associated with some degree of conjunctivitis. A few drops of 1% amethocaine are instilled and the foreign body is removed with a sharp sterile needle. Antibiotic drops are instilled and the eye is covered with a pad and bandage for 12 hours.

Penetrating Injuries

The most serious injuries are due to penetrating wounds, and a foreign body may remain in the eye.

Treatment

This is on the general lines of that laid down for wounds. Excision of the damaged tissues, removal of the foreign body, and suture, together with appropriate measures to prevent infection, are carried out. Applied to the eye, this consists of:

1. Removal of the foreign body. This may require the use of the giant magnet if the foreign body is magnetic, after it has been localised by X-ray of the eye and orbit.

2. Suture of the wound with fine sutures is necessary after excision of prolapsed intraocular structures.

3. The instillation of atropine and covering the eye.

4. The administration of antibiotics locally and systemically.

If the eyeball is damaged so seriously that conservative measures are likely to be of no avail, excision of the eyeball is necessary as there is the risk of sympathetic ophthalmia in the other eye.

Sympathetic ophthalmia is a severe bilateral panuveitis following perforating injury of one eye. This panuveitis can be so severe as to lose the sight from both eyes. Therefore in severe injury it is often advisable to remove the injured eye prior to the eleventh day after injury, which will prevent the development of sympathetic ophthalmia.

Care of a case of excision of the eye

Immediately postoperatively, a firm pad and bandage are required to reduce swelling and bruising. Subsequently the socket will require the instillation of drops or ointment of a suitable antibiotic until healing has occurred. A plastic shell is worn for 3 to 4 weeks to prevent shrinkage and to shape the socket until an artificial eye is worn.

In most cases, a better cosmetic result is obtained by replacing the excised eye with an implant which forms a movable base for an anteriorly placed prosthesis.

50

Gynaecology

Gynaecology is defined as the study of diseases peculiar to women. Today gynaecology has changed because of alterations in social attitudes. For example, population control is of worldwide concern and the gynaecologist is not only involved with the teaching and practice of contraception but also with the problems which arise as a result of contraception.

The Abortion Act of 1967 has resulted in large numbers of women coming into gynaecological wards for termination of pregnancy and yet in the next bed there might be a woman being investigated for infertility.

The nurse must always be conscious of the patients' feelings, a friendly word and a sympathetic ear will do much to help these patients and allay fears.

ANATOMY

The vulva. The labia majora are two skin folds which bound the vulval cleft and meet anteriorly at the mons pubis.

The labia minora are two smaller skin folds lying between the labia majora. The labia minora enclose the vaginal vestibule and each divides anteriorly to form the prepuce of the clitoris.

The clitoris consists of erectile tissue.

The mons pubis is a cushion of fat lying in front of the pubic bone.

The hymen is a septum which partially closes the vaginal orifice.

Bartholin's glands lie within the substance of the posterior part of each labia majora, the ducts of which open on the inner side of the labia minora.

The urethral orifice lies between the clitoris anteriorly and the vaginal orifice posteriorly.

The perineum is the area between the vagina and anus.

Internal genitalia. The internal genitalia comprise the vagina, uterus, Fallopian tubes and ovaries.

The vagina is a muscular canal extending from the hymen below to the cervix of the uterus above. The cervix projects into the vaginal vault and divides it into four fornices, anterior, posterior and the two lateral fornices. Anterior to the vagina is the urethra and bladder, posterior there is the rectum and pouch of Douglas.

The uterus is a pear-shaped, hollow, muscular organ about 7·5 cm long, lying in the middle of the pelvic cavity supported by ligaments. It is covered by peritoneum, except laterally where the anterior and posterior peritoneal layers pass towards the lateral walls of the pelvis forming the broad ligaments. The Fallopian tubes and the blood and lymphatic vessels of the uterus are enclosed in the broad ligaments. The uterus is divided into the body and the cervix. The part of the body above the insertion of the Fallopian tubes is known as the fundus. The uterus is lined by the endometrium, which is composed of tubular glands of columnar epithelium. The cervix, which is the lower part of the uterus, is 2.5 cm in length and projects into the top of the vagina.

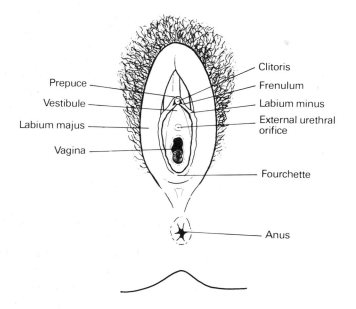

Fig. 50.1 Female external genital organs.

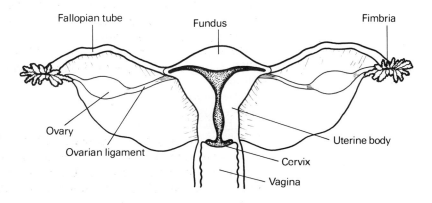

Fig. 50.2 Section through the uterus.

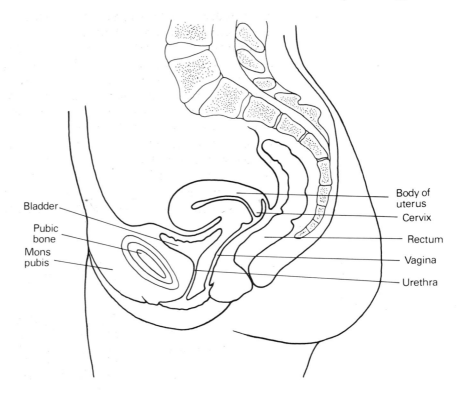

Fig. 50.3 Internal female genitalia.

The Fallopian tubes are a pair of thin muscular canals extending out-wards from each side of the fundus of the uterus. The outer ends, which are fimbriated, project into the peritoneal cavity. The tubes transmit the shed ovum to the uterine cavity, and are lined by ciliated epithelium.

The ovaries are a pair of greyish-white almond-shaped structures, lying in the pelvis, attached to the back of the broad ligaments. They contain numerous ova, or egg cells.

Pelvic floor. This is a diaphragm which bridges across the cavity of the bony pelvis and maintains the pelvic organs in the normal position. Its main constituent is the levator ani muscles but it also consists of pelvic fascia, the perineal body, superficial perineal muscles and pelvic peritoneum. It is perforated by the urethra, vagina and anal canal. Weakness of the pelvic floor gives rise to prolapse.

PHYSIOLOGY

Puberty usually occurs between 12 and 15 years of age. The general body configuration assumes that of an adult woman. Secondary sex characteristics develop such as breast enlargement, pubic hair, subcutaneous fat becomes of adult distribution, and the bony pelvis develops typically female characteristics.

From puberty to the menopause menstruation occurs.

Menstrual cycle. The periods are often irregular for some months after puberty but eventually settle into a regular cycle of between 25 to 35 days. The duration of loss varies widely between one and eight days.

The regularity of the cycle is controlled by hormones. A pituitary hormone, follicular stimulating hormone (FSH), stimulates the ripening of an ovarian follicle; as the follicle ripens it secretes oestrogens which cause the endometrium to proliferate. When the follicle ruptures at midcycle the pituitary gland then secretes luteinising hormone (LH) instead of FSH. The LH maintains the corpus luteum, which has formed from the ruptured follicle. The corpus luteum secretes progesterone, which causes the endometrium to enter a secretory phase which is ready to receive a fertilised ovum.

When the ovum passes through the tube without being fertilised, the corpus luteum regresses and the progesterone level falls off; as the hormone level falls, so menstruation occurs at about the 28th day. If fertilisation occurs, this takes place in the Fallopian tube; the fertilised ovum reaches the uterus approximately four days after ovulation and implants in the endometrium.

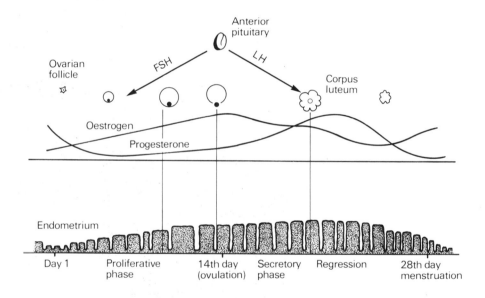

Fig. 50.4 The menstrual cycle.

The menopause (change of life) occurs when the ovaries cease to function at about the age of 50 years.

First, ovulation fails and the ovaries then gradually cease to produce oestrogen and progesterone. The gonadotrophins from the pituitary initially increase and then diminish. Atrophy of the genital organs gradually occurs. Symptoms such as hot flushes, headaches and depression may occur. These symptoms can be relieved by hormone replacement therapy; this is the cyclical administration of oestrogens.

EXAMINATION OF PATIENT

A gynaecological examination consists of inspection and palpation of the abdomen; examination of the breasts should also be routine. This is followed by inspection of the vulva and a bimanual examination, which may be carried out either in the left lateral or dorsal position depending on the preference of the gynaecologist.

The labia are separated and the vulva inspected. The fore-finger and middle finger are then inserted into the vagina and passed up the vagina into the anterior fornix; the other hand is placed on the patient's abdomen just above the symphysis pubis. It is then possible to palpate the body of the uterus between the two hands. The vaginal fingers are then placed in the lateral fornices, and the ovaries and tubes are similarly palpated.

The vagina and cervix are then visualised by inserting a vaginal speculum into the vagina; any lesions of the cervix or vagina will then be seen, and it is at the time of visualising the cervix that a cervical smear should be taken. Swabs are taken from the cervix, the vagina and the vulva when there are signs of inflammatory disease.

Other special investigations are estimation of the pituitary, the ovarian and the adrenal hormones when indicated. A midstream specimen of urine is also frequently indicated when there are urinary symptoms.

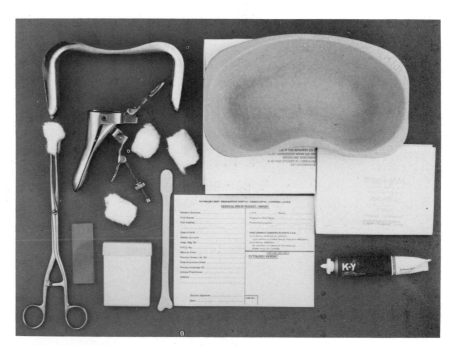

Fig. 50.5 Requirements for Papanicolaou cervical smear.

1 Sponge holder	Container for slide with alcohol ether
1 Vaginal speculum	3 Wool balls
1 Ayre's spatula	1 Disposable glove
1 Glass slide	Bag for discard
1 laboratory form	Tube of lubricant.

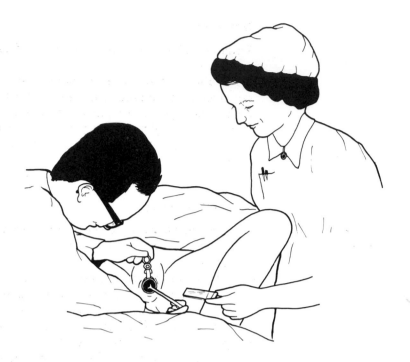

Fig. 50.6 Method of taking cervical smear.

DISORDERS OF MENSTRUATION

Amenorrhoea

Amenorrhoea is the absence of menstruation. Amenorrhoea may be true amenorrhoea or false amenorrhoea (cryptomenorrhoea).

1. True amenorrhoea may be:

(a) *Physiological*. Before puberty and after the menopause, during pregnancy and lactation.

(b) *Pathological*.

(i) Primary—when menstruation has never occurred. Primary amenorrhoea may have general causes such as severe chronic systemic disease i.e. tuberculosis, nephritis, heart disease, endocrine disorders or there may be local causes such as absence or underdevelopment of the uterus or ovaries.

(ii) Secondary—when menstruation has occurred for a time and has then ceased.

Secondary amenorrhoea may have general causes such as a general systemic disease, including any severe illness; endocrine disorders; obesity and malnutrition; contraceptive pills; irradiation or removal of both ovaries; hysterectomy; psychological causes such as shock, grief, change of environment.

Treatment

Treatment of amenorrhoea consists in finding the cause and if possible treating it.

2. False amenorrhoea (cryptomenorrhoea) is where the patient has commenced her menses but there is no external bleeding. This is due to an imperforate hymen or imperfect canalisation of the vagina. The blood collects in the vagina forming a haematocolpos, and in neglected cases blood fills the uterus (haematometra) and even the tubes (haematosalpinges).

Abnormal bleeding

1. Menorrhagia. Excessive or prolonged blood loss.

2. Epimenorrhagia. The periods occur at frequent intervals and are excessively heavy.

3. Epimenorrhoea. The periods occur at frequent intervals.

4. Metrorrhagia. Bleeding between periods.

The above types of bleeding may be caused by:

(a) Hormonal disorders, either an imbalance between oestrogen and progesterone or an excess of oestrogen.

(b) Local disease, uterine growths such as fibroids or polyps, pelvic inflammatory disease.

Treatment. Find the cause and treat it.

5. Postmenopausal bleeding. This is bleeding from the genital tract that occurs after the menopause. The cause must always be diagnosed as it may be due to malignancy; other causes are oestrogen hormonal therapy, urethral caruncle, vaginitis, polyps, ovarian tumours.

Treatment. Find the cause and treat it.

Dysmenorrhoea

Dysmenorrhoea is painful, incapacitating menstruation; there are two main types — primary and secondary dysmenorrhoea.

1. Primary. Occurs in girls and young women. It is a spasmodic pain in the pelvis, lower abdomen and back. Nausea, vomiting and fainting may occur. It commences at the beginning of a period and lasts 12–24 hours. It occurs only when the ovary is ovulating.

Treatment. Adequate analgesics, reassurance and encouragement to continue one's normal activities and, if this is unsuccessful, suppression of ovulation by hormones, the oral contraceptive pill being ideal. Dilatation of the cervix has fallen into disrepute because of the cervix becoming incompetent and causing habitual abortions.

2. Secondary. This is associated with pelvic disease, i.e. fibroids, inflammatory disease. There is a history of regular, painless menses for some years before the onset of dysmenorrhoea. The pain may commence before the menstrual flow.

Treatment. Find the cause and treat it.

DISORDERS ASSOCIATED WITH PREGNANCY

ABORTION

Definition

The termination of pregnancy before the 28th week, the foetus showing no signs of life.

It occurs spontaneously in 10–15 per cent of all pregnancies. It is caused by many factors: foetal abnormality, uterine abnormalities, hormonal disturbances, severe acute or chronic maternal disease.

Types of abortion

1. Threatened abortion. Vaginal bleeding occurs but the cervical canal remains closed and there are no painful uterine contractions and no part of the pregnancy sac is expelled. Treatment is by rest in bed and sedation. If progesterone deficiency can be demonstrated progestogens may be given.

2. Inevitable abortion. There is severe bleeding with painful uterine contractions. The cervix dilates. Treatment is to evacuate the uterus by surgical operation. Blood transfusion may be required.

3. Incomplete abortion. There is severe bleeding with painful uterine contractions. The cervix dilates and part of the pregnancy sac is expelled. Treatment is surgical evacuation of the uterus. Blood transfusion may be required.

4. Complete abortion. This is the same as an incomplete abortion but the pregnancy sac has been expelled complete and, therefore, surgical evacuation of the uterus is not required. Blood transfusion may be required.

5. Missed abortion. This is where the pregnancy dies but is not expelled from the uterus. The uterus should be encouraged to empty itself by administering either an oxytocic or prostaglandin infusion intravenously, or alternatively it may be removed by surgical evacuation if the size of the uterus is not too large.

6. Habitual abortion is where three or more successive abortions have occurred. This is usually associated with a uterine abnormality, i.e. congenital malformations, incompetent internal cervical os, or it may be due to hormonal imbalance. Investigate to discover the cause and treat it.

7. Septic abortion. Any type of abortion which is complicated by infection of the genital tract. The infection is controlled with the appropriate antibiotic followed by surgical evacuation of uterus.

8. Therapeutic abortion. The induction of abortion carried out for medical indications. The Abortion Act 1967 states that if, in the opinion of two registered medical practitioners, the continuation of the pregnancy is likely to endanger the life of the pregnant woman or involve risk to her mental or physical health or that of her existing family or if there is a substantial risk of foetal abnormality, then abortion may be carried out.

The uterus may be evacuated vaginally by aspiration curetage up to the 12th week; after the 12th week abdominal hysterotomy may be performed, or the uterus emptied by medical means such as intra-amniotic hypertonic saline or prostaglandin intravenous infusion.

Ectopic pregnancy

An ectopic pregnancy is where the fertilised ovum becomes implanted elsewhere than in the endometrium of the uterine body. It may occur in the ovary, peritoneal cavity or Fallopian tube. The commonest site is in the Fallopian tube (Fig. 50.7).

In a tubal pregnancy, as the ovum develops, either rupture of the tube or extrusion of the developing ovum into the peritoneal cavity occurs. Both processes are associated with abdominal pain, haemorrhage into the peritoneal cavity and shock.

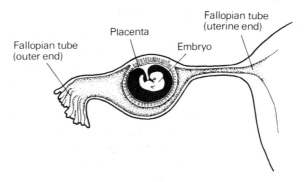

Fig. 50.7 Ectopic pregnancy in the Fallopian tube.

Symptoms and signs

There is usually a history of amenorrhoea and maybe early subjective symptoms of pregnancy. When tubal rupture or tubal abortion occurs there is lower abdominal pain and in half the cases there is some vaginal bleeding. The associated internal haemorrhage can cause referred pain to the shoulder tip and also can lead to pallor, shock, and collapse characterised by a rapid pulse and low blood pressure. On examination the abdomen is tender with some fullness and muscle guarding; free fluid may be demonstrated. Vaginal examination is often inconclusive because of extreme tenderness and pain on movement of the cervix.

Treatment

Resuscitation by blood transfusion followed by laparotomy and removal of the damaged tube. If the diagnosis is in doubt laparoscopy may be carried out before laparotomy.

Hydatidiform mole

This condition is produced by degeneration of the chorion in early pregnancy; the foetus dies and disappears. The chorion is converted into a mass of small cysts often growing at a rapid rate.

It gives rise to severe morning sickness and symptoms of preeclampsia (raised blood pressure, oedema and proteinuria). Vaginal bleeding occurs and vesicles may be expelled. On examination the uterus is frequently larger than dates, but neither palpation, X-ray nor ultrasound scanning reveal a foetus. Pregnancy tests are positive in high dilutions due to the presence of excess chorionic gonadotrophins.

Treatment

The uterus is encouraged to abort the mole by either an oxytocic or prostaglandin infusion. Following abortion of the mole a curettage is performed under anaesthesia to remove any retained products.

A careful follow-up is imperative because of the risks of developing choriocarcinoma. (p. 585).

INFERTILITY

Infertility is where a woman of reproductive age is unable to become pregnant, it may be primary infertility where she has never been pregnant or it may be secondary when she has had a previous pregnancy.

It must be remembered that both the male and the female should be investigated.

Causes of infertility

1. Male. Low sperm count (oligozoospermia) or absent sperms (azoospermia).

2. Female

(a) Failure of ovulation; this might be due to pituitary failure causing lack of gonadotrophins or it might be an ovarian failure.

(b) Blocked or damaged Fallopian tubes.

(c) Infections of the endometrium, especially an infection by tuberculosis.

(d) Poor penetration of the cervical mucus by the sperms.

(e) High serum prolactin levels.

Investigations

1. Male. Semen analysis is performed. A specimen of the seminal fluid is obtained and a sperm count is done, the motility of the sperms and the number of abnormal forms is noted.

2. Female

(a) It was thought that ovulation could be demonstrated by obtaining secretory endometrium in the second half of the menstrual cycle by performing an D. and C. This is now thought to be unreliable and ovulation is now demonstrated by serial estimations of either the serum oestrogen and progestogen content or the oestrid and pregnanedia excretion rates in the urine.

A more simple but far less reliable method of demonstrating ovulation is for the patient to take her temperature each day, ovulation is preceeded by a slight drop in temperature and followed by a slight rise.

(b) Pituitary activity can be assessed by serial estimations of the follicular stimulating hormone (F.S.H.) and the luteinising hormone (L.H.) levels in the blood.

(c) Tubal patency can be demonstrated by either injecting a radio-opaque fluid through the cervix, it then passes through the uterus and tubes, an X-ray is taken and the uterus and tubes visualised and any spill of the fluid from the fimbrial ends of the tube denotes patency. This technique is known as hysterosalpingography. Tubal patency can also be demonstrated by laparoscopy and again injecting a dye through the cervix. If the tubes are patent dye can be seen spilling from the fimbrial ends of the tubes.

(d) Infections of the endometrium are recognised by performing a D. and C., part of the specimen of endometrium is sent for histology and part for special culture to recognise an infection by tuberculosis.

(e) A specimen of the cervical mucus is obtained approximately one hour following intercourse, it is then examined under a microscope and the depth of penetration of the sperms noted.

(f) Serum prolactin levels are estimated.

Treatment

1. Male. Sometimes a testicular biopsy is required to determine whether the testes are capable of forming sperms. If the capability is present the sperm count may be improved by treatment with clomiphene citrate. This is a synthetic drug which acts as a gonadtrophin.

2. Female. If there is a failure of ovulation and the ovaries are normal ovulation can be induced by either clomiphene citrate (see above) or by human gonadrophins (Pergonal). These drugs must be carefully controlled because of the danger of multiple pregnancies.

Blocked tubes are treated by tubal surgery. The success rate is poor and even if successful can predispose to ectopic pregnancies.

Infections of the endometrium are treated with the appropriate antibiotic.

Poor penetration of the cervical mucus by the sperms is now thought to be due to the women developing antibodies against the sperms and treatment so far is unsuccessful. High serum prolactin levels are treated by a course of bromocriptine.

Artificial insemination

Artificial insemination is done with the husband's seminal fluid (A.I.H.) where he is unable to achieve intercourse because of impotency. It is also done with a donor's seminal fluid (A.I.D.) where the husband has oligo or azoospermia.

THE GENITAL TRACT

INFECTIONS OF THE GENITAL TRACT

1. Vulvovaginitis. Infections of the vulva are usually associated with infections of the vagina and they are considered together as vulvovaginitis. The signs and symptoms of vulvovaginitis are a vaginal discharge and irritation of the vulva (pruritus vulvae). The commonest causes of vulvovaginitis are listed below.

(a) *Trichomonas vaginalis*, a small unicellular organism, causes trichomoniasis. The woman can infect herself from the anal canal but it can also be spread by sexual intercourse; it is usually asymptomatic in the male.

It is characterised by a yellow discharge containing small bubbles of gas and the vaginal walls are reddened; there is vulval irritation.

Diagnosis is confirmed by examining a drop of the discharge under a microscope when the actual organisms can be seen.

Treatment is metronidazole tablets (Flagyl) 200 mg orally three times a day for 10 days. If reinfection occurs the husband should be treated also.

(b) *Candida albicans* (*Monilia*) causes a fungal infection (moniliasis, or thrush) and is especially common in diabetics. The discharge is thick and white and there is intense irritation. The diagnosis is confirmed by culture of a vaginal swab; the fungus can then be indentified by mircoscopy.

Treatment is by nystatin pessaries, one to be inserted in the vagina morning and night for 14 days.

(c) *Gonorrhoea*. This infection by the *Gonococcus* is again becoming more prevalent. It is a venereal disease and manifests itself by a vulvovaginitis; it can also cause infection of Bartholin's glands, cervicitis and urethritis. The discharge is yellow and there may be accompanying dysuria.

Diagnosis is by cervical and urethral smears which show the gonococci; these may be grown on culture.

A course of an appropriate antibiotic cures the infection.

(d) *Non-specific infections*. Many bacteria can cause vulvovaginitis, and diagnosis is made by culturing a vaginal swab, indentifying the bacteria and giving the appropriate antibiotic.

If this occurs in elderly patients after the menopause it is called senile vaginitis, and is due to the reduction of oestrogen causing the vagina to contain less lactic acid and, therefore, to be more easily infected. Treatment is by giving small doses of oestrogen either orally or in pessary form.

2. Cervicitis. This is an acute infection of the cervix, commonly due to the gonococcus but can follow puerperal sepsis or even arise from a vulvovaginitis.

There is a purulent vaginal discharge and pus can be seen exuding through the external cervical os.

The organisms should be indentified from a swab and the appropriate antibiotic given.

3. Endometritis. This due to infection of the endometrium of the body of the uterus.

Acute endometritis usually occurs after abortion or childbirth. It causes a raised temperature and pulse rate and, a bloodstained purulent discharge. The treatment is to identify the bacteria by a swab and give the appropriate antibiotic.

Chronic endometritis may be due to tuberculosis and is diagnosed by endometrial biopsy. It can also occur where there is blockage of the cervical canal. The uterus distends with retained pus and forms a pyometra. The most frequent cause in an elderly patient is a carcinoma either of the body of the uterus or the cervix.

4. Salpingitis. This condition should be more correctly referred to as salpingo-oophoritis as both the tubes and ovaries are usually involved. It may be acute or chronic.

Acute salpingo-oophoritis. This may be gonococcal, may follow infection at childbirth or abortion, or may spread from an abdominal focus, e.g. the appendix.

The patient complains of severe lower abdominal pain, the temperature and pulse rise, tenderness and rigidity of the lower abdomen may be present. There may be a purulent vaginal discharge.

On examination the lower abdomen is found to be acutely tender; on pelvic examination movement of the cervix causes pain and palpation through the fornices is extremely painful. A leucocytosis develops.

Treatment

A cervical swab should be taken to indentify the bacteria and then the appropriate antibiotic is given.

Complications

(a) Pyosalpinx—the tube becomes sealed and distended with pus.
(b) Tubo-ovarian abscess—a large abscess cavity forms involving both tube and ovary.
(c) Pelvic abscess.
(d) Narrowing of the tube due to adhesions and subsequently an ectopic pregnancy.
(e) Infertility due to blocked tubes.

Chronic salpingo-oophoritis. This can follow acute salpingo-oophoritis or it may be due to tuberculous infection. The patient presents with general ill-health, lower abdominal pain, menstrual irregularities, vaginal discharge, and infertility. The majority of cases resolve with antibiotic therapy or short-wave pelvic diathermy. In cases which do not resolve with treatment surgery is required for removal of the infected tubes. If the patient is over 40 years old then hysterectomy with removal of both tubes and ovaries is the best treatment.

DISPLACEMENT OF THE GENITAL TRACT

1. Prolapse. Uterovaginal prolapse is where the supports of the vagina and uterus are weakened so that the walls of the vagina bulge into the cavity of the vagina and may protrude through the vaginal introitus. The uterus may also descend down the vagina and emerge at the vaginal introitus.

The vaginal and uterine supports are weakened by child-bearing, and also after the menopause there is atrophy of these supports. There are various types of uterovaginal prolapse.

(a) *Cystocele*. This is prolapse of the anterior vaginal wall together with the base of the bladder.

(b) *Rectocele*. This is prolapse of the lower part of the posterior vaginal wall together with the rectum.

(c) *Enterocele*. This is prolapse of the upper part of the posterior vagina wall together with the pouch of Douglas.

(d) *Uterovaginal prolapse, first degree* — the uterus descends the vaginal until the cervix reaches the introitus.

(e) *Uterovaginal prolapse, second degree* — the cervix protrudes outside the introitus.

(f) *Uterovaginal prolapse, third degree* — the whole uterine body lies outside the introitus; this is sometimes known as a procidentia.

Clinical features

(i) The patient may complain of a lump in the vagina or a feeling of 'something is coming down'.

(ii) Backache and a bearing-down sensation.

(iii) Disturbances of micturition, frequency and dysuria, stress incontinence.

(iv) Bleeding due to the protruding prolapse becoming ulcerated.

(v) Difficulty in defaecation.

Treatment

The treatment of choice is a surgical repair of the prolapse. This consists essentially of excising the redundant parts of the vaginal walls and tightening-up the supporting fascia and pelvic muscles.

(a) Cystocele. This is repaired by anterior colporrhaphy.

(b) Rectocele. This is repaired by combining a posterior colporrhaphy with reconstituting a new perineal body by an operation known as a perineorrhaphy; the operation is, therefore, known as posterior colpoperineorrhaphy.

(c) Enterocele. This is repaired at the same time as the posterior colpoperineorrhaphy.

(d) Uterovaginal prolapse. The minor degrees are repaired by anterior colporrhaphy and posterior colpoperineorrhaphy, and the Mackenrodt ligaments are tightened combined with amputation of the cervix; this is known as a Fothergill's operation, or a Manchester repair.

The major degrees are better treated by a vaginal hysterectomy followed by an anterior colporrhaphy and posterior colpoperineorrhaphy.

If patients are unfit or unwilling to have an operation a pliable ring pessary made from polythene or vinyl is squeezed and inserted into the vagina: when it opens out it takes up the slack in the vaginal walls. The patient is not cured but her symptoms are relieved; however, she must attend a clinic at approximately 3-monthly intervals for the vagina to be inspected for infection or ulceration and for the ring to be changed.

2. Retroversion and retroflexion. Backward displacement is usually a combination of retroversion and retroflexion (Fig. 50.8). The condition occurs normally in approximately 15 per cent of women and is usually symptomless.

It may first occur in the puerperium as the uterus involutes, or it may be drawn backwards by fibrosis from infections or endometriosis, or may be pushed backwards by tumours such as a fibroid or ovarian tumour.

It is now thought that the retroversion is symptomless and any existing symptoms, i.e. backache, menorrhagia, dysmenorrhoea, infertility and abortion, are symptoms of the associated condition.

If, however, the ovaries prolapse into the pouch of Douglas, dyspareunia can result and is an indication to perform one of the uterine suspension operations.

There is very little place for treatment by a pessary.

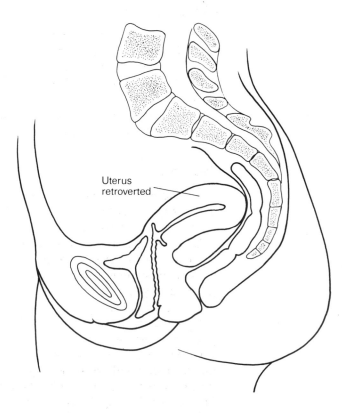

Uterus
retroverted

Fig. 50.8 Retroversion of uterus.

TUMOURS

1. Vulval tumours

Benign

Bartholin's cyst is caused by blockage of the duct of Bartholin's gland and contains mucoid fluid (Fig. 50.9). It is treated by marsupialisation (incision into the cyst and suturing its lining to the skin leaving a permanent stoma).

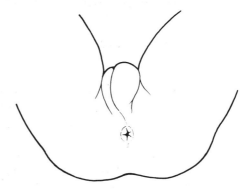

Fig. 50.9 Bartholin's cyst.

Fibromas, lipomas and papillomas. These should be excised.

Malignant

Squamous celled carcinoma of the vulva usually arises in women past the menopause and can be predisposed to by leucoplakia; it presents an ulcer with everted edges. The inguinal lymph glands are involved in the course of the disease.

Treatment is by excision of the vulva and removal of the inguinal, femoral and iliac glands (radical vulvectomy). Radiotherapy is usually reserved for recurrences.

Urethral tumours

Benign

Urethral caruncle. This is a small pedunculated swelling of the posterior lip of the urethral meatus; it is very tender, may cause dysuria and slight bleeding. It consists of adenomatous vascular tissue.

Treatment is by excision, frequently done by diathermy.

Malignant

Carcinoma of the urethra is very rare.

Vaginal tumours

Benign

Vaginal cysts. These are usually asymptomatic and found on routine examination. If causing symptoms they are excised.

Malignant

Primary carcinoma of the vagina is rare and is treated by radiotherapy. **Secondary carcinoma** may follow uterine carcinoma.

Uterine Tumours

Benign tumours

Polyps can arise in the uterine cavity or cervical canal. They cause menorrhagia, intermenstrual bleeding, postcoital bleeding and post-menopausal bleeding.

Treatment. The uterine cavity polyps are curetted away and the cervical ones removed by twisting them off.

Fibromyomas. These are more commonly know as fibroids (Fig. 50.10). They occur usually after the age of 30 years and never arise for the first time after the menopause. They are more common in women who have not had children. Fibroids are more likely to arise in the body of the uterus than the cervix. They are composed of muscle and fibrous tissue, may be single or multiple and can be from a pinhead size to enormous size. They can lie under the peritoneal surface (subperitoneal) or protrude into the

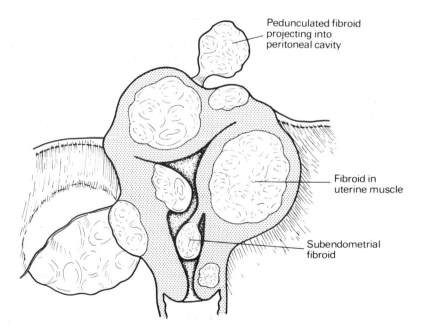

Pedunculated fibroid projecting into peritoneal cavity

Fibroid in uterine muscle

Subendometrial fibroid

Fig. 50.10 A fibroid uterus showing the various sites from which the growths may arise.

cavity (submucous) or be in the wall of the uterus (interstitial). They may also develop pedicles (pedunculated).

Fibroids may be symptomless, but the common symptoms are menorrhagia, and pressure symptoms due to their weight. Pain is due to complications such as degeneration of the fibroids or torsion of a pedunculated fibroid. Enlargement of the abdomen may be the only complaint.

Treatment. Small asymptomatic fibroids do not require any treatment. Myomectomy is performed if the woman is of child-bearing age and has no children or is desirous of further children. Abdominal hysterectomy is performed if the woman is past child-bearing age or has completed her family.

Malignant tumours

Carcinoma of the cervix (Fig. 50.11). This can arise at any age but is more common between the age of 40 and 50 years. There is evidence to suggest that the causative factor is transmitted by coitus; it is more common in people who commence coitus early in life and have many sexual partners. As it is rare in Jews, it is also suggested that it may be related to coitus with uncircumcised partners. There are various stages of carcinoma of the cervix.

Stage O. This is often known as either pre-invasive carcinoma or carcinoma in situ. This stage precedes the development of many cases of invasive carcinoma. It is asymptomatic and can only be discovered by a

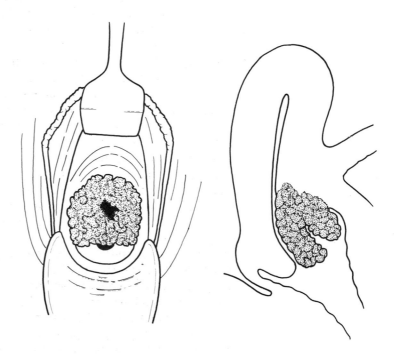

Fig. 50.11 Carcinoma of the cervix. A large carcinoma as seen through a vaginal speculum. Note that the bladder is already invaded by the growth.

vaginal smear followed by biopsies. Not all cases progress to invasive carcinoma.

Stage I. Invasive carcinoma confined to cervix.

Stage IIa. Spread to vaginal vault.

Stage IIb. Spread to parametrium but cervix not fixed.

Stage III. Spread to lower two-thirds vagina or parametrial spread and cervix fixed.

Stage IV. Involvement of bladder and rectum or metastases outside the pelvis.

Symptoms

(i) A watery discharge which may be bloodstained and offensive.

(ii) Irregular vaginal bleeding.

(iii) Postcoital bleeding.

(iv) Pain; this is a late symptom signifying involvement of other organs.

(v) Incontinence of urine or faeces due to fistulae formation.

Diagnosis. Cervical cytology by routine cervical smear in all women over 30 years at regular intervals yields about five positive smears per 1000. These are followed up by biopsy of the whole squamocolumnar junction (cone biopsy).

Treatment. If the biopsy shows the carcinoma to be pre-invasive and it is completely excised the case may be followed up by repeated smears, otherwise total hysterectomy is the treatment of choice. A more recent and developing form of treatment for pre-invasive lesions is to identify the lesion by staining with an iodine preparation and examining the cervix with a colp-microscope and destroying the lesion with a laser beam. If the biopsy shows it to be invasive then the choice is between radiotherapy and surgery in operable cases, the results being much the same. Most gynaecologists these days favour radiotherapy.

If surgery is decided upon, Wertheim's hysterectomy is done. This is a total hysterectomy and bilateral salpingo-oophorectomy; the upper third of the vagina is removed and also the pelvic lymph glands.

Prognosis. The five-year survival rates are:

Stage I   75 per cent

Stage II   50 per cent

Stage III and IV 10 per cent

Carcinoma of the body of the uterus. Usually occurs in women past the menopause but can occur before. Occurs equally in women who have had children and those who have not. It is an important cause of post-menopausal bleeding.

Symptoms. Intermenstrual bleeding and postmenopausal bleeding. There may be some uterine enlargement.

Diagnosis is by diagnostic curettage of the uterus.

Treatment. Total hysterectomy and bilateral salpingo-oophorectomy and removal of a wide cuff of the vagina.

Some gynaecologists give postoperative radiotherapy to reduce the risks of recurrence at the vaginal vault. Radiotherapy can be used in inoperable cases as can progestogens in large doses.

Choriocarcinoma (chorion-epithelioma). The highly malignant tumour follows a hydatidiform mole. It is treated by total hysterectomy and bilateral salpingo-oophorectomy. Any metastases will respond to folic acid antagonists such as methotrexate. This may be combined with a cytotoxic drug.

Ovary

Ovarian tumours are often referred to as ovarian cysts but it must be remembered that many of them are solid tumours. They can arise in any age group. There are many different types of tumour arising from different types of tissue. They can be benign or highly malignant; they may even be a secondary tumour to a primary in the stomach, colon or breast.

Symptoms are few. Uncomplicated cysts are often symptomless; swelling of the abdomen may be the only complaint. Menstrual upset is rare. Pain can occur if complications such as torsion (Fig. 50.12), rupture or infection arise or if the tumour is malignant. Pressure symptoms such as oedema of the legs or dyspnoea may occur.

Treatment. If benign, the tumour is resected leaving part of the ovary. Malignant tumours if operable are treated by total hysterectomy and bilateral salpingo-oophorectomy. If inoperable radiotherapy is unlikely to help but cytotoxic drugs, i.e. cyclophosphamide, may cause temporary regression.

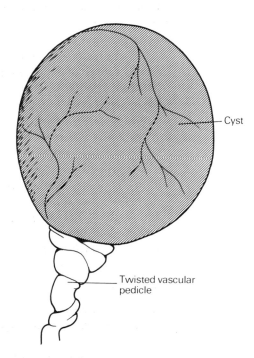

Cyst

Twisted vascular pedicle

Fig. 50.12 Torsion of an ovarian cyst.

Fallopian tubes

Tumours of the Fallopian tubes both benign and malignant are extremely rare.

Endometriosis

This is a condition where endometrial tissue occurs in ectopic situations such as ovaries, myometrium and other pelvic organs. It is benign.

Symptoms. Endometriosis only occurs during reproductive life. It causes infertility, secondary dysmenorrhoea, menstrual upsets, and dyspareunia.

Endometriosis causes the formation of tender, bilateral masses involving the tubes and ovaries. These are known as 'chocolate cysts' as they contain a chocolate-like fluid. The uterus can become enlarged.

Treatment. In young women the affected tissue is excised attempting to conserve some ovarian tissue. Prolonged hormone therapy with progestogens for six to 12 months causes the endometriosis to regress. In older patients total hysterectomy and bilateral salpingo-oophorectomy is performed.

PREPARATION AND POSTOPERATIVE CARE OF PATIENTS

Prior to any operative procedure the patient must be suitably prepared. The patient is admitted to hospital 1 or 2 days before operation.

1. Routine observations are made on admission: temperature, pulse, blood pressure.

2. Urinalysis.

3. Vaginal swab if any evidence of infection.

4. General medical examination.

5. Haemoglobin checked, blood grouped and cross-matched if considered necessary.

6. Consent form signed.

7. Patient's abdomen or perineum shaved for major operations.

8. Bowel preparation is important, enemas or suppositories are necessary in some cases.

9. A bath or bedbath is necessary the evening before operation and the morning of surgery.

10. Night sedatives are given to ensure that the patient has a good sleep before surgery.

11. Food is withheld for 6 hours before operation.

Postoperative care

(a) Minor cases

(i) Immediate postoperative care is the same as for any postoperative theatre case.

(ii) Minor cases are allowed up and about as soon as they are able to manage.

(iii) Vaginal blood loss is observed.

(b) Major cases

(i) Immediate postoperative care is as for any postoperative theatre case.

(ii) Observation of pulse, temperature, blood pressure, wound condition and vaginal loss are made and recorded.

(iii) Analgesics are given as prescribed.

(iv) Intravenous therapy may be ordered.

(v) Fluid intake and output is recorded.

(vi) The patient should be seen by the physiotherapist as soon as possible after surgery.

(vii) Early mobilisation is extremely important to prevent deep venous thrombosis.

(viii) Haemoglobin estimation is carried out on the second postoperative day.

(ix) On the seventh to tenth day abdominal sutures or clips are removed.

(x) Patients are usually discharged from hospital on the tenth to 14th postoperative day and are subsequently seen in the follow-up clinic.

Following major vaginal surgery there is frequently a vaginal pack inserted to prevent bleeding; this often causes difficulty in micturition and, therefore, a catheter is also inserted. The pack is usually removed in 24 hours and the catheter in 48 hours. Following the removal of the catheter the patient is often catheterised on subsequent days to determine whether there is any residual urine following micturition.

GYNAECOLOGICAL OPERATIONS

D and C. This stands for dilatation of the cervix and curettage of the uterus. This is usually done for diagnostic reasons, the curettings being examined histologically. Curettage can be therapeutic in cases such as incomplete abortion.

Abdominal hysterectomy. A total hysterectomy is where the complete uterus is removed. A subtotal hysterectomy is where only the body of the uterus is removed and the cervix left behind; this is not often carried out except where there are technical difficulties in removing the cervix.

Salpingo-oophorectomy is removal of one or both Fallopian tubes and ovaries. This may be carried out for ovarian or tubal disease; it is often combined with hysterectomy.

Ovarian cystectomy. This is removal of a benign ovarian cyst by shelling it out of its capsule and reconstructing the remains of the ovary into its normal shape.

Salpingostomy and reimplantation of tubes. These are performed in cases of infertility where tubal blockage has been demonstrated.

Wertheim's hysterectomy. This is performed for carcinoma of the cervix and is described under that heading.

Pelvic floor repair and vaginal hysterectomy. These are performed for prolapse and are described under that heading.

Simple vulvectomy and radical vulvectomy. These are performed for malignant tumours of the vulva.

Sterilisation is an operation carried out to prevent further pregnancies.

Many methods are used but most are based on dividing the tube, separating and ligating the cut ends.

Laparoscopy. This is the insertion of a laparoscope through the abdominal wall to visualise the pelvic organs. It is principally a diagnostic procedure but sterilisation can also be performed in this way by diathermising the tubes or constricting the tubes with small rubber rings or metal clips.

Myomectomy. The removal of fibroids from the uterus and reconstruction of the uterus.

Shirodkhar's operation. This operation is the insertion of a purse-string suture around the cervix to prevent habitual abortions due to an incompetent internal cervical os.

Vacuum curettage. This is to terminate a pregnancy in the first 12 weeks.

Colposcopy. This is the insertion of an instrument into the vagina to visualise the cervix, frequently a microscope is attached and it is then known as colpo-microscopy.

FAMILY PLANNING

A nurse should know something of the methods available and where expert help and advice can be obtained.

Male contraception

1. *Coitus interruptus.* This is withdrawal of the penis from the vagina immediately before ejaculation and is one of the oldest methods used. It is unsafe and psychological strain can be placed on both partners.

2. *Condom or sheath* (French letter). They are worn over the penis during intercourse to prevent the seminal fluid being deposited in the vagina. It is reasonably effective but may be made safer by the use of a spermicidal agent.

Female contraception

1. *Rhythm method (safe period).* This is the only method acceptable to some people. It is based on the fact that in a regular menstrual cycle ovulation occurs 13 to 15 days prior to the next period, and fertilisation is possible up to five days before or 2 days after ovulation; allowing for an extra day at either end, intercourse should be avoided for these 12 days of the cycle. It is an unreliable form of contraception.

2. *Occlusive caps (diaphragm (Dutch cap), cervical cap).* These are devices which cover the cervix and mechanically obstruct the entrance of spermatozoa. If used with a spermicidal cream or jelly it is a good form of contraception.

3. *Chemical contraceptives.* These are all chemical agents which kill spermatozoa. They are incorporated in jellies, creams, pessaries and aerosol foams. They are relatively unsafe when used alone but should be combined with a mechanical barrier, i.e. sheath or diaphragm.

4. *Intrauterine contraceptive devices (IUCD).* I.U.C.D's are small plastic

devices which are inserted into the uterine cavity. There are many designs, i.e. Lippes loop, Saf-T-Coil, etc. Some have copper wire round the stem which is in the cervical canal, the copper is supposed to react with the cervical mucus and repel the sperms. The mode of actions of I.U.C.D's is uncertain but it is now thought that conception takes place but the fertilised ovum cannot become implanted in the uterine cavity. They are not ideal as they cause menstrual upsets, dysmenorrhoea, pelvic infections, ectopic pregnancies. They can also perforate the uterus and enter the peritoneal cavity. Also pregnancies can occur with them in place and it is, therefore, recommended that they be used in conjunction with a spermicidal agent.

Oral contraception. Oral contraceptives are usually a combination of oestrogen and progesterone and act several ways; ovulation is inhibited; the cervical mucus is rendered hostile to sperms which are, therefore, unable to penetrate the cervical mucus; and lastly the endometrium is not suitable for implantation of any fertilised ovum.

It is a reliable form of contraception and with the newer low dose pills the side effects are minimal. It is contraindicated in certain circumstances, i.e. known thrombotic disease, liver damage, etc.

Sterilisation. This is by tubal ligation in the female or ligation of the vas deferens in the male. It is a permanent method of contraception.

51

Iatrogenic disorders

There were always conditions which arose directly or indirectly from treatment. Admission to hospital has always exposed the patient to the risk of infection and the simplest and apparently most innocuous treatment may produce artificial conditions. Something is restricted, prohibited or added in the form of diet or drugs. The whole of the patient's metabolic processes may be altered. As physiological processes are better understood there is a constant stimulus to design new operations or to invent new drugs and machines which take over temporarily or permanently certain bodily functions.

Radioactive material is used in an ever-increasing variety of forms to investigate function and to treat disease. It is not surprising that many side effects occur and some are so important as to constitute a group of diseases induced by or directly attributable to therapy. Others are minor but none the less troublesome. All, however, are iatrogenic conditions.

In some instances mishaps occur which could easily have been avoided. In other cases a condition arises which could not have been foreseen. Here are considered together conditions arising from treatment whether preventable or otherwise.

They may be:
1. Physical injuries from surgical apparatus or a surgical environment.
2. Chemical injuries.
3. Drug toxicity and idiosyncrasy.
4. Direct operative complications.
5. The effects of surgical ablation.

PHYSICAL INJURIES

These are numerous and fairly obvious. They include:

Burns

These may occur from:
   1. Chemicals used on the wrong tissue or in too concentrated a strength.

There is no substitute for a personal check of the label on the container.

2. Hot-water bottles. These burns can be avoided by not using hot-water bottles. They are unnecessary.

3. Surgical diathermy incorrectly used. A high-frequency current generates heat passing through the body but does not cause an electric shock. This has already been considered in detail (Ch. 10).

Explosions

See Chapter 10.

Scalds

Loss of foreign bodies

See Chapter 10.

Pressure and traction

These injuries may arise from:

1. Tourniquets. Their use is rarely required for control of haemorrhage and if used to provide a bloodless operation field they must be removed by the person who applied them.

2. Plaster casts and splints. If too tight, plaster casts and splints act as tourniquets with the most devasting effects.

3. Pressure sores. These may occur from the roughened edges of a plaster. Even more important are sores in which the body weight is one factor. Others are loss of sensation, incontinence, excessive sweating, oedema and an impaired circulation.

4. Nerve paresis. This is particularly liable to occur if the brachial plexus is stretched or the radial nerve suffers pressure from lying on the edge of the table. The lateral popliteal nerve may be damaged by severe pressure or may be stretched from traction over the neck of the fibula. Drug injection into the radial or sciatic nerves may also cause paresis.

Confinement to bed

This may cause no special trouble, but it may initiate a chain reaction giving rise to conditions such as:

1. Thrombosis and embolism. The incidence of these is diminishing but not abolished by early postoperative ambulation and the measures mentioned in Chapter 13.

2. Diminished blood volume. This occurs from confinement to bed and, in general, patients should be up and about before operation or, if this is impossible, the blood volume should be restored preoperatively. If it is not, drugs used for the induction of anaesthesia which cause vasodilation may bring on early circulatory collapse. A small amount of bleeding will cause a similar effect.

3. Retention of urine. This is commonly due to some degree of prostatic obstruction, particularly in elderly men.

    4. Pressure sores and deformities, such as drop foot.

    5. Faecal impaction.

The surgical environment

The best surgical environment is that in which the access of infective organisms to wounds is prevented. This ideal is rarely achieved completely.

DRUGS AND THERAPEUTIC SUBSTANCES

A few general principles are important. They are:

1. Identification

This is fundamental. If a drug is to be injected the solution must be drawn into the syringe after the label has been read by two people one of whom is a qualified nurse or a doctor. The same care is essential with fluid for infusion. Mixtures dangerous for infusion should be coloured, for example, sodium citrate for use in the bladder.

    Blood is particularly important. The most essential precaution is that the correct cross-matched bottle for the patient is the one being handled. Then it should be checked that:

    (a) It is the correct group.

    (b) The Rh typing is correct.

    (c) That it is not out of date.

    Most important of all a careful watch should be kept that the first 50–100 ml are causing no reaction.

2. Drug therapy in progress when surgery is necessary

This should be reviewed in the light of possible consequences. Particularly important are:

    (a) Anticoagulant therapy. This must always be temporarily reversed by the intravenous administration of protamine sulphate for heparin, or of vitamin K in the case of warfarin.

    (b) Corticosteroid therapy. This delays healing, but if the dosage is reduced too rapidly the original condition for which the patient is being treated may flare up in a fulminating form. Therefore before surgery corticosteroid therapy must be increased so that the response to injury (Ch. 24) can occur. Afterwards it is reduced gradually.

    Drug reactions. There are many complications of steroid therapy which may be of surgical importance. The commonest are:

    (i) Reactivation of quiescent pulmonary tuberculosis.

    (ii) Bleeding from a peptic ulcer.

    (iii) Development of fulminating infections, such as appendicitis, which progress silently.

(iv) The rapid development of cardiac failure.

Other complications include thrombosis, osteoporosis, psychosis, myopathies and skin reactions such as acne and hirsutism.

(c) The correct drug by the wrong route. This may cause great harm. Thiopentone, so effective intravenously, causes arterial thrombosis with gangrene of the hand if given into the brachial artery.

(d) The correct rate. This must be determined for any substance given intravenously.

Complications of drug therapy:

Sensitivity in some individuals is almost inevitable; there is almost no drug to which some individual may not be sensitive. This may vary from a severe anaphylactic reaction to a mild skin rash.

Resistant organisms may develop.

Normally suppressed organisms may proliferate.

Anaemia and damage to the blood-forming tissues may occur. Chloramphenicol, the sulphonamides and most of the cytotoxic drugs used in malignant disease, as well as radiotherapy, are particularly notable.

Crystallisation in the kidney may occur from some sulphonamides associated with an inadequate fluid intake, particularly with an acid urine.

Damage to the nucleus of the VIIIth cranial nerve is almost always due to the aminoglycosides (streptomycin, neomycin).

Vitamin B deficiency is most liable to occur from alteration of the intestinal flora by the tetracycline group of antibiotics.

Jaundice may occur from blood plasma (infective) or drugs. Notable are:

Halothane — used in anaesthesia.

Methyldopa — used for hypertension.

Chlorpromazine — an anxiolytic drug.

Phenylbutazone — an anti-inflammatory agent.

Ampicillin   }
Tetracycline } — antibiotics.

Intestinal ulceration with stricture formation may result from enteric-coated diuretic capsules containing potassium chloride.

Gastric erosions are common from the irritation of aspirin as well as phenylbutazone.

Coma and respiratory failure may be quite alarming following small doses of morphia in a sensitive patient.

Abdominal pain may be severe from excessive dosage of vitamin D, while constipation may result from ganglion-blocking drugs used in the treatment of hypertension.

Sclerosing peritonitis is a complication of practolol.

Retrolental fibroplasia may result from the administration of oxygen in excess of 35 per cent, to the newborn.

Gangrene may result from severe spasm produced by ergot.

Glaucoma is aggravated by atropine.

Citrate intoxication after massive blood transfusion. In addition to causing reduction of serum calcium stored blood contains excess of potassium ions.

DIRECT AND INDIRECT OPERATIVE COMPLICATIONS

These are similar to the general processes outlined in this work.
1. Direct damage from trauma.
2. Obstruction postoperatively.
3. Fluid leakage from the (i) blood vessels, (ii) the suture line in visceral anastomosis.
4. Metabolic changes from surgical intervention. Re-operation may be indicated for (a) fluid leakage (including haemorrhage) and (b) obstruction.
5. Infections.

Operative ablation

The effects which arise from operative ablation depend on the extent of the ablation, to what extent the functional reserves of the body are adequate and to what degree, if any, disability can be overcome or minimised by artificial means. Many of the physiological consequences which arise take time to manifest themselves. The longer the results of many ablations are studied, the more wide-reaching their effects are discovered to be.

Miscellaneous iatrogenic lesions

The obvious sequelae of amputation of the limbs or the breast need no special stress except the importance of ensuring that such mutilation is undertaken only for compelling indications.

Even where the functional reserve is adequate, as in the kidneys, the ovaries or the testes, a conservative attitude to removal is essential, since time may bring similar or more severe disease to the contralateral organ.

Ductless gland ablation can be largely overcome by administration of the appropriate hormone if its removal causes a deficiency. More difficult and more complicated are the effects of extirpation of large amounts of gastrointestinal tract.

Physiological and anatomical shortening of the digestive tract

The stomach. The greatest effects in proportion to the amount removed are seen after gastrectomy, partly due to anatomical and physiological exclusion of the duodenum. The main effects are:
1. Limited intake of food.
2. Anaemia.
3. Vitamin deficiency.
4. Intestinal hurry.
5. Defective absorption.
6. Enterocolitis (possibly from achlorhydria).
7. Other syndromes:
    (a) Face flushing.
    (b) Hypoglycaemia.
    (c) Bilious vomiting.
8. Osteoporosis.

The small intestine. Resection of large lengths of the small intestine results in loss of weight and some frequency of stools.

Intestinal hurry occurs in all conditions of physiological shortening of which gastrectomy is one of the most important examples.

The large intestine. This has a considerable functional reserve and more than half can be removed without any great effect.

The gall-bladder. Cholecystectomy results in dilute bile dribbling into the duodenum as it is formed. Most patients after cholecystectomy have no great disability although there may be a certain amount of windy discomfort and a bowel action which is freer than usual.

After removal of the gall-bladder the patient should be able to eat a reasonable amount of fat but not excessive quantities. In the immediate postoperative phase fat should be liberally supplied to encourage biliary drainage and to avoid further colic from inspissated mucus or a tiny fragment of gravel which may form the nidus of a further stone.

The pancreas. Pancreatectomy, which is usually undertaken for neoplasm, causes:

1. Diabetes, control of which presents no great difficulty.
2. Steatorrhoea, diminished by giving pancreatic enzymes.
3. Diminished calcium absorption.
4. Fat and protein absorption is also disturbed.

Most operative procedures produce after-effects which are usually of a minor nature. The more seriously ill the patient beforehand the more ready he is to accept these discomforts, but where preoperative symptoms, and especially pain, have been slight the less tolerant the patient is likely to be later of postoperative symptoms. It is rightly said that the bad results of operations for peptic ulceration are more frequently the results of bad selection of patients than of bad surgery.

SOME BIOGRAPHICAL NOTES

Hippocrates (460–370 BC) is considered to be the father of modern medicine for he severed medicine from witchcraft and superstition and transformed it into a science based on observation. He travelled widely throughout Greece setting up teaching centres and left model clinical records for posterity (his descriptions of epilepsy and puerperal septicaemia could be found in any modern textbook). His work was assisted by his emphasis on good nursing and a balanced diet. The Hippocratic oath is a tribute to the high ethical standards he brought to the profession.

Galen (AD 130–200). Prior to 1500, Galen was second only to Hippocrates in medicine, and his theories, both correct and erroneous, were accepted without question. After serving the Roman Emperor Marcus Aurelius as personal physician, he retired to write and to study. He was the first experimental physiologist and discovered that the arteries contained blood and that contraction of muscle occurred independently of the nerve supply. Among his other important discoveries were his explanations of respiration and inflammation. His work on anatomy was less successful for he based all his findings on the dissection of animals. As a physician he placed great reliance on drugs, notably opium, sugar and alcohol. While some of his teaching misled, his collection of 80 books preserved much that was finest in ancient medicine throughout the Dark Ages.

Ambroise Paré (1510–90). By his own skill and personality, Paré raised the status of surgery from a despised mechanical art to that of a major profession, using the new discoveries in anatomy to advance surgery. By the discovery that gunshot wounds were not poisonous and required soothing applications rather than boiling oil and by his advocacy of artificial limbs for wounded soldiers, he brought much relief to the surgery of the battlefield. To prevent bleeding after amputation, he replaced the indiscriminate use of a red hot cautery with a simple ligature. Among his other work was the invention of artery forceps, detailed discussion of the treatment of fractures and dislocations and the suggestion that syphilis was the cause of aneurysm. He established himself in a position of great authority as surgeon to four French kings, and riled the established physicians of the time by scorning such remedies as powdered mummy and a unicorn's head.

Andreas Vesalius (1514–64). By freeing anatomy from many of Galen's errors, Vesalius laid the foundation on which many subsequent advances in medicine and surgery could take place. At the age of 23 he was Professor of Anatomy at Padua University and his great work, the *Fabrica*, published in 1543, corrected Galen on many points, completely destroying Galen's osteology and muscle anatomy. For instance, he found the lower jaw consisted of a single bone, that loss of the spleen was compatible with life, and he destroyed such fallacies as the double bile duct and the five-lobed liver. His work on the spinal cord showed the means by which the brain acts on the various muscles of the limbs and trunk. By 1555 he had laid the basis of Harvey's discovery of the circulation by denying the existence of interventricular pores and by noting the existence of valves in the vein without appreciating their significance. His later years were spent as physician to the Emperor Charles V.

St Vincent De Paul (1576–1660) was the founder of the Sisters of Charity. Destined for the Church he was sold into slavery on his capture by pirates. After his release he returned to Paris to fight against poverty, ignorance and infection. Initially 120 well-to-do ladies would visit the poor in teams of four but no nursing was undertaken until St Vincent widened the membership of the Order to include peasant women, known as Sisters of Charity, who were taught simple nursing procedures. The ladies and Sisters of Charity were then amalgamated and the first Nursing Order had been formed, performing heroically on the battlefields of seventeenth-century France. After St Vincent's death the Order waned because it failed to follow the advances in surgery and medicine, but at the time of the Crimean War the Sisters of Charity inspired Florence Nightingale to provide a similar standard of nursing of British soldiers in the Crimea.

William Harvey (1578–1657). It was as Lumelian lecturer that William Harvey delivered the following statement in 1616 which revolutionised the whole of medical science: 'The movement of the blood is constantly in a circle and is brought about by the beat of the heart.' With a sound knowledge of anatomy, Harvey saw that the valves in the veins would permit the blood to pass only to the heart while those in the great arteries permitted blood to flow only away from the heart. He then calculated that the quantity and velocity of the blood was such as made it physically impossible for the blood to do other than return by a venous route. His conclusions were published in his famous book *De Motu Cordis*. His *De Generatione Animalium*, published in 1651, was the first English work on embryology, also containing the first chapters in English on obstetrics. As a staunch Royalist, Harvey compared the heart to his king, Charles I — 'the centre of all strength and power'.

John Hunter (1728–93) was not only one of the foremost surgeons of all time but the most versatile of scientists. He raised surgery to a technical science firmly grounded in physiology and surgical pathology. To assist him in his work he founded a great menagerie of 13 000 specimens and it was his study of the capillary system of the deer which led to his treatment for aneurysm which is still in use today. Among his other discoveries were the arterial supply of the gravid uterus, the olfactory nerve in the nose and many features of the lymphatic system. As a surgical pathologist his descriptions of phlebitis, pyaemia and shock were revolutionary and his technical inventions, such as artificial feeding by a tube in the stomach and apparatus for forced respiration, were of the highest order. As a biologist his work led him to the principle that functional activities in the lower forms of life were simplifications of those in the higher. His love of science caused his death which was as a result of a mistaken inoculation of syphilis and gonorrhoea. A certain incoherence in writing was more than compensated for by his work as a teacher, as three famous doctors (Jenner, Abernethy and Astley Cooper) were his pupils.

Edward Jenner (1749–1823) was a country doctor in Berkeley, Gloucestershire, who noticed that those who had had cowpox (a mild form of pox contracted by milkmaids from cows) never became infected with smallpox. In May 1796 he conducted a crucial experiment by vaccinating an 8-year-old boy with pus from the hand of a dairymaid infected with cowpox. The boy failed to develop smallpox following inoculation eight weeks later. Cowpox was technically known as vaccinia so it was inevitable that Jenner's process became known as vaccination. Not only was one of the most terrible diseases banished from this country but a principle had been established which eventually led to the immunisation of man against many infectious diseases.

James Blundell (1790–1877) was the pioneer in the field of blood transfusion. He discovered the value of transfusion by injection of the blood of a dog into the circulation of another dog but discovered that a dog would die if injected with the blood of a sheep. This established the incompatibility of the blood of different species and prevented the practice of injecting animal blood into human beings. By further experiment he showed that a smaller quantity of blood than the amount lost would resuscitate an animal. The first transfusion of human blood took place on 12 December 1818 on a patient who was fatally ill. His first successful recovery was for a postpartum haemorrhage for which the patient received 8 oz of blood, recorded in the *Lancet* of 1829. Blundell showed, contrary to existing belief, that the blood was not injured by its passage through instruments and that a few air bubbles in the circulation were quite harmless. The problem of coagulation proved difficult and later led to his invention of a special apparatus enabling the blood to be transferred from donor to recipient with minimal physical interference.

Theodor Fliedner (1800–64) was a Lutheran clergyman responsible for the experiment which began nursing reform. In 1826 he founded an association to help discharged prisoners and relieve the sick poor of his parish. This association led in 1836 to the development of a new hospital which was founded at Kaiserswerth, where Fliedner trained women called deaconesses to help him in his work. It was the first nursing experiment to exist independently of a religious order. The deaconesses were examined in medicine and pharmacy but, unlike the nursing training of Florence Nightingale, this was more on the lines of a comprehensive social service including training in cooking, laundering and gardening. Kaiserswerth was the first school of nursing and left a lasting impression with its spirit of dedicated service. At the time of Fliedner's death 1600 deaconesses were nursing as far apart as Turkey and the U.S.A.

William Thomas Morton (1819–68) was a dental partner of Horace Wells (1815–48), whose career was ruined when he gave an unsuccessful public demonstration using nitrous oxide to anaesthetise a patient. A Boston chemist recommended to Morton the use of sulphuric ether and the first successful public demonstration was given at the Massachusetts General Hospital on 16 October 1846 when an operation for a vascular tumour was successfully performed. Morton ruined his reputation by attempting to patent the drug and made no further contribution to the subject.

James Simpson (1811–70). In Edinburgh, the Professor of Midwifery, James Simpson, found ether unsatisfactory in midwifery and used a new drug, chloroform. His first experiment was upon himself and, on recovering consciousness, rightly remarked, 'This is far stronger than ether.' The drug was first administered on a child for an operation for osteomyelitis on 15 November 1847. More powerful and pleasant than ether, chloroform became the standard anaesthetic drug in Britain for the next 50 years and the new medical science of anaesthetics was born with far-reaching effects for the development of surgery.

Florence Nightingale (1820–1910) was the first outstanding figure in the history of nursing. Before she went to the Crimea nursing did not exist as a profession of high ethical and technical standards. She was able to overcome the social barriers which prevented women entering nursing. In 1854 she was able to go to the Crimea where, amid the filth of the hospitals in Scutari, she courageously fought her own battle for cleanliness and care of the patients. She never ceased to fight for sanitary conditions in the army medical service, being influential in later Royal Commissions. Her *Notes on Nursing* and *Notes on Hospitals* emphasise the principles of personal and communal hygiene as well as administrative efficiency.

By 1860 a grateful nation had contributed £50 000 to the Nightingale Fund which was used to establish a nursing school at St Thomas's Hospital London. The great medical advantages of this period could only be of benefit to mankind with trained and educated nurses. Her most notable administrative reform was the removal of nurses from the supervision of the medical staff to that of the matron. She set a standard of nursing education which was a model for all subsequent English and Commonwealth schools. After choosing the probationers herself, she ensured that they would be instructed in the basic sciences by the medical staff and would receive practical instruction in the wards under the supervison of the sisters. In later years she pressed for many reforms in workhouse nursing and was responsible for the grant of a Royal Charter to the Royal British Nursing Association in 1893.

Louis Pasteur (1822–95) is considered to be the founder of modern bacteriology for by extensive study of milk and beer he proved that organisms naturally present in the air are alive and can produce putrefaction, but on heating lose their power and are killed — a discovery fundamental to aseptic surgery. By injecting anthrax bacilli, greatly reduced in strength, into a sheep, he was able to immunise it against subsequent infection by the virulent bacillus. This, and similar experiments, led him to conclude that the origin or extinction of infectious disease in the past may have simply been due to the strengthening or weakening of its virulence by external conditions, and the principle was applied with success in the case of preventive vaccination against hydrophobia. In 1885 the Pasteur Institute was opened and Pasteur surrounded himself with brilliant pupils — among them:

Emile Roux, responsible for epoch-making work on the diphtheria antitoxin;

Yersin, who found a vaccination against plague, and

Calmette, who discovered preventive inoculation against snake bites.

Truly Pasteur was one of the pioneers of modern preventive inoculation.

Lord Lister (1827–1912) was the greatest surgical figure of modern times. As Professor of Surgery in Glasgow, he studied the work of Pasteur from which he deduced that infection in wounds was analogous to putrefaction in wine, and selected carbolic acid as a means of destroying the organisms in the wound. Thus Lister discovered the principle involving the prevention and cure of sepsis in wounds. He insisted that everything touching the wounds should be treated with antiseptic and sought constantly to improve his dressings, eventually deciding on a gauze containing the oxides of mercury and zinc. The effects of the new principle were shown by a dramatic drop in the mortality rate of amputations and compound fractures. Abdominal, cranial and chest surgery date from the invention of the antiseptic system which had made possible the surgery of the hollow cavities of the body. Lister's antiseptic principle was later developed into an aseptic system by Halsted and Spencer Wells.

Among Lister's other achievements were the invention of the sinus forceps, probe pointed scissors and the catgut ligature. He further showed that an uninfected clot if undisturbed can be organised into living tissue, and a piece of dead bone may be absorbed in an aseptic wound.

He was President of the Royal Society 1895–1900 and became the first medical peer in 1897.

Hugh Owen Thomas (1834–91) spent his whole professional life in the poorer areas of nineteenth-century Liverpool, but no one did more to advance the treatment of bones and joints. In his day excision and amputation were the remedies for the chronic diseases of the joints but, instead, Thomas applied the principle of complete rest for the treatment of tuberculous joints and this prevented many amputations. To ensure that the diseased part was not compressed or the circulation of the blood impaired, Thomas invented his famous fracture splint, now known as the Thomas splint. His other inventions included a wrench for the reduction of fractures and an osteoclast to break deformed bones before reseting them. The effect of the Thomas splint was not seen until World War I when it was responsible for the reduction of the mortality rate of fracture of the femur from 80 per cent in 1916 to 7 per cent in 1918 — only now was Thomas seen as a great pioneer. His work was continued by his nephew, Sir Robert Jones, who developed the modern methods of tendon transplantation and bone grafting.

Robert Koch (1843–1910). When he delivered his paper on the anthrax bacillus in 1876, Robert Koch had produced the greatest discovery in bacteriology for he had proved that an infectious disease can often be caused by a specific micro-organism. He also showed how to fix and stain bacteria. In 1882 he announced the discovery of the tubercle bacillus which made possible all subsequent work on the cure for tuberculosis. On his visits to India and Egypt as the head of the German cholera Commission of 1883 he discovered the cause of cholera—the *Vibrio cholerae*—and its transmission by water and food. His work on rinderpest, tropical malaria and bubonic plague was extremely valuable and for his services to medicine he was awarded the Nobel Prize in 1905.

Wilhelm Conrad Roentgen (1845–1923) was Professor of Physics at Würzburgh who, while working with a Crooke's tube, discovered that shadows were forming on a photographic plate. After careful experiment he found that, by making his tube light-proof, a greenish fluorescent light would be thrown on a platino-barium screen 9 feet away. These rays passed through substances ordinarily opaque, such as the soft parts of the body, revealing the bones. He read his paper to the Würzburg Society and when Professor Kolliker submitted his own hand to be photographed all doubts were allayed, Kolliker suggesting the new rays, which had been called X-rays, be known as Roentgen rays.

Among the many honours he was to receive for this discovery were the Rumford Gold Medal of the Royal Society and the Nobel Prize.

Sir Alexander Fleming (1881–1955) was responsible for the greatest contribution to the science of medical treatment made in the first half of the twentieth century—the development of antibiotics. In 1928, on examining one of his culture plants in his laboratory at London University, he found that the growth of the mould was the same as on other culture plates but the microbes near the mould, instead of forming into a yellow opaque mould, had dissolved. He then placed various microbes near the mould with different effects—for instance the diphtheria microbe was among those destroyed whilst the typhoid and influenza microbes were not so affected. Thus an antibiotic had been discovered—something alive in the mould was killing other living microbes. Fleming called this substance penicillin and it has been responsible for inhibiting the growth of the causative organisms of many common infectious diseases. During the Second World War it was used to great effect in the treatment of war wounds and gas gangrene.

Fleming was knighted in 1944 and received the Nobel Prize in 1945.

TABLE OF APPROXIMATE NORMAL VALUES

Haematology

Haemoglobin — 14·6 g/100 ml or 100 per cent
Red cells — 5 million/mm³
White cells —
    Adults — 4 to 10 000/mm³
    Infants — 10 000 to 25 000/mm³
Differentiated white cell count —
    Polymorphs 40 to 75 per cent
    Lymphocytes 20 to 50 per cent
    Monocytes 1 to 6 per cent
    Eosinophils 1 to 6 per cent
    Basophils 1 per cent
Platelets — 150 000 to 350 000/mm³
Bleeding time — 1 to 5 minutes
Coagulation time (capillary) — 2 to 8 minutes
Erythrocyte sedimentation rate (ESR) —
    Men 0 to 10 mm/hour
    Women 0 to 20 mm/hour
    Blood viscosity — 1·50–1·75 cp (centipoise)

Blood chemistry

Electrolytes —
    Serum sodium (Na^+) 136–144 mmol/litre
    Serum potassium (K^+) 3·5–4·5 mmol/litre (3·5 to 4·5 mEq/litre)
    Serum chloride (Cl') 100 mmol/litre (100 mEq/litre)
Acid/Base balance —
    Plasma alkali reserve (or carbondioxide combining power) — 50 to 75 ml
      CO_2/100 ml plasma, often referred to as 50 to 75 volumes per cent
        or 20–30 mmol/l
    Arterial pCO_2 — 35 to 45 mmHg
    Standard bicarbonate 21 to 25 mEq/litre
    Base excess of blood — ± 2 mmol/l
pH — 7:35 to 7:42.
Blood urea — 2·50–6·5 mmol/litre
Blood glucose — 4·44–6·67 mmol/litre
Serum calcium — 2·25–2·62 mmol/litre
Serum phosphate — 0·81–1·4 mmol/litre
Serum cholesterol — 3·35–6·46 mmol/litre
Plasma uric acid — 0·12–0·40 mmol/litre
Serum amylase — 75 to 150 Somogyi units/100 ml
Serum acid phosphatase — 1 to 3 K.A. units/100 ml
Serum alkaline phosphatase — 5 to 11 K.A. units/100 ml
Serum proteins —
    Total — 60–80 g/litre
    Albumin — 36–50 g/litre
    Globulin — 20–30 g/litre

Liver function tests —
    Serum bilirubin — 1·7–15·4 μmol/litre
    Thymol turbidity — 0·4 units
    Serum thyroxine — 3·0 to 7·5 μg/100 ml
Serum transaminases —
    Glutamate oxalacetate transaminase (SGOT) — 10 to 35 units/ml
    Glutamate pyruvate transaminase (SGPT) — 0 to 35 units/ml

Cerebrospinal fluid
Protein — 200–400 mmol/litre
Chloride — 119–126 mmol/litre
Glucose — 2·2–4·4 mmol/litre
White cells — 0 to 5/mm³

Index